Fibre-rich and wholegrain foods

Related titles:

Breadmaking (ISBN 978-0-85709-060-7)

Functional foods (ISBN 978-1-84569-690-0)

Cereal grains (ISBN 978-1-84569-563-7)

Details of these books and a complete list of titles from Woodhead Publishing can be obtained by:

- visiting our web site at www.woodheadpublishing.com
- contacting Customer Services (e-mail: sales@woodheadpublishing.com; fax: +44 (0) 1223 832819; tel.: +44 (0) 1223 499140 ext. 130; address: Woodhead Publishing Limited, 80, High Street, Sawston, Cambridge CB22 3HJ, UK)
- in North America, contacting our US office (e-mail: usmarketing@woodheadpublishing.com; tel.: (215) 928 9112; address: Woodhead Publishing, 1518 Walnut Street, Suite 1100, Philadelphia, PA 19102–3406, USA

If you would like e-versions of our content, please visit our online platform: www.woodheadpublishingonline.com. Please recommend it to your librarian so that everyone in your institution can benefit from the wealth of content on the site.

We are always happy to receive suggestions for new books from potential editors. To enquire about contributing to our Food Science, Technology and Nutrition series, please send your name, contact address and details of the topic/s you are interested in to nell.holden@woodheadpublishing.com. We look forward to hearing from you.

The Woodhead team responsible for publishing this book:
Commissioning Editor: Nell Holden
Publications Coordinator: Adam Davies
Project Editor: Sarah Lynch
Editorial and Production Manager: Mary Campbell
Production Editor: Richard Fairclough
Freelance Project Manager: Annette Wiseman
Copyeditor: Sue Clements
Proofreader: Jessica Mnatzaganian
Cover Designer: Terry Callanan

Woodhead Publishing Series in Food Science, Technology and Nutrition:
Number 237

Fibre-rich and wholegrain foods

Improving quality

Edited by
Jan A. Delcour and Kaisa Poutanen

WOODHEAD PUBLISHING

Oxford Cambridge Philadelphia New Delhi

Published by Woodhead Publishing Limited,
80 High Street, Sawston, Cambridge CB22 3HJ, UK
www.woodheadpublishing.com
www.woodheadpublishingonline.com

Woodhead Publishing, 1518 Walnut Street, Suite 1100, Philadelphia,
PA 19102–3406, USA

Woodhead Publishing India Private Limited, G-2, Vardaan House, 7/28 Ansari Road,
Daryaganj, New Delhi – 110002, India
www.woodheadpublishingindia.com

First published 2013, Woodhead Publishing Limited

British Library Cataloguing in Publication Data
A catalogue record for this book is available from the British Library.

Library of Congress Control Number: 2012954754

ISBN 978-0-85709-038-6 (print)
ISBN 978-0-85709-578-7 (online)
ISSN 2042-8049 Woodhead Publishing Series in Food Science, Technology and Nutrition (print)
ISSN 2042-8057 Woodhead Publishing Series in Food Science, Technology and Nutrition (online)

The publisher's policy is to use permanent paper from mills that operate a sustainable forestry policy, and which has been manufactured from pulp which is processed using acid-free and elemental chlorine-free practices. Furthermore, the publisher ensures that the text paper and cover board used have met acceptable environmental accreditation standards.

Cover image courtesy of Ulla Holopainen, VTT Technical Research Centre, Finland

Typeset by RefineCatch Limited, Bungay, Suffolk, UK
Printed by MPG Printgroup

Contents

Contributor contact details .... *xiii*
Woodhead Publishing Series in Food Science, Technology and Nutrition .... *xix*

Part I Introductory issues **1**

1 Definitions, regulations and health claims associated with dietary fibre and wholegrain foods **3**
J. W. Van der Kamp, TNO, The Netherlands, and J. Lupton, Texas A&M University, USA
1.1 Introduction 3
1.2 Defining dietary fibre and wholegrain 4
1.3 Analysing the dietary fibre and wholegrain content of food 10
1.4 Labelling 12
1.5 Recommendations and guidelines for dietary fibre and wholegrain intake 16
1.6 Health claims for dietary fibre and wholegrain 18
1.7 References 22

2 Dietary fibre analysis in foods **25**
B. V. McCleary, A. Draga, and N. Sloane, Megazyme International Ireland Limited, Ireland
2.1 Introduction 25
2.2 An integrated procedure for the measurement of total dietary fibre, including resistant starch and non-digestible oligosaccharides 34
2.3 Updates of the original integrated total dietary fibre procedure 47
2.4 Interlaboratory evaluation of integrated total dietary fibre procedures 52

2.5 Progress in acceptance of dietary fibre methodology by Codex Alimentarius ... 53
2.6 References ... 58

3 Health aspects of dietary fibre ... 61
J. Slavin, University of Minnesota, USA
3.1 Introduction ... 61
3.2 Fibre: definitions, measurement and intake ... 62
3.3 Characterization and digestive impact of fibre ... 64
3.4 Dietary fibre (DF) and disease ... 67
3.5 Fibre and obesity ... 68
3.6 Dietary fibre (DF) and microbiota ... 71
3.7 Future trends ... 72
3.8 Sources of further information and advice ... 73
3.9 References ... 73

4 Wholegrain foods and health ... 76
J. Lappi, H. Mykkänen and M. Kolehmainen, University of Eastern Finland, Finland, and K. Poutanen, VTT Technical Research Centre of Finland, Finland
4.1 Introduction ... 76
4.2 Epidemiological studies ... 77
4.3 Human interventions ... 81
4.4 Food factors important for the health effects of wholegrain foods ... 87
4.5 Conclusion and future trends ... 89
4.6 References ... 90

5 The range of dietary fibre ingredients and a comparison of their technical functionality ... 96
S. W. Cui, Y. Wu and H. Ding, Agriculture and Agri-food Canada, Canada
5.1 Introduction ... 96
5.2 Technical functionalities of dietary fibre ingredients ... 97
5.3 Insoluble dietary fibre ingredients ... 100
5.4 Soluble high molecular weight dietary fibre ingredients ... 101
5.5 Soluble low molecular weight dietary fibre ingredients ... 109
5.6 Resistant starch ... 111
5.7 Conclusion ... 111
5.8 References ... 116

6 Consumption and consumer challenges of wholegrain foods **120**
K. W. Dammann, Cargill, Incorporated, USA, D. Hauge, Grains for Health Foundation, USA, R. A. Rosen, Independent Consultant, USA, N. Schroeder, Johns Hopkins University, USA, and L. Marquart, Grains for Health Foundation and University of Minnesota, USA
6.1 Introduction 120
6.2 Whole grain and fiber consumption 121
6.3 Wholegrain foods and consumer challenges: internal (personal) factors 125
6.4 Wholegrain foods and consumer challenges: external factors 132
6.5 Approaches to introducing wholegrain foods 136
6.6 Future trends 139
6.7 Sources of further information and advice 142
6.8 References 142

Part II Dietary fibre sources **151**

7 Improving the content and composition of dietary fibre in wheat **153**
P. R. Shewry, Rothamsted Research, UK, and University of Reading, UK
7.1 Introduction 153
7.2 Fibre content and composition of wheat fractions 154
7.3 Genetic variation in arabinoxylan (AX) amount, structure and composition 157
7.4 Specific effects of agronomy and environment on arabinoxylan (AX) and β-glucan content and composition 162
7.5 Heritability and genetic analysis of arabinoxylan (AX) and β-glucan content 163
7.6 Exploitation of genetic variation in grain dietary fibre in plant breeding 165
7.7 Conclusion 166
7.8 Acknowledgements 166
7.9 References 167

8 Cereal brans as dietary fibre ingredients **170**
J. Sibakov, P. Lehtinen and K. Poutanen, VTT Technical Research Centre of Finland, Finland
8.1 Introduction 170
8.2 Cereal cell walls as dietary fibre 171
8.3 Cereal bran production technology 172
8.4 Technologies to improve the properties of cereal brans as source of dietary fibre 180

8.5 Food applications of cereal fibre ingredients 181
8.6 Conclusion and future trends 183
8.7 References 183

9 Vegetable, fruit and potato fibres 193
M. Nyman and L. Haskå, Lund University, Sweden
9.1 Introduction 193
9.2 Fruits and vegetables as sources of dietary fibre 194
9.3 Effects of processing on fruit and vegetable dietary fibre 198
9.4 Conclusion 203
9.5 References 203

Part III Improving the quality of fibre-rich and wholegrain foods: cereal products 209

10 Fibre-enriched and wholegrain breads 211
A. Rakha, National Institute of Food Science & Technology, Pakistan, P. Åman and R. Andersson, Swedish University of Agricultural Sciences, Sweden
10.1 Introduction 211
10.2 Fibre enrichment of breads 216
10.3 Processing 221
10.4 Properties of dietary fibre-enriched dough and breads 228
10.5 Conclusion 230
10.6 References 230

11 Performance of resistant starches in baking: a case study on fibre-rich and wholegrain muffins 236
A. Salvador and S. Fiszman, Instituto de Agroquímica y Tecnología de Alimentos (CSIC), Spain
11.1 Introduction 236
11.2 Muffin batter 238
11.3 Muffin properties 244
11.4 Sensory shelf life of muffins 249
11.5 Sensory characteristics of muffins 250
11.6 Conclusion 252
11.7 Acknowledgements 253
11.8 References 253

12 Fibre in extruded products 256
N. Sozer and K. Poutanen, VTT Technical Research Centre of Finland, Finland
12.1 Introduction 256
12.2 Extrusion cooking 257

12.3 Effects of dietary fibre (DF) on the extrusion process and product quality 260
12.4 Effects of extrusion on dietary fibre (DF) properties 265
12.5 Conclusion and future trends 267
12.6 References 268

13 Fibre-enriched and wholewheat pasta 273
C. S. Brennan, Lincoln University, New Zealand
13.1 Introduction 273
13.2 Process variables affecting pasta production 277
13.3 Enrichment of pasta with whole grains or dietary fibre 281
13.4 Relationship between ingredient selection, processing and nutrition 283
13.5 Conclusion and future trends 285
13.6 References 286

14 Fibre-enriched and wholewheat noodles 291
A. S. Ross, Oregon State University, USA
14.1 Introduction 291
14.2 Noodle quality attributes 293
14.3 Wholewheat noodles 295
14.4 Fiber-enriched wheat flour noodles 297
14.5 Wheat flour noodles and resistant starch 301
14.6 Wholegrain and fiber-enriched noodles from other botanical sources 302
14.7 Conclusion 304
14.8 References 305

Part IV Improving the quality of fibre-enriched foods: other products 309

15 Fibre-enriched dairy products 311
H. D. Goff, University of Guelph, Canada
15.1 Introduction 311
15.2 Dairy product categories and formulations 312
15.3 Challenges of fibre enrichment 314
15.4 Potential dietary fibre supplements for dairy products 316
15.5 Potential product applications 319
15.6 Future trends 325
15.7 References 326

16 Fibre-enriched meat products **329**
F. Jiménez-Colmenero and G. Delgado-Pando, Instituto de Ciencia y Tecnología de Alimentos y Nutrición (ICTAN-CSIC) (formerly Instituto del Frío), Spain
16.1 Introduction 329
16.2 Strategies for the development of healthier meat products 331
16.3 Fibre as an ingredient in meat product formulation 332
16.4 Dietary fibre in meat products 333
16.5 Future trends 342
16.6 Acknowledgements 343
16.7 References 343

17 Fibre-enriched seafood **348**
A. J. Borderías and M. Pérez-Mateos, Instituto de Ciencia y Tecnología de Alimentos y Nutrición (ICTAN-CSIC) (formerly Instituto del Frío), Spain, and I. Sánchez-Alonso, Instituto de Estructura de la Materia (IEM-CSIC), Spain
17.1 Introduction 348
17.2 Fortification with dietary fibres of aquatic origin 349
17.3 Fortification with dietary fibres of terrestrial origin 354
17.4 Conclusion 362
17.5 Future trends 362
17.6 Sources of further information and advice 363
17.7 Acknowledgements 364
17.8 References 364

18 Fibre-enriched beverages **369**
L. Viscione, Dupont Nutrition and Health (formerly Danisco UK Ltd), UK
18.1 Introduction 369
18.2 Adding fibres into drinks 370
18.3 Types of fibres suitable for fortifying non-dairy drinks: gums and beta-glucans 373
18.4 Types of fibres suitable for fortifying non-dairy drinks: fructans and glucose products 378
18.5 Typical beverage formulations containing fibre 383
18.6 Troubleshooting 384
18.7 Future trends 384
18.8 References 385

19 Fibre-enriched snack foods **389**
V. Stojceska, The Manchester Metropolitan University, UK
19.1 Introduction 389
19.2 Extrusion processing of ready-to-eat snacks 390
19.3 Nutritional benefits of extruded whole grains 392
19.4 Cereal by-products as a new source of dietary fibre 399
19.5 Improving the quality of extruded products 399
19.6 Conclusion 402
19.7 Future trends 402
19.8 References 403

20 Companion animal nutrition as affected by dietary fibre inclusion **407**
M. C. Rossoni Serão and G. C. Fahey Jr, University of Illinois, USA
20.1 Introduction 407
20.2 Effects of dietary fibre on food intake and gastric and small intestinal function in companion animals 408
20.3 Effects of dietary fibre on intestinal function of companion animals 412
20.4 Clinical significance of dietary fibres in companion animal diets 415
20.5 Strategies for incorporating fibre into companion animal diets 417
20.6 Conclusion 418
20.7 References 418

21 Soluble and insoluble fibre in infant nutrition **421**
G. Boehm, Danone Research, Centre for Specialised Nutrition, Germany
21.1 Introduction 421
21.2 Non-digestible carbohydrates in human milk 423
21.3 Soluble non-digestible carbohydrates of non-human milk origin 426
21.4 Insoluble non-digestible carbohydrates 436
21.5 Conclusion 438
21.6 References 439

Index *451*

Contributor contact details

(* = main contact)

Editors

Dr Jan A. Delcour
Laboratory of Food Chemistry and Biochemistry
KU Leuven
Kasteelpark Arenberg 20
3001 Leuven
Belgium

E-mail: jan.delcour@biw.kuleuven.be

Professor Kaisa Poutanen
VTT Biotekniikka
Tietotie 2
02044 Espoo
Finland

E-mail: Kaisa.Poutanen@vtt.fi

Chapter 1

Jan Willem Van der Kamp*
TNO Food and Nutrition
P.O. Box 360
3700 AJ ZEIST
The Netherlands

E-mail: jan-willem.vanderkamp@tno.nl

Joanne Lupton
Texas A&M University
USA

Chapter 2

Barry V. McCleary,* Anna Draga and N. Sloane
Megazyme International Ireland Limited
Bray Business Park
Southern Cross Road
Bray
County Wicklow
Ireland

E-mail: barry@megazyme.com; barrymcleary@me.com

Chapter 3

Joanne Slavin
Department of Food Science and Nutrition
University of Minnesota
1334 Eckles Avenue
St Paul
Minnesota 55108
USA

E-mail: jslavin@umn.edu; jslavin@g-mx.umn.edu

Chapter 4

Jenni Lappi,* Hannu Mykkänen and Marjukka Kolehmainen
Institute of Public Health and Clinical Nutrition
School of Medicine
University of Eastern Finland
P.O. Box 1627
FI-70211 Kuopio
Finland

E-mail: jenni.lappi@uef.fi, hannu.mykkanen@uef.fi, marjukka.kolehmainen@uef.fi

Kaisa Poutanen
VTT Technical Research Centre of Finland
Tietotie 2
02044 Espoo
Finland

E-mail: Kaisa.Poutanen@vtt.fi

Chapter 5

Steve W. Cui,* Ying Wu and Huihuang Ding
Guelph Food Research Centre
Agriculture and Agri-food Canada
Canada

E-mail: steve.cui@agr.gc.ca

Chapter 6

Kristen W. Dammann
Regulatory Senior Scientist
Scientific and Regulatory Affairs
Food Ingredients and Systems North America
Cargill Incorporated
Wayzata, Minnesota
USA

Denise Hauge, MS
Director
Grains for Health Foundation
St Louis Park, Minnesota
USA

Renee A. Rosen
Independent Consultant
Plymouth, Minnesota
USA

Natalia Schroeder
Postdoctoral Fellow
Johns Hopkins University
Bloomberg School of Public Health
Baltimore, Maryland
USA

Len Marquart*
President
Grains for Health Foundation
St Louis Park, MN

and

Associate Professor
University of Minnesota
St Paul, Minnesota
USA

E-mail: lmarquar@umn.edu

Chapter 7

Peter R. Shewry
Distinguished Research Fellow
Department of Plant Science
Rothamsted Research
Harpenden
Hertfordshire
AL5 2JQ
UK

E-mail: peter.shewry@rothamsted.ac.uk

and

Professor of Crops and Food
School of Agriculture, Policy and Development
University of Reading
Agriculture Building
Earley Gate
Whiteknights Road
P.O. Box 237
Reading
RG6 6AR
UK

Email: p.r.shewry@reading.ac.uk

Chapter 8

J. Sibakov,* P. Lehtinen and K. Poutanen
VTT Technical Research Centre of Finland
P.O. Box 1000
FI-02044 VTT
Finland

E-mail: Juhani.Sibakov@vtt.fi; Pekka.Lehtinen@vtt.fi

Chapter 9

Margareta Nyman* and Lina Haskå
Applied Nutrition and Food Chemistry
Department of Food Technology, Engineering and Nutrition
Kemicentrum
Lund University
P.O. Box 124
SE-22100 Lund
Sweden

E-mail: Margareta.Nyman@appliednutrition.lth.se

Chapter 10

A. Rakha
National Institute of Food Science & Technology
University of Agriculture
Faisalabad
Pakistan

P. Åman* and R. Andersson
Department of Food Science
Swedish University of Agricultural Sciences
SE-750 07
Uppsala
Sweden

E-mail: per.aman@slu.se

Chapter 11

Ana Salvador* and S. Fiszman
Instituto de Agroquímica y Tecnología de Alimentos (CSIC)
Avda Agustín Escardino 7
46980 Paterna (Valencia)
Spain

Email: asalvador@iata.csic.es; sfiszman@iata.csic.es

Chapter 12

Nesli Sozer* and Kaisa Poutanen
VTT Technical Research Centre of Finland
P.O. Box 1000
FI-02044 VTT
Finland

E-mail: Nesli.SozerAykal@vtt.fi; Kaisa.Poutanen@vtt.fi

Chapter 13

Charles Brennan
Professor of Food Science
Department of Wine, Food and Molecular Biosciences
Commerce Building 109
P.O. Box 84
Lincoln University
Lincoln
7647 Christchurch
New Zealand

E-mail: charles.brennan@lincoln.ac.nz

Chapter 14

Andrew S. Ross
Department of Crop and Soil Science

and

Department of Food Science and Technology
Oregon State University
Corvallis
Oregon 97331
USA

E-mail: rossan@coas.oregonstate.edu

Chapter 15

H. Douglas Goff
Department of Food Science
University of Guelph
Guelph
Ontario N1G 2W1
Canada

E-mail: dgoff@uoguelph.ca

Chapter 16

F. Jiménez-Colmenero* and G. Delgado-Pando
Department of Products
Meat and Meat Products Laboratory
Instituto de Ciencia y Tecnología de Alimentos y Nutrición (ICTAN-CSIC) (formerly Instituto del Frío)
C/ Jose Antonio Novais 10
Ciudad Universitaria
28040 Madrid
Spain

E-mail: fjimenez@ictan.csic.es

Chapter 17

A. J. Borderías* and M. Pérez-Mateos
Instituto de Ciencia y Tecnología de Alimentos y Nutrición (ICTAN-CSIC) (formerly Instituto del Frío)
C/ José Antonio Novais 10
28040 Madrid
Spain

E-mail: jborderias@ictan.csic.es

I. Sánchez-Alonso
Instituto de Estructura de la Materia (IEM-CSIC)
C/ Serrano 121
28006 Madrid
Spain

Chapter 18

Luisa Viscione
Dupont Nutrition and Health (formerly Danisco UK Ltd)
Reigate Place
43 London Road
Reigate
Surrey
RH2 9PW
UK

E-mail: luisa.viscione@dupont.com

Chapter 19

Valentina Stojceska
The Manchester Metropolitan University
Hollings Campus
Old Hall Lane
Manchester
M33 7LD
UK

E-mail: V.Stojceska@mmu.ac.uk

Chapter 20

Mariana C. Rossoni Serão*
Postdoctoral Research Associate
Comparative Nutrition – University of Illinois
Department of Animal Sciences
118 Animal Sciences Laboratory
1207 West Gregory Drive
Urbana
Illinois 61801
USA

E-mail: mrossoni@illinois.edu

George C. Fahey, Jr
Professor Emeritus of Animal Sciences and Nutritional Sciences
Comparative Nutrition – University of Illinois
Department of Animal Sciences
166 Animal Sciences Laboratory
1207 West Gregory Drive
Urbana
Illinois 61801
USA

E-mail: gcfahey@illinois.edu

Chapter 21

Gunther Boehm
Danone Research, Centre for Specialised Nutrition
Germany

Woodhead Publishing Series in Food Science, Technology and Nutrition

1 **Chilled foods: a comprehensive guide** *Edited by C. Dennis and M. Stringer*
2 **Yoghurt: science and technology** *A. Y. Tamime and R. K. Robinson*
3 **Food processing technology: principles and practice** *P. J. Fellows*
4 **Bender's dictionary of nutrition and food technology Sixth edition** *D. A. Bender*
5 **Determination of veterinary residues in food** *Edited by N. T. Crosby*
6 **Food contaminants: sources and surveillance** *Edited by C. Creaser and R. Purchase*
7 **Nitrates and nitrites in food and water** *Edited by M. J. Hill*
8 **Pesticide chemistry and bioscience: the food-environment challenge** *Edited by G. T. Brooks and T. Roberts*
9 **Pesticides: developments, impacts and controls** *Edited by G. A. Best and A. D. Ruthven*
10 **Dietary fibre: chemical and biological aspects** *Edited by D. A. T. Southgate, K. W. Waldron, I. T. Johnson and G. R. Fenwick*
11 **Vitamins and minerals in health and nutrition** *M. Tolonen*
12 **Technology of biscuits, crackers and cookies Second edition** *D. Manley*
13 **Instrumentation and sensors for the food industry** *Edited by E. Kress-Rogers*
14 **Food and cancer prevention: chemical and biological aspects** *Edited by K. W. Waldron, I. T. Johnson and G. R. Fenwick*
15 **Food colloids: proteins, lipids and polysaccharides** *Edited by E. Dickinson and B. Bergenstahl*
16 **Food emulsions and foams** *Edited by E. Dickinson*
17 **Maillard reactions in chemistry, food and health** *Edited by T. P. Labuza, V. Monnier, J. Baynes and J. O'Brien*
18 **The Maillard reaction in foods and medicine** *Edited by J. O'Brien, H. E. Nursten, M. J. Crabbe and J. M. Ames*
19 **Encapsulation and controlled release** *Edited by D. R. Karsa and R. A. Stephenson*
20 **Flavours and fragrances** *Edited by A. D. Swift*
21 **Feta and related cheeses** *Edited by A. Y. Tamime and R. K. Robinson*

22 **Biochemistry of milk products** *Edited by A. T. Andrews and J. R. Varley*
23 **Physical properties of foods and food processing systems** *M. J. Lewis*
24 **Food irradiation: a reference guide** *V. M. Wilkinson and G. Gould*
25 **Kent's technology of cereals: an introduction for students of food science and agriculture Fourth edition** *N. L. Kent and A. D. Evers*
26 **Biosensors for food analysis** *Edited by A. O. Scott*
27 **Separation processes in the food and biotechnology industries: principles and applications** *Edited by A. S. Grandison and M. J. Lewis*
28 **Handbook of indices of food quality and authenticity** *R. S. Singhal, P. K. Kulkarni and D. V. Rege*
29 **Principles and practices for the safe processing of foods** *D. A. Shapton and N. F. Shapton*
30 **Biscuit, cookie and cracker manufacturing manuals Volume 1: ingredients** *D. Manley*
31 **Biscuit, cookie and cracker manufacturing manuals Volume 2: biscuit doughs** *D. Manley*
32 **Biscuit, cookie and cracker manufacturing manuals Volume 3: biscuit dough piece forming** *D. Manley*
33 **Biscuit, cookie and cracker manufacturing manuals Volume 4: baking and cooling of biscuits** *D. Manley*
34 **Biscuit, cookie and cracker manufacturing manuals Volume 5: secondary processing in biscuit manufacturing** *D. Manley*
35 **Biscuit, cookie and cracker manufacturing manuals Volume 6: biscuit packaging and storage** *D. Manley*
36 **Practical dehydration Second edition** *M. Greensmith*
37 **Lawrie's meat science Sixth edition** *R. A. Lawrie*
38 **Yoghurt: science and technology Second edition** *A. Y. Tamime and R. K. Robinson*
39 **New ingredients in food processing: biochemistry and agriculture** *G. Linden and D. Lorient*
40 **Benders' dictionary of nutrition and food technology Seventh edition** *D. A. Bender and A. E. Bender*
41 **Technology of biscuits, crackers and cookies Third edition** *D. Manley*
42 **Food processing technology: principles and practice Second edition** *P. J. Fellows*
43 **Managing frozen foods** *Edited by C. J. Kennedy*
44 **Handbook of hydrocolloids** *Edited by G. O. Phillips and P. A. Williams*
45 **Food labelling** *Edited by J. R. Blanchfield*
46 **Cereal biotechnology** *Edited by P. C. Morris and J. H. Bryce*
47 **Food intolerance and the food industry** *Edited by T. Dean*
48 **The stability and shelf-life of food** *Edited by D. Kilcast and P. Subramaniam*
49 **Functional foods: concept to product** *Edited by G. R. Gibson and C. M. Williams*
50 **Chilled foods: a comprehensive guide Second edition** *Edited by M. Stringer and C. Dennis*
51 **HACCP in the meat industry** *Edited by M. Brown*
52 **Biscuit, cracker and cookie recipes for the food industry** *D. Manley*
53 **Cereals processing technology** *Edited by G. Owens*
54 **Baking problems solved** *S. P. Cauvain and L. S. Young*
55 **Thermal technologies in food processing** *Edited by P. Richardson*
56 **Frying: improving quality** *Edited by J. B. Rossell*
57 **Food chemical safety Volume 1: contaminants** *Edited by D. Watson*

58 **Making the most of HACCP: learning from others' experience** *Edited by T. Mayes and S. Mortimore*
59 **Food process modelling** *Edited by L. M. M. Tijskens, M. L. A. T. M. Hertog and B. M. Nicolaï*
60 **EU food law: a practical guide** *Edited by K. Goodburn*
61 **Extrusion cooking: technologies and applications** *Edited by R. Guy*
62 **Auditing in the food industry: from safety and quality to environmental and other audits** *Edited by M. Dillon and C. Griffith*
63 **Handbook of herbs and spices Volume 1** *Edited by K. V. Peter*
64 **Food product development: maximising success** *M. Earle, R. Earle and A. Anderson*
65 **Instrumentation and sensors for the food industry Second edition** *Edited by E. Kress-Rogers and C. J. B. Brimelow*
66 **Food chemical safety Volume 2: additives** *Edited by D. Watson*
67 **Fruit and vegetable biotechnology** *Edited by V. Valpuesta*
68 **Foodborne pathogens: hazards, risk analysis and control** *Edited by C. de W. Blackburn and P. J. McClure*
69 **Meat refrigeration** *S. J. James and C. James*
70 **Lockhart and Wiseman's crop husbandry Eighth edition** *H. J. S. Finch, A. M. Samuel and G. P. F. Lane*
71 **Safety and quality issues in fish processing** *Edited by H. A. Bremner*
72 **Minimal processing technologies in the food industries** *Edited by T. Ohlsson and N. Bengtsson*
73 **Fruit and vegetable processing: improving quality** *Edited by W. Jongen*
74 **The nutrition handbook for food processors** *Edited by C. J. K. Henry and C. Chapman*
75 **Colour in food: improving quality** *Edited by D. MacDougall*
76 **Meat processing: improving quality** *Edited by J. P. Kerry, J. F. Kerry and D. A. Ledward*
77 **Microbiological risk assessment in food processing** *Edited by M. Brown and M. Stringer*
78 **Performance functional foods** *Edited by D. Watson*
79 **Functional dairy products Volume 1** *Edited by T. Mattila-Sandholm and M. Saarela*
80 **Taints and off-flavours in foods** *Edited by B. Baigrie*
81 **Yeasts in food** *Edited by T. Boekhout and V. Robert*
82 **Phytochemical functional foods** *Edited by I. T. Johnson and G. Williamson*
83 **Novel food packaging techniques** *Edited by R. Ahvenainen*
84 **Detecting pathogens in food** *Edited by T. A. McMeekin*
85 **Natural antimicrobials for the minimal processing of foods** *Edited by S. Roller*
86 **Texture in food Volume 1: semi-solid foods** *Edited by B. M. McKenna*
87 **Dairy processing: improving quality** *Edited by G. Smit*
88 **Hygiene in food processing: principles and practice** *Edited by H. L. M. Lelieveld, M. A. Mostert, B. White and J. Holah*
89 **Rapid and on-line instrumentation for food quality assurance** *Edited by I. Tothill*
90 **Sausage manufacture: principles and practice** *E. Essien*
91 **Environmentally-friendly food processing** *Edited by B. Mattsson and U. Sonesson*
92 **Bread making: improving quality** *Edited by S. P. Cauvain*
93 **Food preservation techniques** *Edited by P. Zeuthen and L. Bøgh-Sørensen*
94 **Food authenticity and traceability** *Edited by M. Lees*

95 **Analytical methods for food additives** *R. Wood, L. Foster, A. Damant and P. Key*
96 **Handbook of herbs and spices Volume 2** *Edited by K. V. Peter*
97 **Texture in food Volume 2: solid foods** *Edited by D. Kilcast*
98 **Proteins in food processing** *Edited by R. Yada*
99 **Detecting foreign bodies in food** *Edited by M. Edwards*
100 **Understanding and measuring the shelf-life of food** *Edited by R. Steele*
101 **Poultry meat processing and quality** *Edited by G. Mead*
102 **Functional foods, ageing and degenerative disease** *Edited by C. Remacle and B. Reusens*
103 **Mycotoxins in food: detection and control** *Edited by N. Magan and M. Olsen*
104 **Improving the thermal processing of foods** *Edited by P. Richardson*
105 **Pesticide, veterinary and other residues in food** *Edited by D. Watson*
106 **Starch in food: structure, functions and applications** *Edited by A.-C. Eliasson*
107 **Functional foods, cardiovascular disease and diabetes** *Edited by A. Arnoldi*
108 **Brewing: science and practice** *D. E. Briggs, P. A. Brookes, R. Stevens and C. A. Boulton*
109 **Using cereal science and technology for the benefit of consumers: proceedings of the 12th International ICC Cereal and Bread Congress, 24 – 26th May, 2004, Harrogate, UK** *Edited by S. P. Cauvain, L. S. Young and S. Salmon*
110 **Improving the safety of fresh meat** *Edited by J. Sofos*
111 **Understanding pathogen behaviour: virulence, stress response and resistance** *Edited by M. Griffiths*
112 **The microwave processing of foods** *Edited by H. Schubert and M. Regier*
113 **Food safety control in the poultry industry** *Edited by G. Mead*
114 **Improving the safety of fresh fruit and vegetables** *Edited by W. Jongen*
115 **Food, diet and obesity** *Edited by D. Mela*
116 **Handbook of hygiene control in the food industry** *Edited by H. L. M. Lelieveld, M. A. Mostert and J. Holah*
117 **Detecting allergens in food** *Edited by S. Koppelman and S. Hefle*
118 **Improving the fat content of foods** *Edited by C. Williams and J. Buttriss*
119 **Improving traceability in food processing and distribution** *Edited by I. Smith and A. Furness*
120 **Flavour in food** *Edited by A. Voilley and P. Etievant*
121 **The Chorleywood bread process** *S. P. Cauvain and L. S. Young*
122 **Food spoilage microorganisms** *Edited by C. de W. Blackburn*
123 **Emerging foodborne pathogens** *Edited by Y. Motarjemi and M. Adams*
124 **Benders' dictionary of nutrition and food technology Eighth edition** *D. A. Bender*
125 **Optimising sweet taste in foods** *Edited by W. J. Spillane*
126 **Brewing: new technologies** *Edited by C. Bamforth*
127 **Handbook of herbs and spices Volume 3** *Edited by K. V. Peter*
128 **Lawrie's meat science Seventh edition** *R. A. Lawrie in collaboration with D. A. Ledward*
129 **Modifying lipids for use in food** *Edited by F. Gunstone*
130 **Meat products handbook: practical science and technology** *G. Feiner*
131 **Food consumption and disease risk: consumer–pathogen interactions** *Edited by M. Potter*
132 **Acrylamide and other hazardous compounds in heat-treated foods** *Edited by K. Skog and J. Alexander*

133 **Managing allergens in food** *Edited by C. Mills, H. Wichers and K. Hoffman-Sommergruber*
134 **Microbiological analysis of red meat, poultry and eggs** *Edited by G. Mead*
135 **Maximising the value of marine by-products** *Edited by F. Shahidi*
136 **Chemical migration and food contact materials** *Edited by K. Barnes, R. Sinclair and D. Watson*
137 **Understanding consumers of food products** *Edited by L. Frewer and H. van Trijp*
138 **Reducing salt in foods: practical strategies** *Edited by D. Kilcast and F. Angus*
139 **Modelling microorganisms in food** *Edited by S. Brul, S. Van Gerwen and M. Zwietering*
140 **Tamime and Robinson's Yoghurt: science and technology Third edition** *A. Y. Tamime and R. K. Robinson*
141 **Handbook of waste management and co-product recovery in food processing Volume 1** *Edited by K. W. Waldron*
142 **Improving the flavour of cheese** *Edited by B. Weimer*
143 **Novel food ingredients for weight control** *Edited by C. J. K. Henry*
144 **Consumer-led food product development** *Edited by H. MacFie*
145 **Functional dairy products Volume 2** *Edited by M. Saarela*
146 **Modifying flavour in food** *Edited by A. J. Taylor and J. Hort*
147 **Cheese problems solved** *Edited by P. L. H. McSweeney*
148 **Handbook of organic food safety and quality** *Edited by J. Cooper, C. Leifert and U. Niggli*
149 **Understanding and controlling the microstructure of complex foods** *Edited by D. J. McClements*
150 **Novel enzyme technology for food applications** *Edited by R. Rastall*
151 **Food preservation by pulsed electric fields: from research to application** *Edited by H. L. M. Lelieveld and S. W. H. de Haan*
152 **Technology of functional cereal products** *Edited by B. R. Hamaker*
153 **Case studies in food product development** *Edited by M. Earle and R. Earle*
154 **Delivery and controlled release of bioactives in foods and nutraceuticals** *Edited by N. Garti*
155 **Fruit and vegetable flavour: recent advances and future prospects** *Edited by B. Brückner and S. G. Wyllie*
156 **Food fortification and supplementation: technological, safety and regulatory aspects** *Edited by P. Berry Ottaway*
157 **Improving the health-promoting properties of fruit and vegetable products** *Edited by F. A. Tomás-Barberán and M. I. Gil*
158 **Improving seafood products for the consumer** *Edited by T. Børresen*
159 **In-pack processed foods: improving quality** *Edited by P. Richardson*
160 **Handbook of water and energy management in food processing** *Edited by J. Klemeš, R. Smith and J.-K. Kim*
161 **Environmentally compatible food packaging** *Edited by E. Chiellini*
162 **Improving farmed fish quality and safety** *Edited by Ø. Lie*
163 **Carbohydrate-active enzymes** *Edited by K.-H. Park*
164 **Chilled foods: a comprehensive guide Third edition** *Edited by M. Brown*
165 **Food for the ageing population** *Edited by M. M. Raats, C. P. G. M. de Groot and W. A. Van Staveren*
166 **Improving the sensory and nutritional quality of fresh meat** *Edited by J. P. Kerry and D. A. Ledward*

167 **Shellfish safety and quality** *Edited by S. E. Shumway and G. E. Rodrick*
168 **Functional and speciality beverage technology** *Edited by P. Paquin*
169 **Functional foods: principles and technology** *M. Guo*
170 **Endocrine-disrupting chemicals in food** *Edited by I. Shaw*
171 **Meals in science and practice: interdisciplinary research and business applications** *Edited by H. L. Meiselman*
172 **Food constituents and oral health: current status and future prospects** *Edited by M. Wilson*
173 **Handbook of hydrocolloids Second edition** *Edited by G. O. Phillips and P. A. Williams*
174 **Food processing technology: principles and practice Third edition** *P. J. Fellows*
175 **Science and technology of enrobed and filled chocolate, confectionery and bakery products** *Edited by G. Talbot*
176 **Foodborne pathogens: hazards, risk analysis and control Second edition** *Edited by C. de W. Blackburn and P. J. McClure*
177 **Designing functional foods: measuring and controlling food structure breakdown and absorption** *Edited by D. J. McClements and E. A. Decker*
178 **New technologies in aquaculture: improving production efficiency, quality and environmental management** *Edited by G. Burnell and G. Allan*
179 **More baking problems solved** *S. P. Cauvain and L. S. Young*
180 **Soft drink and fruit juice problems solved** *P. Ashurst and R. Hargitt*
181 **Biofilms in the food and beverage industries** *Edited by P. M. Fratamico, B. A. Annous and N. W. Gunther*
182 **Dairy-derived ingredients: food and nutraceutical uses** *Edited by M. Corredig*
183 **Handbook of waste management and co-product recovery in food processing Volume 2** *Edited by K. W. Waldron*
184 **Innovations in food labelling** *Edited by J. Albert*
185 **Delivering performance in food supply chains** *Edited by C. Mena and G. Stevens*
186 **Chemical deterioration and physical instability of food and beverages** *Edited by L. H. Skibsted, J. Risbo and M. L. Andersen*
187 **Managing wine quality Volume 1: viticulture and wine quality** *Edited by A. G. Reynolds*
188 **Improving the safety and quality of milk Volume 1: milk production and processing** *Edited by M. Griffiths*
189 **Improving the safety and quality of milk Volume 2: improving quality in milk products** *Edited by M. Griffiths*
190 **Cereal grains: assessing and managing quality** *Edited by C. Wrigley and I. Batey*
191 **Sensory analysis for food and beverage quality control: a practical guide** *Edited by D. Kilcast*
192 **Managing wine quality Volume 2: oenology and wine quality** *Edited by A. G. Reynolds*
193 **Winemaking problems solved** *Edited by C. E. Butzke*
194 **Environmental assessment and management in the food industry** *Edited by U. Sonesson, J. Berlin and F. Ziegler*
195 **Consumer-driven innovation in food and personal care products** *Edited by S. R. Jaeger and H. MacFie*
196 **Tracing pathogens in the food chain** *Edited by S. Brul, P. M. Fratamico and T. A. McMeekin*

197 **Case studies in novel food processing technologies: innovations in processing, packaging, and predictive modelling** *Edited by C. J. Doona, K. Kustin and F. E. Feeherry*
198 **Freeze-drying of pharmaceutical and food products** *T.-C. Hua, B.-L. Liu and H. Zhang*
199 **Oxidation in foods and beverages and antioxidant applications Volume 1: understanding mechanisms of oxidation and antioxidant activity** *Edited by E. A. Decker, R. J. Elias and D. J. McClements*
200 **Oxidation in foods and beverages and antioxidant applications Volume 2: management in different industry sectors** *Edited by E. A. Decker, R. J. Elias and D. J. McClements*
201 **Protective cultures, antimicrobial metabolites and bacteriophages for food and beverage biopreservation** *Edited by C. Lacroix*
202 **Separation, extraction and concentration processes in the food, beverage and nutraceutical industries** *Edited by S. S. H. Rizvi*
203 **Determining mycotoxins and mycotoxigenic fungi in food and feed** *Edited by S. De Saeger*
204 **Developing children's food products** *Edited by D. Kilcast and F. Angus*
205 **Functional foods: concept to product Second edition** *Edited by M. Saarela*
206 **Postharvest biology and technology of tropical and subtropical fruits Volume 1: fundamental issues** *Edited by E. M. Yahia*
207 **Postharvest biology and technology of tropical and subtropical fruits Volume 2: açai to citrus** *Edited by E. M. Yahia*
208 **Postharvest biology and technology of tropical and subtropical fruits Volume 3: cocona to mango** *Edited by E. M. Yahia*
209 **Postharvest biology and technology of tropical and subtropical fruits Volume 4: mangosteen to white sapote** *Edited by E. M. Yahia*
210 **Food and beverage stability and shelf life** *Edited by D. Kilcast and P. Subramaniam*
211 **Processed meats: improving safety, nutrition and quality** *Edited by J. P. Kerry and J. F. Kerry*
212 **Food chain integrity: a holistic approach to food traceability, safety, quality and authenticity** *Edited by J. Hoorfar, K. Jordan, F. Butler and R. Prugger*
213 **Improving the safety and quality of eggs and egg products Volume 1** *Edited by Y. Nys, M. Bain and F. Van Immerseel*
214 **Improving the safety and quality of eggs and egg products Volume 2** *Edited by F. Van Immerseel, Y. Nys and M. Bain*
215 **Animal feed contamination: effects on livestock and food safety** *Edited by J. Fink-Gremmels*
216 **Hygienic design of food factories** *Edited by J. Holah and H. L. M. Lelieveld*
217 **Manley's technology of biscuits, crackers and cookies Fourth edition** *Edited by D. Manley*
218 **Nanotechnology in the food, beverage and nutraceutical industries** *Edited by Q. Huang*
219 **Rice quality: a guide to rice properties and analysis** *K. R. Bhattacharya*
220 **Advances in meat, poultry and seafood packaging** *Edited by J. P. Kerry*
221 **Reducing saturated fats in foods** *Edited by G. Talbot*
222 **Handbook of food proteins** *Edited by G. O. Phillips and P. A. Williams*

223 **Lifetime nutritional influences on cognition, behaviour and psychiatric illness** *Edited by D. Benton*
224 **Food machinery for the production of cereal foods, snack foods and confectionery** *L.-M. Cheng*
225 **Alcoholic beverages: sensory evaluation and consumer research** *Edited by J. Piggott*
226 **Extrusion problems solved: food, pet food and feed** *M. N. Riaz and G. J. Rokey*
227 **Handbook of herbs and spices Second edition Volume 1** *Edited by K. V. Peter*
228 **Handbook of herbs and spices Second edition Volume 2** *Edited by K. V. Peter*
229 **Breadmaking: improving quality Second edition** *Edited by S. P. Cauvain*
230 **Emerging food packaging technologies: principles and practice** *Edited by K. L. Yam and D. S. Lee*
231 **Infectious disease in aquaculture: prevention and control** *Edited by B. Austin*
232 **Diet, immunity and inflammation** *Edited by P. C. Calder and P. Yaqoob*
233 **Natural food additives, ingredients and flavourings** *Edited by D. Baines and R. Seal*
234 **Microbial decontamination in the food industry: novel methods and applications** *Edited by A. Demirci and M. O. Ngadi*
235 **Chemical contaminants and residues in foods** *Edited by D. Schrenk*
236 **Robotics and automation in the food industry: current and future technologies** *Edited by D. G. Caldwell*
237 **Fibre-rich and wholegrain foods: improving quality** *Edited by J. A. Delcour and K. Poutanen*
238 **Computer vision technology in the food and beverage industries** *Edited by D.-W. Sun*
239 **Encapsulation technologies and delivery systems for food ingredients and nutraceuticals** *Edited by N. Garti and D. J. McClements*
240 **Case studies in food safety and authenticity** *Edited by J. Hoorfar*
241 **Heat treatment for insect control: developments and applications** *D. Hammond*
242 **Advances in aquaculture hatchery technology** *Edited by G. Allan and G. Burnell*
243 **Open innovation in the food and beverage industry: concepts and case studies** *Edited by M. Garcia Martinez*
244 **Trends in packaging of food, beverages and other fast-moving consumer goods (FMCG)** *Edited by N. J. Farmer*
245 **New analytical approaches for verifying the origin of food** *Edited by P. Brereton*
246 **Microbial production of food ingredients, enzymes and nutraceuticals** *Edited by B. McNeil, D. Archer, I. Giavasis and L. Harvey*
247 **Persistent organic pollutants and toxic metals in foods** *Edited by M. Rose and A. Fernandes*
248 **Cereal grains for the food and beverage industries** *E. Arendt and E. Zannini*
249 **Viruses in food and water: risks, surveillance and control** *Edited by N. Cook*
250 **Improving the safety and quality of nuts** *Edited by L. J. Harris*
251 **Metabolomics in food and nutrition** *Edited by B. Weimer and C. Slupsky*
252 **Food enrichment with omega-3 fatty acids** *Edited by C. Jacobsen, N. Skall Nielsen, A. Frisenfeldt Horn and A.-D. Moltke Sørensen*
253 **Instrumental assessment of food sensory quality: a practical guide** *Edited by D. Kilcast*
254 **Food microstructures: microscopy, measurement and modelling** *Edited by V. J. Morris and K. Groves*

255 **Handbook of food powders: processes and properties** *Edited by B. R. Bhandari, N. Bansal, M. Zhang and P. Schuck*
256 **Functional ingredients from algae for foods and nutraceuticals** *Edited by H. Domínguez*
257 **Satiation, satiety and the control of food intake: theory and practice** *Edited by J. E. Blundell and F. Bellisle*
258 **Hygiene in food processing: principles and practice Second edition** *Edited by H. L. M. Lelieveld, J. Holah and D. Napper*

Part I

Introductory issues

1

Definitions, regulations and health claims associated with dietary fibre and wholegrain foods

J. W. Van der Kamp, TNO, The Netherlands, and J. Lupton, Texas A&M University, USA

DOI: 10.1533/9780857095787.1.3

Abstract: Consumers worldwide are becoming increasingly interested in healthy eating, and have consequently (re)discovered the value of wholegrain-based and fibre-rich products. Governments and industry associations are developing regulations and guidelines for labelling, while authorities and scientific bodies are issuing and renewing dietary guidelines for recommended intake and assessing the numerous health claim proposals submitted by the industry. After a short outline on definitions and related analytical methods, this chapter presents an overview of the current state of affairs.

Key words: dietary fibre, wholegrain, labelling, dietary recommendations, health claims.

1.1 Introduction

For the past century, most cereal products have been based on flour that consists mainly of the endosperm, that is, after removal of the outer parts of the kernel, bran and germ: the two parts containing most of the dietary fibre and other bioactive components such as micronutrients and phytochemicals. Levels of these substances in wholewheat flour are 2.5 to more than five times higher than those in refined white flour.

Consumers worldwide are becoming increasingly interested in healthy eating, and have consequently (re)discovered the value of wholegrain-based products. As a response, the food industry is developing a growing number of products associated with health benefits, including products high in dietary fibre and whole grains, and consumption of wholegrain products is growing, both in countries

Table 1.1 Wholegrain new product launches by category

Category	2000	2002	2004	2006	2008	2010	2011
Baby food	3	7	8	29	55	86	102
Bakery	84	158	337	639	1092	1248	1228
Breakfast cereals	37	74	175	414	824	971	1039
Meals and entrees	7	11	25	71	127	116	129
Side dishes	18	47	49	127	250	277	287
Snacks	2	17	57	286	435	485	484
Other	13	7	23	35	100	89	109
Total	164	321	674	1601	2883	3272	3378

Source: Whole Grains Council.
http://www.wholegrainscouncil.org/newsroom/whole-grain-statistics.

with a wholegrain tradition, such as those in northern Europe, and in countries where wholegrain was previously scarcely known. Table 1.1 shows how the launches of new wholegrain products have grown exponentially over the past decade.

Governments and industry associations are developing regulations and guidelines for labelling, while authorities and scientific bodies are issuing and renewing dietary guidelines for recommended intake and assessing the numerous health claim proposals submitted by the industry.

1.2 Defining dietary fibre and wholegrain

For several decades, no worldwide agreement on the definition of dietary fibre or wholegrain could be obtained. For dietary fibre, most parties involved endorsed a definition covering all carbohydrates that are non-digestible in the small intestine, but others wanted to include only remnants of edible plant cells, polysaccharide, lignin and associated substances, as being naturally present in plant-based foods. Similarly, for wholegrain, many countries only have very brief definitions dating back some years, such as 'Wholegrain products include the entire germ, endosperm and bran. Grains that have been subjected to processing such as milling are also included.'

As a basis for both the information given to consumers and the regulations relating to wholegrain and dietary fibre, internationally agreed definitions and regulations in this area need to be established. This section outlines the definitions that have been drawn up in recent years for dietary fibre and wholegrain and adopted by a number of countries.

1.2.1 Definitions of dietary fibre

In 2009, Codex Alimentarius adopted the following definition of dietary fibre:

> Dietary fibre consists of carbohydrate polymers[a] with ten or more monomeric units[b], which are not hydrolyzed by the endogenous enzymes in the small intestine of humans and belong to the following categories:
>
> - Edible carbohydrate polymers naturally occurring in the food as consumed;
> - Carbohydrate polymers which have been obtained from food raw material by physical, enzymatic or chemical means and which have been shown to have a physiological effect of benefit to health as demonstrated by generally accepted scientific evidence to competent authorities, and;
> - Synthetic carbohydrate polymers which have been shown to have a physiological effect of benefit to health as demonstrated by generally accepted scientific evidence to competent authorities.
>
> [a] When derived from a plant origin, dietary fibre may include fractions of lignin and/or other compounds when associated with polysaccharides in the plant cell walls and if these compounds are quantified by the American Association of Analytical Chemists (AOAC) gravimetric analytical method for dietary fibre analysis: Fractions of lignin and the other compounds (proteic fractions, phenolic compounds, waxes, saponins, phytates, cutin, phytosterols, etc.) intimately "associated" with plant polysaccharides in the AOAC 991.43 method.
>
> [b] Decision on whether to include carbohydrates of 3 to 9 monomeric units should be left up to national authorities.
>
> (Codex Alimentarius, 2011)

Prior to this, in November 2008 the European Union had also agreed on a definition of dietary fibre, which was similar to the Codex definition. The EU has decided to include all carbohydrates with three or more monomeric units (EU, 2008). A range of other countries, including China, Japan and Canada, have also chosen to include non-digestible carbohydrates with degree of polymerisation (DP) >2.

In the debates surrounding the definition of dietary fibre, the health benefits of fibres present in foods such as fruit, vegetables, potatoes and wholegrain products were considered as generally accepted, whereas questions were raised about the health benefits of isolated and synthetic non-digestible carbohydrates. Therefore for these categories the Codex Alimentarius definition includes the requirement that these must 'have been shown to have a physiological effect of benefit to health as demonstrated by generally accepted scientific evidence to competent authorities'. The same requirement has also been included in most other recent definitions.

1.2.2 Definitions of wholegrain

In addition to the short definitions of some decades ago, recently more comprehensive definitions have been developed in a number of countries, including items such as a positive list of the grains included and specifications of allowed processes. Characteristics of a number of these definitions are given in Table 1.2.

Table 1.2 Definitions of wholegrain

Who and what	What qualifies as a whole grain?	Which grains are included?
Germany, 1961 DIN #10355 Mahlerzeugnisse (considered a standard definition but not a law) USA 1999 AACC International	Wholemeal flour and wholemeal break flour must include all components of the cleaned kernels, including the germ. The pericarp of the grain kernels can be removed before the processing. Whole grains shall consist of the intact, ground, cracked or flaked caryopsis, whose principal anatomical components – the starchy endosperm, germ and bran – are present in the same relative proportions as they exist in the intact caryopsis.	All plants from the *Poaceae* (*Gramineae*) family plus the pseudocereals amaranth, buckwheat, and quinoa.
USA, 2004 Whole Grains Council (Whole Grains Council, 2004)	Whole grains or foods made from them contain all the essential parts and naturally-occurring nutrients of the entire grain seed. If the grain has been processed (e.g., cracked, crushed, rolled, extruded, and/or cooked), the food product should deliver approximately the same rich balance of nutrients that are found in the original grain seed.	All plants from the *Poaceae* (*Gramineae*) family plus the pseudocereals amaranth, buckwheat, and quinoa. *Note: This list is not meant to be comprehensive, but to include those grains most familiar to consumers. Other cereal grasses from the Poaceae (or Gramineous) family, such as canary seed, Job's tears, Montina, Timothy, fonio, etc. are also whole grains when consumed with all of their bran, germ and endosperm.*
UK 2010 The Institute of Grocery Distribution (IGD, 2007)	[Whole grain] refers to the edible entire grain after removal of inedible parts such as the hull and glume. It must include the entire germ, endosperm and bran. Temporary separation of whole grain constituents during processing for later recombination is acceptable provided the proportions of the germ, endosperm and bran are the same or virtually the same as in the original grain. Simply adding together these three whole grain constituents as separate ingredients does not constitute a whole grain and making a claim that it does could be misleading to consumers.	Amaranth, barley, buckwheat, maize, millet, oats, quinoa, rye, sorghum, teff, triticale, brown rice, wheat, wild rice.

Denmark, 2007 Danish National Food Institute (www.food.dtu.dk) (Whole Grains Council, 2007a)	Wholegrain is defined as intact and processed (dehulled, ground, cracked, flaked or the like) grains, where the components endosperm, bran and germ are present in the same proportions as in the intact grain.	Includes grain seeds from the following genera of the grass family *Gramineae*: barley (*Hordeum*), oat (*Avena*), wheat (*Triticum*), rye (*Secale*), rice (*Oryza*), millet (*Panicum*), maize (*Zea*; only as dried maize) and sorghum (*Sorgum*) (no wild rice and no pseudocereals).
Scandinavian keyhole	A whole grain is defined as intact and processed (dehulled, ground, cracked, flaked, or the like) products where endosperm, germ, and bran are present in the same proportions as in the intact grain. If these fractions are separated under processing, they should be added back so that the final product has approximately the same relative proportions of the three parts as in the intact grain.	The whole grain definition includes the following wholegrain cereals: wheat, rye, oats, barley, maize (dry seeds), rice, millet, and sorghum. Wild rice, quinoa, amaranth, and buckwheat are not included.
EU, 2010 HEALTHGRAIN (HEALTHGRAIN, 2010)	Whole grains shall consist of the intact, ground, cracked or flaked kernel after the removal of inedible parts such as the hull and husk. The principal anatomical components – the starchy endosperm, germ and bran – are present in the same relative proportions as they exist in the intact kernel. Small losses of components – that is, less than 2% of the grain/10% of the bran – that occur through processing methods consistent with safety and quality are allowed.	The same grains as in the AACC/FDA definition.
Australia New Zealand Food Standards Code	Wholegrain means the intact grain or the dehulled, ground, milled, cracked or flaked grain where the constituents – endosperm, germ and bran – are present in such proportions that represent the typical ratio of those fractions occurring in the whole cereal, and includes wholemeal. Wholemeal means the product containing all the milled constituents of the grain in such proportions that it represents the typical ratio of those fractions occurring in the whole cereal.	

Grains included

All definitions of wholegrain are restricted to cereal and pseudo-cereal grains, that is, the grains where, generally, the outer layers (the bran and endosperm) can be removed. The UK IGD Guideline (2007) and the HEALTHGRAIN (2010) definition adopted the list of grains included given in the American Association of Cereal Chemists (AACC) definition above. The definition proposed by the Whole Grains Council included this in a more flexible way by stating: 'this list is not meant to be comprehensive, but to include those grains most familiar to consumers. Other cereal grasses from the *Poaceae* (or Gramineous) family, such as canary seed, Job's tears, Montina, Timothy, fonio, etc. are also whole grains when consumed with all of their bran, germ and endosperm' (Whole Grains Council, 2004).

The grains included in the AACC definition are also included in the Food and Drugs Administration (FDA) whole grain health claim. However, the HEALTHGRAIN definition, including the same grains as the AACC definition, explicitly states: 'This whole grain definition is expected to be useful in the context of nutrition recommendations and guidelines and nutrition claims. Health claims, on the other hand, must be based on documentation of specific effects of grains or grain components in the diet.' Also, in the UK and Scandinavia a larger set of grains is included in definitions made for labelling purposes than in those made for the purpose of health claims used before the EU adopted Regulation 1924/2006 on nutrition and health claims (EU Corrigendum, 2006). Starting from the public health perspective, products prepared with whole grains or wholemeal flours of all cereal and pseudo-cereal grains are to be preferred over their counterparts based on refined grains. Within this context broad definitions, such as those of AACC, HEALTHGRAIN and IGD, are appropriate. However, with strict regulations, as in the EU, these broad definitions are not applicable for health claims. Also, when consumption of whole grains is mentioned as a preferred way for realising an adequate intake of dietary fibre, as is recommended, for example, by the World Health Organization (WHO) (2003) and the Health Council of the Netherlands (2006), only a more restricted list of grains will qualify.

Processing

The Australia New Zealand Food Standards Code restricts the use of the term wholegrain to products made with intact grain kernels. For other products the term 'wholemeal' should be used instead. Other definitions use wholegrain to refer to processed grains as well, including ground, milled and flaked grains. Germanic languages, like German, Dutch, Danish and Swedish, use terms like Vollkorn (German) and Fuldkorn (Danish) to describe both intact and processed kernels.

Over 90% of the wholegrain wheat, corn and rye flour in food supply chains is created through milling processes in which kernels are broken, separated into milling streams containing endosperm-rich (white) flour, germ and various bran fractions, and recombined in fixed ratios. For flour with a long shelf life, rancidity-promoting enzymes in the germ are inactivated by heat treatment of the germ fraction. This 'modern milling' process ensures a longer shelf life and constant flour quality in terms of composition and processability compared with the traditional stone-ground process, in which grain is milled without separation and recombination. Recombination may take place both at the flour mill and during production of the final product. With this production process the recombined flour may be composed of white flour, germ and bran originating from different batches of the grain.

In the HEALTHGRAIN (2010) definition small losses of components – that is, less than 2% of the grain / 10% of the bran – that occur through processing methods consistent with safety and quality are allowed. This option is included because the very outer pericarp layer is removed in order to decrease levels of contaminants that may be concentrated in this layer, such as mycotoxins or agrochemicals. Similar losses are also allowed in definitions used in Switzerland and Germany, but not in other definitions.

Occasionally the question is raised whether recombination should be allowed for wholegrain products, since the final composition may be not exactly the same as that of wholemeal flour produced by stone-ground processing. This issue was discussed in depth when the most recent definition, issued by HEALTHGRAIN, was drafted. The reasons put forward for including recombination were:

- The great majority of the research supporting the health benefits of whole grains has been based on consumption of foods made with recombined whole grains. This holds for all epidemiology studies, since recombination is being applied for (almost) all commonly consumed products and also for most clinical trials.
- The composition of wholegrain flour of one type of grain shows major variations. Studies before HEALTHGRAIN, and in HEALTHGRAIN with a focus on wheat, have shown that the composition of wholegrain is affected by both genetic (cultivar) and environmental factors. In the HEALTHGRAIN studies (Ward *et al.*, 2008), cultivars could be differentiated according to high and low levels of fibre and other bioactive substances: i) high fibre, high bioactives; ii) high fibre, low bioactives; iii) low fibre, high bioactives; and iv) low fibre, low bioactives. One may assume that wholemeal flours made by the recombination of fixed ratios of milling streams will ensure a more consistent composition than that observed in flours made by stone-grinding of individual batches and cultivars.

When applied responsibly, recombination may produce a more consistent wholemeal composition; however, incorrect application may result in 'wholemeal' flours with levels of germ and/or bran far below the acceptable range. The HEALTHGRAIN definition therefore states that production of wholegrain flours and products must follow appropriate quality systems (Good Manufacturing Processes, and so on). The Whole Grains Council requires any company seeking to use the Whole Grain Stamp based on any reconstituted ingredients to sign a legal form attesting that all of the bran, germ and endosperm are present in their original proportions, in line with the FDA definition of whole grain (FDA, 2006).

Future developments in wholegrain definitions
Since a Codex agreement for a definition can markedly contribute to international harmonisation, several parties asked Codex for a definition of wholegrain, as had been provided for dietary fibre (outlined in Section 1.2.1). However, the Codex Committee on Nutrition and Foods for Special Dietary Uses decided in its 2010 session that it would not be involved in defining wholegrain (CCNFSDU, 2010). The HEALTHGRAIN Forum – the association established in 2010 after the end of the HEALTHGRAIN EU project – is aiming to have the HEALTHGRAIN definition accepted as the EU definition.

The current definitions of wholegrain cover a large set of cereal grains: however, there is a growing need to establish wholegrain criteria and/or definitions for individual cereal grains, due to the request by food inspection agencies for analytical criteria for wholegrain flours and products. In Europe, the European Food Safety Authority (EFSA) requires a well-defined composition for any ingredients, foods or food categories claimed to have health benefits before these claims are approved.

1.3 Analysing the dietary fibre and wholegrain content of food

1.3.1 Analysis of dietary fibre content

Since the early 1980s, dietary fibre has been analysed predominantly by using the AOAC Official Method 985.29 and its modified version AOAC 991.43, using organic buffers instead of phosphate buffers. These methods have been used for the great majority of fibre values listed in food composition databases. In a number of countries fibre is even defined as the sum of compounds analysed as such with the AOAC 985.29 method.

In the UK, fibre was traditionally analysed with the Englyst method (Englyst and Hudson, 1996). This method mainly measures non-starch polysaccharide (NSP), giving lower estimates of dietary fibre values in products with resistant starch, lignin and oligosaccharides. In more recent years a shift towards the AOAC methods mentioned above can be noticed.

As is outlined in more detail in Chapter 2, AOAC 985.29 does not determine all resistant starch (only the fraction resistant to the enzymes used in the assay, which includes mainly retrograded amylose, known as RS3), while other, mainly low molecular, types of fibre are measured only for a minor part or not at all. The combination of AOAC 985.29 with methods that measure the missing parts creates the problem of double counting (McCleary, 2007).

The integrated procedure for Total Dietary Fibre, the AOAC Official Method 2009.01 – described in detail in Chapter 2 – has been adopted by Codex Alimentarius as a type 1 method in the 32nd Session of the Codex Committee on Methods of Analysis and Sampling, March 2011 (CCMAS, 2011). High molecular weight and low molecular weight non-digestible saccharides are measured separately in this method, so fibre levels including and excluding oligosaccharides with DP3–9 can be determined.

The first results from the analysis of fibre in bakery products using AOAC 2009.01 show significantly higher levels than those determined using AOAC 985.29: for example, for white bread > 4% vs. < 3%, for wheat flour ~ 6% vs. ~2.5% and for wholemeal bread > 8% instead of ~ 7%. The increase is mainly due to the inclusion of low molecular weight saccharides (Brunt, 2011). About one-third of this increase is due to the incorrect counting of a minor part of digestible starch as low molecular weight non-digestible oligosaccharides (Brunt, 2011; Brunt and Sanders, 2012). Another flaw in the method is the lack of quantitative analysis of DP3 oligofructose, a significant part of inulin fibre products. With such a diverse mixture of analytes as total dietary fibre such flaws are not unexpected when experienced analysts are starting to use this new method. As indicated by Brunt, these flaws can be corrected by minor adaptations of AOAC 2009.01. When these corrections are being incorporated in a new version, this improved version of AOAC 2009.01 is the logical candidate for becoming the new legally endorsed method of analysis for dietary fibre in the EU and abroad.

In addition to the 2009.01 method, the AOAC and AACC International have also launched the Official method AOAC 2011.25, measuring total dietary fibre as the sum of insoluble and soluble fibre. However, EFSA and Food and Agriculture Organization of the United states (FAO)/WHO are considering this differentiation as method-dependent, and solubility does not always predict physiological effects. Therefore, Food and Agricultive Organization of the United States (FAO)/WHO proposed that the distinction between soluble and insoluble fibre should be phased out (FAO/WHO, 1998).

1.3.2 Analysis of wholegrain content

All wholegrain flours have significantly higher levels of fibre and other bioactive compounds than their refined counterparts without bran and germ. Levels vary due to genetic and environmental factors. Results from HEALTHGRAIN for 150 wheat cultivars showed variation in the level of fibre with a factor of 2 and of some other bioactive components with factors ranging from 1.5 to 5 (Ward *et al.*, 2008). Although variations in commercially available cultivars are expected to be somewhat smaller, they are far from negligible; for example, dietary fibre levels of wheat cultivars grown in Germany ranged from 9 to 15% in a period of ten years (Dr Lindhauer, Max Rubner Institute, Detmold, personal communication).

Good methods for determining the percentage of wholegrain in a flour or a product are not currently available. Chen *et al.* (2004) found a good correlation between calculated and analysed alkylresorcinol (AR) levels in cereal foods (R^2 = 0.91), and concluded that it is possible to estimate the proportion of wholegrain wheat and/or rye in a given cereal product on the basis of AR content and C17:0/C21:0 ratio. Levels of alkylresorcinols are being used successfully in nutrition studies for estimating wholegrain intake. Since alkylresorcinols are present in the bran but not in the germ, measurement of alkylresorcinol levels cannot be considered as a suitable method for analysis for quality control purposes.

The absence of good methods should not lead to the abandonment of any analytical control, however. A practical approach may be achieved if the following steps are undertaken:

- Agreement on average compositions and allowed deviations for wholegrain (flour); such agreements may be preferably obtained at international level, but also agreements at national levels can contribute to a more constant composition of wholegrain flours.
- Initial analysis of fibre and total lipids with well-established routine methods in order to detect major deviations.
- Subsequent analysis of alkylresorcinols, and possibly also of selected other components, when a more sophisticated approach is required.

As another step in achieving recombined wholegrain products with consistent composition, the development of protocols for good manufacturing practice, including the establishment of preferred recombination ratios of white flour/bran/germ, may be considered.

1.4 Labelling

1.4.1 Dietary fibre labelling

Wide international agreement exists regarding the minimum levels of fibre that are required for labelling a product as a source of fibre or as high in fibre. The wording used by Codex is given below.

1 Source of fibre: min. 3 g/100 g or min. 1.5 g/100 kcal, or at least 10% of daily reference value per serving.
2 High in fibre: min. 6 g/100g, or min. 3g/100 kcal, or at least 20% of daily reference value per serving.

(Codex Alimentarius, 1997)

Conditions for nutrient content claims for dietary fibre in liquid foods, along with serving sizes and daily reference values, need to be determined at national level. In the minimum levels adopted by the EU only levels of fibre per 100 g and 100 kcal are mentioned (EFSA, 2007).

1.4.2 Wholegrain labelling

In labelling practices according to Quantitative Ingredient Declaration (QUID) the percentage of wholegrain flour is usually mentioned. However, for front of pack announcements – such as ‘wholegrain xxx (name of product)’, ‘source of wholegrain’ and ‘high in wholegrain’ – a wide variety of regulations and recommendations exist. Examples are given in Table 1.3. However, in many countries and for many product types there is no regulation relating to labelling.

Table 1.3 What qualifies as a wholegrain (WG) food?

Where and when	Who and what	What qualifies as a wholegrain food?	Other restrictions
USA August 2006	WG Council Whole Grain Stamp, USDA Food Safety and Inspection Service (FSIS) version (Whole Grains Council, 2006)	At least 8 g WG per serving and at least 51% of the grain is WG (Basic Stamp) At least 16g WG per serving, and all the grain is WG (100% Stamp).	None.
UK November 2007	IGD *UK Whole Grain Guidance Report* (IGD, 2007)	For packaged foods wishing to communicate the presence of WG, for example, by stating 'contains whole grains' or 'with whole grains' on pack and in brand communications, the IGD Working Group recommend that foods should contain a minimum level of 8 g WG per serving (based on final batch load proportions).	Foods calling attention to their WG content will need to make a Quantitative Ingredient Declaration (QUID).
Canada December 2007	WG Council Whole Grain Stamp, Canadian version (Whole Grains Council, 2007b)	At least 8 g WG per serving (Basic Stamp) At least 16 g WG per serving, and all the ingredients are WG (100% Stamp in Canada).	None.
USA December 2007	U.S. Department of Agriculture (USDA)/ USDA Food and Nutrition Service (FNS) Special supplemental nutrition program for Women, Infants and Children (WIC) (USDA, 2007)	In general, WG must be the first ingredient and the food must qualify for the FDA Whole Grain Health Claim (i.e. 51% of weight is WG).	Only certain grain products qualify; no added sugar, salt, or oil allowed in rice, barley, bulgur or oatmeal; sugar restriction and iron requirement for breakfast cereals.

(*Continued overleaf.*)

Table 1.3 (Continued)

Where and when	Who and what	What qualifies as a wholegrain food?	Other restrictions
Denmark 2007	Danish National Food Institute (Whole Grains Council, 2007a)	Calculated on dry matter, the whole grains shall be the specified percentage or more of the total grains, for each category: 100% for flour, grains, rice 50% for bread (AND 30% of total weight) 60% for crispbread, breakfast cereal, pasta.	Only the foods listed here can be called WG – so no WG cookies, cakes, waffles, etc.!
Sweden – 1989 Denmark – 2009 Norway – 2009	Livsmedelsverket Natl. Food Admin. Keyhole Symbol	Calculated on dry matter, the whole grains shall be the specified percentage or more of the total grains, for each category: 100% for flour, meal, grains 50% for crispbread, porridge, pasta (unfilled) 25% for bread, sandwiches, wraps 15% for pizzas, pierogis, other savoury pies.	Only the categories listed here are eligible. Limits on fats, sugars and sodium; minimum of fibre in some categories. http://www.noeglehullet.dk/NR/rdonlyres/BF547063-9C1D-4E7F-AFF4-FD4BE315A982/0/MicrosoftWordStatutoryordertheKeyholelabel.pdf.
USA October 2009	Institute of Medicine of the National Academies (IOM) *School Meals: Building Blocks for Healthy Children* report (Institute of Medicine, 2009)	Calls for schools to serve 'WG-rich' foods; to qualify, a food must meet ONE of the following: a. contain at least 8 g of WG content per serving OR b. qualify for the FDA WG health claim (51% WG by weight) OR c. have a whole grain as the first ingredient by weight for non-mixed dishes (e.g., breads, cereals) or as the first *grain* ingredient by weight for mixed dishes (e.g., pizza, corn dogs).	Must qualify as a Grain/Bread serving in the Food Buying Guide for Child Nutrition Programs (minimum of 14.75 g of grain, in most cases). Note: The report recommends raising the standard to more than 8g as time goes on.

Germany		Foods must have a certain baker's percent of WG to use the name WG: 90% WG for wheat and rye bread 100% WG for pasta.	
Netherlands	*Warenwetbesluit meel en brood* (1998) and information from Netherlands Bakery Centre (NBC)	Breads can only legally be called WG if 100% of the grain is WG. There is no law for other foods, but common practice is to 'use the 50% rule' and call products WG if at least half of the grain in a product is WG.	Terms such as 20%, 30%, 50% or 80% WG on packaging are not used (and for bread legally not allowed).
France	Association of biscuit manufacturers	'Source of WG' 15–40% of WG in product 'Rich in WG' > 40% in product	Requirements (proposed) • 40% cereals • < 35 % calorific value from fat • < 35 of saturated fat • No trans fat • < 40g/100g total sugars

The basic principles of most regulations and recommendations are:

- at least 50% of the grain (or flour) should be wholegrain;
- a portion or serving should contain a significant amount of wholegrain.

The 50% principle was not applied in the French guideline for biscuits, since a sudden transition from the common white flour-based products to products with >50% wholegrain would result in very low consumer acceptance.

Eight grams per serving is often seen as a significant amount. For bread this is delivered in a 28 g slice made with 50% wholemeal wheat flour, resulting in ~30 g whole grain/100 g.

In some regulations and recommendations maximum levels are set for (saturated) fat and sugars, but in other cases this issue is left to generic regulations for nutrition profiling, namely those drawn up to prevent nutrition and health statements on products whose overall composition is unhealthy. Ambitious regulations (those requiring high levels of wholegrain and (very) low levels of fat and sugar) may on the one hand stimulate research into the development of attractive products that meet these criteria, but may on the other hand lead to the abandonment of any effort in this area, because the requirements are seen as too demanding.

The option offered by the use of the wholegrain stamp issued by the Whole Grains Council and the clear listing of the amount of wholegrain in g/100 g product may be a good solution for:

- allowing flexibility for the differences between countries and regions;
- stimulating marketing and R&D for raising the amount to values higher than those of competitors;
- conveying a clear wholegrain signal to consumers by using one type of logo.

1.5 Recommendations and guidelines for dietary fibre and wholegrain intake

1.5.1 Recommended dietary fibre intake

A number of bodies have issued recommendations for dietary fibre intake. A selection is presented in Table 1.4.

The WHO report (2003) sets no precise population goal for the intake of total dietary fibre, but at least 25 g per day should be provided from fruit, vegetables and wholegrain foods. This population goal is based on evidence linking high intake of dietary fibre (from fruit, vegetables and wholegrain foods) with decreased risk of weight gain (convincing), type 2 diabetes (probable) and cardiovascular diseases (probable). This recommendation was supported by the recent FAO/WHO Scientific Update on carbohydrate in the human diet (Mann *et al.*, 2007).

EFSA (2010a) considers a fibre intake of 25 g/day to be adequate for normal laxation in adults. The EFSA Panel notes that there is evidence in adults of benefit to health associated with consumption of diets rich in fibre-containing foods at dietary fibre intakes greater than 25 g per day, for example reduced risk of coronary

Table 1.4 Recommended dietary fibre intakes for adults

	USA[a] (IOM, 2005)	Nordic Countries (NNR, 2004)	WHO (2003)	Netherlands (GR, 2001 and 2006)	France, (AFSSA, 2001)	Germany, Austria, Switzerland (D-A-CH, 2008)	UK (DoH, 1991)	EFSA (2010a)
DF g/day	w: 25 m: 38	25–35	>25[a]	30–40[b]	25–30	30	18[c]	>25[d]
g/MJ	3.4	3		3.4		w: 3 m: 2.4		

[a] Total dietary fibre from wholegrain cereals, fruit and vegetables.
[b] Dietary fibre intake via products not enriched with isolated and purified dietary fibre.
[c] Refers to non-starch polysaccharides.
[d] Intake of 25 g/day is adequate for normal laxation in adults There is evidence of benefit to health associated with consumption of diets rich in fibre-containing foods at dietary fibre intakes >25 g/day.

Source: adapted from EFSA (2010).

Notes: Such evidence should be considered when developing food-based dietary guidelines. AFSSA, Agence Française de Sécurité Sanitaire des Aliments; DoH, UK Committee on Medical Aspects of Food Policy; m, men; NNR, Nordic Nutrition Recommendations; w, women.

heart disease and type 2 diabetes and improved weight maintenance. Such evidence should be considered when developing food-based dietary guidelines. A fibre intake of 2 g/MJ is considered adequate for normal laxation in children from the age of one year. Although EFSA mentions one intake level, the effects of different fibre types on faecal weight show marked differences: 5.4 g stool/g fibre from wheat bran, 4.9 g/g from fruits and vegetables, 3 g/g from isolated cellulose and 1.3g/g from isolated pectin (Cummings 1993). Therefore, the EFSA recommendation may also be seen as being in favour of consumption of fruits, vegetables and wholegrain products.

The Institute of Medicine (2005) and the Health Council of the Netherlands recommended 3.4 g fibre/MJ for adults, corresponding to 25 to 40 g fibre/day, depending on the energy delivered in the daily diet. This higher level, compared with those recommended by WHO and EFSA, was chosen taking into account not only laxation but also the reduced risk for coronary heart diseases. The Health Council of the Netherlands did not issue a dietary reference intake level for fibre, but a guideline, mentioning that the recommended level refers to intake of fibre as present in (non-enriched) food products, such as fruits, vegetables and wholegrain products; this approach was chosen since observational studies show that beneficial effects may be obtained from the consumption of such foods, which contain both fibre and bioactive co-passengers, and that both the fibre and the co-passengers may play a role.

The current recommended levels of fibre are based on measurements using the AOAC Official methods 985.29 or 991.43. However, as noted in Section 1.3.1, measurements taken using AOAC 2009.01 are significantly higher for bread and a range of other products. If AOAC 2009.01 in the current or an improved version will become the new standard method for total dietary fibre, the currently recommended levels for intake of dietary fibre should be reassessed.

1.5.2 Recommended wholegrain intake

Dietary guidelines for wholegrain intake are provided by government-linked organisations and also by 'disease' associations (such as the American Heart Association). The consumption of wholegrain products is recommended in many guidelines all over the world. Recommendations can be qualitative or quantitative, for example: 'starchy food such as bread, cereals rice, pasta and potatoes are a really important part of a healthy diet. Try to choose wholegrain varieties whenever you can' (FSA, 1999) or 'consume 3 or more ounce-equivalent servings of wholegrain products per day' (USDA, 2010). The latter recommendation is based on the results of epidemiology studies, showing that people who eat at least 48 g of whole grains each day can reduce the risk of coronary heart disease and diabetes by between 20 and 40% (Montonen *et al.*, 2003; Venn and Mann, 2004; Flight and Clifton, 2006; Mellen *et al.*, 2008; de Munter *et al.*, 2007). Serving sizes may vary, but in the case of wholegrain consumption one serving is usually a slice of bread (1 ounce, 28 g), delivering ~16 g whole grain. Pereira *et al.*'s (2004) meta-analysis indicated that each increase of 10 g per day in the consumption of dietary fibre from cereals was associated with a 25% decrease in the risk of fatal coronary heart disease.

Among the quantitative recommendations, 48 g wholegrain/day is the lowest. In Denmark the recently established recommendation is 75 g/day, while in The Netherlands the recommended diet for adults includes about six slices of bread, preferably wholegrain, which corresponds to ~115 g wholegrain/day. Forty-eight grams of wholegrain consumed as three slices of wholegrain bread (fibre level 6.8%, USDA food composition database) delivers 5.7 g fibre, which represents only 23% of the 25 g fibre/day that is often recommended, and only 16% when 35 g/day fibre is recommended.

When the average daily fibre intake from cereal products is ~ 50% (Netherlands, Hulshof *et al.*, 2004) or higher (Nordic Europe), a recommended wholegrain intake of 48 g/day is only about half the amount required for a proportional contribution to a recommended fibre intake of 25 g/day. From this fibre perspective, the 75 g wholegrain recommended in Denmark is also too low. More generally, unless the percentage of fibre intake from cereal products is below 25%, a daily 48 g wholegrain intake, although helpful for reducing the risk of heart diseases and diabetes, does not proportionally contribute to widely accepted recommended (minimum) levels for intake of dietary fibre.

1.6 Health claims for dietary fibre and wholegrain

More than a decade ago, national authorities began to implement regulations for nutrition or health claims for foods. Claims submitted by companies or other interested parties can be accepted or rejected by competent authorities.

EFSA has completed the assessment of over 4000 proposed Article 13.1 'general function' health claims, submitted by companies and others from all 27 EU member states. These refer to the role of a nutrient or substance in growth, development and body functions; psychological and behavioural functions; slimming and weight control, satiety or reduction of available energy from the diet. These claims do not include those related to child development or health or disease risk reduction. EFSA's conclusions have been adopted by the EU and the list of permitted health claims has been published (EU, 2012).

An overview of permitted health claims related to cereals and fibre and some of the rejected claims is given in Table 1.5.

Table 1.5 EFSA Scientific Opinions on fibre-related health claims

Material	Claimed effect	EFSA opinion/conditions of use	*EFSA Journal* number
Rye fibre	Contributes to normal bowel function.	The claim may be used only for food which is high in that fibre as referred to in the claim HIGH FIBRE.	2011; 9(6): 2249
Barley grain fibre	Contributes to an increase in faecal bulk.	The claim may be used only for food which is high in that fibre as referred to in the claim HIGH FIBRE.	2011; 9(6): 2249
Oat grain fibre	Contributes to an increase in faecal bulk.	The claim may be used only for food which is high in that fibre as referred to in the claim HIGH FIBRE.	2011; 9(6): 2249
Wheat bran fibre	Contributes to an increase in faecal bulk.	The claim may be used only for food which is high in that fibre as referred to in the claim HIGH FIBRE.	2010; 8(10): 1817
Wheat bran fibre	Contributes to an acceleration of intestinal transit.	Information shall be given to the consumer that the claimed effect is obtained with a daily intake of ≥ 10 g of wheat bran fibre.	2010; 8(10): 1817
Arabinoxylan (AX) produced from wheat endosperm (wheat grain fibre, mainly soluble)	Consumption of AX as part of a meal contributes to a reduction of the blood glucose rise after that meal.	May be used only for food which contains at least 8 g AX-rich fibre produced from wheat endosperm (≥ 60% AX) per 100 g of available carbohydrates in a quantified portion as part of the meal.	2011; 9(6): 2205

(*Continued overleaf.*)

Table 1.5 (Continued)

Material	Claimed effect	EFSA opinion/conditions of use	*EFSA Journal* number
Beta-glucans from oats and barley	Consumption of beta-glucans from oats or barley as part of a meal contributes to the reduction of the blood glucose rise after that meal.	The claim may be used only for food which contains ≥ 4 g of beta-glucans from oats or barley for each 30 g of available carbohydrates in a quantified portion as part of the meal. In order to bear the claim information shall be given to the consumer that the beneficial effect is obtained by consuming the beta-glucans from oats or barley as part of the meal.	2011; 9(6): 2207
Beta-glucans	Contribute to the maintenance of normal blood cholesterol levels.	The claim may be used only for food which contains ≥ 1 g of beta-glucans from oats, oat bran, barley, barley bran, or from mixtures of these sources per quantified portion. In order to bear the claim information shall be given to the consumer that the beneficial effect is obtained with a daily intake of 3 g.	2009; 7(9): 1254 2011; 9(6): 2207
Resistant starch	Replacing digestible starches with resistant starch in a meal contributes to a reduction in the blood glucose rise after that meal.	The claim may be used only for food in which digestible starch has been replaced by resistant starch so that the final content of resistant starch is at least 14 % of total starch.	2011; 9(4): 2024
Wholegrain (WG) WG flour WG foods Diets rich in WG	Gut health / bowel function, weight control, blood glucose/insulin levels, weight management, blood cholesterol, satiety, glycaemic index, digestive function and cardiovascular health.	The food constituent, wholegrain, which is the subject of this opinion is not sufficiently characterised in relation to the claimed effects.	2010; 8(10): 176
Dietary fibre (DF), rich in DF and 'soluble fibre'	Wide range of claims.	The food constituent, dietary fibre, which is the subject of this opinion, is not sufficiently characterised in relation to the claimed effects.	2010; 8(10): 1735

Two important criteria strictly maintained in EFSA's evaluations are:

- the sufficient characterisation of the product;
- the establishment of a cause–effect relationship.

The EFSA criteria for a positive assessment of a health claim largely correspond with those for convincing evidence (WHO, 2003). For dietary recommendations, both EFSA and many other authoritative bodies are accepting probable – and sometimes also possible – evidence as sufficient.

1.6.1 Health claims for dietary fibre

EFSA rejected many of the submitted health claims for dietary fibre:

- Health claims for total and soluble dietary fibre – due to insufficient characterisation of the material;
- All health claims covering pre- and probiotic effects;
- Many health claims for fibres obtained by isolation and further processing of fibres, including claims for wheat-based resistant maltodextrins and for inulins.

1.6.2 Health claims for wholegrain

The association between wholegrain consumption and reduced risk of cardiovascular diseases has resulted in the following claims being made for wholegrain:

- USA: 'Diets rich in whole grain foods and other plant foods and low in total fat, saturated fat, and cholesterol may reduce the risk of heart disease and some cancers' (FDA, 1999).
- UK: 'People with a healthy heart tend to eat more wholegrain foods as part of a healthy lifestyle' (JHCI, 2002).
- Sweden: 'A healthy lifestyle and a balanced diet rich in wholegrain products reduce the risk for (coronary) heart disease' (see Frølich and Åman, 2010). For this health claim, approved in 2003, only grains high in fibre commonly used in Sweden were included: wheat, rye, barley and oats.

In November 2010, EFSA (2010b) did not approve health claims submitted for wholegrains related to the following claimed effects: 'gut health'/'bowel function', 'weight control', 'blood glucose'/'insulin levels', 'weight management', 'blood cholesterol', 'satiety', 'glycaemic index', 'digestive function' and 'cardiovascular health'. The EFSA panel concluded that the food constituent, wholegrain, is not sufficiently characterised in relation to the claimed effects. Due to this non-approval the current claims in the UK and Sweden will have to be withdrawn.

As observed for dietary fibre, the absence of an approved health claim does not impede the development and maintenance of dietary recommendations for wholegrain. A possible option for obtaining approval for wholegrain health claims may be the submission of claims restricted to a single cereal grain and its products.

1.7 References

BRUNT K. (2011) Dietary fibre levels in bread according to AOAC 985.29 and AOAC 2009.01 method. First results. 9th International Food data Conference, 14–17 September 2011, Norwich, UK, http://www.eurofir.net/9th_ifdc/oral_presentations (Accessed 1 October 2012).

BRUNT K. and SANDERS P. (2012) Improvement of the AOAC 2009.01 total dietary fibre method for bread and other high starch containing matrices. *Food Chemistry*. http://dx.doi.org/10.1016/j.foodchem.2012.10.109.

CCMAS (2011) 32nd session of the Codex Committee on Methods of Analysis and Sampling, report available at www.codexalimentarius.net/download/report/757/REP11_MAe.pdf (Accessed 1 October 2012).

CCNFSDU (2010) '32nd Session of the Codex Committee on Nutrition and Foods for Special Dietary Uses', summary available at https://www.ccnfsdu.de/index.php?id=569 (Accessed 1 October 2012).

CHEN Y., ROSS A. B., AMAN P. and KAMAL-ELDIN A. (2004) Alkylresorcinols as markers of whole grain wheat and rye in cereal products. *Journal of Agricultural and Food Chemistry* **52** (26), 8242–6.

CODEX ALIMENTARIUS (1997) Guidelines for Use of Nutrition and Health Claims (CAC/GL 23-1997), available at www.codexalimentarius.net/download/standards/351/CXG_023e.pdf (Accessed 1 October).

CODEX ALIMENTARIUS (2011) *Guidelines on Nutrition Labelling* (adopted in 1985; revised in 1993 and 2011; amendments in 2003, 2006, 2009 and 2010; annex adopted in 2011), available at www.codexalimentarius.net/download/standards/34/CXG_002e.pdf (Accessed 1 October 2012).

CUMMINGS J. H. (1993) The effect of dietary fiber on faecal weight and composition. In: SPILLER GA, editor. *CRC Handbook of Dietary Fiber in Human Nutrition*. Boca Raton, FL, USA: CRC Press; 1993: 263–349.

DE MUNTER J. S. L., HU F. B., SPIEGELMAN D., FRANZ M. and VAN DAM R. M. (2007) Whole Grain, Bran, and Germ Intake and Risk of Type 2 Diabetes: A Prospective Cohort Study and Systematic Review. *PLoS Medicine* **4** (8), e261. DOI: 10.1371/journal.pmed.0040261.

EFSA (2007) Statement of the Scientific Panel on Dietetic Products, Nutrition and Allergies on a request from the Commission related to dietary fibre, available at http://www.efsa.europa.eu/en/efsajournal/doc/1060.pdf (Accessed 1 October 2012). DOI: 10.2903/j.efsa.2007.1060.

EFSA (2010a) Scientific Opinion on Dietary Reference Values for carbohydrates and dietary fibre. *EFSA Journal* **8** (3), 1462, available at http://www.efsa.europa.eu/de/efsajournal/pub/1462.htm (Accessed 1 October 2012). DOI 10.2903/j.efsa.2010.1462.

EFSA (2010b) Scientific Opinion on the substantiation of health claims related to whole grain (ID 831, 832, 833, 1126, 1268, 1269, 1270, 1271, 1431) pursuant to Article **13**(1) of Regulation (EC) No 1924/2006. *EFSA Journal* **8** (10), 1766, available at http://www.efsa.europa.eu/en/efsajournal/pub/1766.htm (Accessed 1 October 2012). DOI 10.2903/j.efsa.2010.1766.

ENGLYST H. N. and HUDSON G. J. (1996) The classification and measurement of dietary carbohydrates. *Food Chemistry* **57**, 15–21.

EU (2006) Corrigendum to Regulation (EC) No. 1924/2006 of the European Parliament and of the Council of 20 December 2006 on nutrition and health claims made on foods (OJ L 404, 30.12.2006). *Official Journal of the European Union* L012, 18 January 2007, 0003–0018.

EU (2008) Commission Directive 2008/100/EC: Annex II, available at http://eur-lex.europa.eu/LexUriServ/LexUriServ.do?uri=OJ:L:2008:285:0009:0012:EN:PDF (Accessed 1 October 2012).

EU (2012) COMMISSION REGULATION (EU) No. 432/2012 of 16 May 2012 establishing a list of permitted health claims made on foods, other than those referring to the reduction of disease risk and to children's development and health (OJ L 136 1–38 25 May 2012).

FAO/WHO (1998) *Carbohydrates in human nutrition. Report of a Joint FAO/WHO expert consultation.* FAO Food and Nutrition Paper – 66, Rome.

FDA (2006), US Food and Drug Administration Whole Grain Label Statements, available at http://www.fda.gov/Food/GuidanceComplianceRegulatoryInformation/GuidanceDocuments/FoodLabelingNutrition/ucm059088.htm (Accessed 1 October 2012).

FDA (1999) Appendix C: Health Claims in *Guidance for Industry: A Food Labeling Guide*, available at http://www.fda.gov/Food/GuidanceComplianceRegulatoryInformation/GuidanceDocuments/FoodLabelingNutrition/FoodLabelingGuide/ucm064919.htm (Accessed 1 October 2012).

FLIGHT I. and CLIFTON P. (2006) Cereal grains and legumes in the prevention of coronary heart disease and stroke: a review of the literature. *European Journal of Clinical Nutrition* **60**, 1145–59. DOI:10.1038/sj.ejcn.1602435.

FRØLICH W. and ÅMAN P. (2010) Whole grain for whom and why? *Food & Nutrition Research* **54**, 5056. DOI: 10.3402/fnr.v54i0.5056.

FOOD STANDARDS AGENCY (2010) EatWell, your guide to healthy eating. www.food.gov.uk/multimedia/.../eatwell0708.pdf

HEALTH COUNCIL OF THE NETHERLANDS (2006) *Guideline for dietary fibre intake.* Publication no. 2006/03, Health Council of the Netherlands, The Hague.

HEALTHGRAIN (2010) Whole Grain Definition, available at http://www.healthgrain.org/webfm_send/44 (Accessed 1 October 2012).

HULSHOF, K. F. A. M., OCKÉ, M. C., VAN ROSSUM, C. T. M., BUURMA-RETHANS, E. J. M., BRANTS, H. A. M. *et al.* (2004) RIVM rapport 350030002/2004 Resultaten van de Voedselconsumptiepeiling 2003.

IGD (2007) *UK Whole Grain Guidance*, available at http://www.igd.com/index.asp?id=1&fid=1&sid=4&tid=54&cid=169 (Accessed 1 October 2012).

INSTITUTE OF MEDICINE (2005) *Dietary reference intakes for energy, carbohydrate, fiber, fat, fatty acids, cholesterol, protein, and amino acids.* Washington, DC: National Academies Press.

INSTITUTE OF MEDICINE (2009) *School Meals: Building Blocks for Healthy Children*, available at http://www.iom.edu/Reports/2009/School-Meals-Building-Blocks-for-Healthy-Children.aspx (Accessed 1 October 2012).

JHCI (2002) Joint Health Claims Initiative, *Generic claims: Wholegrain foods and heart health, final report.* Available at http://www.jhci.org.uk/approv/wgrainh.htm (Accessed 1 October 2012).

MANN J., CUMMINGS J. H., ENGLYST H. N., KEY T., LIU S. *et al.* (2007) FAO/WHO Scientific Update on carbohydrates in human nutrition: conclusions. *European Journal of Clinical Nutrition* **61** (Suppl. 1), S132–7. DOI:10.1038/sj.ejcn.1602943.

MCCLEARY B. V. (2007) An integrated procedure for the measurement of total dietary fibre (including resistant starch) non-digestible oligosaccharides and available carbohydrates. *Analytical and Bioanalytical Chemistry* **389** (1), 291–308. DOI: 10.1007/s00216-007-1389-6.

MELLEN P. B., WALSH T. F. and HERRINGTON D. M. (2008) Whole grain intake and cardiovascular disease: A meta-analysis. *Nutrition, Metabolism and Cardiovascular Diseases* **18**, 283–90.

MONTONEN J., KNEKT P., JARVINEN R., AROMAA A. and REUNANEN A. (2003) Whole grain and fiber intake and the incidence of type 2 diabetes. *American Journal of Clinical Nutrition* **77** (3), 622–9.

PEREIRA M. A., O'REILLY E., AUGUSTSSON K., FRASER G. E., GOLDBOURT U. *et al.* (2004) Dietary Fiber and Risk of Coronary Heart Disease: A Pooled Analysis of Cohort Studies. *Archives of Internal Medicine* **164**, 370–6.

USDA (2007) *Special Supplemental Nutrition Program for Women, Infants and Children (WIC): Revisions in the WIC Food Packages; Interim Rule*, available at http://www.fns.usda.gov/wic/regspublished/wicfoodpkginterimrulepdf.pdf (Accessed 1 October 2012).

USDA (2005) Dietary Guidelines for Americans 2005 http://www.health.gov/dietaryguidelines/dga2005/document/html/chapter5.htm.

USDA (2011) *USDA National Nutrient Database for Standard Reference*, available at http://ndb.nal.usda.gov/.

VENN B. J. and MANN J. I. (2004) Cereal grains, legumes and diabetes. *European Journal of Clinical Nutrition* **58**, 1443–61.

WARENWETBESLUIT MEEL EN BROOD (1998) Staatsblad 1998 **341** 1–8 available at https://zoek.officielebekendmakingen.nl/stb-1998-341.html.

WARD J. L., POUTANEN K., GEBRUERS K., PIIRONEN V., LAMPI A.-M., *et al.* (2008) The HEALTHGRAIN cereal diversity screen: concept, results, and prospects. *Journal of Agricultural and Food Chemistry* **56**, 9699–709.

WHO (2003) *Diet, nutrition and the prevention of chronic diseases*. Report of a Joint WHO/FAO Expert Consultation. WHO Technical Report Series 916, Geneva.

WHOLE GRAINS COUNCIL (2004) *Definition of Whole Grains*, available at http://wholegrainscouncil.org/whole-grains-101/definition-of-whole-grains (Accessed 1 October 2012).

WHOLE GRAINS COUNCIL (2006) *FSIS Stamp Usage Guide for the Whole Grain Stamp*, available at http://www.wholegrainscouncil.org/files/US_FSIS_StampUsageGuide2012.pdf (Accessed 1 October 2012).

WHOLE GRAINS COUNCIL (2007a) *Whole Grains in Denmark*, available at http://wholegrainscouncil.org/files/WholeGrainsinDenmark.pdf.

WHOLE GRAINS COUNCIL (2007b) *Canadian Whole Grain Stamp*, available at http://www.wholegrainscouncil.org/whole-grain-stamp/canadian-stamp.

2

Dietary fibre analysis in foods

B. V. McCleary, A. Draga, and N. Sloane, Megazyme International Ireland Limited, Ireland

DOI: 10.1533/9780857095787.1.25

Abstract: The concept of dietary fibre has been evolving over the past 20 years from a chemical to a physiological focus. This has led to changes in the definition of dietary fibre and the inclusion of carbohydrate components that previously were not considered to be dietary fibre, and, consequently, were not measured, or were partially measured. The inclusion of resistant starch and non-digestible oligosaccharides (e.g. fructo-oligosaccharides, arabino-xylosaccharides, galacto-oligosaccharides, resistant maltodextrins and Polydextrose) has required the development of improved, all-inclusive analytical methodology to service the definition. In this chapter, the current status concerning definition of dietary fibre and methodology to service this definition will be discussed. More specifically, an integrated procedure for the measurement of total dietary fibre as defined by Codex Alimentarius is described in detail.

Key words: total dietary fibre, resistant starch, non-digestible oligosaccharides, SDFP, SDFS, FOS, AXOS, Codex Alimentarius, analysis of fibre.

2.1 Introduction

> The definition and analysis of dietary fibre are intimately related. Analysis methods have to be developed in accordance with the conceptual definitions, but, in practice, compromises must be accepted due to constraints of cost and time. All types of dietary components can be separated at different levels of complexity and determined separately for research purposes, though short-hand methods are needed for labelling and control purposes (Asp, 2001).

Interest in dietary fibre is a consequence of the belief that dietary fibre contributes positively to the health / quality of life of the consumer. The physiological effects of dietary fibre are what makes it of interest to the consumer, food nutritionists and regulators (DeVries, 2004). Because dietary fibre is a multi-component mixture, it is essential that there is a clear definition and that there is methodology to allow measurement of the defined components.

A physiological basis for the definition of dietary fibre is necessary. If it were not for the physiological effects of dietary fibre, there would be no interest in the subject on the part of researchers, consumers, regulators and manufacturers. The term 'dietary fibre' was coined and its definition refined based on observations of positive health effects related to consumption of diets rich in this component. Aspects of the definition, physiological relevance, health benefits and analytical aspects of dietary fibre have been reviewed by Champ *et al.* (2003).

The term 'dietary fibre' first appeared in 1953, and referred to the non-digestible constituents of plants that make up the plant cell wall, known to include cellulose, hemicellulose and lignin (Hipsley, 1953). The aim was to define some property of the constituent of the food that could be related to physiological behaviour in the human small intestine. Later, Burkitt *et al.* (1972) recommended that individuals should increase their dietary fibre intake in order to increase their stool volume and softness. In 1974, Trowell published a definition of dietary fibre, and this definition was broadened in 1976 (Trowell *et al.*, 1976) to include all indigestible polysaccharides such as gums, modified celluloses, mucilages, oligosaccharides and pectins. The definition remained primarily physiological, identifying dietary fibre on the basis of edibility and resistance to digestion, but was broadened to reflect research findings obtained in the interim years. Some of the non-digestible polysaccharides were included because they were found to have the physiological actions attributed to dietary fibre but could not necessarily be chemically identified as having their origins in the plant cell wall. This broadened definition quickly gained widespread acceptance.

Efforts directed towards developing a method to meet these analytical requirements focused on the removal of starch and protein (Theander and Aman, 1982). It was essential that the enzymes employed were sufficiently active, as well as being devoid of contaminating activities acting on dietary fibre components. Following extensive international collaboration, the method that evolved was AOAC Official Method 985.29 'Total Dietary Fibre in Foods; Enzymatic-Gravimetric Method' (Prosky *et al.*, 1985; AOAC Official Methods of Analysis, 2010; American Association of Cereal Chemists (AACC) Method 32–05). This method employed thermostable α-amylase and amyloglucosidase (AMG) to hydrolyse starch to glucose and dextrins and protease to depolymerize protein to peptides. Ethanol is added to samples to precipitate high molecular weight soluble dietary fibre (HMWSDF) from the soluble protein and starch fragments. This method was subsequently extended to allow measurement of total, soluble and insoluble dietary fibre in foods (AOAC Official Method 991.43) (Lee *et al.*, 1992; AOAC Method 991.43). Other methods for measurement of fibre components have been developed, evaluated and subsequently approved by AOAC International. A number of these methods have recently been accepted by the Codex Committee on Methods of Analysis and Sampling (Joint Food and Agricultural Organization / World Health Organization (FAO/WHO) Food Standards Programme), as detailed in Table 2.1. In this table, dietary fibre components that are or are not measured by the particular method are shown.

Table 2.1 Methods of analysis of dietary fibre as approved by CCMAS (March 2011), showing official validation and exactly what is measured and what is not measured by the method

Method	What is measured	What is not measured	Codex type
AOAC 985.29 (AACCI 32–05.01) (Prosky) Enzymic/gravimetric (AACCI 32–05.01)	High molecular weight dietary fibre (insoluble and soluble), including: 1. Insoluble dietary fibre 2. Some resistant starch (RS2 and RS3) 3. Chemically modified starch (RS4) (overestimated) 4. Only high molecular weight soluble dietary fibre that precipitates in 4 volumes (~76%) ethanol 5. Some inulin, Polydextrose and Fibersol 2	Most resistant starch Most non-digestible oligosaccharides (e.g. FOS and galacto-oligosaccharides) Most of inulin, Polydextrose and Fibersol 2	I
AOAC 991.43 (AACCI 32–07.01) (NMKL 129, 2003) (Lee modification of Prosky.) Enzymic/gravimetric	A. Insoluble dietary fibre (including some resistant starch); and separately, B. Only high molecular weight soluble dietary fibre that precipitates in 4 volumes (~76%) ethanol, including: 1. High molecular weight soluble polysaccharides such as beta-glucan, arabinoxylan, psyllium gum, arabinogalactan 2. Some inulin, Polydextrose and Fibersol 2	Most resistant starch Most non-digestible oligosaccharides (e.g. FOS and galacto-oligosaccharides) Most of inulin, Polydextrose and Fibersol 2	I
AOAC 993.21 (Applicable to food and food products that contain more than 10% dietary fibre and less than 2% starch.)	High molecular weight dietary fibre (insoluble and soluble), including: 1. Insoluble dietary fibre 2. Some resistant starch (RS3 and RS2) 3. Chemically modified starch (RS4) (overestimated) 4. Only high molecular weight soluble dietary fibre that precipitates in 4 volumes (~76%) ethanol 5. Some inulin, Polydextrose and Fibersol 2	Non-digestible oligosaccharides (e.g. FOS and galacto-oligosaccharides) Most of inulin, Polydextrose and Fibersol 2	I

(*Continued overleaf.*)

Table 2.1 (Continued)

Method	What is measured	What is not measured	Codex type
AOAC 994.13 (AACCI 32–25.01) (NMKL 162, 1998) (Uppsala method) Enzymic/gravimetry/ Spectrophotometry Provides sugar composition and Klason lignin content	High molecular weight dietary fibre (insoluble and soluble), including: 1. Insoluble dietary fibre 2. Some resistant starch (RS2 and RS3) 3. Chemically modified starch (RS4) (overestimated) 4. Only high molecular weight soluble dietary fibre that precipitates in 4 volumes (~76%) ethanol 5. Some inulin, Polydextrose and Fibersol 2	Most resistant starch Most non-digestible oligosaccharides (e.g. FOS and galacto-oligosaccharides) Most of Inulin, Polydextrose and Fibersol 2	I
2001.03 (Suitable for all foods where resistant starches are not present.) (AACCI 32–41.01)	A. High molecular weight dietary fibre (insoluble and soluble), including: 1. Insoluble dietary fibre 2. Some resistant starch (RS3 and RS2) 3. Chemically modified starch (RS4) (overestimated) 4. Only high molecular weight soluble dietary fibre that precipitates in 4 volumes (~76%) ethanol 5. Some inulin, Polydextrose and Fibersol 2 B. Lower molecular weight soluble dietary fibre that is soluble in 4 volumes (~76%) ethanol, including: 1. Remainder of inulin, Polydextrose and Fibersol 2 2. Remainder of the non-digestible oligosaccharides (e.g. FOS and galacto-oligosaccharides)	Most resistant starch	I
2009.01 (Incubation with alpha-amylase and Amyloglucosidase (AMG) at physiological temperature.) (AACCI 32–45.01)	All dietary fibre, including: A. High molecular weight dietary fibre (insoluble and soluble), including all resistant starch B. Lower molecular weight soluble dietary fibre	Nothing	I

AOAC 991.42 (AACCI 32–20.01)	Insoluble dietary fibre	A. High molecular weight soluble fibre B. Low molecular weight soluble dietary fibre	I
AOAC 993.19	Only high molecular weight soluble dietary fibre that precipitates in 4 volumes (~76%) ethanol	A. Insoluble dietary fibre B. Lower molecular weight soluble dietary fibre	I
AOAC 995.16 (AACCI 32–23.01)	(1–3)(1–4) Beta-D-Glucans	Everything else	II
AOAC 997.08 (AACCI 32–31.01)	Fructans (Inulin, reducing and non-reducing FOS)	Everything else	II
AOAC 999.03 (AACCI 32–32.01)	Fructans (Inulin, and non-reducing FOS; reducing FOS are slightly underestimated)	Everything else	III
AOAC 2000.11 (AACCI 32–28.01)	Polydextrose	Everything else	II
AOAC 2001.02 (AACCI 32–33.01)	Trans-galacto-oligosaccharides	Everything else	II
AOAC 2002.02 (AACCI 32–40.01)	Resistant starch	Everything else	II

Other methods, namely those for the measurement of insoluble glucans and mannans of yeast cell wall, non-starch polysaccharides and an alternative method for fructo-oligosaccharides, have been accepted by Codex Alimentarius as Type IV methods (i.e. methods that have not been subjected to rigorous interlaboratory evaluation through AOAC International).

The AACC undertook a critical review of the status of dietary fibre science and definition in 1998. Over the course of a year, the committee held three workshops and provided an international website, available to all web users worldwide, to receive comments. After due deliberation, an updated definition of dietary fibre was delivered to the AACC Board of Directors for adoption in early 2000, and published (Anon, 2001):

> Dietary fibre is the edible parts of plants or analogous carbohydrates that are resistant to digestion and absorption in the human small intestine with complete or partial fermentation in the large intestine. Dietary fibre includes polysaccharides, oligosaccharides, lignin, and associated plant substances. Dietary fibres promote beneficial physiological effects including laxation, and/or blood cholesterol attenuation, and/or blood glucose attenuation. (Anon, 2001)

Concurrently, in the UK, Englyst and colleagues (Englyst and Cummings, 1984; Englyst and Hudson, 1987) developed methods for the measurement of non-starch polysaccharides (NSP), based on the original work of Southgate (1969; 1982). These NSP procedures measure only non-starch polysaccharides; resistant starch (RS) and non-digestible oligosaccharides (NDO) are excluded. Starch in the sample is dissolved in hot dimethyl sulphoxide (DMSO), diluted in buffer and depolymerized with thermostable α-amylase followed by pullulanase. The recovered NSP is acid hydrolysed to monosaccharides, which are measured by high-performance liquid chromatography (HPLC) by gas liquid chromatography (after derivatization) or colorimetrically.

Several definitions of dietary fibre (DF) have appeared over the past decade. The Food Nutrition Board (FNB) of the Institute of Medicine of the National Academies (USA) (2001) defined dietary fibre as follows: 'Dietary fibre consists of non-digestible carbohydrates and lignin that are intrinsic and intact in plants. Added fibre consists of isolated, non-digestible carbohydrates that have beneficial physiological effects in humans. Total fibre is the sum of dietary fibre and added fibre.'

The need for a clear definition of dietary fibre to support nutrition claims has been an agenda item for the Codex Alimentarius commission since 1992. This effort was led by the Codex Committee on Nutrition and Foods for Special Dietary Uses (CCNFSDU). The definition of dietary fibre that arose from the 27th Session of CCNFSDU (ALINORM 06/29/26), in Bonn, Germany, 21–25 November 2005 (Codex, 2005), was similar in many respects to that proposed by AACC, but with no reference to physiological effects, namely:

> Dietary fibre means carbohydrate polymers with a degree of polymerization (DP) not lower than 3 which are neither digested nor absorbed in the small intestine. A degree of polymerization not lower than 3 is intended to exclude mono- and

disaccharides. It is not intended to reflect the average DP of the mixture. Dietary fibre consists of one or more of:

- Edible carbohydrate polymers naturally occurring in the food as consumed;
- Carbohydrate polymers which have been obtained from raw materials by physical, enzymatic or chemical means;
- Synthetic carbohydrate polymers.

At the 30th session of CCNFSDU (Codex, 2008) the committee agreed on the following definition of dietary fibre:

Dietary fibre means carbohydrate polymers[a] with ten or more monomeric units[b], which are not hydrolyzed by the endogenous enzymes in the human small intestine and belong to the following categories;

- Edible carbohydrate polymers naturally occurring in the food as consumed.
- Carbohydrate polymers which have been obtained from raw materials by physical, enzymatic or chemical means and which have been shown to have a physiological effect of benefit to health as demonstrated by generally accepted scientific evidence to competent authorities;
- Synthetic carbohydrate polymers which have been shown to have a physiological effect of benefit to health as demonstrated by generally accepted scientific evidence to competent authorities.

a. When derived from a plant origin, dietary fibre may include fractions of lignin and/or other compounds when associated with the polysaccharides in the plant cell walls and if these compounds are quantified by the AOAC gravimetric analytical method for dietary fibre analysis. Fractions of lignin and the other compounds (proteic fractions, phenolic compounds, waxes, saponins, phytates, cutin, phytosterols, etc.) intimately 'associated' with plant polysaccharides are often extracted with the polysaccharides in AOAC 991.43 method. These substances are included in the definition of fibre insofar as they are actually associated with the poly- or oligosaccharidic fraction of fibre. However when extracted or even reintroduced into a food containing non-digestible polysaccharides, they cannot be defined as dietary fibre. When combined with polysaccharides, these associated substances may provide additional beneficial effects (pending adoption of Section on Methods of Analysis and Sampling).

b. Decision on whether to include carbohydrates from 3 to 9 monomeric units should be left to national authorities.

The European situation (Commission Directive L 285/9) is as follows:

Definition of the material constituting fibre

For the purposes of this Directive 'fibre' means carbohydrate polymers with three or more monomeric units, which are neither digested nor absorbed in the human small intestine and belong to the following categories:

— edible carbohydrate polymers naturally occurring in the food as consumed;
— edible carbohydrate polymers which have been obtained from food raw material by physical, enzymatic or chemical means and which have a beneficial physiological effect demonstrated by generally accepted scientific evidence;
— edible synthetic carbohydrate polymers which have a beneficial physiological effect demonstrated by generally accepted scientific evidence.

The fact that the AOAC procedures for measurement of dietary fibre (e.g. AOAC Methods 985.29 and 991.43) do not quantitatively measure resistant starch and, in general, measure little of the NDO (Fig. 2.1) is well known to researchers and analysts in the field. Methods have thus been developed for measurement of some specific NDO: fructo-oligosaccharides, AOAC Methods 997.08 (Hoebregs, 1997) and 999.03 (McCleary *et al.*, 2000); Polydextrose, AOAC Method 2000.11 (Craig *et al.*, 2001); Fibresol 2, AOAC Method 2001.03 (Gordon and Okuma, 2002); galacto-oligosaccharides, AOAC Method 2001.02 (de Slegte, 2002). At present, there is no specific procedure for arabino-xylo-saccharides (AXOS) (Grootaert *et al.*, 2007). Methods for the specific and accurate measurement of *β*-glucan, AOAC Method 995.16 (McCleary and Codd, 1991) and resistant starch, AOAC Method 2002.02 (McCleary and Monaghan, 2002; McCleary *et al.*, 2002) have also been developed and validated. The need for an integrated procedure for the measurement of dietary fibre (including resistant starch), and of all of the NDO as a group, was discussed in a methods group meeting at the conference 'Dietary Fibre 2006', Helsinki, 11–14 June 2006 (Dietary Fibre Conference, 2006). Various approaches aimed at resolving this

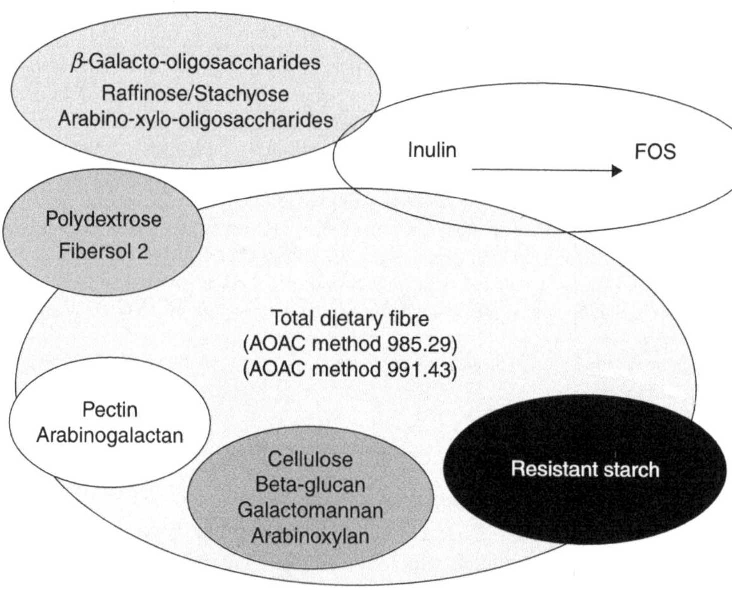

Fig. 2.1 Schematic representation of dietary fibre components measured, and not measured, by AOAC Official Methods 985.29 and 991.43. Also depicted are the problems of partial measurement of RS, Polydextrose® and resistant maltodextrins by current AOAC total dietary fibre methods. Most of the low molecular weight soluble dietary fibre (LMWSDF; galacto-oligosaccharides, fructo-oligosaccharides, etc.) are not measured. The currently described integrated total dietary fibre procedure measures all components shown, with no double counting (from McCleary *et al.*, 2010).

analytical challenge were proposed, and the method described in this chapter is one of these approaches.

An integrated method for the measurement of total dietary fibre was published in 2007 (McCleary, 2007). This method allows the accurate measurement of insoluble dietary fibre (IDF) (including resistant starch), high molecular weight soluble dietary fibre (HMWSDF; also now referred to as SDFP (soluble dietary fibre which precipitates in the presence of 76% aqueous ethanol)) and low molecular weight soluble dietary fibre (LMWSDF), also referred to as non-digestible oligosaccharides (NDO) or as soluble dietary fibre which does not precipitate in the presence of 76% aqueous ethanol (SDFS). Details of this procedure are outlined in Fig. 2.2. The use of pancreatic α-amylase at 37°C and pH 6.0 more closely simulates digestion in the human digestive tract and yields RS values in line with those obtained with AOAC Official Method 2002.02 (Table 2.2) and with results from ileostomy patients (Champ *et al.*, 2001). This method was successfully subjected to interlaboratory evaluation (McCleary *et al.*, 2010) and accepted as AOAC Official Method 2009.01. In this study, total high molecular weight dietary fibre (HMWDF) and SDFS are measured. In an Association of Official Analytical Chemists International/American Association of Cereal Chemists International (AOACI/AACCI) interlaboratory study just completed (McCleary *et al.*, 2012), the method has been evaluated for the measurement of IDF, SDFP and SDFS.

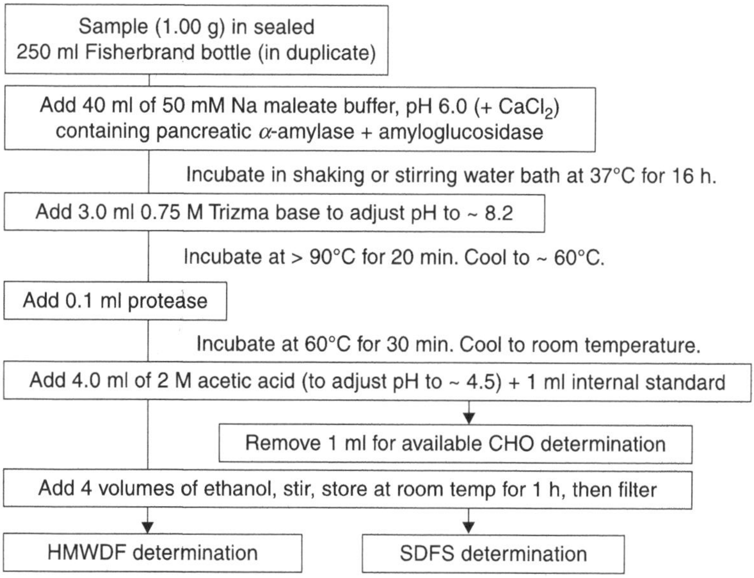

Fig. 2.2 Schematic representation of the integrated total dietary fibre (TDF) assay procedure, also showing where samples can be removed for determination of available carbohydrates.

Table 2.2 Resistant starch values determined for a number of samples using AOAC Official Methods 2002.02 and 2009.01

Sample details	Resistant starch % w/w (as is basis)	
	AOAC Method 2002.02	New TDF/RS Method
Native potato starch	64.9	56.8
Actistar®	58.0	48.8
Hylon VII®	50.0	48.6
Novelose 240®	48.4	44.2
Novelose 330®	38.8	38.7
Hi Maize 1043®	41.0	41.7
CrystaLean®	39.8	37.9
Amylose (potato)	38.2	36.6
Regular maize starch	0.5	0.8
Pinto beans (dry milled)	39.4	35.6
Haricot beans (dry milled)	36.9	31.2
Red kidney beans[a]	5.0	5.3
Red lentils (dry milled)	7.6	6.1
Flagelot beans (freeze-dried)[a]	5.3	4.5
Cooked/cooled potato	4.0	3.2
Corn flakes	2.2	2.4

Notes: Hylon VII® is native high amylose maize starch. Novelose 240®, Novelose 330®, Hi Maize 1043® and Crystalean® are retrograded high amylose maize starches.[a]

Samples were freeze-dried with a final moisture content of approx. 2–3%.

2.2 An integrated procedure for the measurement of total dietary fibre, including resistant starch and non-digestible oligosaccharides

2.2.1 Principle

An integrated procedure (AOAC Method 2009.01) is described for the measurement of total dietary fibre, including RS and SDFS (i.e. NDO) of DP ≥ 3. This method combines the key attributes of AOAC Official Methods of Analysis 2002.02, 985.29, 991.43 and 2001.03. A modification of this method to allow separate measurement of IDF and SDFP is also described. Duplicate test portions are incubated with pancreatic α-amylase (PAA) and amyloglucosidase (AMG) for 16 h at 37°C in sealed 250 ml bottles in a shaking water bath while mixing with sufficient vigour to maintain continuous suspension. Alternatively, the solutions can be stirred using a 2mag Mixdrive 15® submersible magnetic stirrer with a 30 × 7 mm stirrer bar and a stir rate of 170 rpm (Fig. 2.3) (http://www.2mag.de/english/stirrer/multiple/stirrer_multiple_04_mixdrive6_15.html). During this step, non-resistant starch is solubilized and hydrolysed to D-glucose, maltose and small levels of non-hydrolysed maltodextrins by the combined action of the two enzymes. The reaction is terminated by pH adjustment followed by temporary heating. Protein in the sample is denatured and digested with protease. Specific dietary fibre fractions are measured as follows.

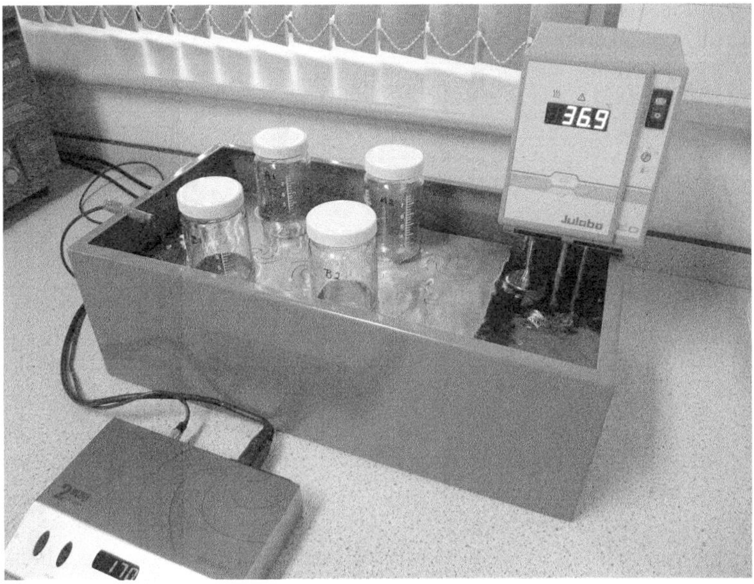

Fig. 2.3 Arrangements for mixing or stirring of suspensions of dietary fibre-containing samples in a 2mag Mixdrive 15® submersible magnetic stirrer with a 30 × 7 mm stirrer bar.

Insoluble dietary fibre (IDF), higher molecular weight soluble dietary fibre (soluble in water but insoluble in 76% aqueous ethanol; SDFP) and lower molecular weight soluble dietary fibre (soluble in 76% aqueous ethanol; SDFS) determination

IDF is recovered by filtration of the aqueous reaction mixture and the residue is washed, dried and weighed. SDFP in the filtrate is precipitated with ethanol or industrial methylated spirits (IMS), recovered, dried and weighed. Both the IDF and SDFP residues are corrected for protein, ash and blank values for the final calculation of the IDF and SDFP values. The aqueous ethanol filtrate from the soluble dietary fibre (SDF) fraction is concentrated, adjusted to ~ pH 4.5 and incubated with AMG (Brunt, 2011), heated to 100°C, desalted, reconcentrated and analysed by HPLC for SDFS.

Total high molecular weight dietary fibre (HMWDF) and SDFS determination

Four volumes of 95% ethanol are added to the incubation mixture and stirred. SDFP is precipitated from the incubation mixture and the suspension is filtered. The HMWDF (comprising IDF and SDFP) recovered on the crucible is washed, dried and weighed. This residue weight is corrected for protein, ash and the blank value for the final calculation. The aqueous ethanol filtrate is concentrated, incubated with AMG, heated to 100°C, desalted, reconcentrated and analysed by HPLC for SDFS.

Table 2.3 Total dietary fibre values determined for a range of samples that have been traditionally used as standards in TDF assays

Sample details	Total dietary fibre, % w/w (as is basis)	
	AOAC Method 991.43	New TDF/RS Method
β-Glucan	98.0	96.0
Casein	0	0
Pectin	86.5	87
Wheat starch	0.1	0.1
Larch arabinogalactan	83.5	84.0
High amylose maize starch	29.3	46.5
Wheat arabinoxylan	95.0	94.5

The enzymes used in the current method are of very high purity; they are effectively devoid of contaminants active on β-glucan, pectin and arabinoxylan. SDFS such as fructo-oligosaccharides (FOS) and galacto-oligosaccharides (GOS) are not hydrolysed, and the degree of hydrolysis of Polydextrose® and Fibresol-2® is in line with the information provided by the suppliers.

To ensure the presence of the appropriate enzyme activity and absence of undesirable enzyme activity, the materials listed in Table 2.3 (available in the kit, K-TDFC from Megazyme) are analysed using the entire procedure. Each new lot of enzymes should be tested, as should enzymes that have not been tested in the previous six months.

2.2.2 Apparatus

1 Grinding mill – Centrifugal, with 12-tooth rotor and 0.5 mm sieve, or similar device. Alternatively, a cyclone mill can be used for small test laboratory samples provided the mill has sufficient air flow or other cooling to avoid overheating of samples.
2 Digestion bottles – 250 ml Fisherbrand® soda glass, wide mouth bottles with polyvinyl lined cap (cat. no. FB73219) (https://extranet.fisher.co.uk/insight2_uk/mainSearch.do?keywords=FB73219&utm_source=fisher_web&utm_medium=product_page&utm_campaign=all_product_promote; accessed 4 October 2012).
3 Fritted crucible – Gooch, fritted disk, Pyrex® 50 ml, pore size coarse, ASTM 40–60 mm, Corning® No. 32940–50C, or equivalent.
4 Prepare as follows:

(i) Ash overnight at 525°C in muffle furnace, cool furnace to 130°C before removing crucibles to minimize breakage.
(ii) Remove any residual Celite® and ash material by using a vacuum.
(iii) Soak in 2% cleaning solution (2.2.3(15)) at room temperature for 1 h.
(iv) Rinse crucibles with water and deionized water.

(v) For final rinse, use 15 ml acetone and air dry.
(vi) Add approximately 1.0 g Celite® to dried crucibles and dry at 130°C to constant weight.
(vii) Cool crucible in desiccator for approximately 1 h and record mass of crucible containing Celite®.

5 Filtering flask – heavy-walled, 1–l Büchner flask (Fig. 2.4).
6 Rubber ring adaptors.– for use to join crucibles with filtering flasks (Fig. 2.4).
7 Vacuum source – vacuum pump or aspirator with regulator capable of regulating vacuum (e.g. Edwards XDS 10; single-phase 115/230V; product code: A726–01–903).
8 Water bath(s) – rotary motion (150 rpm), large-capacity (20–24 l) with covers; capable of maintaining temperature of 37 ± 1°C and 60 ± 1°C (e.g. Grant® OLS 200 shaking incubation bath). Alternatively, use a 2mag Mixdrive 15® submersible magnetic stirrer with a 30 × 7 mm stirrer bar, set at 170 rpm (Fig. 2.3).
9 Balance – 0.1 mg readability, accuracy and precision.
10 Ovens – Two, mechanical convection, set at 103 ± 2°C and 130 ± 3°C.
11 Timer.
12 Desiccator – Airtight, with silica gel or equivalent desiccant. Desiccant dried biweekly overnight in 130°C oven.

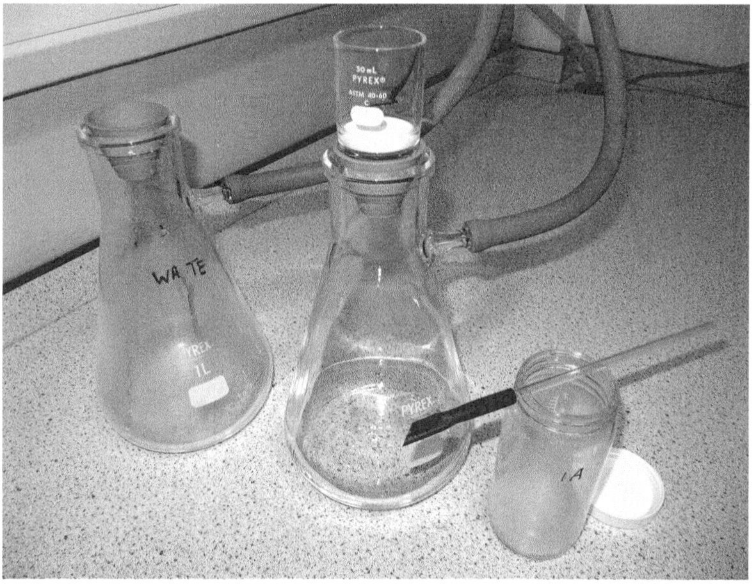

Fig. 2.4 Heavy-walled, 1 l Büchner flask with rubber ring adaptors; 250 ml Fisherbrand® soda glass, wide mouth bottles with polyvinyl lined cap; and rubber policeman spatula.

13 pH meter.
14 Thermometer – Capable of measuring to 110°C.
15 Positive displacement pipettor – e.g. Eppendorf Multipette®

   (a) with 25 ml Combitip® (to dispense 3 ml aliquots of 0.75 M Trizma® Base solution and 4 ml aliquots of 2 M acetic acid).
   (b) with 5.0 ml Combitip® (to dispense 0.3 ml aliquots of AMG and 0.1 ml of AMG and protease solutions).

16 Cylinder – Graduated, 100 ml and 500 ml.
17 Magnetic stirrers and stirring bars – (7 × 30 mm; plain magnetic stirrer bars; cat. no. 442–0269, VWR Dublin, Ireland).
18 Rubber policeman spatulas – VWR International (cat. no. 53801–008) (Fig. 2.4).
19 Muffle furnace – 525 ± 5°C.
20 Polypropylene columns – Bio-Rad, Econo-Pac™ Disposable Chromatography Columns (cat. no. 732–1010) with an Alltech One-Way Stopcock (cat. no. 211524) (Fig. 2.5).
21 Liquid chromatograph (LC) – With oven to maintain a column temperature of 90°C and a 50 μl injection loop. System must separate maltose from maltotriose.
22 Guard column (or pre-column) – Waters Guard Pak® LC pre-column inserts (Waters part no. WAT015209) or equivalent.

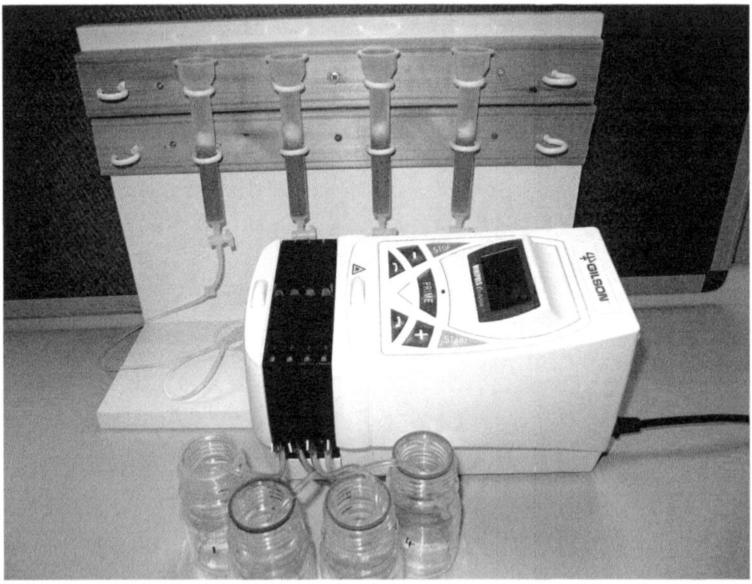

Fig. 2.5 Deionization of samples with mixed bed resin (~4 g Amberlite® FPA53 (OH^-) and ~4 g Ambersep® 200 (H^+)) in Bio-Rad, Econo-Pac® Disposable Chromatography Columns connected to a Gilson Minipuls® Evolution pump.

23 LC column – Waters Sugar-Pak® 6.5 × 300 mm column (part no. WAT085188) or equivalent. Mobile phase distilled water plus ethylene diamine tetraacetic acid disodium calcium salt ($Na_2CaEDTA$) (50 mg/l); flow rate 0.5 ml/min; column temp. 90°C; run time 30 min to assure column cleaned out.
24 Detector – Refractive index (RI); maintained at 50°C.
25 Data integrator or computer – For peak area measurement.
26 Filters for disposable syringe – Millipore Millex® Syringe Driven Filter Unit 0.45 mm (low protein binding Durapore PVDF), 25 mm or 13 mm or equivalent.
27 Filters for water – Millipore, 0.45 mm Durapore® Membrane Filters type HVLP, 47 mm.
28 Filter apparatus – To hold 47 mm, 0.45 mm filter (2.2.2(27)); to filter larger volumes of water.
29 Syringes –10 ml, disposable, plastic.
30 Syringes – Hamilton® 100 μl, 710SNR syringe.
31 Rotary evaporator – Heidolph Laborota® 4000 or equivalent.

2.2.3 Reagents

1 Ethanol (or IMS) 95% v/v.
2 Ethanol (or IMS) 78% v/v – Place 180 ml deionized water into 1 l volumetric flask. Dilute to volume with 95% v/v ethanol (or IMS). Mix.
3 Acetone, reagent grade.
4 Stock amyloglucosidase (AMG) solution (Megazyme cat. no. K-INTDF), 3300 Units/ml in 50% v/v glycerol – Solution is viscous; dispense using a positive displacement dispenser. AMG solution is stable for approx. 3 years when stored at 4°C. (Note: one unit of enzyme activity is the amount of enzyme required to release 1 micromole of D-glucose from soluble starch per minute at 40°C and pH 4.5). AMG solution should be essentially devoid of β-glucanase, β-xylanase and detectable levels of free D-glucose. Stable for > 4 years at −20°C.
5 Pancreatic α-amylase (50 units/ml)/AMG (3.4 units/ml) – Immediately before use, dissolve 0.10 g of purified porcine pancreatic α-amylase (150 000 units/g; AOAC Method 2009.01) (Megazyme cat. no. K-INTDF) in 290 ml of sodium maleate buffer (50 mM, pH 6.0 plus 2 mM $CaCl_2$ and 0.02% sodium azide) (2.2.3(14)) and stir for 5 min. Add 0.3 ml of AMG (2.2.3(4)). Stable for > 2 years at −20°C.
6 Protease (50 mg/ml; 350 tyrosine units/ml) in 50% v/v glycerol (Megazyme cat. no. K-INTDF) – Solution is viscous; dispense using a positive displacement dispenser. Protease must be devoid of α-amylase and essentially devoid of β-glucanase and β-xylanase. Use as supplied. Stable for > 3 years at 4°C.
7 LC retention time standard – Standard having the distribution of oligosaccharides (DP >3) corn syrup solids (DE 25; Matsutani Chemical

Industry Co., Ltd, Itami City, Hyogo, Japan; www.matsutani.com) analysed by LC plus maltose in a ratio of 4:1 (w/w). Dissolve 2.5 g of oligosaccharide mixture in 80 ml of 0.02% sodium azide solution (2.2.3(13)) and transfer to 100 ml volumetric flask. Pipette 10 ml of internal standard (2.2.3(8)) into the flask. Bring to volume with 0.02% sodium azide solution (2.2.3(13)). Transfer solutions to 50 ml polypropylene storage bottles®. Stable for > 1 year at room temperature. Stable for > 4 years at −20°C.

8 D-Sorbitol. (Internal standard for Sugar-Pak® column) – 100 mg/ml containing sodium azide (0.02% w/v). Weigh 10 g of analytical grade (> 99%) D-sorbitol into a 100 ml volumetric flask. Dissolve in 80 ml of 0.02% (w/v) sodium azide solution (2.2.3(13)) and adjust to volume with 0.02% sodium azide solution. Mix well. Stable for > 2 years at room temperature. Stable for > 4 years at −20°C. (Note: handle sodium azide with caution, only after reviewing material safety data sheet, using appropriate personal protective gear and laboratory hood.)

9 D-Glucose LC standards (5, 10, 20 mg/ml) – Accurately weigh 0.5, 1.0 and 2.0 g portions of high purity (> 99.5%) D-glucose (Sigma Chemical Company; cat. no. 5767) and transfer to three separate 100 ml volumetric flasks. To each flask pipette 10 ml of internal standard (2.2.3(8)). Bring to volume with 0.02% sodium azide solution (2.2.3(13)). Transfer solutions to 100 ml Duran® bottles. Stable at room temperature for 1 year.

10 Sodium maleate buffer – 50 mM, pH 6.0 plus 2 mM $CaCl_2$ and 0.02% sodium azide. Dissolve 11.6 g of maleic acid in 1600 ml of deionized water and adjust the pH to 6.0 with 4 M (160 g/l) NaOH solution. Add 0.6 g of calcium chloride ($CaCl_2.2H_2O$) and 0.4 g of sodium azide and adjust the volume to 2 l. Stable for > 1 year at 4°C. (Note: do not add the sodium azide until the pH has been adjusted. Acidification of sodium azide releases a poisonous gas. Handle sodium azide and maleic acid with caution, only after reviewing Materials Safety Data Sheet (MSDS), using appropriate personal protective gear and laboratory hood.)

11 Trizma Base® (Sigma cat. no. T-1503), 0.75 M – Add 90.8 g of Trizma® base to approx. 800 ml of deionized water and dissolve. Adjust volume to 1 l. Stable for > 1 year at room temperature.

12 Acetic acid solution, 2 M – Add 115 ml of glacial acetic acid (Fluka 45731) to a 1 l volumetric flask. Dilute to 1 l with deionized water. Stable for > 1 year at room temperature.

13 Sodium azide solution (0.02% w/v) – Add 0.2 g of sodium azide to 1 l of deionized water and dissolve by stirring. (Note: do not add sodium azide to solutions of low pH. Acidification of sodium azide releases a poisonous gas. Handle sodium azide with caution, only after reviewing MSDS, using appropriate personal protective gear and laboratory hood.) Stable at room temperature for > 2 years.

14 Deionized water containing $Na_2CaEDTA$ (50 mg/l) – Weigh 50 mg of $Na_2CaEDTA$ into a 1 l Duran bottle and dissolve in 1 l distilled water. Prepare fresh weekly; filter through 0.45 mm filter (2.2.2(27)) before use.

15 Cleaning solution – Micro-90® (International Products Corp., USA (www.ipcol.com/shopexd.asp?id=15) (accessed 4 October 2012). Make a 2% solution with deionized water.
16 pH standards – Buffer solutions at pH 4.0, 7.0 and 10.0.
17 Celite® – acid-washed, pre-ashed (Megazyme G-CEL100 or G-CEL500).
18 Mixed-bed ion exchange resins for each test portion –

(a) m-1. – approx. 4 g Amberlite® FPA53 (OH^-) resin (Rohm and Haas, France S.A.S.) (see also Megazyme cat. no. G-AMBOH), ion exchange capacity 1.6 meq/ml (min) or equivalent (R-OH exchange capacity data supplied by manufacturer) and
(b) m-2. – approx. 4 g Ambersep® 200 (H^+) resin or equivalent (Rohm and Haas, France S.A.S.) (see also Megazyme cat. no. G-AMBH), ion exchange capacity: 1.6 meq/ml (minimum). Mix the two resins just prior to use and pack in column (2.2.2(20), Bio-Rad disposable chromatography column) for analysis of each test portion (see Fig. 2.5). After mixing and packing, add a small cotton wool plug and wash with 20 ml of deionized water. If using other resins and there is a concern that carbohydrates may be retained on the resin, prepare a test solution consisting of 1 ml of 100 mg/ml internal standard (2.2.3(8)) and 2.5 ml of 10 mg/ml fructo-oligosaccharides diluted to 10 ml. Proceed to step 2.2.9(1b) 'Deionization of sample'. Recovery of the internal standards and fructo-oligosaccharides should match that of the solution injected directly onto the LC (Fig. 2.6).

2.2.4 Preparation of test samples

Collect and prepare samples as intended to be eaten (i.e. baking mixes should be prepared and baked, pasta should be cooked, etc.). De-fat per AOAC 985.29 if >10% fat. For high moisture samples (>25%) it may be desirable to freeze dry. Grind ~50 g in a grinding mill (2.2.2(1)) to pass a 0.5 mm sieve. Transfer all material to a wide mouthed plastic jar, seal, and mix well by shaking and inversion. Store in the presence of a desiccant.

2.2.5 Enzyme purity

To ensure absence of undesirable enzymatic activities and effectiveness of desirable enzymatic activities, run standards (Megazyme cat. no. K-TDFC) each time the enzyme lot changes or after the enzyme has been stored for more than 6 months.

2.2.6 Enzyme digestion of samples

1 **Blanks.** With each assay, run two blanks along with samples to measure any contribution from reagents to residue.

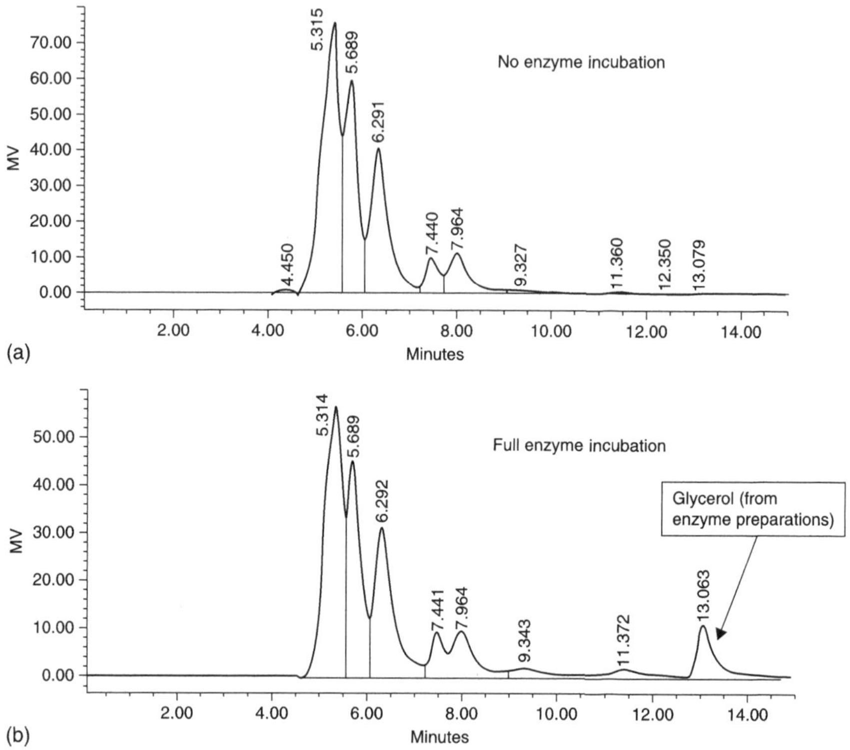

Fig. 2.6 High-performance liquid chromatography (HPLC) trace for Raftilose P-95® dissolved in water and analysed directly, compared with Raftilose P-95® recovered as NDO after running through the current integrated TDF procedure. Column: Waters Sugar-Pak® (6.5 mm × 300 mm). Solvent: distilled water containing EDTA (50 mg/l). Flow rate: 0.5 ml/min. Temperature: 90°C. (a) No enzyme incubation. (b) Full enzyme incubation.

2 Samples

(a) Weigh-duplicate 1.000 ± 0.005 g samples accurately into 250 ml Fisherbrand® soda glass, wide mouth bottles (2.2.2(2)).

(b) Addition of enzymes – Wet the sample with 1.0 ml of ethanol and add 40 ml of pancreatic α-amylase/AMG mixture (2.2.3(5)) to each bottle. Cap the bottles. Transfer the bottles to a Grant OLS 200 shaking incubation bath (or similar) (2.2.2(8)) and secure the bottles in place with the springs in the shaker frame. Alternatively, use a 2mag Mixdrive 15® submersible magnetic stirrer (2.2.2(8)) with 7 × 30 mm stirrer bars (Fig. 2.3).

(c) Incubation with pancreatic α-amylase/AMG – Incubate the reaction solutions at 37°C and 150 rpm in orbital motion in a shaking water bath (2.2.2(8)) or at 170 rpm on a 2mag Mixdrive 15® submersible magnetic stirrer (to ensure complete suspension) for exactly 16 h (e.g. 5.00 pm to 9.00 am).

(d) Adjustment of pH to approx. 8.2 (pH 7.9–8.4) and inactivation of α-amylase and AMG – After 16 h, remove all sample bottles from the shaking water bath and immediately add 3.0 ml of 0.75 M Trizma® base solution (2.2.3(11)) to terminate the reaction. (At the same time, if only one shaker bath is available, increase the temperature of the shaking incubation bath to 60°C in readiness for the protease incubation step.) Slightly loosen the caps of the sample bottles and immediately place the bottles in a water bath (non-shaking) at 95–100°C, and incubate for 20 min with occasional shaking (by hand). Using a thermometer, ensure that the final temperature of the bottle contents is > 90°C (checking of just one bottle is adequate).
(e) Cool – Remove all sample bottles from the hot water bath (use appropriate gloves) and cool to approx. 60°C.
(f) Protease treatment – Add 0.1 ml of protease solution (2.2.3(6)) with a positive displacement dispenser (solution is viscous). Incubate at 60°C for 30 min.
(g) pH adjustment – Add 4.0 ml of 2 M acetic acid (2.2.3(12)) to each bottle and mix. This gives a final pH of approx. 4.3.
(h) Internal standard – Add 1.0 ml of D-sorbitol internal standard solution (100 mg/ml) (2.2.3(8)) to each bottle and mix well.

3 Proceed to step 2.2.7(1) for determination of HMWDF/SDFS; or to step 2.2.8(2a) for determination of IDF/SDFP/SDFS.

2.2.7 Determination of HMWDF (IDF plus SDFP)

1 Precipitation SDFP – Preheat the sample to 60°C and add 192 ml (measured at room temperature) of 95% (v/v) ethanol (or IMS) pre-heated to 60°C. Mix thoroughly and allow the precipitate to form at room temperature for 60 min.
2 Filtration setup – Tare crucible containing Celite® (from 2.2.2(3)) to the nearest 0.1 mg. Wet and redistribute the bed of Celite® in the crucible, using 15 ml of 78% (v/v) ethanol or IMS from wash bottle. Apply suction to crucible to draw Celite® onto fritted glass as an even mat (Fig. 2.4).
3 Filtration – Using vacuum, filter precipitated enzyme digest (2.2.7(1)) through crucible. Using a wash bottle with 78% (v/v) ethanol (or IMS) (2.2.3(2)), quantitatively transfer all remaining particles to crucible. Retain filtrate and washings and proceed to step 2.2.9(1a) for determination of SDFS.
4 Wash – Using a vacuum, wash residue sequentially with two 15 ml portions of the following: 78% (v/v) ethanol (or IMS), 95% (v/v) ethanol (or IMS) and acetone.
5 Dry crucibles containing residue overnight in 105°C oven. If a forced air oven is used, loosely cover the crucibles with aluminium foil to prevent loss of dried sample.
6 Cool crucible in desiccator for approx. 1 h. Weigh crucible containing dietary fibre residue and Celite® to nearest 0.1 mg. To obtain residue mass, subtract tare weight, i.e. weight of dried crucible and Celite®.

7 Protein and ash determination – The residue from one crucible is analysed for protein, and the second residue of the duplicate is analysed for ash. Perform protein analysis on residue using Kjeldahl or combustion methods. (Caution should be exercised when using a combustion analyser for protein in the residue. Celite® volatilized from the sample can clog the transfer lines of the unit.) Use 6.25 factor for all cases to calculate mg of protein. For ash analysis, incinerate the second residue for 5 h at 525°C. Cool in desiccator and weigh to nearest 0.1 mg. Subtract crucible and Celite® weight to determine ash.
8 Determination of HMWDF – Subtract ash and protein from average residue weight and proceed to step 2.2.10 for calculation of HMWDF.

2.2.8 Determination of IDF, SDFP and SDFS

1 IDF

(a) Filtration setup – Tare crucible containing Celite® (2.2.2(4)) to nearest 0.1 mg. Wet and redistribute the bed of Celite® in the crucible, using 15 ml of 78% (v/v) EtOH (or IMS) (2.2.3(2)) from wash bottle. Apply suction to crucible to draw Celite® onto the fritted glass as an even mat (Fig. 2.4).
(b) Filtration – Using vacuum, filter the enzyme digest from step 2.2.6(2) through the crucible. Using a wash bottle with 60°C deionized water, rinse the incubation bottle with a minimum volume of water (approx. 10 ml) and use a rubber policeman (spatula) to dislodge all particles from the walls of the container. Transfer this suspension to the crucible. Wash the bottle with a further 10 ml of water at 60°C and again transfer to the crucible. Collect the combined filtrate and washings and adjust the volume to 70 ml and retain this for determination of SDFP (2.2.8(2a)) and SDFS (2.2.9(1a)).
(c) Wash – Using a vacuum, wash the residue successively with two 15 ml portions of the following: 78% (v/v) ethanol (or IMS), 95% (v/v) ethanol (or IMS) and acetone. Discard the washings.
(d) Dry crucibles containing residue overnight in 105°C oven.
(e) Cool crucibles in desiccators for approximately 1 h. Weigh crucible containing insoluble dietary fibre residue and Celite® to nearest 0.1 mg. To obtain residue mass, subtract tare weight, i.e. weight of dried crucible and Celite®. Calculate IDF; step 2.2.10.

2 SDFP

(a) Precipitation of SDFP – Pre-heat the filtrate of each sample (approx. 70 ml) to 60°C and add 280 ml (measured at room temperature) of 95% (v/v) ethanol (or IMS) (2.2.3(1)) preheated to 60°C and mix thoroughly. Allow the precipitate to form at room temperature for 60 min.
(b) Recovery of SDFP and SDFS – Proceed according to steps 2.2.7(3) to 2.2.7(8). For determination of SDFS – Proceed according to steps 2.2.9(1a) to 2.2.9(2b).

2.2.9 Determination of SDFS

Note: Proper deionization is an essential part of obtaining quality chromatographic data on SDFS. To obtain familiarity regarding the appearance of salt peaks in the SDFS chromatograms, dissolve 10 mg of sodium chloride in 9 ml of deionized water and add 1 ml of 100 mg/ml LC internal standard (2.2.3(8)) and proceed to step 2.2.9(1c) at 'Transfer the solution to a 10 ml disposable . . .'. To assure the resins being used are of adequate deionizing capacity, dissolve 10 mg of sodium chloride in 1 ml of deionized water. Add 1 ml of 100 mg/ml LC internal standard (2.2.3(8)), and proceed to step 2.2.9(1b) at 'Transfer 2 ml of this solution to the top of . . .'. The LC chromatogram of this solution should show no peaks in the time range corresponding to carbohydrates of DP3 or greater.

1 Extraction and chromatography procedure

(a) Filtrate recovery – Set aside the filtrate from one of the sample duplicates (2.2.7(3)) to use in case of spills or if duplicate SDFS data are desired. Transfer one half of filtrate (2.2.7(3)) of the other sample duplicate to a 500 ml evaporator flask and evaporate to dryness under vacuum at 60°C.

(b) Deionization of sample and AMG incubation – Add 5 ml of 150 mM HCl to the evaporator flask and swirl the flask for approx. 2 min to dissolve the sample (this adjusts the pH to ~ 4.5). Transfer the solution to a sealable polypropylene 20 ml container, add 0.1 ml of AMG (2.2.3(4)) and incubate at 60°C for 1 h. Then heat the solution at 100°C for 5 min. Transfer 2 ml of this solution to the top of the Bio-Rad disposable column containing 4 g each of freshly prepared and thoroughly mixed Amberlite FPA 53 (OH^-) (2.2.3(18)) and Ambersep 200 (H^+) (2.2.3(18)) (Fig. 2.5). Elute the column at a rate of 1.0 ml/min into a 100 ml Duran® bottle. When the sample has entered the resin, add 2 ml of distilled water to the resin and allow this to percolate in. Then add approximately 20 ml of deionized water to the top of the column and continue to elute at a rate of 1.0 ml/min. Transfer the eluate to a 250 ml round bottom rotary evaporator flask and evaporate to dryness under vacuum at 60°C. Add 2 ml of deionized water to the flask and redissolve the sugars by swirling the flask for approx. 2 min. Using a Pasteur pipette, transfer the solution to a polypropylene storage container.

(c) Preparation of samples for LC analyses – Transfer the solution to a 10 ml disposable syringe (2.2.2(29)), and filter through a 0.45 μm filter (2.2.2(26)). Use a 100 ml LC glass syringe (2.2.2(30)) to fill the 50 ml injection loop on the LC (2.2.2(21)). Perform this analysis in duplicate. Column: Waters Sugar-Pak® (6.5 × 300 mm). Solvent: distilled water containing Na_2Ca-EDTA (50 mg/l). Flow rate: 0.5 ml/min. Temperature: 90°C.

(d) Determine the response factor for D-glucose – Since D-glucose provides an LC refractive index (RI) response equivalent to the response factor for the non-digestible oligosaccharides that make up SDFS, the LC is calibrated using D-glucose, and the response factor is used for determining the mass of SDFS. Use a 100 μl LC syringe to fill a 50 μl injection loop for each standard D-sorbitol/D-glucose solution. Inject in triplicate.

2 Obtain the values for the peak areas of D-glucose and internal standard from the three chromatograms. The reciprocal of the slope obtained by comparing the ratio of peak area of D-glucose / peak area of D-sorbitol internal standard (y-axis) to the ratio of the mass of D-glucose / mass of D-sorbitol (x-axis) is the 'response factor'. Determine the average response factor (typically 0.97 for D-sorbitol).

Response factor (Rf) = (PA-IS) /(PA-Glu) × (Wt-Glu / Wt-IS)

where:

PA-IS = peak area internal standard (D-sorbitol);
PA-Glu = peak area D-glucose;
Wt-Glu = mass of D-glucose in standard;
Wt-IS = mass of D-sorbitol in standard.

(a) Calibrate the area of chromatogram to be measured for SDFS – Use a 100 ml LC syringe (2.2.2(30)) to fill the 50 ml injection loop with retention time standard (2.2.3(7)). Inject in duplicate. Determine demarcation point between DP 2 and DP 3 oligosaccharides (disaccharides maltose versus higher oligosaccharides) (Fig. 2.7).

(b) Determine peak area of SDFS (PA-SDFS) and internal standard (PA-IS) in chromatograms of sample extracts – Inject sample extracts (2.2.9(1c)) on LC. Record area of all peaks of DP greater than the DP2/DP3 demarcation point as PA-SDFS. Record the peak area of internal standard as PA-IS.

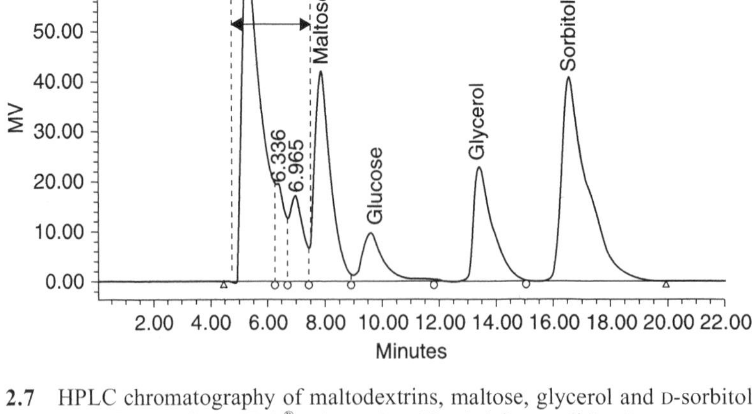

Fig. 2.7 HPLC chromatography of maltodextrins, maltose, glycerol and D-sorbitol on a Waters Sugar-Pak® column (see Fig. 2.6 for conditions).

2.2.10 Calculations for HMWDF, IDF and SDFP

Blank (B) determination (mg):

$$= (BR_1 + BR_2)/2 - P_B - A_B$$

where:

BR_1 and BR_2 = residue mass (mg) for duplicate blank determinations, respectively, and P_B and A_B = mass (mg) of protein and ash, respectively, determined on first and second blank residues.

HMWDF, IDF or SDFP (mg/100 g)

$$= \{[(R_1 = R_2)/2 - P_B - P_A - B] / (M_1 + M_2)/2\} \times 100$$

where:

R_1 = residue mass 1 from M1 in mg;
R_2 = residue mass 2 from M2 in mg;
M_1 = test portion mass 1 in g; M_2 = test portion mass 2 in g;
P_A = ash mass from R_1 in mg: P_B = protein mass from R_2 in mg.
HMWDF (%) = HMWDF (mg/100 g)/1000
IDF (%) = IDF (mg/100 g)/1000
SDFP (%) = SDFP (mg/100 g)/1000

2.2.11 Calculations for SDFS

SDFS (mg/100 g)

$$= Rf \times (Wt\text{-}IS, mg) \times (PA\text{-}SDFS)/(PA\text{-}IS) \times 100/M$$

where:

Rf is the response factor.

Wt-IS is weight in mg of internal standard contained in 1 ml of internal standard solution pipetted into sample mixture (100 mg).

PA-SDFS is the peak area of the SDFS.

PA-IS is the peak area of the internal standard (D-sorbitol).

M is the test portion mass (M_1 or M_2) in grams of the sample whose filtrate was concentrated and analysed by LC.

2.2.12 Calculation of integrated TDF

Integrated TDF (%) = HMWDF (%) + SDFS (%)

2.3 Updates of the original integrated total dietary fibre procedure

The original integrated procedure for the measurement of total dietary fibre (TDF) was published in 2007 (McCleary). Since then, efforts have been made to simplify the method and to allow the processing of a larger number of samples in a given time. Several aspects of the assay have been re-evaluated, including the incubation conditions, desalting format and choice of internal standard and LC chromatographic columns.

2.3.1 Incubation conditions

The incubation conditions for the integrated dietary fibre procedure are modelled on those used in AOAC Official Method 2002.02 (resistant starch). In that procedure, incubations were designed to give hydrolysis of non-resistant starch only. The method was developed using a set of resistant starch-containing samples that had been characterized through studies with ileostomy patients. In contrast to the resistant starch method, in the integrated dietary fibre method it is necessary to include an incubation step at approx. 100°C for the denaturation of protein; otherwise, protein is not degraded by protease. During this step, some of the resistant starch is solubilized. To ensure that none of this is depolymerized by α-amylase and AMG, these enzymes must be inactivated or denatured before the resistant starch is solubilized. This is achieved using a combination of pH and temperature conditions. As a result, most of the solubilized resistant starch precipitates from solution on addition of ethanol (to 76% concentration) and recovered as HMWDF. Lower degree of polymerization starch fragments that are resistant to hydrolysis by AMG and pancreatic α-amylase in the assay, but are not resistant to the α-glucosidases in the small intestine, are removed by incubating the SDFS fraction with much higher levels of AMG before desalting the SDFS sample.

To ensure that resistant starch is not solubilized during the 16 h incubation period, reactions were initially performed in bottles in which the contents were suspended by rotary shaking in a shaking water bath. More recently, it has been found that stirring of the contents, either with a suspended magnetic stirrer bar or with a stirrer bar in the reaction bottle, gave similar values for most samples. The results obtained for three types of starch are shown in Fig. 2.8. Dietary fibre values obtained for regular maize starch and high amylose maize starch were the same. With native potato starch granules, similar values were obtained when samples were incubated in the shaking water bath or were stirred with a suspended stirrer. When a stirrer bar is added into the incubation bottle, values for potato starch drop dramatically. This is thought to be due to the physical damage caused to the starch granules by the stirrer bar. This type of stirring had little or no effect on the determined resistant starch (and dietary fibre) in kidney beans, green bananas and various high amylose starch samples. Consequently, stirring of the reaction mixture in bottles with a stirrer bar can be performed using a device such as a Mixdrive 15® submersible magnetic stirrer.

2.3.2 Internal standards

Since AOAC Official Method 2001.03 'Total dietary fiber in foods containing resistant maltodextrins – enzymatic-gravimetric method and liquid chromatography determination" (Gordon and Okuma, 2002) employs gel permeation

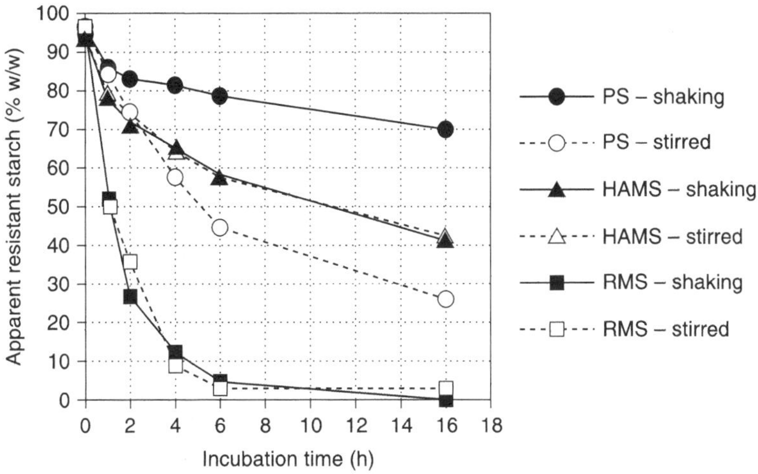

Fig. 2.8 Effect of shaking, suspended stirring and stirring with a magnetic stirrer bar added to the incubation bottle on the time course of hydrolysis of regular maize starch (RMS), high amylose maize starch (HAMS) and native potato starch (PS).

chromatography (TSK-GEL G2500PWXL®) rather than ion exchange as with the Waters Sugar-Pak column, attempts were made to find an internal standard that would work in both systems. Glycerol was considered to be non-ideal because glycerol occurs in a lot of processed food products and is also used as a stabilizer in the enzymes employed in the incubations. D-Sorbitol works well with the Sugar-Pak column, but it chromatographs with D-glucose on the TSK gel permeation columns. Numerous other compounds including sugars, sugar alcohols, diols and glycols were evaluated. Of these, 1,2-pentanediol, 1,5-pentanediol, diethylene glycol and triethylene glycol were the best based on chromatography in the two systems. However, 1,2-pentanediol showed significant loss in handling. Of the remainder, diethylene glycol was the preferred compound. However, even with this compound, if the samples were taken to dryness on rotary evaporation, a small percentage of the diethylene glycol was lost (presumably coating to the inside of the flask). Of the potential internal standards with acceptable chromatography properties, the only one suitable for the Waters Sugar Pak® column was D-sorbitol.

D-Sorbitol itself is not an ideal internal standard. The commercial fibre product Polydextrose® contains approx. 2% D-sorbitol and it is thought that this will interfere with analysis of products containing this product. However, it is unlikely that any food product will contain more than 10% Polydextrose®, in which case the level of D-sorbitol is approx. 0.2%, which will have insignificant effect on the assay. Also, if D-sorbitol is thought to be present in the sample, analysis can be performed without addition of the internal standard or, alternatively, calculations can simply be performed using the external standard assay format. Also, in such cases, the use of diethylene glycol as the internal standard could be considered (Fig. 2.9), knowing that samples should not be taken to dryness on rotary evaporation.

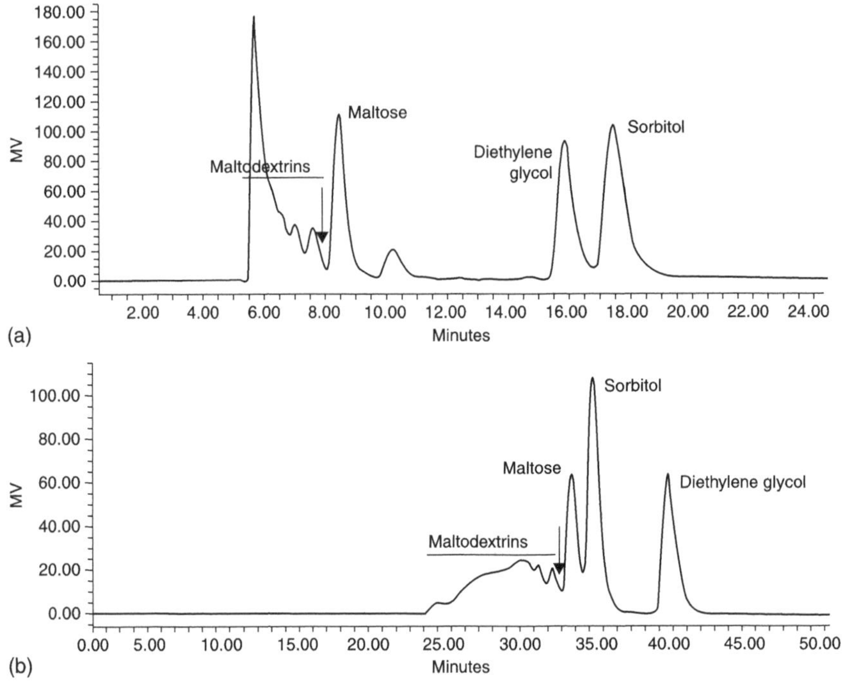

Fig. 2.9 Chromatography of a mixture of maltodextrins, maltose, diethylene glycol and D-sorbitol on: (a) a Waters Sugar-Pak® (6.5 × 300 mm, part no. WAT085188) column. Solvent: distilled water containing EDTA (50 mg/l); flow rate: 0.5 ml/min; temperature 90°C; or (b) on two TSK® gel filtration columns (G2500PWXL) in series. Solvent: distilled water; flow rate 0.5 ml/min; temperature 80°C. The arrows show demarcation between DP 2 (maltose) and DP 3 (higher maltodextrins).

2.3.3 Desalting of samples for HPLC

In the original integrated dietary procedure, the desalting conditions recommended in AOAC Official Method 2001.03 were employed, in which 25 g each of Amberlite cation and anion exchange resins were mixed and packed into a chromatography column. Subsequently, the amount of resin was halved, along with sample size. More recently, with the use of an internal standard that was completely recovered (D-sorbitol), it has been possible to reduce the amount of sample handled, along with the amounts of desalting resins to approximately 20% of that originally recommended. There are several advantages in this modification. First, all evaporations are reduced to 20%, which is a major time saving. Second, cheap, easy to use plastic columns (Bio-Rad, Econo-Pac™ Disposable Chromatography Columns) can be used. These are large enough to hold the 8 g of mixed bed resin and to accommodate the volume (20 ml) of deionized/distilled water used to elute the sugars from the column (Fig. 2.5). Essentially all sugar is eluted with this volume of water (Fig. 2.10). Also, the rates of elution of the sugars in the sample and the D-sorbitol internal standard are the same.

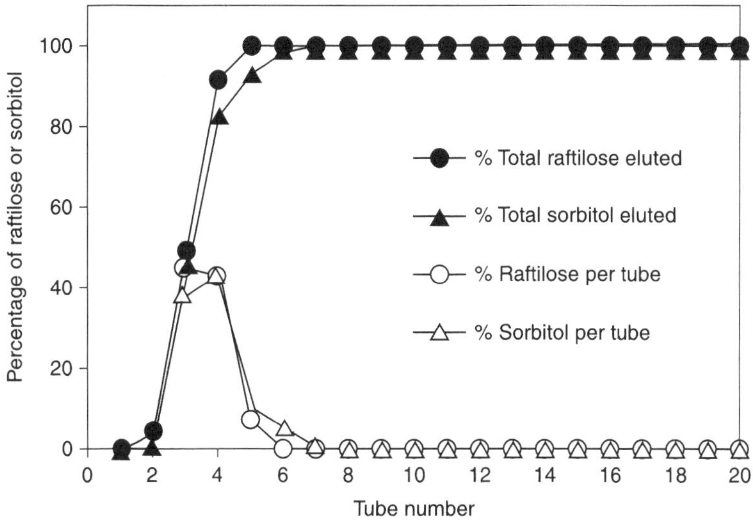

Fig. 2.10 Elution of D-sorbitol and fructo-oligosaccharides from a mixed bed resin column (Amberlite® FPA53 (OH–) plus Ambersep® 200). Note that the rate of elution of the D-sorbitol and fructo-oligosaccharides is the same and that essentially all carbohydrate is eluted with 20 ml of water.

Alternatively, samples can be desalted/de-ashed using cation and anion exchange guard columns, H^+ and CO_2^{3-} forms, respectively (BioRad Labs Catalogue # 125–0118) (Post *et al.*, 2010). In this case, the aqueous ethanolic solution is concentrated by rotary evaporation, redissolved in distilled water, adjusted to volume, clarified and injected directly onto the HPLC via the de-ashing guard columns. This procedure simplifies sample preparation for LC, and it is possible to monitor exhaustion of the de-ashing columns. A major consideration is the cost of the disposable de-ashing guard columns and the need for a separate pump for the HPLC.

2.3.4 Analysis of difficult samples

For most samples analysed to date, chromatography on a Waters Sugar-Pak® column gives effective separation of disaccharides and trisaccharides. The one exception noted is the fructosyl-trisaccharide (F3) (inulotriose) obtained on depolymerization of inulin. From Fig. 2.11, it can be seen that this compound elutes after the disaccharides sucrose and maltose, and partially overlaps them. In fact, it chromatographs at the same point as lactose. In handling oligosaccharide mixtures containing this compound, there are two possible options. Compounds can be separated using TSK gel permeation chromatography (TSK-GEL G2500PWXL®) rather than ion exchange as with the Waters Sugar-Pak®, but without the option of using D-sorbitol as an internal standard. Alternatively, an aliquot of the sample prepared for HPLC can be incubated with a mixture

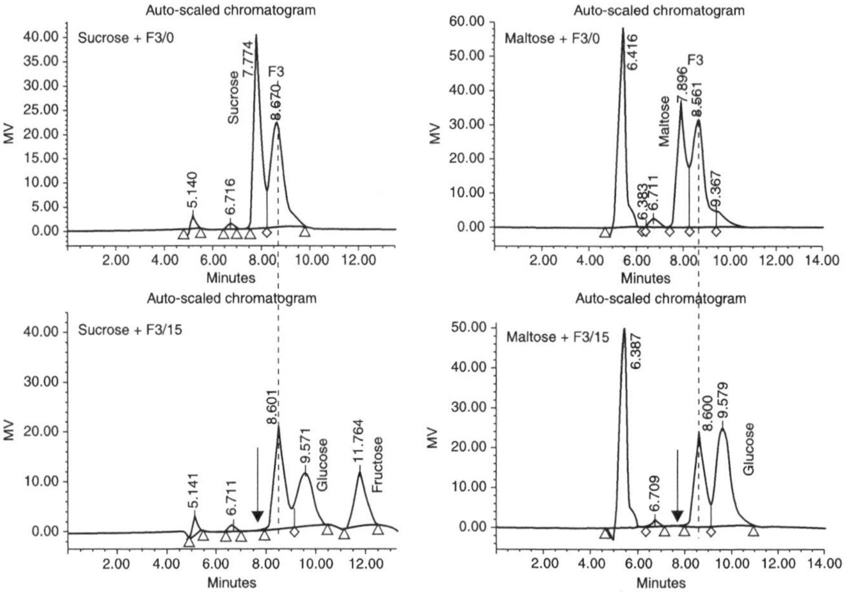

Fig. 2.11 Hydrolysis of sucrose and maltose with thermostable α-glucosidase. One millilitre of a mixture of F3 (5 mg/ml) with either sucrose or maltose (5 mg/ml) was incubated with 0.1 ml of thermostable α-glucosidase (500 U/ml) in 10 mM sodium maleate buffer (pH 6.0) at 50°C for 15 min. Reaction tube was incubated at 100°C for 5 min. The solution was centrifuged in a microfuge at 12 000 rpm for 5 min and the sample directly applied to the HPLC column.

of thermostable α-glucosidase (to hydrolyse the sucrose and maltose) and β-galactosidase (to hydrolyse lactose) and chromatographed again to measure F3 (by reference to the D-sorbitol internal standard). This value can simply be added to the value obtained for the oligosaccharide mixture of DP $\geq$ 3 obtained for the sample before α-glucosidase/β-galactosidase treatment.

Samples containing highly viscous/gelatinous dietary fibre (e.g. psyllium gum) are very difficult to filter through crucibles. Such samples may be better handled by recovering the various fractions by high-speed centrifugation. Work in this area is urgently required.

2.4 Interlaboratory evaluation of integrated total dietary fibre procedures

The integrated total dietary fibre assay procedure has been subjected to two major interlaboratory studies under the auspices of AOAC International. In the first study (McCleary *et al.*, 2010), total HMWDF and SDFS were measured. HMWDF was not fractionated into IDF and SDFP. On the basis of the results from this study, the method was accepted as AOAC Official Method 2009.01. In the second

Table 2.4 Statistical data for total dietary fibre (HMWDF plus LMWSDF) determined using the modification of AOAC Official Method 2009.01

Sample/ Parameter	Cabbage	Apple flakes	Chocolate	Biscuits	Cookies	Peanuts	Oat bran	Bread
# of Labs	15	15	15	15	14	13	14	13
Mean %	29.90	10.45	26.55	11.79	21.37	16.39	23.71	18.40
S_r	0.86	0.47	1.39	0.49	0.52	1.41	0.87	0.64
S_R	2.05	0.95	2.74	1.10	1.72	2.37	3.14	1.56
RSD_r	2.88	4.51	5.25	4.17	2.43	8.60	3.65	3.47
RSD_R	6.85	9.11	10.31	9.30	8.04	14.48	13.23	8.47
HORRAT	2.85	3.24	4.22	3.37	3.19	5.51	5.33	3.28

Source: McCleary *et al.*, 2012.

Note: Sr = within laboratory repeatability; SR = between laboratory variability; RSDr = within laboratory relative repeatability; RSDR = between laboratory relative variability; HORRAT = The ratio of the reproducibility standard deviation calculated from the data to the predicted relative standard deviation.

study, IDF, SDFP and SDFS were measured separately (McCleary *et al.*, 2012). On the basis of the results from that study, the method has recently been accepted as AOAC Official Method 2011.25. A summary of the results for TDF is shown in Table 2.4. The statistics compare favourably with those obtained for other interlaboratory evaluations of dietary fibre methods (Table 2.5) (McCleary *et al.*, 2010). Of particular interest is the fact that TDF values determined by summing HMWDF and SDFS are very similar to those obtained by summing IDF, SDFP and SDFS (Table 2.6).

2.5 Progress in acceptance of dietary fibre methodology by Codex Alimentarius

At the 30th session of CCNFSDU (2008), the Committee agreed on a definition of dietary fibre (detailed above). However, the Committee also agreed on the establishment of an Electronic Working Group (eWG) led by the Delegation of France, open to all Codex members. The specific role of this eWG was to: a) review and update, as appropriate, the list of methods available for dietary fibre analysis, taking into account the new provisions in the draft definition of dietary fibre that would require the selection of methods of analysis, and possible information on new available methods; b) consider how the results from different methods specific to different types of dietary fibre could be combined together to arrive at the total dietary fibre content in a food; c) evaluate the performance of methods in measuring different types of dietary fibre; d) make recommendations for methods of analysis for dietary fibre in different food matrices; e) consider the footnote in the accepted definition that relates to oligosaccharides of degree of polymerization (DP) of 3–9, and to prepare a recommendation as to its revision with regard to the methods of analysis, if necessary.

Table 2.5 Statistical details for various dietary fibre methods run through AOAC International interlaboratory evaluations

Method number	Title	S_r	RSD_r	S_R	RSD_R	HORRAT
985.29	Total Dietary Fiber in Foods	0.15–0.99	0.56–66.25	0.27–1.36	1.58–66.25	0.76–17.46
991.42	Insoluble Dietary Fiber in Food and Food Products	0.41–2.82	0.86–10.38	0.62–9.49	3.68–19.44	1.73–8.68
991.43*	Insoluble Dietary Fiber in Food and Food Products	0.36–1.06	1.50–6.62	0.85–2.06	1.58–12.17	0.74–4.66
992.16	Total Dietary Fiber	0.18–1.01	1.48–14.73	0.22–2.06	4.13–17.94	1.84–4.62
993.19	Soluble Dietary Fiber in Food and Food Products	0.49–1.15	1.74–5.93	0.79–2.05	2.41–7.01	1.13–2.83
994.13	Total Dietary Fiber (Determined as Neutral Sugar Residues, Uronic Acid Residues, and Klason Lignin)	0.32–2.88	1.80–6.96	0.52–4.90	4.80–11.30	2.32–4.20
2001.03	Dietary Fiber Containing Supplemented Resistant Maltodextrin (RMD)	0.02–1.63	1.33–6.10	0.04–2.37	1.79–9.39	0.77–3.32
2002.02	Resistant Starch in Starch and Plant Materials	0.08–2.66	1.97–4.12	0.21–3.87	4.58–10.90	1.44–3.74
2009.01	Total Dietary Fiber in Foods	0.41–1.43	1.65–12.34	1.18–5.44	4.70–17.97	1.91–6.49

Source: McCleary *et al.*, 2012.
Notes: *Samples that were not dried and/or desugared only.

Table 2.6 Collaborative study data for total dietary fibre (% TDF) as measured directly versus the sum of IDF and SDF reported by laboratories who ran both methods

Sample Lab #	Cabbage		Apple flakes		Chocolate		Biscuits		Cookies		Peanuts		Oat bran		Bread	
1 Direct	28.51	29.58	9.78	9.51	25.80	25.30	11.51	11.52	20.50	19.85	14.81	14.11	20.90	23.16	17.69	17.70
1 Sum	28.90	27.82	9.87	9.80	27.05	28.32	11.78	12.02	21.03	20.22	17.12	17.35	22.90	23.04	17.25	17.81
2 Direct	27.42	27.86	10.09	9.53	23.49	23.06	11.75	11.71	19.10	19.02	15.25	15.71	19.65	20.23	17.13	17.46
2 Sum	27.93	29.32	10.61	10.04	24.01	23.56	12.26	12.21	19.62	19.53	15.76	16.85	20.17	20.74	17.64	17.97
3 Direct	27.56	27.32	9.74	10.10	23.69	24.84	8.49	8.89	20.98	22.15	14.62	15.69	22.48	22.68	17.50	17.50
3 Sum	28.87	28.75	9.39	9.95	25.97	29.51	10.06	10.23	24.15	24.94	19.63	21.29	34.48	21.49	22.79	20.47
4 Direct	28.07	27.76	11.89	12.88	27.88	29.34	13.13	14.01	23.10	21.77	29.09	27.29	23.25	20.89	17.10	13.19
4 Sum	27.07	26.45	9.67	10.10	21.97	21.00	12.02	13.31	19.24	18.31	13.95	13.41	20.52	17.38	16.22	16.43
5 Direct	27.79	29.04	9.02	8.55	23.24	23.30	10.12	10.40	19.75	19.97	14.68	14.17	20.74	19.90	11.86	11.73
5 Sum	28.12	29.59	9.24	9.02	23.34	23.54	10.25	10.01	20.63	20.67	*	*	20.40	20.30	12.15	11.53

Source: McCleary *et al.*, 2012.
Notes: *Laboratory reported no result for this sample.

In their draft document (Alinorm, 2009), the eWG noted that the Official AOAC methods are widely accepted globally for general labelling of nutrient content in foods as well as for health and nutrition claims. The AOAC methods are designed to be accurate, cost effective, and reproducible in various analytical environments on which industry relies. They are the most studied and validated methods available for the quantification of food components. Their use in routine analysis presents no insurmountable difficulty. These methods have passed the rigour of scientific substantiation to achieve the status of reference methods. The eWG also noted that (at that time) no one AOAC validated method could measure all non-digestible carbohydrates in foods. AOAC 991.43 (Lee *et al.*, 1992) is one of the most widely used 'total' dietary fibre methods. Both this method and AOAC 985.29 (Prosky *et al.*, 1985) will measure insoluble polysaccharides and soluble high molecular weight components (i.e. those that are precipitated by alcohol (SDFP)). However, neither fully measures the resistant starch fraction, nor do they recover the non-digestible oligosaccharide components included in the definition of dietary fibre. They quantify only part of the total resistant starch, inulin, Polydextrose (Craig *et al.*, 2000), fructo-oligosaccharides and resistant maltodextrin, all of which have relevant physiological functions. Furthermore, some oligosaccharides are not measured at all. The eWG also noted that, due to the complexity of the molecular structure of fibres, additional AOAC methods were subsequently developed to validate labelling declarations and claims by measuring specific dietary fibre components in foods that have been shown to exert physiological benefit. Maintaining these methods (e.g. AOAC 999.03 (McCleary *et al.*, 2000) for fructans) has a number of advantages. By focusing on one component the method is more specific, resulting in higher specificity and accuracy needed to detect fibre present in food products. Equally important, these component-specific methods facilitate routine, cost-effective analysis.

The eWG concluded (draft document) that the NSP method does not accurately quantify total dietary fibre. It is inappropriate as a routine technique given its inability to support the now agreed upon Codex definition of dietary fibre. Methods measuring NSP alone give lower estimates than methods for total dietary fibre in foods containing resistant starch, resistant oligosaccharides and/or lignin. The eWG did not recommend the inclusion of methods where there is as yet no publication about protocol and relevant validation data.

The eWG also noted that the definition encompasses a range of different types of carbohydrate polymers that are recovered to varying extents by different analytical methods. This creates potential problems of double accounting when a carbohydrate fraction is partially or completely measured by more than one method. Examples of this are high molecular weight inulin, which, in addition to being measured specifically by enzymatic–chemical fructan methods, is also partially recovered in the residue of enzymatic–gravimetric methods (Quemener *et al.*, 1993; 1997). The enzymatic–gravimetric methods AOAC 991.43 and 985.29 also recover some, but not all, resistant starch (McCleary and Rossiter, 2004), which can create a double accounting problem if these data are then combined with that obtained by a separate specific determination of resistant starch. There is also the potential for obtaining a lower than expected value if there is under-recovery of a specific fraction by particular methods. The high degree of specificity associated with most direct chemical methods generally means that the problems of combining results from different methods are diminished.

The eWG noted (draft document) that the lack of a validated procedure to combine AOAC methods to determine total fibre content has repeatedly raised concerns during the lengthy process to finalize the definition of dietary fibre. It also noted that, in response to this gap in methodology, a new integrated method of analysis of total dietary fibre has been developed by McCleary (2007) which measures total dietary fibre (including resistant starch), non-digestible oligosaccharides and available carbohydrates. This new integrated method is based principally on existing official AOAC methods 2002.02 and 991.43 and AOAC method 2001.03 (Gordon and Okuma, 2002). A process similar to that described in AOAC Official Method 2001.03 allows the measurement of non-digestible oligosaccharides in the range from DP 3 to approx. DP 10.

The eWG concluded that 'this new integrated method provides a path forward for analysing the full range of dietary fibres included in the scope of the Codex definition, in a manner that better reflects overall the fiber that is physiologically relevant. This method is in the stage of collaborative study analysis and is likely to achieve AOAC approval'. In addition, the eWG suggested that the Committee should consider the inclusion of the new method of analysis for total dietary fibre (McCleary, 2007), once AOAC validation has been completed.

In the 34th session of CCNFSDU (Geneva, Switzerland, 4–9 July 2011), the outcome of the 32nd meeting in Santiago, Chile (1–5 November 2010) was reported as follows:

> **Method of analysis of dietary fibre**
>
> 14. The Committee recalled that the 31st Session of CCMAS had indicated that most of the methods of analysis for dietary fibre were empirical and some of them might be overlapping, and therefore had agreed that they could be endorsed as Type IV in order to make them available as Codex methods and asked the CCNFSDU to define their scope more precisely.
>
> 15. The Committee agreed to change the provisions for six general methods of analysis to describe them more precisely and proposed them as Type I methods. Regarding eight methods that measure individual specific components, the Committee agreed to propose them as Type II methods (one of these was subsequently changed to a Type III method). Regarding the three 'other methods', the Committee agreed to propose that they should be maintained as Type IV methods (See Appendix VI). Some delegations indicated that they were unable to comment at this stage and would make their comments to the CCMAS.
>
> 16. In reply to the proposal of CCMAS to delete the AOAC 2001.03 method, the Committee agreed to keep it because it was applicable when resistant starches are not present and AOAC 2009.01 was applicable to food that may, or may not, contain resistant starches.

These agreements are summarized in Table 2.1 (see page 27).

After many years of debate within the working groups of Codex Alimentarius, finally, a consensus opinion on a definition of dietary fibre has been agreed. With the recent agreements on dietary fibre methodology and Codex Alimentarius typing (CCMAS, Budapest, March 2011), a clear guideline has been given to food manufacturers, analysts and regulators.

2.6 References

AACC Method 32–05, Total Dietary Fiber. *Approved Methods of the American Association of Cereal Chemists*, 9th ed. The Association, St Paul, MN, 1995.

ALINORM 09/32/26, http://www.codexalimentarius.net/web/archives.jsp?year=09.

ALINORM REP11/NFSDU, http://www.codexalimentarius.net/web/archives.jsp?year=11.

ANON (2001) The definition of dietary fiber. *Cereal Foods World* **46**:112–26.

AOAC Method 991.43, Total, Insoluble and Soluble Dietary Fiber in Food—Enzymatic-Gravimetric Method, MES-TRIS Buffer. *Official Methods of Analysis*, 16th ed. AOAC International, Gaithersburg, MD, 1995.

AOAC (2010) *Official Methods of analysis of AOAC International* (W. HORWITZ, Ed.), 18th ed., revision 3, 2010; AOAC International, Gaithersberg, USA.

ASP, N.-G. (2001) *Advanced Dietary Fibre Technology* (B. V. MCCLEARY and L. PROSKY, Eds), Blackwell Science Publishers, Oxford, UK.

BRUNT, K. (2011) Dietary fiber levels in bread according to AOAC 985.29 and AOAC 2009.01 method. *Proceedings of the 9th International Food Data Conference*, Norwich, UK, 15–17 September 2011, http://www.eurofir.net/sites/default/files/9th%20IFDC/Presentations/Brunt.pdf.

BURKITT, D. P., WALKER, A. R. P. and PAINTER, N. S. (1972) Effect of dietary fibre on stools and transit times and its role in the causation of disease. *Lancet* ii:1408.

CHAMP, M., KOZLOWSKI, F. and LECANNU, G. (2001) *In vivo* and *in vitro* methods for resistant starch measurement. In *Advanced Dietary Fibre Technology* (B. V. MCCLEARY and L. PROSKY, Eds), Blackwell Science Ltd, Oxford, UK, pp. 106–19.

CHAMP, M., LANGKILDE, A.-M., BROUNS, F., KETTLITZ, B. and COLLET, Y. (2003) Advances in dietary fibre characterisation. 1. Definition of dietary fibre, physiological relevance, health benefits and analytical aspects. *Nut. Res. Rev.* **16**:71–8.

CODEX COMMITTEE ON NUTRITION AND FOODS FOR SPECIAL DIETARY USES (CCNFSD; ALINORM 06/29/26), 27th Session, Bonn, Germany, 21–25 November 2005.

CODEX COMMITTEE ON NUTRITION AND FOODS FOR SPECIAL DIETARY USES (CCNFSDU), 30th Session, Cape Town, South Africa, 3–7 November 2008.

CRAIG, S. A., HOLDEN, J. F. and KHALED, M. Y. (2001) Determination of polydextrose in foods by ion chromatography: collaborative study. *J AOAC Int.* **84**:472–8.

DE SLEGTE, J. (2002) Determination of trans-galactooligosaccharides in selected food products by ion-exchange chromatography: collaborative study. *J AOAC Int.* **85**:417–23.

DEVRIES, J. W. (2004) Dietary fiber: the influence of definition on analysis and regulation. *J AOAC Int.* **87**:682–706.

DIETARY FIBRE CONFERENCE (2006), Helsinki, 11–14 June 2006.

ENGLYST, H. N. and CUMMINGS, J. H. (1984) Simplified method for the measurement of non-starch polysaccharides by gas-liquid chromatography of constituent sugars as alditol acetates. *Analyst* **109**:937–42.

ENGLYST, H. N. AND HUDSON, G. J. (1987) Colorimetric method for the routine measurement of dietary fibre as non-starch polysaccharides. A comparison with gas-liquid chromatography. *Food Chemistry* **24**:63–7.

GORDON, D. T. and OKUMA, K. (2002) Determination of total dietary fibre in selected foods containing resistant maltodextrin by enzymatic-gravimetric method and liquid chromatography: collaborative study. *J AOAC Int.* **85**:435–44.

GROOTAERT, C., DELCOUR, J. A., COURTIN, C. M., BROEKAERT, W. F., VERSTRAETE, W. and VAN DE WIELE, T. (2007) Microbial metabolism and prebiotic potency of arabinoxylan oligosaccharides in the human intestine. *Trends in Food Science and Technology*, **18**:64–71.

HIPSLEY, E. H. (1953) Dietary 'fibre' and pregnancy toxaemia. *British Medical Journal*, **2**:420–2.

HOEBREGS, H. (1997) Fructans in foods and food products, ion exchange chromatographic method: collaborative study, *Journal of AOAC International*, **80**(5): 1029–37; AOAC Official Method 997.08, Fructans in food products, ion exchange chromatography. In: *Official Methods of Analysis*, 16th ed., AOAC International, Arlington.

INSTITUTE OF MEDICINE (2001) in *Dietary reference intakes: Energy, Carbohydrates, Fiber, Fat, Fatty Acids, Cholesterol, Protein and Amino Acids*, National Academies Press, Washington, DC.

LEE, S. C., PROSKY, L. and DEVRIES, J. W. (1992) Determination of total, soluble, and insoluble dietary fiber in foods-Enzymatic-gravimetric method, MES-TRIS buffer: Collaborative study. *Journal of the Association of Official Analytical Chemists* **75**:395–416.

MCCLEARY, B. V. (2007) An integrated procedure for the measurement of total dietary fibre (including resistant starch), non-digestible oligosaccharides and available carbohydrates. *Anal. Bioanal. Chem.* **389**:291–308.

MCCLEARY, B. V. and CODD, R. (1991). Measurement of (1–3)(1–4)-b-D-glucan in barley and oats: a streamlined enzymic procedure. *J. Fd Sci Agriculture*, **55**:303–12.

MCCLEARY, B. V. and MONAGHAN, D. A. (2002) Measurement of resistant starch. *J. AOAC Int.* **85**:665–75.

MCCLEARY, B. V. AND ROSSITER, P. (2004) Measurement of novel dietary fibres. *J. AOAC Int.* **87**:707–17.

MCCLEARY, B. V., MURPHY, A. and MUGFORD, D. C. (2000) Determination of oligofructans and fructan polysaccharides in foodstuffs by an enzymatic/spectrophotometric method: collaborative study, *J AOAC Int.* **83**:356–64; AOAC Official Method 999.03, Measurement of oligofructans and fructan polysaccharides in foodstuffs by an enzymatic/spectrophotometric method. In: *Official Methods of Analysis*, 16th ed., AOAC International, Arlington.

MCCLEARY, B. V., MCNALLY, M. and ROSSITER, P. (2002) Measurement of resistant starch by enzymic digestion in starch samples and selected plant materials: collaborative study. *J. AOAC Int.* **85**:1103–11.

MCCLEARY, B. V., DEVRIES, J. W., RADER, J. I., COHEN, G., PROSKY, L., *et al.* (2010) Determination of total dietary fiber (CODEX definition) by enzymatic-gravimetric method and liquid chromatography: collaborative study. *J. AOAC Int.* **93**:221–33.

MCCLEARY, B. V., DEVRIES, J. W., RADER, J. I., COHEN, G., PROSKY, L., *et al.* (2012) Determination of insoluble, soluble and total dietary fiber (CODEX definition) by enzymatic-gravimetric method and liquid chromatography: collaborative study. *J. AOAC Int.* **95**:824–44.

POST, B. E., MARSHAK, M. R. and DEVRIES, J. W. (2010) Simultaneous ion removal and quantitation of low-molecular-weight dietary fiber from high-molecular weight dietary fiber filtrates using liquid chromatography. *J. AOAC Int.* **93**:234–42.

PROSKY, L., ASP, N.-G., FURDA, I., DEVRIES, J. W., SCHWEIZER, T. F. and HARLAND, B. F. (1985) Determination of total dietary fiber in foods and food products: collaborative study. *J. AOAC Int.* **68**:677–9.

QUEMENER, B., THIBAULT, J.-F. and COUSSEMENT, P. (1993) Determination of inulin and oligofructose in food products, and integration in the AOAC method for measurement of total dietary fibre. *Lebensm.-Wiss. U. Technol.* **27**:125–32.

QUEMENER, B., THIBAULT, J.-F. and COUSSEMENT, P. (1997) Integration of inulin determination in the AOAC method for measurement of total dietary fibre. *Int. J. Biol. Macromol.* **21**:175–8.

SOUTHGATE, D. A. T. (1969) Determination of carbohydrates in foods. II. Unavailable carbohydrates. *J. Sci. Fd Agric.* **20**:326–30.

SOUTHGATE, D. A. T. (1982) Definition and terminology of dietary fiber. In: *Dietary Fiber in Health and Disease* (G. V. VAHOUNY and D. KRITCHEVSKY, Eds), Plenum Press, New York, pp. 1–7.

THEANDER, O. and AMAN, P. (1982) Studies on dietary fiber: A method for the analysis and chemical characterization of total dietary fiber. *J. Sci. Fd Agric.* **33**:340–4.

TROWELL, H. C. (1974) Definition of dietary fibre. *Lancet* **1**:503.

TROWELL, H. C., SOUTHGATE, D. A. T., WOLEVER, T. M. S., LEEDS, A. R., GASSULL, M. A. and JENKINS, D. J. A. (1976) Dietary fiber redefined. *Lancet* **1**:967.

3

Health aspects of dietary fibre

J. Slavin, University of Minnesota, USA

DOI: 10.1533/9780857095787.1.61

Abstract: Intakes of dietary fibre are linked to improved health outcomes. Dietary fibre is difficult to define and measure and not all dietary fibre is alike. Generally most physiological effects are found with traditional fibres such as cereal brans and vegetables. Some isolated soluble fibres, including oats and barley, are particularly good at lowering blood lipids. Usual intakes of dietary fibre are about half recommended levels, so there is a need to increase consumption of fibre from all sources.

Key words: dietary fibre, fermentation, obesity, cardiovascular disease, satiety.

3.1 Introduction

Fibre is not an essential nutrient in the usual way we consider essential nutrients. Unlike traditional nutrients, the benefits of fibre are linked to its lack of digestion and absorption in the upper gastrointestinal tract. Fibre has additional physiological effects in the colon, where it can survive transit and increase stool size or be fermented by intestinal bacteria. This fermentation in the gut decreases pH, promotes growth of microbiota, and produces short-chain fatty acids and gut metabolites that may play a role in disease prevention. Short-chain fatty acids are also absorbed in the colon and are a potential energy source. Therefore, fibre is not just an inert substance that travels through the digestive tract, but plays many roles in digestion and absorption.

Additionally, dietary fibre intake has been linked to the prevention and management of many diseases. Epidemiologic studies support that higher intakes of fibre from all sources are associated with less incidence of cardiovascular disease. Additionally, fibre's role in enhancement of satiety and prevention of obesity continues to be supported by research trials. The protectiveness of fibre for diabetes and different types of cancer is less consistent, but plant-based, higher fibre diets are recommended in the prevention of chronic diseases across the world.

The role of isolated fibres, as compared with plant foods high in fibre, whole grains, legumes, and to a lesser extent vegetables and fruits, continues to be debated. Plant-based diets high in fibre have known health benefits, but isolated fibres including β-glucan, psyllium, and inulin modify biomarkers in human subjects, such as lipid lowering, improved gut function, and blood glucose stabilization. In fact, there are more published data on the effectiveness of isolated fibres on health biomarkers than intact plant foods.

3.2 Fibre: definitions, measurement and intake

Traditionally, fibre is measured as chemical components, such as cellulose, hemicellulose, pectin, and lignin. Currently the United States relies on an 'analytical approach' to determine what is or is not considered fibre for purposes of listing fibre content on food labels. In 2001 the Institute of Medicine (IOM) developed the following set of working definitions for fibre in the food supply:

> Dietary Fiber consists of nondigestible carbohydrates and lignin that are intrinsic and intact in plants.
> Functional Fiber consists of isolated, nondigestible carbohydrates that have beneficial physiological effects in humans.
> Total Fiber is the sum of Dietary Fiber and Functional Fiber. (IOM, 2001)

These definitions recognize the diversity of non-digestible carbohydrates in the food supply. Fibre definitions and measurement continue to be debated. Most definitions suggest that fibre is plant material not digested by mammalian enzymes. But some consider limiting fibre to 'plant material' to be too restrictive. Some would include chitosan, which forms the exoskeleton of crustaceans, or certain heat-treated animal proteins that are not readily digestible by mammalian enzymes and thus reach the large intestine relatively intact. Others include in their definition of fibre 'resistant starch', which may not be digested and absorbed in the small intestine and thus may have characteristics similar to those of fibre, under certain circumstances. Resistant starches occur in some foods. But resistant starch can also be manufactured or produced during food processing. Whether oligosaccharides present in beans and other vegetables (raffinose, stachyose and verbacose) and fructans (storage poly- and oligosaccharides) in vegetables and fruits such as onions and artichokes are fibre has also been debated. The alcohol precipitation steps used in fibre analytical techniques exclude these substances, yet they have biological effects similar to those of other non-digested polysaccharides.

Another point of discussion is whether dietary fibre has to be intact in the food to be characterized as dietary fibre, or whether it can be isolated from carbohydrates and still be considered fibre. The IOM definition of fibre says that dietary fibre comes from food – whole grains, legumes, vegetables, fruits and nuts – while functional fibre is isolated fibre with a documented health benefit. The basis for this division is that the epidemiological data describing physiological effects and potential health benefits from fibre were generated from food frequency instruments that measure the fibre content of foods. Whether the same benefits would come from consuming isolated or manufactured fibres is unknown. Certain isolated fibres, such as oat bran and psyllium, are particularly effective in the lowering of serum lipids, but other isolated fibres do not lower serum lipids.

Carbohydrate chemists prefer a chemical, rather than a physiological, definition of fibre, as well as a simple, universally accepted analytical method for dietary fibre to allow compliance and enforcement of fibre labelling laws. As the range of fibres in foods varies greatly, it is difficult to find a simple, universally accepted method to measure fibre.

The botanical categories of fibre are cellulose, hemicellulose, pectic substances, gums, mucilage, algal polysaccharides and lignin. With the exception of lignin (a polyphenol), all fibres are complex polysaccharides. They differ from each other in the sugar residues making up the polysaccharide and in the arrangement of the residues. The principal residues in fibres are glucose, galactose, mannose and certain pentoses. Cellulose is the most widely distributed fibre in the plant kingdom. It is the only truly 'fibrous' fibre. Hemicelluloses include a wide variety of polysaccharides, which contain both pentoses and hexoses. Although these compounds are called hemicellulose, they are chemically unrelated to cellulose. Pectic substances are water-soluble polysaccharides rich in galacturonic acid. Gums are secreted by plants in response to injury, and as such are not part of the plant cell wall. However, gums are classified as dietary fibre because of the way in which mammalian systems use and respond to them. Mucilages are similar to gums in that they are polysaccharides that form viscous solutions. Because of the water-retaining ability of mucilages, they protect seeds from desiccation. Algal polysaccharides are extracted from algae and represent a diverse group of fibres. Lignin, a polyphenolic compound, is found in the woody parts of plants, such as the stem.

Arrangement of the sugar residues in the polysaccharide is often more important to the physiological effect of the fibre than are the residues themselves. Branching and substitutions on the primary carbohydrate chain can have major consequences with respect to physical properties. In addition to the primary structure of fibre, which is determined by the bonds between residues, the molecule's secondary structure also can affect digestibility. For example, the α-1,4 glucose linkage in starch is readily cleaved by mammalian enzymes. However, modification of the same starch molecule to produce a different three-dimensional organization may render it resistant to human digestive enzymes. In other words, the packing or arrangement of the molecule can restrict access of enzymes to the bonds they normally hydrolyse. This is why starch can become 'resistant' to enzymatic hydrolysis and act like dietary fibre. Raw starches, such as raw potato and banana starch, are almost completely resistant to pancreatic amylase and thus reach the colon relatively intact.

The location of fibre components within the plant, and whether or not fibre is extracted from the plant or eaten intact, may have significant physiological consequences. Fibre contained within an intact cell wall must first be disrupted for the physiological effects of the particular fibres to be exerted. Resistance to breakage of the cell wall depends on the structure of the cell wall and its degree of lignification. The number of plant cells per particle ingested (particle size) also may determine the accessibility of the cell wall to digestive enzymes (Slavin, 2003), as may cooking, processing and mastication of the food (Bjorck *et al.*, 1994).

In establishing the dietary recommended intakes, the IOM (2002) recommended an adequate intake (AI) level of 14 g of fibre for each 1000 kcal of energy consumed for all individuals from 1 year of age throughout the remainder of their lives. On the basis of median energy intakes, this equates to 25 g/day for women and 38 g/day for men aged 19 to 50. The AI was set at 21 g/day and 30 g/day, respectively, for women and men aged 51 and older based on lower median energy intakes for older adults. There are no data suggesting that pregnant or lactating women would benefit from increased fibre intake, yet, because energy intakes increase for these two groups, the recommended AIs are 28 g/day and 29 g/day for pregnant and lactating women, respectively.

Recommendations are not provided for infants younger than 1 year of age. An AI was not developed for this age group because milk, which contains no fibre, is the primary recommended food source until 6 months of age, and there are no data on fibre intake in infants until after 1 year of age. On the basis of median energy intakes, the AI for children from 1 to 3 years was set at 19 g/day and for children from 4 to 8 years at 25 g/day. Once children reach 9 years of age, the energy intake between boys and girls differs sufficiently that their AI levels are also different. Therefore, the AI for boys aged 9 to 13 years is 31 g/day, and the AI for boys aged 14 to 18 years is 38 g/day. The AI for girls aged 9 to 18 is 26 g/day.

Americans consume only 15 g of fibre per day, which is far short of the suggested AI levels (Slavin, 2008). However, it is possible to meet the recommended AI levels without drastically altering food choices (IOM, 2002). Often, the limitation that prevents people from meeting these goals is that they do not know which foods provide desirable levels of dietary fibre. Food sources of fibre include whole grain products, legumes, vegetables, and dried fruits. Most common foods consumed contain between 1 and 3 grams of fibre per serving. The major sources of dietary fibre in the American diets are white flour and potatoes, not because they are concentrated fibre sources but because they are widely consumed (Slavin, 2008). Comparing fibre intakes across countries is difficult as national databases for fibre content of foods are not measured by standard methods. Cust *et al.* (2009) compared fibre intakes in the European Prospective Investigation into Cancer and Nutrition (EPIC) study. Total fibre intakes were highest in the UK health-conscious cohort and lowest in Sweden. Bread, fruits and vegetables represented the largest sources of fibre, but food sources varied considerably between countries. Total fibre intakes ranged from 15 g/day to 32 g/day, although most intakes were in the 20–25 g/day range.

3.3 Characterization and digestive impact of fibre

3.3.1 Physiological characterization

Fibres are also categorized by their physiological effects. The primary physiological categories have been soluble versus insoluble. However, more recently fibres have been characterized as being viscous versus non-viscous, or fermentable versus non-fermentable (IOM, 2002). In general, the structural fibres (cellulose, lignin and some hemicelluloses) are insoluble, non-viscous and less fermentable. In contrast, the gel-forming fibres (pectins, gums, mucilages and the remaining hemicelluloses) are soluble, viscous and more fermentable, and these fibres exert effects on digestion and absorption in the upper gastrointestinal tract. Although these generalizations are useful, there are many exceptions to these generalizations. Gum arabic, for example, is a soluble fibre that does not form a viscous solution. Therefore current trends are no longer to characterize fibres based on solubility, but to characterize them based on their functionality, which is more dependent on viscosity and fermentability.

The role that fibre plays within the gastrointestinal tract depends on the fibre's physical and chemical attributes. One of the neurological pathways involved in the feeling of satiety is that of distention or physical fullness. Because fibres are resistant to breakdown in the stomach, the bulk they add to the diet produces a feeling of fullness. Therefore, even though caloric intake may be similar, distention resulting from an increased fibre intake leads to a feeling of satiety. The viscosity of polysaccharides and their ability to form gels in the stomach may slow gastric emptying. Therefore gel-forming fibres further contribute towards a feeling of satiety by maintaining a feeling of fullness for a longer period after a meal (IOM, 2002). In contrast, fibres that do not form gels (such as wheat bran and cellulose) have less effect on the rate at which the meal exits from the stomach.

Polysaccharides that produce a viscous solution can delay and even interfere with the absorption of nutrients such as carbohydrates, lipids and proteins from the small intestine. The reasons for this effect on absorption include delayed gastric emptying, entrapment of nutrients in the gel-like structure, interference with micelle formation, and decreased access of enzymes to the nutrients. Positive benefits of delayed nutrient absorption include an improvement of glucose tolerance and a lowering of serum cholesterol levels. Delayed absorption of carbohydrate results in a lower postprandial glucose level. In general, the more viscous the fibre, the greater the effect on blood glucose, although data on this topic are conflicting (Slavin, 2008). When glucose is absorbed in small amounts over an extended period, as seen with viscous fibres, the insulin response is theoretically attenuated. Because of the flattened glucose curves seen with ingestion of viscous fibres, these fibres are often recommended for diabetics, who typically have lipid profiles that indicate an elevated risk of cardiovascular disease.

Certain viscous fibres lower serum cholesterol, including guar gum, pectin, psyllium, and oat and barley. The mechanism by which fibres lower serum cholesterol is multifactorial. Alternatively, different fibres may work by different mechanisms (Gunness and Gidley, 2010). These hypotheses include the binding of bile acids to fibre, which then interferes with their enterohepatic recirculation. By this hypothesis, more bile acids are excreted in the faeces, requiring additional synthesis of bile acids from cholesterol, thus lowering the body's cholesterol pool. An additional consequence of binding bile acids is that they would be less available for micelle formation, which in turn could interfere with the absorption of cholesterol and triacylglycerols. A different mechanism, which remains controversial, is the production of the short-chain fatty acid propionate from fermentation of fibre in the colon. Propionate is absorbed from the colon, through the portal vein, and has been shown by some investigators to inhibit HMG-CoA reductase 3-hydroxy-3-methyl-glutary-CoA reductase, the rate-limiting enzyme for cholesterol biosynthesis.

Large amounts of dietary fibre may interfere with mineral bioavailability. Because the charged groups on polysaccharides are usually negatively charged, the tendency of dietary fibre is to bind cations such as calcium, magnesium, sodium and potassium. This may limit the absorption of these minerals from the small intestine. This is not generally considered a public health concern, but it may be pertinent in certain cases when individuals have very high-fibre diets and low intakes of minerals such as calcium and magnesium. On the other hand, some data suggest that inulin, a fructo-oligosaccharide, can enhance absorption of calcium in the large intestine due to the lowered pH produced by fermentation (Scholz-Ahrens *et al.*, 2007).

Fibre is metabolized by the colonic microflora in an anaerobic process with the production of short-chain fatty acids, hydrogen, carbon dioxide and biomass. The short-chain fatty acids are the major carbon products of fermentation. Acetate is rapidly absorbed from the colonic lumen into the portal blood and then goes to the liver before entering the general circulation. Acetate is used as an energy source by most non-hepatic tissues in the body. Propionate, like acetate, is also rapidly absorbed and enters the portal vein, by which it is transported to the liver. In contrast to acetate, however, propionate is used by the liver. Some studies show that propionate inhibits HMG-CoA reductase activity. Butyrate is unique in that it is the preferred energy source for colonocytes (epithelial cells lining the colon) (Wong *et al.*, 2006). Colonocytes metabolize butyrate to CO_2, which in part spares the use of glucose.

Different fibres have different bulking properties, depending on their degree of fermentation. Naturally, as a fibre is fermented, it is no longer available to contribute directly to faecal bulk. Fermentation can, however, increase bacterial mass, which will bind water and increase faecal weight. Other factors that affect the colonocytes and are subject to dilution by dietary fibres include bile acids, diacylglycerols, long-chain fatty acids and ammonia. The responses to increased fibre intake may explain the reduction in colon cancer incidence observed in the EPIC study (Bingham *et al.*, 2003).

As a fibre is fermented to short-chain fatty acids, the pH of luminal contents decreases. This is significant because many bacterial reactions are pH-sensitive. For example, the bacterial enzyme responsible for forming secondary bile acids from primary bile acids (7α-dehydroxylase) is inactivated below a pH of 6.5. Colon contents often can reach this pH when fibre is fermented.

3.3.2 Transit time and constipation

Colonic motility is the largest determinant of overall gastrointestinal transit times. Gastric emptying averages between 2 and 5 hours, and small intestinal emptying time averages between 3 and 6 hours, compared with 40 to 70 hours for residue from a particular meal to make its way through the lower portion of the gastrointestinal tract (Hillemeier, 1995). Fibre can delay absorption of some nutrients in the small intestine because of the dilution potential that fibres have, which reduces exposure to and absorption of nutrients by epithelial cells.

Not all fibres are equally effective in speeding gastrointestinal transit time. Dietary fibre has been described as 'normalizing' transit time. Fibres are also effective in binding water and speeding transit and are the active ingredient in many laxative products (Slavin, 2008). Constipation is a persistent condition in which defecation is difficult or infrequent. Most cases of constipation are attributed to unknown causes, and many of these individuals can be treated by increasing hydration, exercise and fibre intake. Approximately 1% of individuals may have intractable constipation, meaning it is not easily managed or cured.

3.3.3 Calorific content of fibre

Because fibres may be fermented to short-chain fatty acids, which can be absorbed from the colon and utilized for metabolism, the concept that dietary fibre contributes no energy is clearly wrong. However, assigning a caloric value to dietary fibre is difficult. The best estimate of energy yield generated by fibre fermentation in humans is between 6.2 and 10.4 kJ/g (1.5 and 2.5 kcal/g) of fibre (IOM, 2002), compared with 16.7 kJ/g (4.0 kcal/g) for starch.

3.4 Dietary fibre (DF) and disease

The incidences of heart disease, colon cancer and obesity in populations consuming a Western-type diet are typically much higher, partly because of lower intake of fibre-rich foods, than are observed in most developing countries. Many difficulties are associated with the study of fibre intake and health, and with interpretation of the results of published studies. The major problem is that of defining what type of fibre is being consumed and then adequately describing how much is being consumed and how much is utilized within the intestinal tract. In addition, it is difficult to separate the effect of a change in dietary fibre from the accompanying changes in nutrient density and nutrient intake that accompany the addition of fibre sources to a diet. A comparison of a high-fibre versus low-fibre diet usually indicates an alteration in the caloric density of the diet and often results in a lower intake of energy sources and other nutrients, unless the bulk quantity of diet consumed is increased. In addition, a high-fibre diet may imply the intake of additional biologically active compounds such as phytochemicals that are not present in the low-fibre diet. Experimental diets should be designed to contain the same amount of all nutrients and non-nutrient compounds other than the fibre sources chosen for comparison. The simplest design involves use of purified fibre sources, but purified fibre sources may not have the same effect as intact food sources. Therefore, much more research must be performed under tightly controlled protocols before the real value of dietary fibre can be fully evaluated.

3.4.1 Dietary fibre and cardiovascular disease

The American Dietetic Association (ADA) published a position paper, which presents the findings of the ADA Evidence Analysis Library systematic review on the health implications of dietary fibre (Slavin, 2008). This review found fair evidence that dietary fibre from whole foods may lower blood pressure, improve serum lipids and reduce inflammation. Other recent studies reported a range of cardiovascular benefits associated with dietary fibre. Flint *et al.* (2009) reported that cereal fibre was associated with reduced blood pressure in adults.

3.4.2 Dietary fibre and type 2 diabetes

The ADA position paper on the health implications of dietary fibre (Slavin, 2008) concluded that limited evidence suggested that 'diets providing 30–50g fibre per day from whole food sources consistently produce lower serum glucose levels compared to a low fibre diet.' Hopping *et al.* (2010) examined the association between dietary fibre and type 2 diabetes in a large multiethnic cohort in Hawaii over a 14-year period. Subjects in the top quintile of grain fibre intake had a 10% reduction in diabetes risk, while diabetes risk was reduced by 22% among men in the highest quintile of vegetable fibre intake.

Effects of isolated fibres on blood glucose and insulin are inconsistent, at best. It is generally accepted that more soluble, viscous fibres are most effective in lowering glucose and insulin response, although many studies find conflicting results (Mathern *et al.*, 2009). Willis *et al.* (2011a) found no relationship between intake of mixed fibres and blood glucose and insulin response. Dietary fibre is often recommended in the treatment of type 2 diabetes, although controversies exist on how to count the carbohydrate content of fibre supplements given to diabetics (Post *et al.*, 2012).

3.4.3 Dietary fibre and bowel health

In developed countries chronic constipation is a common disorder for adults and children. Dietary fibre from whole foods increases stool weight and improves transit time, thereby reducing constipation. The ADA systematic review of the health implications of dietary fibre concluded that there was a lack of data examining the impact of fibre from whole foods on outcomes in gastrointestinal diseases. This may be due to the complexity and cost of these studies (Slavin, 2008).

3.5 Fibre and obesity

There is strong epidemiological support that high fibre intakes are linked to lower body weight and less weight gain over time. Biologically plausible mechanisms exist to help explain why fibre would be linked to lower body weight:

- changes in hormones including glucose, insulin and gut hormones;

- physical effects of fibre in the diet, leading to increased chewing, increased viscosity in the digestive tract and lower palatability;
- gut effects of fibre, including fermentation to short-chain fatty acids and changes in the microbiota.

Despite strong interest in these mechanisms, few published human studies link intake of isolated fibres to biological mechanisms. In general, high amounts of fibre are needed to show physiological changes (often 30 g per dose or more). As all fibres are chemically and physiologically different, no conclusions can be drawn that a given amount or type of fibre will have any effect on body weight, weight maintenance or satiety. As concluded in the Dietary Reference Intakes (DRIs), 'there is no overwhelming evidence that Dietary Fiber has an effect on satiety or weight maintenance, therefore this endpoint is not used to set a recommended intake level.'

Observational studies suggest that fibre intake is inversely associated with body weight (Liu *et al.*, 2003). The strongest data supporting a relationship between fibre and weight maintenance come from epidemiological studies that find dietary fibre intake is lower for obese men and women than for lean men and women. Studies in which human subjects are fed low and high fibre diets suggest that humans tend to eat about 10% fewer calories when high fibre diets are consumed (Howarth *et al.*, 2001). When these studies were conducted, the additional fibres added to foods were not particularly tasty, and therefore perhaps reduced food intake was because of palatability, rather than a physiological mechanism related to fibre.

There are many potential mechanisms for how increased intake of dietary fibre can affect weight maintenance, and no one mechanism is widely accepted. Generally, mechanisms include: a) hormonal, including changes in glucose, insulin and gut hormones; b) physical, including effects on chewing, diet dilution and food form; c) gastrointestinal, such as changes in gut transit, nutrient digestibility, and changes in products of fermentation, including short-chain fatty acids, and microbiota. Thus, each fibre source may affect energy balance via many different mechanisms, and few fibres have been systematically studied for effects on body weight.

Tucker and Thomas (2009) reported that, in a 20-month period, every 1 g increase in total fibre consumed per day decreased body weight by 0.25 kg. Foods high in dietary fibre were measured in this study, and no functional fibre alone was added to the diet. In fact, no functional fibre, whether insoluble, soluble, viscous or fermentable, has been conclusively shown to alter biomarkers of interest in weight management. Du *et al.* (2010) found that total fibre and cereal fibre were inversely associated with subsequent increases in weight and waist circumference. Fruit and vegetable fibre was also inversely associated with waist circumference change, but not with weight change.

Satiation and satiety are controlled by a cascade of factors that begins when a food is consumed and continues as food enters the gastrointestinal tract and is digested and absorbed (Benelam, 2009). As food moves down the digestive tract, signals are sent to the brain, and gut hormones are produced that affect energy balance in a variety of ways, including slowing gastric emptying, acting as neurotransmitters, and reducing gastrointestinal secretions. The terms satiety and satiation are often used differently in the literature, and many methods exist to measure each.

The most common study design for satiety studies uses a test preload in which variables of interest are carefully controlled. Generally subjects rate aspects of their appetite sensations, such as fullness or hunger, at intervals and then, after a predetermined time interval, consume a test meal at which energy intake is measured. Longer-term studies typically provide foods or drinks of known composition to be consumed ad libitum and use measures of energy intake and/or appetite ratings as indicators of satiety. Measurement of satiety is complicated because many internal signals also influence appetite, such body weight, age, sex, habitual diet, exercise and dietary restraint. It is extremely difficult to conduct satiety studies in free-living individuals, so most studies are conducted in a laboratory setting. Usually visual analogue scales are used to monitor hunger, fullness and motivation to eat.

Fibre includes a wide range of compounds and, although fibre generally affects satiety, not all fibres are equally effective in changing satiety (Slavin and Green, 2007). Typically a large dose of fibre is required, such as 10 g or more in a serving of food. Viscous fibres, such as guar gum, oat bran and psyllium, are generally more effective, although insoluble fibres that survive gut transit, such as wheat bran and cellulose, also are known to alter satiety.

Willis *et al.* (2009) compared the satiety response when four different muffins were fed at breakfast. Resistant starch and corn bran had the most positive impact on satiety, whereas polydextrose had little effect and behaved like the low-fibre muffin. Generally, whole foods that naturally contain fibre are satiating. Flood-Obbagy and Rolls (2008) compared the effect of fruit in different forms on energy intake and satiety at a meal. Results showed that eating apple reduced lunch energy intake by 15 per cent compared with control. Fullness ratings differed significantly after preload consumption, with apple being the most satiating, followed by apple sauce, then apple juice, then the control food. The addition of a pectin fibre to the apple juice did not alter satiety.

Other fibres added to drinks do change satiety. Pelkman *et al.* (2007) added low doses of a gelling pectin-alginate fibre to drinks and measured satiety. The drinks were consumed twice a day over 7 days and energy intake at the evening meal was recorded. The 2.8 g dose of pectin alginate caused a decrease of 10 per cent in energy intake at the evening meal. Thus, it generally found that high-fibre foods are more satiating and that certain isolated fibres affect satiety while others are not effective. Clinical studies are needed to assess the effectiveness of isolated fibres on satiety, as there are no measures of fibre chemistry (solubility, structure, etc.) that can predict this effect.

Improved satiety and decreased food intake are common theories used to describe why increased fibre intake may be associated with a lower body weight.

Few studies have evaluated how various doses of the same fibre influence satiety in the same subject population. In each of these studies, the higher fibre dose was more satiating than the low- or no-fibre dose. Mathern *et al.* (2009) studied the effects of 0, 4 and 8 g of viscous fenugreek fibre on a variety of appetite sensations. They found that 8 g of fenugreek mixed into orange juice was significantly more satiating than 0 or 4 g. Similarly, Gustafsson *et al.* (1994) found that portions of carrots containing 6 and 9 g of fibre were significantly more satiating than portions containing 3 g of fibre, when incorporated into a mixed meal.

Studies that use lower doses of fibre generally find no effect on satiety. For example, Mattes (2007) found no difference in satiety when subjects consumed a snack bar with 4 g of mixed fibre and a bar with 1 g of fibre. Similarly, Hlebowicz *et al.* (2007) found no differences in appetite ratings after subjects consumed a control cereal and cereals with 1.5 to 7 g of fibre. Lastly, a third study found snack bars with 4 to 10 g of added fibre had no influence on appetitive sensations compared with a 2 g fibre control (Peters *et al.*, 2009). Collectively, the results of these studies suggest that higher fibre doses may be needed to induce satiety. Willis *et al.* (2010) found that increasing doses of mixed fibre, fed in muffins for breakfast, did not influence short-term satiety. Hess *et al.* (2011) reported that short-chain fructo-oligosaccharides given as 0, 5, or 8 g per dose did not enhance acute satiety or hunger.

Gut hormones are also proposed as important factors for the control of appetite and satiety. Ghrelin has been shown to be positively correlated with hunger, while glucagon-like peptide-1 (GLP-1) and peptide YY3–36 (PYY3–36) are believed to be inversely correlated. There is some evidence, however, that fibre intake may inhibit ghrelin suppression. Compared with low- or no-fibre foods, ghrelin suppression was inhibited following meals containing high doses of psyllium, viscous fibres and wheat fibre. Willis *et al.* (2010) found that ghrelin was higher after the 12 g fibre muffin, while GLP-1 was higher after the fibre-free dose as compared with the fibre treatments.

Juvonen *et al.* (2009) compared high- and low-viscosity beverages with equivalent fibre content and found that the high-viscosity beverage significantly slowed gastric emptying and suppressed GLP-1 release compared with the equivalent low-viscosity beverage. Willis *et al.* (2011b) found that a solid meal with naturally occurring fibre from oatmeal and whole fruits increased gastric emptying time and decreased hunger more than a liquid meal with added resistant maltodextrin fibre. Monsivais *et al.* (2011) reported that soluble fibre dextrin improved short-term energy intake in beverages, while soluble corn fibre, polydextrose and resistant starch did not, when beverages were supplemented with about 12 g of fibre.

3.6 Dietary fibre (DF) and microbiota

Evidence that the intestinal microbiota are linked with overall health is emerging (Davis and Milner, 2009). The adult human gut contains 100 trillion microbial organisms, which are referred to as the microbiota. Although the importance of the microbiota has been accepted for diseases of the large intestine, it is now thought that the microbiota play a role in obesity control and other chronic diseases, ranging to autism. Because of these new ideas, interest in measuring the microbiota in clinical trials is high.

Prebiotics are defined as 'a non-digestible food ingredient that beneficially affects the host by selectively stimulating the growth and/or activity of one or a limited number of bacteria in the colon, and thus improves host health' (De Vrese and Schrezenmeir, 2008). Some oligosaccharides, such as fructo-oligosaccharides and galacto-oligosaccharides, are generally accepted as prebiotics and are often added to infant formula and other food products. All prebiotics are dietary fibres, but not all dietary fibres are prebiotics. Recommended intakes of dietary fibre can provide prebiotics to the diet.

Some of the proposed health benefits of prebiotics include reduction in diarrhoea incidence, improvements in gut health, elimination of allergies and prevention of infections. It is accepted that the gut microflora have a potential role in immune function, but studies showing an improvement in immunity with consumption of either prebiotics or probiotics are limited. Despite the continued interest in enhancing the gut environment, there are no cohort studies in which faecal samples have been collected and higher levels of bifidobacteria or lactobacillus in faeces linked to improved health status.

The effect of prebiotics on immune function, infection and inflammation was reviewed (Lomax and Calder, 2009). Results are mixed in human trials. Ten trials involving infants and children have mostly reported benefits on infectious outcomes, while in 15 adult trials little effect was seen.

3.7 Future trends

Hippocrates wrote in 430 BC that 'wholemeal bread clears out the gut and passes through as excrement,' supporting that physiological benefits of fibre have been long appreciated. Fibre interest peaked in the early 1970s with the publications of Burkitt and colleagues (1974) extolling the virtues of unrefined diets high in fibre and the lack of diseases in rural African populations. These are wonderful stories, but would not pass the rigorous scientific standards of today's evidence-based reviews.

In an evidence-based review, the relationship between dietary fibre and disease receives only moderate and limited support, since many prospective, epidemiologic studies do not find significant relationships between intake of fibre and disease incidence. These studies are limited by low consumption of dietary fibre in most cohorts. Generally grain fibre is more protective than either vegetable or fruit fibre, while intake of legume fibre is too low to determine accurately.

Fibre science is likely to stall out again unless agreement can be reached on definitions for dietary fibre and methods to measure dietary fibre. Isolated fibres vary greatly in chemical composition and physiological effect, and clinical studies are needed to show that these fibres provide some physiological effectiveness.

Current interest in fibre is high, although much interest is focused on vegetarian eating patterns including fruits, vegetables and whole grains. Support for the health benefits of these eating patterns is also quite weak when an evidence-based review is conducted. Additionally, if these foods are found to have protective properties, then it could be the dietary fibre, vitamins, minerals or phytochemicals in plant-based foods that provide the protective benefits.

Dietary fibre does have accepted physiological benefits, especially in the area of bowel health. Although the scientific data may be inconsistent, the booming sales of over-the-counter fibre supplements sold as laxatives supports that many consumers know that dietary fibre aids digestive health and they rely on fibre supplements for regularity.

Public health messages to increase intake of plants high in fibre, whole grains, legumes, vegetables and fruits are appropriate. Despite much talk about the importance of fibre in the diet, intakes of fibre continue to be about half recommended levels. Consumption of fibre as supplements or as an additive in foods or drinks may be necessary if consumers are to reach recommended intakes of fibre.

3.8 Sources of further information and advice

INSTITUTE OF MEDICINE (2001) *Dietary Reference Intakes: Proposed Definition of Dietary Fibre*. National Academy Press, Washington, DC.

INSTITUTE OF MEDICINE (2002) Dietary, functional, and total fibre. In: *Dietary Reference Intakes for Energy, Carbohydrate, Fibre, Fat, Fatty Acids, Cholesterol, Protein, and Amino Acids*. National Academy Press, Washington, DC, pp. 7-1–7-69.

PILCH SM (ed.) (1987) *Physiological Effects and Health Consequences of Dietary Fibre*. Federation of American Societies for Experimental Biology, Bethesda, MD.

3.9 References

BENELAM B (2009) Satiation, satiety and their effects on eating behaviour. *Nutr Bul* **34**: 126–73.

BINGHAM SA, DAY NE, LUBEN R, FERRARI P, SLIMANI N, *et al.* (2003) Dietary fibre in food and protection against colorectal cancer in the European Prospective Investigation into cancer and nutrition (EPIC): an observational study. *Lancet* **361**:1496–501.

BJORCK I, GRANFELDT Y, LILJEBERG H, TOVAR J and ASP NG (1994) Food properties affecting the digestion and absorption of carbohydrates. *Am J Clin Nutr* **59**(Suppl 3):699S–705S.

BURKITT DP, WALKER ARP and PAINTER NS (1974) Dietary fibre and disease. *J Am Med Assoc* **229**:1068–72.

CUST AE, SKILTON MR, VAN BAKEL MME, HALKJAER J, OLSEN A, *et al.* (2009) Total dietary carbohydrate, sugar, starch and fibre intakes in the European prospective Investigation into Cancer and Nutrition. *Eur J Clin Nutr* **63**:537–60.

DAVIS CD and MILNER JA (2009) Gastrointestinal microflora, food components and colon cancer prevention. *J Nutr Biochem* **20**:743–52.

DE VRESE M and SCHREZENMEIR J (2008) Probiotics, prebiotics, and synbiotics. *Adv Biochem Engin/Biotechnol* **111**:1–66.

DU H, VAN DER A DL, BOSHUIZEN HC, FOROUHI NG, WAREMAN NJ, *et al.* (2010) Dietary fibre and subsequent changes in body weight and waist circumference in European men and women. *Am J Clin Nutr* **91**:329–36.

FLINT AJ, HU FB, GLYN RJ, JENSEN MK, FRANZ M, *et al.* (2009) Whole grains and incident hypertension in man. *Am J Clin Nutr* **90**:493–8.

FLOOD-OBBAGY JE and ROLLS BJ (2008) The effect of fruit in different forms on energy intake and satiety at a meal. *Appetite* **52**:416–22.

GUNNESS P and GIDLEY MJ (2010) Mechanisms underlying the cholesterol-lowering properties of soluble dietary fibre polysaccharides. *Food Funct* **1**:149–55.

GUSTAFSSON K, ASP NG, HAGANDER B and NYMAN M (1994) Dose-response effects of boiled carrots and effects of carrots in lactic acid in mixed meals on glycaemic response and satiety. *Eur J Clin Nutr* **48**:386–96.

HESS J, BIRKETT A, THOMAS W and SLAVIN J (2011) Effects of short-chain fructooligosaccharides on satiety responses in healthy men and women. *Appetite* **56**:128–34.

HILLEMEIER C (1995) An overview of the effects of dietary fibre on gastrointestinal transit. *Pediatrics* **96**:997–9.

HLEBOWICZ J, WICKENBERG J, FAHLSTROM R, BJORGELL O, ALMER LO and DARWICHE G (2007) Effect of commercial breakfast fibre cereals compared with corn flakes on postprandial blood glucose, gastric emptying and satiety in healthy subjects: A randomized blinded crossover trial. *Nutr J* **6**:22.

HOPPING BN, ERBER E, GRANDINETTI A, VERHEUS M, KOLONEL LN and MASKARINEC G (2010) Dietary fibre, magnesium, and glycemic load alter risk of type 2 diabetes in a multiethnic cohort in Hawaii. *J Nutr* **140**:68–74.

HOWARTH NC, SALTZMAN E and ROBERTS SB (2001) Dietary fibre and weight regulation. *Nutr Rev* **59**:129–39.

INSTITUTE OF MEDICINE (2001) *Dietary Reference Intakes: Proposed Definition of Dietary Fibre*. National Academy Press, Washington, DC.

INSTITUTE OF MEDICINE (2002) Dietary, functional, and total fibre. In: *Dietary Reference Intakes for Energy, Carbohydrate, Fibre, Fat, Fatty Acids, Cholesterol, Protein, and Amino Acids*. National Academy Press, Washington, DC, pp 7-1–7-69.

JUVONEN KR, PURHONEN AK, SALMENKALLIO-MARTTILA M, LAHTEENMAKI L, LAAKSONEN DE, *et al.* (2009) Viscosity of oat bran-enriched beverages influences gastrointestinal hormonal responses in healthy humans. *J Nutr* **139**:461–6.

LIU S, WILLETT WC, MANSON JE, HU FB, ROSNER B and COLDITZ G (2003) Relation between changes in intakes of dietary fibre and grain products and changes in weight and development of obesity among middle-aged women. *Am J Clin Nutr* **78**:920–7.

LOMAX AR and CALDER PC (2009) Prebiotics, immune function, infection and inflammation: a review of the evidence. *Br J Nutr* **101**:633–8.

MATHERN JR, RAATZ SK, THOMAS W and SLAVIN JL (2009) Effect of fenugreek fibre on satiety, blood glucose and insulin response and energy intake in obese subjects. *Phytother Res* **23**:1543–8.

MATTES RD (2007) Effects of a combination fibre system on appetite and energy intake in overweight humans. *Physiol Behav* **90**:705–11.

MONSIVAIS P, CARTER BE, CHRISTIANSEN M, PERRIQUE MM and DREWNOWSKI A (2011) Soluble fibre dextrin enhances the satiating power of beverages. *Appetite* **56**:9–14.

PELKMAN CI, NAVIA JL, MILLER AE and POHLE RJ (2007) Novel calcium-gelled pectin beverage reduced energy intake in non-reducing overweight and obese women: interaction with dietary restraint status. *Am J Clin Nutr* **86**:1595–602.

PETERS HP, BOERS HM, HADDEMAN E, MELNIKOV SM and QVYJT F (2009) No effect of added beta-glucan or of fructooligosaccharide on appetite or energy intake. *Am J Clin Nutr* **89**:58–63.

POST RE, MAINOUS AG, KING DE and SIMPTON KN (2012) Dietary fibre for the treatment of type 2 diabetes mellitus: a meta-analysis. *J Am Board Fam Med* **25**:16–23.

SCHOLZ-AHRENS KE, ADA P, MARTEN B, WEBER P, TIMM W, *et al.* (2007) Prebiotics, probiotics, and synbiotics affect mineral absorption, bone mineral content, and bone structure. *J Nutr* **137**(3Suppl.2):838S–846S.

SLAVIN J (2003) Why whole grains are protective: biological mechanisms. *Proc Nutr Soc* **62**:129–34.

SLAVIN JL (2008) Position of the American Dietetic Association: Health implications of dietary fibre. *J Am Diet Assoc* **108**:1716–31.

SLAVIN J and GREEN H (2007) Dietary fibre and satiety. *Nutr Bul* 32(Suppl.1):**32**–42.

TUCKER LA and THOMAS KS (2009) Increasing total fibre intake reduces risk of weight and fat gains in women. *J Nutr* **139**:576–81.

WILLIS HJ, ELDRIDGE AL, BEISEIGEL J, THOMAS W and SLAVIN JL (2009) Greater satiety response with resistant starch and corn bran in human subjects. *Nutr Res* **29**:100–5.

WILLIS HJ, THOMAS W, ELDRIDGE AL, HARKNESS L, GREEN H and SLAVIN JL (2010) Increasing doses of fibre do not influence short-term satiety or food intake and are inconsistently linked to gut hormones levels. *Food Nutr Res* **54**:5135. DOI: 10.3402/fnrv54.5135.

WILLIS HJ, THOMAS W, ELDRIDGE AL, HARKNESS L, GREEN H and SLAVIN JL (2011a) Glucose and insulin do not decrease in a dose-dependent manner after increasing doses of mixed fibres are consumed in muffins for breakfast. *Nutr Res* **31**:42–7.

WILLIS HJ, THOMAS W, WILLIS DJ and SLAVIN JL (2011b) Feasibility of measuring gastric emptying time, with a wireless motility device, after subjects consume fibre-matched liquid and solid breakfasts. *Appetite* **57**:38–44.

WONG JM, DE SOUZA R, KENDALL CW, EMAM A and JENKINS DJ (2006) Colonic health: fermentation and short chain fatty acids. *J Clin Gastroenterol* **40**:235–43.

4

Wholegrain foods and health

J. Lappi, H. Mykkänen and M. Kolehmainen, University of Eastern Finland, Finland, and K. Poutanen, VTT Technical Research Centre of Finland, Finland

DOI: 10.1533/9780857095787.1.76

Abstract: Epidemiological evidence shows that consumption of wholegrain foods decreases the risk of chronic diseases such as type 2 diabetes. However, it is unclear whether the beneficial effects are due to whole grains or, in fact, to cereal dietary fibre. Despite the convincing evidence of epidemiological studies, intervention studies do not consistently confirm the benefits of whole grains as compared with refined grains. This may be due to limitations on intervention studies such as study population, control of intervention diet, and outcome measures. Food factors, such as chemical composition and structure of foods, should also be taken into account when considering the health effects of wholegrain foods.

Key words: wholegrain foods, type 2 diabetes, epidemiological, cereal dietary fibre, food factor.

4.1 Introduction

Intake of wholegrain foods, like that of fruit and vegetables, is increasingly recommended as a part of a healthy diet. Dietary Guidelines for Americans 2010 recommend increasing the consumption of whole grain foods and limiting that of refined grain foods (US Department of Agriculture and US Department of Health and Human Services). Refined grains should be replaced with whole grains so that at least half of the grains consumed are whole grains.

In the United States, the first wholegrain health claim was accepted in July 1999 for foods containing 51% or more wholegrain ingredients (Food and Drug Administration (FDA) 1999). According to the health claim, the risk of heart disease and certain cancers may be reduced by diets rich in wholegrain foods and other plant foods and low in total and saturated fat and cholesterol. Wholegrain health claims related to heart disease were later approved in the UK (Joint Health

Claims Initiative (JHCI) 2002) and in Sweden (Swedish code 2003). These health claims on whole grains are based on scientific evidence from epidemiological studies. In autumn 2010, the European Food Safety Authority (EFSA) rejected the wholegrain health claim in Europe, stating that wholegrain foods are not sufficiently characterized and a cause and effect relationship is inadequate to support the health claim (European Food Safety Authority (EFSA) 2010a).

In this chapter, the health effects of wholegrain foods are discussed with the main emphasis on type 2 diabetes. It is not easy to distinguish the effects of whole grains from those of cereal fibre. In addition to convincing epidemiological studies, health effects of wholegrain foods as compared with refined grain foods have been tested in human intervention studies with contradictory results. Possible reasons for the inconsistent results and food factors important for health effects will also be discussed.

4.2 Epidemiological studies

4.2.1 Protective effects of wholegrain foods

Epidemiological studies show that increased consumption of wholegrain foods is associated with decreased risk of type 2 diabetes and metabolic syndrome (Table 4.1), and cardiovascular disease (CVD) outcomes such as coronary heart disease, stroke and fatal CVD (Anderson *et al.* 2000, Mellen *et al.* 2008). Furthermore, increasing the intake of whole grains is associated, although not consistently, with improvement in several risk factors for type 2 diabetes and CVD: total cholesterol (Jensen *et al.* 2006, Newby *et al.* 2007) and low density lipoprotein (LDL)-cholesterol concentration (Newby *et al.* 2007, McKeown *et al.* 2002), homocysteine concentration (Jensen *et al.* 2006, Lutsey *et al.* 2007), insulin sensitivity (Liese *et al.* 2003, Steffen *et al.* 2003), fasting insulin concentration (McKeown *et al.* 2002), C-peptide and leptin concentration (Jensen *et al.* 2006), and 2-hour glucose concentration (Newby *et al.* 2007). Regarding cancer, recent studies have shown a protective effect of whole grains and cereal fibre on the risk of colorectal cancer (Larsson *et al.* 2005, Schatzkin *et al.* 2007) but also opposite results have been reported (Park *et al.* 2005).

A diet including wholegrain foods seems to be associated with a lower risk of being overweight, and can slightly help to reduce weight gain (Williams *et al.* 2008). There is some evidence that whole grains affect fat accumulation in the body: consumption of whole grains lowered the volume of visceral adipose tissue, whereas the volume was increased by consumption of refined grains (McKeown *et al.* 2010).

4.2.2 Whole grains and cereal dietary fibre

Current evidence supports the role of wholegrain foods in the decreased risk of type 2 diabetes. However, based on the epidemiological studies reported, it is not possible to conclude whether the observed effects are due to intake of wholegrain

Table 4.1 Reported consumption of wholegrain foods in epidemiological studies showing a decreased risk of type 2 diabetes or metabolic syndrome

Wholegrain foods	Intake of whole grain foods/d[1]	Method and year of dietary assessment	Results[2]	Reference and country of study
WG breakfast cereal, dark bread, popcorn, cooked oatmeal, wheat germ, brown rice, bran and other grains (e.g. bulgur, kasha, couscous). Breakfast cereals were regarded as WG if the product contained ≥ 25% WG or bran by weight.	0.1 vs. 2.7 (servings)	126-item FFQ 1984, 1986, 1990	RR of T2D: 0.73 (CI 0.63;0.85) p for trend <0.0001	Liu *et al.* 2000 USA
WG breakfast cereal, dark bread, popcorn, cooked oatmeal, wheat germ, brown rice, bran and other grains (e.g. bulgur, kasha, couscous). Breakfast cereals were regarded as WG if the product contained ≥25% WG or bran by weight.	0.1 vs. 2.9 (servings)	127-item FFQ 1986	RR of T2D: 0.79 (CI 0.65;0.96) p for trend 0.0089	Meyer *et al.* 2000 USA
WG breakfast cereal, dark bread, popcorn, cooked oatmeal, wheat germ, brown rice, bran and other grains (e.g. bulgur, kasha, couscous). Breakfast cereals were regarded as WG if the product contained ≥25% WG or bran by weight.	0.4 vs. 3.2 (servings)	131-item FFQ 1986, 1990, 1994	RR of T2D: 0.70 (CI 0.57;0.85) p for trend 0.0006	Fung *et al.* 2002 USA
Only grains included: rye bread, all WG flours and other products (rye, whole wheat, wheat germ, rolled oats, barley, millet, buckwheat) derived from different grain foods, breads prepared from mixtures of WG and refined grains (proportion of WG flour 25–50%).	79 vs. 302 (g)	dietary history interview, once over time 1966–72	RR of T2D: 0.65 (CI 0.36;1.18) p for trend 0.02	Montonen *et al.* 2003 Finland
WG breakfast cereal, dark bread, popcorn, cooked oatmeal, wheat germ, brown rice, bran and other grains (e.g. bulgur, kasha, couscous). Breakfast cereals were regarded as WG if the product contained ≥25% WG or bran by weight.	0.1 vs. 2.9 (servings)	126-item FFQ once over time 1991–5	OR of metabolic syndrome: 0.67 (CI 0.48;0.91) p for trend 0.01	McKeown *et al.* 2004 USA
Dark breads (Sangak, Barbari, Taftoon), barley bread, popcorn, cornflakes (a wholegrain breakfast cereal), wheat germ, bulgur.	6 vs. 229 (g)	FFQ once in 1999–2000	In the lowest and highest quartiles 28% and 21% of subjects, respectively, had metabolic syndrome	Esmaillzadeh *et al.* 2005 Iran

Total number of grain servings was divided into WG servings on the basis of the proportion of WG and refined-grain ingredients in the food.	0.31 vs. 2.9 (servings)	3-d food records, once over time 1981–4	OR of metabolic syndrome: 0.46 (CI 0.27;0.79) *p* for trend 0.005	Sahyoun *et al.* 2006 USA
Dark breads such as wheat, rye, and pumpernickel bread, high fibre, bran, or granola cereals, shredded wheat.	0.03 vs. 1.29 (servings)	68-item FFQ 1995	HR of T2D: 0.69 (CI 0.60;0.79) *p* for trend < 0.0001	Van Dam *et al.* 2006 USA
Whole wheat and wholewheat flour, whole oats and whole oat flour, whole cornmeal and whole corn flour, brown rice and brown rice flour, whole rye and whole rye flour, whole barley, bulgur, buckwheat, popcorn, amaranth, psyllium.	NHS I: 3.7 vs. 31.2 NHS II: 6.2 vs. 39.9 (g of wholegrain ingredients)	NHS I:126-item FFQ 1984, 1986, 1990, 1994, 1998 NHS II: 131-item FFQ 1991, 1995, 1999	RR of T2D: NHS I: 0.75 (CI 0.68;0.83) *p* for trend <0.001 NHS II: 0.86 (CI 0.72;1.02) *p* for trend 0.03	De Munter *et al.* 2007 USA

Notes: WG, whole grain; FFQ, food frequency questionnaire; RR, risk ratio; T2D, type 2 diabetes; CI, confidence interval; OR, odds ratio; HR, hazard ratio; NHS, Nurses' Health Study.

[1] The lowest vs. the highest quintile/quartile.
[2] RR/OR/HR (the highest vs. the lowest intake quintile/quartile) and the 95% confidence interval.

foods or whether it is, in fact, the bran or cereal dietary fibre mediating the effect. Studies concerning cereal fibre also show that increased consumption of cereal based fibre decreases the risk for type 2 diabetes (Table 4.2). In addition, Fung *et al.* (2002) and McKeown *et al.* (2004) report that the significant association of whole grains with type 2 diabetes or metabolic syndrome was largely explained by cereal fibre. Only one study conducted in Australia shows no reduced risk of type 2 diabetes with increased intake of cereal fibre (Hodge *et al.* 2004).

When the dietary data of epidemiological studies were collected in the 1980s and 1990s, no unambiguous definition of whole grains existed. At present, definitions have been agreed for whole grains and wholegrain foods (as discussed by Van der Kamp and Lupton in Chapter 1 of this book). It is unlikely that the subjects in the epidemiological studies consumed wholegrain foods according to the current definition. In seven of the epidemiological studies conducted in the USA regarding type 2 diabetes, metabolic syndrome, or risk factors for type 2 diabetes, a similar food frequency questionnaire (FFQ) was used to assess the intake of wholegrain foods (Jensen *et al.* 2006, McKeown *et al.* 2002, Steffen *et al.* 2003, Fung *et al.* 2002, McKeown *et al.* 2004, Liu *et al.* 2000, Meyer *et al.*

Table 4.2 Reported intakes of cereal fibre in epidemiological studies showing a decreased risk of type 2 diabetes with increasing intake of cereal fibre

Intake of cereal fibre (g/d)[1]	Method and year of dietary assessment	Results[2]	Reference and country of study
2.5 vs. 10.2	131-item FFQ 1986	0.7 (CI 0.51;0.96) *p* for trend = 0.007	Salmerón *et al.* 1997a USA
2.0 vs. 7.5	134-item FFQ 1986	0.72 (CI 0.58;0.9) *p* for trend = 0.001	Salmerón *et al.* 1997b USA
2.66 vs. 9.43	127-item FFQ 1986	0.64 (0.53;0.79) *p* for trend = 0.0001	Meyer *et al.* 2000 USA
Not reported	66-item FFQ, 1987–9	For whites 0.75 (CI 0.60;0.92) *p* for trend = 0.006 For African-Americans 0.86 (CI 0.65;1.15) *p* for trend = 0.525	Stevens *et al.* 2002 USA
0.47–12.0 vs. 24.5–111	Dietary history interview, 1966–72	0.39 (CI 0.20;0.77) *p* for trend = 0.01	Montonen *et al.* 2003 Finland
3.1 vs. 8.8	133-item FFQ 1991, 1995	0.64 (CI 0.48;0.86) *p* for trend = 0.004	Schulze *et al.* 2004 USA
6.6 vs. 16.6	148-item FFQ, 1994–8	0.72 (CI 0.56;0.93) *p* for trend = 0.02	Schulze *et al.* 2007 Germany

Notes: FFQ, food frequency questionnaire; CI, confidence interval.

[1] The lowest vs. the highest quintile/quartile.

[2] Risk ratio with 95% confidence interval; the highest intake quintile/quartile as compared with the lowest.

2000). In these studies, the wholegrain food category included wholegrain breakfast cereal, dark bread, popcorn, cooked oatmeal, wheat germ, brown rice, bran and other grains (e.g. bulgur, kasha, couscous). Breakfast cereals were regarded as wholegrain if the product contained ≥ 25% whole grains or bran by weight. Also the composition of 'dark bread' remained unspecified.

In other USA studies the classification of the wholegrain food group is more strictly defined. Dark bread was defined as whole wheat, rye, pumpernickel or other high-fibre bread (Lutsey *et al.* 2007, Liese *et al.* 2003, van Dam *et al.* 2006). Jensen *et al.* (2006) are the only investigators who left out dark bread because they did not regard it as a wholegrain food. A wholegrain food was also defined according to the proportion of wholegrain ingredients in the product (Sahyoun *et al.* 2006), or the amount of wholegrain ingredients consumed was calculated from the cereal foods consumed (Jensen *et al.* 2006, Newby *et al.* 2007, de Munter *et al.* 2007). Thus, it is of importance to pay attention to how the whole grains are defined in the study reports: reporting the intake of whole grains as ingredients is a more specified way to report wholegrain intake than reporting servings of unspecified wholegrain foods.

In spite of the differences among the studies defining wholegrain foods and calculation of intake, there are statistically significant inverse associations between wholegrain food intake and the risk of type 2 diabetes, metabolic syndrome, or risk factors for type 2 diabetes. The study by Yoo *et al.* (2004) showed no association between wholegrain consumption and features of the metabolic syndrome, probably because the intake of wholegrain foods among young adults (aged 19–38 years) was very low (< 0.5 servings/d). When the intake is reported as wholegrain ingredients, a beneficial health effect is observed with intake of 31–55 g (on average 44 g) of whole grains a day (Jensen *et al.* 2006, Newby *et al.* 2007, de Munter *et al.* 2007). Wholegrain wheat and rye contain 11.6–17.0% and 15.2–20.9% of total fibre, respectively (Vitaglione *et al.* 2008). Hence, the calculated intake of cereal fibre from the average intake of whole grain ingredients is 6–8 g/d. In the USA, decreased risk of type 2 diabetes is reported with a mean daily intake of 9 g of cereal fibre (Table 4.2); an amount that is close to the above calculated intake of fibre from wholegrain foods. Based on these calculations, it can be stated that the cereal fibre is an important mediator of the health effects of wholegrain foods.

4.3 Human interventions

The intervention studies conducted with mainly wholegrain wheat and rye products show varied outcomes, not always supporting the epidemiological data (Table 4.3). In intervention studies, only the changes in risk factors for type 2 diabetes and other chronic diseases can be detected due to the rather short duration of the interventions. Improved insulin sensitivity and decreased fasting insulin concentration (Pereira *et al.* 2002, Rave *et al.* 2007) or improved acute insulin response (Juntunen *et al.* 2003b, Laaksonen *et al.* 2005) have been detected in

Table 4.3 Human interventions on whole grains vs. refined grains

Reference	Subject characteristics	Study design	Whole grain test products, intake/d	Control products, intake/d	Results[2]
Leinonen *et al.* 2000	22 F, 18 M 43 ± 2 y BMI* 26 ± 1 (M); 24 ± 0.5 (F) Healthy, elevated total cholesterol.	Randomized crossover 2 × 4 wk with 4 wk washout period.	Rye bread M: 219 ± 14.6 g F: 163 ± 5.1 g	White wheat bread M: 200 ± 9.6 g F: 152 ± 5.6 g.	No effect on fasting glucose and insulin. Total and LDL cholesterol decreased in men only. No effect on HDL and triacylglycerol.
Pereira *et al.* 2002	6 F, 5 M 25–56 y BMI 30 ± 1 Hyperinsulinaemia.	Randomized crossover 2 × 6 wk with 6–9 wk washout period.	Breakfast cereal (á 30 g), bread (á 30 g), pasta (á 140 g cooked), muffin (á 75 g), cookies (á 25 g), snacks (á 26 g) 6–10 servings. 80% of consumed grains were wheat, remainder oats, rice, corn, barley, rye; grains were ground to flour.	Refined wheat, rice and corn (no bran, germ, little fibre).	Fasting insulin level decreased. Insulin sensitivity improved[3]. Insulin resistance decreased[4].
Juntunen *et al.* 2003b	20 F 59 ± 6 y BMI 28 ± 3 Healthy, elevated total cholesterol. Three subjects with impaired glucose tolerance.	Randomized crossover 2 × 8 wk with 8 wk washout period.	High fibre rye bread (enriched with rye bran). Minimum of 4–5 portions (á 24.1–28.1 g), i.e. ≥ 96–140 g.	White wheat bread ≥ 83–125 g.	Acute insulin response increased[5]. No effect on insulin sensitivity[5]. No effect on fasting glucose and insulin.
McIntosh *et al.* 2003	28 M 40–65 y BMI 30 ± 1 Glucose metabolism not mentioned, no history or presence of GI, renal or hepatic disease.	Randomized crossover 3 × 4 wk.	Rye WG diet: 135 g wholemeal bread, 22 g crispbread, 50 g breakfast cereal. Wheat WG diet: 135 g wholemeal bread, 42 g crispbread, 50 g breakfast cereal. Amount of WG ingredients in a diet was 88 g.	Low fibre foods: white bread (135 g), refined wheat crispbread (42 g), rice cereal (50 g).	No difference in fasting glucose and insulin responses.

Andersson *et al.* 2007	22 F, 8 M 59 ± 5 y BMI 28 ± 2 Healthy with one or more of the following: elevated fasting insulin or glucose concentration, increased triglycerides, reduced HDL cholesterol, borderline hypertension.	Randomized crossover 2 × 6 wk 6–8 wk washout period.	Three portions of bread (á 45g), 2 portions of crispbread (á 12 g), 1 portion of muesli (á 35 g), 1 portion of pasta (á 70 g). Planned intake of WG ingredients was 112 g of which ≥ 90% was consumed by the subjects. Grains (wheat, rye, oat) contained ≥ 50% WG per dry substance, mainly in milled form.	Refined wheat, rye and corn.	No effect on insulin sensitivity,[3] blood glucose, insulin, lipids, FFA, blood pressure, markers of inflammation.
Katcher *et al.* 2008	23 F, 24 M 45 ± 8 y (in WG group), 47 ± 10 y (in refined grain group). BMI 36 ± 4 (in WG group) 36 ± 5 (in refined grain group). Metabolic syndrome[6].	Randomized parallel, 12 wk. Diets were hypocaloric.	Bread and rolls, ready-to-eat cereal, brown rice, oatmeal, pasta, salty snacks and snack bars (WG was listed as the first ingredient on the food label). About 5 servings. One serving was 1 slice of bread, 28 g of ready-to-eat cereal, or 120 ml of cooked cereal/rice/pasta.	Refined grains < 0.2 servings of WG foods/d.	Body weight decreased in both groups. CRP decreased 38% in the WG group, but there was no change in the refined grain group. Decrease in % body fat in the abdominal region was greater in the WG group than in the refined grain group. No effect of WG on fasting and 2-h glucose and insulin concentrations, glucose and insulin AUCs, insulin sensitivity[7].

(*Continued overleaf*.)

Table 4.3 (Continued)

Reference	Subject characteristics	Study design	Whole grain test products, intake/d	Control products, intake/d	Results[2]
Tighe *et al.* 2010	102 F, 104 M 52 ± 1 y BMI 28 ± 0.5 Healthy or features of metabolic syndrome or moderate hypercholesterolaemia. Sedentary or moderately active (< 2 aerobic sessions/wk). Subjects with high habitual intake of WG foods were excluded.	Randomized parallel, 16 wk including 4 wk run-in on refined grain diet.	Group 1: wholewheat foods, 3 servings (70–80 g wholemeal bread and 30–40 g WG cereals). Group 2: wholewheat foods, 1 serving, and oats, 2 servings.	Refined grain foods.	No effect on insulin sensitivity,[8] insulin resistance,[4] fasting glucose and insulin concentrations Decreased systolic blood pressure with whole wheat and whole wheat + oats diets. No effect on triglycerides, HDL, hsCRP, IL-6; total and LDL cholesterol decreased with refined grain diet.
Giacco *et al.* 2010	3 F, 12 M 55 ± 8 y BMI 27 ± 3.0 Healthy (normal glucose and lipid concentrations).	Randomized crossover 2 × 3 wk.	Wholemeal wheat bread, pasta, rusks, crackers. Content of cereal fibre in the diet 23 g.	The same as WG products but in refined form. Content of cereal fibre in the diet 10 g.	No effect on insulin resistance[4] or fasting plasma glucose, insulin, FFA, hs-CRP, blood pressure. Both diets decreased total and LDL cholesterol, but the WG diet slightly more.

Brownlee *et al.* 2010	266 (about 50% F) 46 ± 10 y BMI 30 ± 4 Healthy Subjects with habitual intake of more than 1.5 servings/d of WG foods were excluded.	Randomized parallel, 16 wk (3 treatment groups).	Subjects freely selected from the provided foods: wholewheat bread, Shredded Wheat, Cheerios, porridge oats, brown basmati rice, wholewheat pasta, Weetabix, oat bar, WG crisps. In all products content of WG was > 50 % except rice and pasta. Intake of WG ingredients was 74 ± 28.5 g in one test group and 115 ± 39.6 g in another test group.	Subjects continued their habitual consumption of a low WG diet. Consumption of refined grain foods was not controlled. Intake of WG ingredients was 19 ± 19.9 g.	No effect on insulin sensitivity[8] or on any other measured outcome (such as anthropometry, lipid profile, inflammatory status). Intake of energy and carbohydrates increased in the treatment groups and decreased in the control group.

Notes: á, one serving or portion; AUC, area under curve; BMI, body mass index; CRP, C-reactive protein; F, female; FFA, free fatty acids; GI, glycaemic index; HDL, high density lipoprotein; hsCRP, high sensitive C-reactive protein; IL-6, interleukin-6; LDL, low density lipoprotein; M, male; WG, whole grain; y, years; *kg/m^2.

[1] Completing the intervention.
[2] Refined grain diet as reference.
[3] Measured by euglycaemic hyperinsulinaemic clamp technique.
[4] Measured by HOMA ('homeostatic model assessment').
[5] Measured by FSIGTT ('frequently sampled intravenous glucose tolerance test').
[6] According to National Cholesterol Education Program Adult Treatment Panel III criteria.
[7] Measured by ISI ('insulin sensitivity index') derived from oral glucose tolerance test (Matsuda and DeFronzo 1999).
[8] Measured by modified QUICKI ('quantitative insulin sensitivity check index').

some intervention studies. Furthermore, a few interventions show beneficial effects on total and LDL cholesterol concentrations, blood pressure, percentage of abdominal fat, and C-reactive protein (CRP) with consumption of wholegrain foods (Leinonen *et al.* 2000, Katcher *et al.* 2008, Giacco *et al.* 2010, Tighe *et al.* 2010). However, several studies have not observed effects on glucose and insulin metabolism or other risk factors for chronic diseases among subjects consuming wholegrain foods (Leinonen *et al.* 2000, Katcher *et al.* 2008, Giacco *et al.* 2010, Tighe *et al.* 2010, McIntosh *et al.* 2003, Andersson *et al.* 2007, Brownlee *et al.* 2010).

There are several possible reasons why the results from the intervention studies are not consistent. First, not all the above mentioned intervention studies were conducted to study the effects of wholegrain foods on the risk factors of type 2 diabetes, such as glucose and insulin metabolism. For example, McIntosh *et al.* (2003) aimed to investigate markers of bowel health and no other risk factors for chronic diseases. Second, the technique to measure glucose and insulin metabolism varies among the studies. Fasting glucose and insulin measurements are not sensitive enough to detect subtle changes in active glucose and insulin metabolism, and especially in an everyday life setting when people mostly are in a postprandial state. Thus, more informative measurements are needed.

Among the intervention studies the way of measuring insulin sensitivity or resistance varies. The euglycaemic hyperinsulinaemic clamp technique, frequently sampled intravenous glucose tolerance test (FSIGTT), and insulin sensitivity index (ISI) derived from the oral glucose tolerance test (Matsuda and DeFronzo, 1999) reflect whole body insulin sensitivity after an insulin and/or glucose challenge (Priebe, 2009). Instead, homeostatic model assessment (HOMA) and quantitative insulin sensitivity check index (QUICKI) only measure hepatic insulin sensitivity in the fasting state. Thus, different ways of measuring insulin sensitivity should be taken into account when interpreting the results.

In some intervention studies wheat or rye has been the sole grain used, but in other studies the intervention diet has consisted of both wheat and rye, and oats, in different proportions. Different types of grains should be studied separately since they may have different effects on the responses. For example, when a rye bread-based diet was compared with a wheat and oat bread-based diet, the acute insulin response was improved (Laaksonen *et al.* 2005) and inflammatory markers decreased (Kallio *et al.* 2008) only with rye bread. Furthermore, not only the type of a grain but also the preservation of the botanical structure are important determinants of the physiological effects of grains. Pereira *et al.* (2002) and Andersson *et al.* (2007) mention that the test products used in their studies were mainly based on milled flour, but other researchers have not provided any description of the milling or particle size of the flour used.

Additional factors that should be taken into account when interpreting the results of the intervention studies are health status of the subjects and controlling of the diets. Whether the subjects have been healthy or had features of the metabolic syndrome may affect the results; changes in biochemical responses may be larger and easier to detect in subjects with abnormalities in the metabolism.

Both the intervention and control diets should be carefully designed and their use controlled to limit confounding by other dietary factors than whole grains. For example, Brownlee *et al.* (2010), who observed no effect in any measured outcome, did not monitor the consumption of refined grains in the control group. Moreover, further analyses of their data revealed that on the wholegrain diet the intake of energy and carbohydrates increased from the baseline, which may have compromised the beneficial effects of whole grains.

Characterization of the food/constituent, use of appropriate outcome measures, conditions of use of the product, and representativeness of the target group are also factors considered when EFSA is evaluating the evidence compiled for substantiation of the health claims. In 2010, EFSA provided draft guidance on scientific requirements for health claims related to gut and immune function, including acceptable outcome measures for appropriate disease risk reductions (European Food Safety Authority (EFSA) 2010b). In the near future, EFSA's aim is to provide more detailed information also on other specific topics such as health claims related to blood glucose control. For planning and preparing clinical interventions on whole grains, EFSA's guidance is worth taking into account.

4.4 Food factors important for the health effects of wholegrain foods

Several explanations have been presented in epidemiological studies for the protective effect of whole grains. Common mechanisms suggested are improved insulin sensitivity (Jensen *et al.* 2006, Fung *et al.* 2002, McKeown *et al.* 2004, van Dam *et al.* 2006) and reduced and slow glycaemic response of wholegrain foods (Fung *et al.* 2002, McKeown *et al.* 2004, Liu *et al.* 2000, Meyer *et al.* 2000, Esmaillzadeh *et al.* 2005), which, however, is affected by the particle size of the flour of the grain products. The epidemiological studies do not provide information about the milled or intact form of the grains. Only Meyer *et al.* (2000) mention that the wholegrain products may have consisted mainly of milled grains, that is, wholemeal flour.

Components of whole grains linked to the protective effects, in addition to fibre, are antioxidants or, in general, phytochemicals associated with grain fibre (Jensen *et al.* 2006, Newby *et al.* 2007, Liese *et al.* 2003, Liu *et al.* 2000, van Dam *et al.* 2006, Sahyoun *et al.* 2006, Esmaillzadeh *et al.* 2005). It is also proposed that production of short chain fatty acids (SCFA) from insoluble fibre in the colon would have an effect on hepatic insulin sensitivity or on enhanced glucose oxidation and insulin clearance (Liese *et al.* 2003). Possible protective mechanisms of whole grains, including gut fermentation of indigestible carbohydrates, are reviewed by Slavin (2004). Despite the suggestions in the epidemiological studies, intervention studies have not been able to elucidate the mechanisms underlying the lowered risk of type 2 diabetes by consumption of wholegrain foods.

The intervention studies on wholegrain foods have unfortunately not taken into account chemical composition and structure of whole grains used in the test products. In the following, the significance of these factors is discussed in more detail.

4.4.1 Chemical composition

Wholegrain raw material differs from refined grain ingredients in containing the bran and embryo. In refined grain foods, the outer part of a grain has been removed, substantially lowering the content of fibre. Grain fibre includes a diverse mixture of cell wall carbohydrate polymers. These polymers are located in different cell wall structures forming three bran layers; pericarp, testa and aleurone (Surget and Barron 2005). The outermost layer, pericarp, contains insoluble fibre and bioactive compounds. The testa, between the pericarp and aleurone layers, is rich in alkylresorcinols. Aleurone contains insoluble and soluble fibre, bioactive compounds, vitamins and minerals. The main fibre components in grains are cellulose, arabinoxylans (AX) and β-glucan (Selvendran 1984). β-Glucan is found in high concentrations in barley and oats (Brennan and Cleary 2005, Andersson *et al.* 2008). The main dietary fibre constituent in wheat and rye is AX (Kamal-Eldin *et al.* 2009). Rye also contains high amounts of fructan (Karppinen *et al.* 2003).

The spectrum of bioactive compounds in grains is diverse. For example, the major bioactive compounds in wheat bran are sulfur compounds, minerals and trace elements, polyphenols (mainly phenolic acids), alkylresorcinols, betaine, choline and phytosterols (Fardet 2010). All these compounds chemically associated with fibre are included in the definition of dietary fibre by the Codex Alimentarius Commission (FAO/WHO Codex Alimentarius Commission 2009) and the European Union (European Union 2008). A comprehensive description of these bioactive compounds and their possible health effects was recently reviewed by Fardet (2010) and Okarter and Liu (2010).

Naturally, there is large chemical heterogeneity among different grains due to the type, variety and growing conditions (Kamal-Eldin *et al.* 2009, Gebruers *et al.* 2010, Shewry *et al.* 2010). Furthermore, it is not only the chemical composition of grains but also how the components are organized in the grain structure that is an important contributor for the physiological effects of grain products.

The presence of fibre-associated bioactive compounds probably has an important role in mediating the physiological effects of grain fibre. These compounds have a wide range of structures but the knowledge of their intakes, bioavailability and metabolism in the human body is incomplete (Saura-Calixto 2011).

4.4.2 Structure

Both the molecular and botanical structures of grains and process-induced food structure affect the physiological responses to grain products. As already pointed out, prevalence of intact botanical structure of grains is an important determinant of glycaemic response. Intact or coarsely ground grains increase postprandial glucose concentration less than finely milled flour due to limited accessibility of α-amylase to starch (Fardet *et al.* 2006, Nilsson *et al.* 2008). Starch in rye bread can also be inaccessible to effective digestion in the small intestine due to the swollen starch granules and outleached amylose, which make the structure of rye bread hard (Juntunen *et al.* 2003a).

In addition to the grain and food structure, the structure and chemical composition of cereal fibre have effects on physiological responses. β-Glucans in oats and barley are viscous cereal fibres that form a gel by binding water in the upper gastrointestinal tract (Dikeman and Fahey 2006). The viscosity in the stomach and small intestine beneficially affects glycaemic responses and blood cholesterol concentrations (Dikeman and Fahey 2006, Jenkins *et al.* 2000). The viscosity is affected by molecular weight of the fibre, and thus physiological responses to viscous fibres may be altered by processing conditions that change the molecular weight and viscosity (Dikeman and Fahey 2006).

Grain fibre with the associated bioactive compounds provides various substrates for large intestinal fermentation. Fermentation is dependent on the type and structure of fibre, which in turn determine the physiological and metabolic effects (Guillon *et al.* 2007). Large and complex polysaccharides and their organization in cell walls may provide an advantage over the more rapidly fermented oligosaccharides since their fermentation takes place slowly and is prolonged further along the large intestine (Glitsø *et al.* 1999, Glitsø *et al.* 2000, Crittenden *et al.* 2002, Le Gall *et al.* 2009). Fermentation of grain fibre produces SCFA, such as acetate, propionate and butyrate, which are absorbed from the large intestine (Wong *et al.* 2006). Evidence based on *in vitro* studies suggests that SCFA might have positive effects on peripheral insulin sensitivity (Denise Robertson 2007). In addition, the phenolic compounds released from the grain fibre complex in the large intestine may partly determine the health benefits of wholegrain foods (Vitaglione *et al.* 2008).

4.5 Conclusion and future trends

Epidemiological evidence suggests that intake of wholegrain foods decreases the risk of several chronic diseases such as type 2 diabetes. This hypothesis has led to several clinical intervention studies in which the effect of consuming wholegrain foods versus refined grain foods has been investigated with respect to risk factors for type 2 diabetes. However, intervention studies have thus far not provided consistent evidence of the advantage of wholegrain foods over refined grain foods.

Intake of wholegrain foods has been assessed by self-reported consumption based on food frequency questionnaires or food records when measuring the consumption of wholegrain foods. In future, fasting plasma concentration of alkylresorcinols could be used as a relatively reliable biomarker of consumption of wholegrain wheat and rye in both epidemiological studies and interventions (Aubertin-Leheudre *et al.* 2008, Landberg *et al.* 2009, Ross *et al.* 2009, Montonen *et al.* 2010). Moreover, by measuring the proportion of different alkyl chain lengths in alkylresorcinols, it is also possible to estimate whether the source of whole grain in the diet has mainly been wheat or rye, or both.

In addition to the need for biomarkers reflecting objective intake of wholegrain foods in intervention studies, more detailed information about intake of cereal fibre during an intervention and about the structure of grain ingredients in intervention products is required. The botanical and molecular structure of the grain most probably has a role in determining the health effects of wholegrain foods.

In general, events mediated via the small intestine, such as glycaemic response or cholesterol absorption, have been considered to explain the effects of grain foods and the role of the large intestine has been largely ignored. The demonstrated beneficial effects of whole grains in the large intestine are restricted to the local effects of dietary fibre such as decreased transit time, increased faecal weight, increased faecal frequency or improved faecal consistency (Pereira *et al.* 2002, McIntosh *et al.* 2003, Grasten *et al.* 2000, Li *et al.* 2003, Bird *et al.* 2008). Recently, however, interest has emerged also in the effects of the large intestinal events elsewhere in the body. It has been suggested that the association of cereal fibre intake with decreased risk of type 2 diabetes is mediated via gut (Weickert and Pfeiffer 2008). The mediating mechanisms most probably include large intestinal fermentation derived from gut microbiota. At the moment, multidisciplinary research is going on in fields such as cereal technology, clinical nutrition, microbiology, molecular biology and metabolomics, aiming to explain the role of the large intestine in the development and prevalence of chronic diseases. The multidisciplinary approach also requires multifactorial data analyses to combine dietary, clinical and microbial data.

In the epidemiological studies, those who consumed the highest amount of wholegrain foods weighed less, were more physically active, smoked less, and consumed less alcohol and fat than those with the lowest consumption of wholegrain foods (Fung *et al.* 2002, Liu *et al.* 2000, Meyer *et al.* 2000, van Dam *et al.* 2006, de Munter *et al.* 2007). A recent systematic review and meta-analysis concluded that dietary patterns characterized by high intake of whole grains, fruit and vegetables, fish and poultry, and by decreased intake of red meat, processed foods, sugar-sweetened beverages and starchy foods, decrease the risk of type 2 diabetes (Esposito *et al.* 2010). For the healthful dietary pattern, choosing wholegrain foods instead of refined grain foods is essential. Thus, a wide selection of wholegrain products on the market would help consumers in building up and following a balanced diet.

4.6 References

ANDERSON J W, HANNA T J, PENG X and KRYSCIO R J (2000), 'Whole grain foods and heart disease risk', *Journal of the American College of Nutrition*, **19**, 291S–299S.

ANDERSSON A, TENGBLAD S, KARLSTRÖM B, KAMAL-ELDIN A, LANDBERG R, *et al.* (2007), 'Whole-grain foods do not affect insulin sensitivity or markers of lipid peroxidation and inflammation in healthy, moderately overweight subjects', *Journal of Nutrition*, **137**, 1401–7.

ANDERSSON A A, LAMPI A M, NYSTROM L, PIIRONEN V, LI L, *et al.* (2008), 'Phytochemical and dietary fiber components in barley varieties in the HEALTHGRAIN Diversity Screen', *Journal of Agricultural and Food Chemistry*, **56**, 9767–76.

AUBERTIN-LEHEUDRE M, KOSKELA A, MARJAMAA A and ADLERCREUTZ H (2008), 'Plasma alkylresorcinols and urinary alkylresorcinol metabolites as biomarkers of cereal fiber intake in Finnish women', *Cancer epidemiology, biomarkers & prevention: a publication of the American Association for Cancer Research, cosponsored by the American Society of Preventive Oncology*, **17**, 2244–8.

BIRD A R, VUARAN M S, KING R A, NOAKES M, KEOGH J, *et al.* (2008), 'Wholegrain foods made from a novel high-amylose barley variety (Himalaya 292) improve indices of bowel health in human subjects', *The British Journal of Nutrition*, **99**, 1032–40.

BRENNAN C S and CLEARY L J (2005), 'The potential use of cereal (1→3,1→4)-*β*-d-glucans as functional food ingredients', *Journal of Cereal Science*, **42**, 1–13.

BROWNLEE I A, MOORE C, CHATFIELD M, RICHARDSON D P, ASHBY P, *et al.* (2010), 'Markers of cardiovascular risk are not changed by increased whole-grain intake: the WHOLEheart study, a randomised, controlled dietary intervention', *The British Journal of Nutrition*, **104**, 125–34.

CRITTENDEN R, KARPPINEN S, OJANEN S, TENKANEN M, FAGERSTRÖM R, *et al.* (2002), 'In vitro fermentation of cereal dietary fibre carbohydrates by probiotic and intestinal bacteria', *Journal of the Science of Food and Agriculture*, **82**, 781–9.

DE MUNTER J S, HU F B, SPIEGELMAN D, FRANZ M and VAN DAM R M (2007), 'Whole grain, bran, and germ intake and risk of type 2 diabetes: a prospective cohort study and systematic review', *PLoS Medicine*, **4**, e261.

DENISE ROBERTSON M (2007), 'Metabolic cross talk between the colon and the periphery: implications for insulin sensitivity', *The Proceedings of the Nutrition Society*, **66**, 351–61.

DIKEMAN C L and FAHEY G C (2006), 'Viscosity as related to dietary fiber: a review', *Critical Reviews in Food Science and Nutrition*, **46**, 649–63.

ESMAILLZADEH A, MIRMIRAN P and AZIZI F (2005), 'Whole-grain consumption and the metabolic syndrome: a favorable association in Tehranian adults', *European Journal of Clinical Nutrition*, **59**, 353–62.

ESPOSITO K, KASTORINI C M, PANAGIOTAKOS D B and GIUGLIANO D (2010), 'Prevention of type 2 diabetes by dietary patterns: a systematic review of prospective studies and meta-analysis', *Metabolic Syndrome and Related Disorders*, **8**, 471–6.

EUROPEAN FOOD SAFETY AUTHORITY (EFSA) (2010a), 'Scientific opinion on the substantiation of health claims related to whole grain (ID 831, 832, 833, 1126, 1268, 1269, 1270, 1271, 1431) pursuant to article 13(1) of Regulation (EC) No 1924/2006', *EFSA Journal*, **8**, 1766.

EUROPEAN FOOD SAFETY AUTHORITY (EFSA) (2010b), *Guidance on the scientific requirements for health claims related to gut and immune function*. Available from www.efsa.europa.eu/en/consultations/call/nda100928.pdf (Accessed 23 March 2011).

EUROPEAN UNION (2008), 'Comission directive 2008/100/EC', *Off J EU*, **L285**, 9–12.

FAO/WHO CODEX ALIMENTARIUS COMMISSION (2009), 'Report of the 30th session of the Codex Committee on nutrition and food for special dietary uses', *ALINORM*, 09/32/26.

FARDET A (2010), 'New hypotheses for the health-protective mechanisms of whole-grain cereals: what is beyond fibre?', *Nutrition Research Reviews*, **23**, 65–134.

FARDET A, LEENHARDT F, LIOGER D, SCALBERT A and REMESY C (2006), 'Parameters controlling the glycaemic response to breads', *Nutrition Research Reviews*, **19**, 18–25.

FOOD AND DRUG ADMINISTRATION (FDA) (1999), *Health claim notification for whole grain foods*. Available from http://www.fda.gov/Food/LabelingNutrition/LabelClaims/FDAModernizationActFDAMAClaims/ucm073639.htm (Accessed 29 March 2011).

FUNG T T, HU F B, PEREIRA M A, LIU S, STAMPFER M J, *et al.* (2002), 'Whole-grain intake and the risk of type 2 diabetes: a prospective study in men', *The American Journal of Clinical Nutrition*, **76**, 535–40.

GEBRUERS K, DORNEZ E, BEDO Z, RAKSZEGI M, FRAS A, *et al.* (2010), 'Environment and genotype effects on the content of dietary fiber and its components in wheat in the HEALTHGRAIN diversity screen', *Journal of Agricultural and Food Chemistry*, **58**, 9353–61.

GIACCO R, CLEMENTE G, CIPRIANO D, LUONGO D, VISCOVO D, *et al.* (2010), 'Effects of the regular consumption of wholemeal wheat foods on cardiovascular risk factors in healthy people', *Nutrition, Metabolism, and Cardiovascular Diseases: NMCD*, **20**, 186–94.

GLITSØ L V, GRUPPEN H, SCHOLS H A, HØJSGAARD S, SANDSTRÖM B and BACH KNUDSEN K E (1999), 'Degradation of rye arabinoxylans in the large intestine of pigs', *Journal of the Science of Food and Agriculture*, **79**, 961–9.

GLITSØ LV, JENSEN B B and BACH KNUDSEN K E (2000), 'In vitro fermentation of rye carbohydrates including arabinoxylans of different structure', *Journal of the Science of Food and Agriculture*, **80**, 1211–18.

GRASTEN S M, JUNTUNEN K S, POUTANEN K S, GYLLING H K, MIETTINEN T A and MYKKANEN H M (2000), 'Rye bread improves bowel function and decreases the concentrations of some compounds that are putative colon cancer risk markers in middle-aged women and men', *The Journal of Nutrition*, **130**, 2215–21.

GUILLON F, SAULNIER L, ROBERT P, THIBAULT J F and CHAMP M (2007), 'Chemical structure and function of cell walls through cereal grains and vegetable samples' in SALOVAARA H, GATES F and TENKANEN M, *Dietary fibre components and functions*, Netherlands, Wageningen Academic Publishers, 31–64.

HODGE A M, ENGLISH D R, O'DEA K AND GILES G G (2004), 'Glycemic index and dietary fiber and the risk of type 2 diabetes', *Diabetes Care*, **27**, 2701–6.

JENKINS D J, KENDALL C W, AXELSEN M, AUGUSTIN L S and VUKSAN V (2000), 'Viscous and nonviscous fibres, nonabsorbable and low glycaemic index carbohydrates, blood lipids and coronary heart disease', *Current Opinion in Lipidology*, **11**, 49–56.

JENSEN M K, KOH-BANERJEE P, FRANZ M, SAMPSON L, GRONBAEK M and RIMM E B (2006), 'Whole grains, bran, and germ in relation to homocysteine and markers of glycemic control, lipids, and inflammation 1', *The American Journal of Clinical Nutrition*, **83**, 275–83.

JOINT HEALTH CLAIMS INITIATIVE (JHCI) (2002). *Generic health claim for wholegrain foods and heart health.* Available from http://www.jhci.org.uk/approv/wgrainh.htm (Accessed 4 October 2012).

JUNTUNEN K S, LAAKSONEN D E, AUTIO K, NISKANEN L K, HOLST J J, *et al.* (2003a), 'Structural differences between rye and wheat breads but not total fiber content may explain the lower postprandial insulin response to rye bread', *The American Journal of Clinical Nutrition*, **78**, 957–64.

JUNTUNEN K S, LAAKSONEN D E, POUTANEN K S, NISKANEN L K and MYKKANEN H M (2003b), 'High-fiber rye bread and insulin secretion and sensitivity in healthy postmenopausal women', *The American Journal of Clinical Nutrition*, **77**, 385–91.

KALLIO P, KOLEHMAINEN M, LAAKSONEN D E, PULKKINEN L, ATALAY M, *et al.* (2008), 'Inflammation markers are modulated by responses to diets differing in postprandial insulin responses in individuals with the metabolic syndrome', *The American Journal of Clinical Nutrition*, **87**, 1497–503.

KAMAL-ELDIN A, LAERKE H N, KNUDSEN K E, LAMPI A M, PIIRONEN V, *et al.* (2009), 'Physical, microscopic and chemical characterisation of industrial rye and wheat brans from the Nordic countries', *Food and Nutrition Research*, **53**, 10.3402/fnr.v53i0.1912.

KARPPINEN S, MYLLYMÄKI O, FORSSELL P and POUTANEN K (2003), 'Fructan content of rye and rye products', *Cereal Chemistry*, **80**, 168–71.

KATCHER H I, LEGRO R S, KUNSELMAN A R, GILLIES P J, DEMERS L M, *et al.* (2008), 'The effects of a whole grain-enriched hypocaloric diet on cardiovascular disease risk factors in men and women with metabolic syndrome', *The American Journal of Clinical Nutrition*, **87**, 79–90.

LAAKSONEN D E, TOPPINEN L K, JUNTUNEN K S, AUTIO K, LIUKKONEN K H, *et al.* (2005), 'Dietary carbohydrate modification enhances insulin secretion in persons with the metabolic syndrome', *The American Journal of Clinical Nutrition*, **82**, 1218–27.

LANDBERG R, KAMAL-ELDIN A, ANDERSSON S O, JOHANSSON J E, ZHANG J X, *et al.* (2009), 'Reproducibility of plasma alkylresorcinols during a 6-week rye intervention study in men with prostate cancer', *The Journal of Nutrition*, **139**, 975–80.

LARSSON S C, GIOVANNUCCI E, BERGKVIST L and WOLK A (2005), 'Whole grain consumption and risk of colorectal cancer: a population-based cohort of 60,000 women', *British Journal of Cancer*, **92**, 1803–7.

LE GALL M, SERENA A, JORGENSEN H, THEIL P K and BACH KNUDSEN K E (2009), 'The role of whole-wheat grain and wheat and rye ingredients on the digestion and fermentation processes in the gut–a model experiment with pigs', *The British Journal of Nutrition*, **102**, 1590–600.

LEINONEN K S, POUTANEN K S and MYKKÄNEN H M (2000), 'Rye bread decreases serum total and LDL cholesterol in men with moderately elevated serum cholesterol', *Journal of Nutrition*, **130**, 164–70.

LI J, KANEKO T, QIN L Q, WANG J AND WANG Y (2003), 'Effects of barley intake on glucose tolerance, lipid metabolism, and bowel function in women', *Nutrition (Burbank, Los Angeles County, Calif.)*, **19**, 926–9.

LIESE A D, ROACH A K, SPARKS K C, MARQUART L, D'AGOSTINO R B JR AND MAYER-DAVIS E J (2003), 'Whole-grain intake and insulin sensitivity: the Insulin Resistance Atherosclerosis Study', *The American Journal of Clinical Nutrition*, **78**, 965–71.

LIU S, MANSON J E, STAMPFER M J, HU F B, GIOVANNUCCI E, *et al.* (2000), 'A prospective study of whole-grain intake and risk of type 2 diabetes mellitus in US women', *American Journal of Public Health*, **90**, 1409–15.

LUTSEY P L, JACOBS D R JR, KORI S, MAYER-DAVIS E, SHEA S, *et al.* (2007), 'Whole grain intake and its cross-sectional association with obesity, insulin resistance, inflammation, diabetes and subclinical CVD: The MESA Study', *The British Journal of Nutrition*, **98**, 397–405.

MATSUDA M and DEFRONZO R A (1999), 'Insulin sensitivity indices obtained from oral glucose tolerance testing: comparison with the euglycemic insulin clamp', *Diabetes Care*, **22**, 1462–70.

MCINTOSH G H, NOAKES M, ROYLE P J and FOSTER P R (2003), 'Whole-grain rye and wheat foods and markers of bowel health in overweight middle-aged men', *The American Journal of Clinical Nutrition*, **77**, 967–74.

MCKEOWN N M, MEIGS J B, LIU S, WILSON P W and JACQUES P F (2002), 'Whole-grain intake is favorably associated with metabolic risk factors for type 2 diabetes and cardiovascular disease in the Framingham Offspring Study', *The American Journal of Clinical Nutrition*, **76**, 390–8.

MCKEOWN N M, MEIGS J B, LIU S, SALTZMAN E, WILSON P W and JACQUES P F (2004), 'Carbohydrate nutrition, insulin resistance, and the prevalence of the metabolic syndrome in the Framingham Offspring Cohort', *Diabetes Care*, **27**, 538–46.

MCKEOWN N M, TROY L M, JACQUES P F, HOFFMANN U, O'DONNELL C J and FOX C S (2010), 'Whole- and refined-grain intakes are differentially associated with abdominal visceral and subcutaneous adiposity in healthy adults: the Framingham Heart Study', *The American Journal of Clinical Nutrition*, **92**, 1165–71.

MELLEN P B, WALSH T F and HERRINGTON D M (2008), 'Whole grain intake and cardiovascular disease: a meta-analysis', *Nutrition, Metabolism, and Cardiovascular Diseases: NMCD*, **18**, 283–90.

MEYER K A, KUSHI L H, JACOBS D R JR, SLAVIN J, SELLERS T A and FOLSOM A R (2000), 'Carbohydrates, dietary fiber, and incident type 2 diabetes in older women', *The American Journal of Clinical Nutrition*, **71**, 921–30.

MONTONEN J, KNEKT P, JÄRVINEN R, AROMAA A and REUNANEN A (2003), 'Whole-grain and fiber intake and the incidence of type 2 diabetes', *The American Journal of Clinical Nutrition*, **77**, 622–9.

MONTONEN J, LANDBERG R, KAMAL-ELDIN A, AMAN P, KNUEPPEL S, *et al.* (2010), 'Reliability of fasting plasma alkylresorcinol concentrations measured 4 months apart', *European Journal of Clinical Nutrition*, **64**, 698–703.

NEWBY P K, MARAS J, BAKUN P, MULLER D, FERRUCCI L and TUCKER K L (2007), 'Intake of whole grains, refined grains, and cereal fiber measured with 7-d diet records and associations with risk factors for chronic disease', *The American Journal of Clinical Nutrition*, **86**, 1745–53.

NILSSON A C, OSTMAN E M, GRANFELDT Y and BJÖRCK I M (2008), 'Effect of cereal test breakfasts differing in glycemic index and content of indigestible carbohydrates on daylong glucose tolerance in healthy subjects', *American Journal of Clinical Nutrition*, **87**, 645.

OKARTER N and LIU R H (2010), 'Health benefits of whole grain phytochemicals', *Critical Reviews in Food Science and Nutrition*, **50**, 193–208.

PARK Y, HUNTER D J, SPIEGELMAN D, BERGKVIST L, BERRINO F, *et al.* (2005), 'Dietary fiber intake and risk of colorectal cancer: a pooled analysis of prospective cohort studies', *JAMA: the journal of the American Medical Association*, **294**, 2849–57.

PEREIRA M A, JACOBS D R JR, PINS J J, RAATZ S K, GROSS M D, *et al.* (2002), 'Effect of whole grains on insulin sensitivity in overweight hyperinsulinemic adults', *The American Journal of Clinical Nutrition*, **75**, 848–55.

PRIEBE M G (2009), *Whole grain foods and the prevention of type 2 diabetes mellitus*, Netherlands, University of Groningen.

RAVE K, ROGGEN K, DELLWEG S, HEISE T and TOM DIECK H (2007), 'Improvement of insulin resistance after diet with a whole-grain based dietary product: results of a randomized, controlled cross-over study in obese subjects with elevated fasting blood glucose', *British Journal of Nutrition*, **98**, 929–36.

ROSS A B, PINEAU N, KOCHHAR S, BOURGEOIS A, BEAUMONT M and DECARLI B (2009), 'Validation of a FFQ for estimating whole-grain cereal food intake', *The British Journal of Nutrition*, **102**, 1547–51.

SAHYOUN N R, JACQUES P F, ZHANG X L, JUAN W and MCKEOWN N M (2006), 'Whole-grain intake is inversely associated with the metabolic syndrome and mortality in older adults', *American Journal of Clinical Nutrition*, **83**, 124–31.

SALMERÓN J, ASCHERIO A, RIMM E B, COLDITZ G A, SPIEGELMAN D, *et al.* (1997a), 'Dietary fiber, glycemic load, and risk of NIDDM in men', *Diabetes Care*, **20**, 545–50.

SALMERÓN J, MANSON J E, STAMPFER M J, COLDITZ G A, WING A L and WILLETT W C (1997b), 'Dietary fiber, glycemic load, and risk of non-insulin-dependent diabetes mellitus in women', *Journal of the American Medical Association*, **277**, 472–7.

SAURA-CALIXTO F (2011), 'Dietary fiber as a carrier of dietary antioxidants: an essential physiological function', *Journal of Agricultural and Food Chemistry*, **59**, 43–9.

SCHATZKIN A, MOUW T, PARK Y, SUBAR A F, KIPNIS V, *et al.* (2007), 'Dietary fiber and whole-grain consumption in relation to colorectal cancer in the NIH-AARP Diet and Health Study', *The American Journal of Clinical Nutrition*, **85**, 1353–60.

SCHULZE M B, LIU S, RIMM E B, MANSON J E, WILLETT W C and HU F B (2004), 'Glycemic index, glycemic load, and dietary fiber intake and incidence of type 2 diabetes in younger and middle-aged women', *American Journal of Clinical Nutrition*, **80**, 348–56.

SCHULZE M B, SCHULZ M, HEIDEMANN C, SCHIENKIEWITZ A, HOFFMANN K and BOEING H (2007), 'Fiber and magnesium intake and incidence of type 2 diabetes: a prospective study and meta-analysis', *Archives of Internal Medicine*, **167**, 956–65.

SELVENDRAN R R (1984), 'The plant cell wall as a source of dietary fiber: chemistry and structure', *The American Journal of Clinical Nutrition*, **39**, 320–37.

SHEWRY P R, PIIRONEN V, LAMPI A M, EDELMANN M, KARILUOTO S, *et al.* (2010), 'Effects of genotype and environment on the content and composition of phytochemicals and dietary fiber components in rye in the HEALTHGRAIN diversity screen', *Journal of Agricultural and Food Chemistry*, **58**, 9372–83.

SLAVIN J (2004), 'Whole grains and human health', *Nutrition Research Reviews*, **17**, 99–110.

STEFFEN L M, JACOBS D R JR, MURTAUGH M A, MORAN A, STEINBERGER J, *et al.* (2003), 'Whole grain intake is associated with lower body mass and greater insulin sensitivity among adolescents', *American Journal of Epidemiology*, **158**, 243–50.

STEVENS J, AHN K, JUHAERI J, HOUSTON D, STEFFAN L and COUPER D (2002), 'Dietary fiber intake and glycemic index and incidence of diabetes in African-American and white adults: the ARIC study', *Diabetes Care*, **25**, 1715–21.

SURGET A and BARRON C (2005), 'Histologie du grain de blé', *Industrie des Céréales*, **145**, 3–7.

Swedish code (2003), 'Health claims', available at http://www.healthgrain.eu/php/chapter-seven.php#UK (Accessed 4 October 2012).

TIGHE P, DUTHIE G, VAUGHAN N, BRITTENDEN J, SIMPSON W G, *et al.* (2010), 'Effect of increased consumption of whole-grain foods on blood pressure and other cardiovascular risk markers in healthy middle-aged persons: a randomized controlled trial', *The American Journal of Clinical Nutrition*, **92**, 733–40.

US DEPARTMENT OF AGRICULTURE AND US DEPARTMENT OF HEALTH AND HUMAN SERVICES (2010), 'Dietary Guidelines for Americans 2010', 7th Edition, Washington, DC: US Government Printing Office, December 2010.

VAN DAM R M, HU F B, ROSENBERG L, KRISHNAN S and PALMER J R (2006), 'Dietary calcium and magnesium, major food sources, and risk of type 2 diabetes in U.S. black women', *Diabetes Care*, **29**, 2238–43.

VITAGLIONE P, NAPOLITANO A and FOGLIANO V (2008), 'Cereal dietary fibre: a natural functional ingredient to deliver phenolic compounds into the gut', *Trends in Food Science and Technology*, **19**, 451–63.

WEICKERT M O and PFEIFFER A F (2008), 'Metabolic effects of dietary fiber consumption and prevention of diabetes', *The Journal of Nutrition*, **138**, 439–42.

WILLIAMS P G, GRAFENAUER S J and O'SHEA J E (2008), 'Cereal grains, legumes, and weight management: a comprehensive review of the scientific evidence', *Nutrition Reviews*, **66**, 171–82.

WONG J M, DE SOUZA R, KENDALL C W, EMAM A and JENKINS D J (2006), 'Colonic health: fermentation and short chain fatty acids', *Journal of Clinical Gastroenterology*, **40**, 235–43.

YOO S, NICKLAS T, BARANOWSKI T, ZAKERI I F, YANG S J, *et al.* (2004), 'Comparison of dietary intakes associated with metabolic syndrome risk factors in young adults: the Bogalusa Heart Study', *The American Journal of Clinical Nutrition*, **80**, 841–8.

5

The range of dietary fibre ingredients and a comparison of their technical functionality

S.W. Cui, Y. Wu and H. Ding, Agriculture and Agri-food Canada, Canada

DOI: 10.1533/9780857095787.1.96

Abstract: This chapter describes the evolving definition of dietary fibres and their technical functionalities when applied in various food products. Dietary fibres can be categorized into three groups, insoluble dietary fibre, soluble dietary fibre and resistant starch. Soluble dietary fibre has been widely used as thickener, emulsifier, stabiliser, fat replacer, suspending and gelling agents, etc. in food and pharmaceutical industry. For each dietary fibre ingredient, the chemical composition, physical and functional properties, and common applications are described in the chapter. Dietary fibres are becoming one of the most important food ingredients for their irreplaceable roles of techno-functional as well as biofunctional purposes in food products. The future trends and challenges of dietary fibre applications are also discussed.

Key words: dietary fibre, food ingredients, thickener, emulsifier, stabiliser, fat replacer, suspending agent, gelling agent, technical functionality, biofunctionality.

5.1 Introduction

The latest version of the definition of dietary fibre was approved by the Codex Alimentarius Commission during the 32nd Session at FAO Headquarters, Rome, 29 June to July 2009 (ALINORM 09/32/A):

> Dietary Fibre means carbohydrate polymers with ten or more monomeric units, which are not hydrolysed by the endogenous enzymes in the small intestine of humans and belong to the following categories:
>
> Edible carbohydrate polymers naturally occurring in the food as consumed;
>
> Carbohydrate polymers, which have been obtained from food raw material by physical, enzymatic or chemical means and which have been shown to have a

physiological effect of benefit to health as demonstrated by general accepted scientific evidence to competent authorities;

Synthetic carbohydrate polymers which have been shown to have a physical effect of benefit to health as demonstrated by general accepted scientific evidence to competent authorities.

When derived from a plant origin, dietary fibre may include fractions of lignin and/or other compounds when associated with polysaccharides in the plant cell walls and if these compounds are quantified by the AOAC gravimetric analytical methods for dietary fibre analysis: fractions of lignin and the other compounds (proteic fractions, phenolic compounds, waxes, saponins, phytates, cutin, phytosterols, etc.) intimately 'associated' with plant polysaccharides in the AOAC 991.43 method.

Decision on whether to include carbohydrates of 3 to 9 monomeric units should be left to national authorities.

The concept of dietary fibre is broad, and many ingredients routinely applied in food chains belong to the category of dietary fibre. These ingredients are widely applied in various kinds of food products.

In this chapter, commonly used ingredients serving as dietary fibre will be described. The dietary fibre ingredients will be categorized into three groups: insoluble dietary fibre, soluble dietary fibre and resistant starch. It is worth noting that some dietary fibres are pure polysaccharides or oligosaccharides, whereas many dietary fibres also contain other compounds (proteic fractions, phenolic compounds, waxes, etc.) after extraction from plant origin. Those compounds are also included in the definition of dietary fibres if they are intimately associated and may exert extra beneficial physiological effects (Phillips and Cui, 2011).

For each dietary fibre ingredient, four areas will be covered in the description: first, chemical composition, including monosaccharide units, linkage pattern and chemical structure; second, physical properties such as appearance as an ingredient, viscosity and/or gelling property, concentration dependency, and interactions with other food components; third, functional properties under various environmental and processing conditions; and, finally, its common applications in food products.

5.2 Technical functionalities of dietary fibre ingredients

This section describes the technical functionalities of dietary fibre ingredients, including hydration and water-holding capacity, viscosity, gel-forming property, emulsification property, fat replacement property, and interaction with other components. These technical functionalities or techno-functional properties are highly influenced by the physicochemical properties of dietary fibres, such as particle size, porosity, molecular weight, and conformation in aqueous solution.

5.2.1 Hydration and water-holding capacity

Hydration is a process wherein the fibres in contact with water start absorbing water molecules due to the hydrophilic nature of dietary fibre. Hydration properties of dietary fibres are related to the chemical structure of the component polysaccharides, and other factors such as porosity, particle size, ionic form (if charged), pH, temperature, ionic strength, type of ions in solution and stresses upon the fibre ingredient (Doublier and Wood, 1995; Elleuch *et al.*, 2011). Water-holding capacity is a measure of the amount of water that can be absorbed, fixed or held by the ingredient after equilibrium of hydration (Cui and Roberts, 2009). The particle size, chemical composition, and structure of dietary fibre influence the water-holding capacity. The water-holding capacity of soluble polysaccharides is usually higher than that of insoluble ones.

Most raw materials containing cereal fibres are ground for better acceptance of the final product, and this process can affect hydration properties. For example, the swelling and water-binding capacity of pea hull fibres was decreased while the water-holding capacity was slightly increased through grinding (Ralet *et al.*, 1993). The kinetics of water uptake was also different: the ground product hydrated instantaneously; in contrast, the unground product reached equilibrium after 30 minutes; this was believed to be related to the differences in their surface area (Ralet *et al.*, 1993). Hydration properties can be changed by processing and heat treatment. For example, for wheat bran- and apple fibre-based products, boiling slightly increased the water-binding capacity, while steam-cooking and roasting showed no significant effects; the kinetics of water uptake was also different for various products (Caprez *et al.*, 1986).

5.2.2 Viscosity

Viscosity is caused by the entanglement of polysaccharide chains in aqueous solution, which creates friction for the flow of liquid. Viscosity is defined as the ratio of shear stress to shear rate, and depends largely on molecular weight, structure and conformation of the polymers in a solution (Wang and Cui, 2005). Polysaccharides contain a large number of hydroxyl groups, oxygen atoms and other groups that may interact with water molecules, mainly through hydrogen bonding. The mobility of water, and even the formation and growth of ice crystals, can be controlled by those interactions, thus exerting significant impacts on the textural and consumer acceptance of foods. Conformation in solution determines the ability to give viscosity. At the same molecular weight, a rigid 'rod-like' conformation such as that of xanthan can give high viscosity at a low concentration, while a random coil-like or globular structure will give low viscosity because the molecules occupy less volume in the solution.

5.2.3 Gel-forming capacity

After mixing with liquid, some dietary fibres can form a gel. The gel-forming capacity and the extent of thickening are affected by the chemical composition, concentration, ionic type and strength, pH, temperature, and so on (Wang and Cui, 2005). The polymer chains are cross-linked via covalent or non-covalent bonds so as to form a three-dimensional polymer network, among which intermolecular interactions, including hydrogen bonding, ionic bonding, hydrophobic interactions and van der Waals attraction, may contribute to the gelation of polysaccharides. Gelling behaviour varies with the type of polysaccharide (Cui and Roberts, 2009).

5.2.4 Emulsification properties

Although polysaccharides are not conventionally used as surface active components due to their hydrophilic properties, they are widely added to emulsions to stabilize the system. One important reason is that polysaccharides can act as thickeners to slow down droplet flocculation and/or creaming. When the concentration is high enough, polysaccharides can form a three-dimensional network through intermolecular entanglements to entrap the oil droplets and effectively inhibit their movement, thus prolonging the stability of the emulsion system (Wang and Cui, 2005; Dickinson, 2009). Several polysaccharides may exhibit surface activity due to possessing hydrophobic groups or containing a certain amount of protein which is difficult to separate. For polysaccharides with surface activities, the addition of polysaccharides to emulsions can reduce the surface tension; a further increase in concentration can result in increased viscosity of the aqueous phase, thus stabilizing the emulsion system.

5.2.5 Fat replacement properties

Some dietary fibres can be used as fat replacers in food due to their excellent water management properties. When fat is removed from food products, additional water will be added to replace it. Some dietary fibres play key roles in controlling this extra added water to prevent change of the original texture. Researchers have focused on the use of soluble dietary fibres in dairy and bakery products, such as the use of inulin, gellan, guar gum or resistant starch in cheese, yogurt, muffin and sausage (Zahn *et al.*, 2010; Ozboy-Ozbas *et al.*, 2010). To retain juiciness and keep the original texture without negative impacts on flavour are the most important characteristics when incorporating dietary fibres as fat replacers into novel healthy food products (Brewer, 2012).

5.2.6 Interaction with other components

Polysaccharides can interact with other food components and lead to enhanced functional properties or adverse effects on nutrient availability. Some of the interactions are exploited in food products. Polysaccharide/protein interactions are used in emulsion systems to give improved emulsification properties. Synergistic interactions between different polysaccharides, such as xanthan/galactoglucomannan, xanthan/carrageenan and xanthan/konjac glucoglucomannan, are also well recognized and used in products (Wang and Cui, 2005; Agoub *et al.*, 2007). Some polysaccharides can bind polar molecules and ions, leading to reduced availability of those molecules (Cui and Roberts, 2009).

5.3 Insoluble dietary fibre ingredients

5.3.1 Cellulose and lignin

Cellulose is the main constituent of plant cell walls, and exists abundantly in vegetables, fruits, cereals and legumes. It coexists with hemicellulose, pectin and lignin. Lignin is not a carbohydrate but a highly cross-linked, complex three-dimensional structure based on phenylpropane units. Since lignin is intimately associated with non-starch polysaccharides (e.g. covalently linked to hemicellulose), it is usually considered as part of insoluble dietary fibre (Phillips and Cui, 2011). Cellulose is composed of β-1,4-linked D-glucose with a variable degree of polymerization (DP) ranging from 1000 to 14 000 and a molecular weight of 162 to 2268 kDa (Cui *et al.*, 2011). Crystalline structures of cellulose can be formed via hydrogen bonding along the chains of glucose, and the crystalline microfibril structure does not dissolve in hot water.

A variety of modified celluloses have been approved as food additives (Murray, 2009). Currently, modified celluloses for food use are limited to hydroxypropyl cellulose, hydroxypropyl methylcellulose, methylcellulose, methylethylcellulose, sodium carboxymethyl-cellulose or their mixtures. They were derived from cellulose pulp (wood pulp or cotton linters) by chemical modification. The preparation procedures are outlined as follows: (1) cellulose pulp is first dispersed in alkali solution to form alkali cellulose; (2) the alkali cellulose is treated with specific reagents (chloromethane, propylene oxide, and/or monochloracetic acid) to substitute the hydroxyl groups to anhydroglucose (β-glucopyranose) units; (3) the substitution reaction is followed by purification and washing to remove by-products and to increase the purity for food application (Izydorczyk *et al.*, 2005). The substitution group, the degree of substitution and the average chain length or DP of the cellulose molecules are the three main factors influencing the properties of modified cellulose. Solutions of modified cellulose are neutral-flavoured, odourless and colourless.

5.3.2 Oat bran

Oat bran can be collected from outer layers of the oat groats. The content of total dietary fibre in oat bran varies from 12 to 24% depending on the cultivar variety, growing location, weather conditions and fertilization (Mälkki and Virtanen, 2001). About half of the total dietary fibre in oat bran is soluble and the other half is insoluble. β-Glucan is the main component of the soluble fibre. The insoluble fibres are mainly cellulose, lignin and some associated hemicelluloses. The insoluble oat fibres act as ideal bulking agents with water hydration capacity from 4.1 to 12.7 (g/g dry substance) (Mälkki, 2001). They can be used as the carrier of minor components associated with fibre, absorbents of various flavour components, and fat replacers in ground beef and pork sausage products (Verma and Banerjee, 2010).

5.3.3 Wheat bran

Wheat bran is a by-product of the milling process of wheat. It usually contains 14–19% of total grain weight. As a rich source of dietary fibre, wheat bran contains

46% of non-starch polysaccharides, including arabinoxylan (70%), cellulose (24%) and beta-glucan (6%), and it also contains minor amounts of glucoglucomannan and arabinogalactan (Carre and Brillouet, 1986; Bertrand *et al.*, 1981).

Depending on composition and particle size, wheat bran fractions may have negative effects on product quality, such as textural properties and loaf volume for bread. Reducing the particle size of wheat bran can influence product quality by increasing interaction surface and releasing reactive intracellular components (Noort *et al.*, 2010).

5.3.4 Legume fibre

Legumes are a rich source of dietary fibre. Legume fibres can be divided into 'inner' and 'outer' fibres. 'Inner' fibres are cotyledon fibres consisting of cell wall polysaccharides with varying degrees of solubility. 'Outer' fibres are from seed coat (hull) containing mainly water-insoluble polysaccharides and some pectin (Brooks *et al.*, 2008). The chemical composition of dietary fibre in legumes varies with the raw material. Fibre fractions can be extracted by various methods such as grinding, milling, sieving or using wet process according to the solubility of fractions in water or ethanol (Tosh and Yada, 2010). Cellulose, xyloglucans, arabinose-rich pectins, and some oligosaccharides are the major components in the fibre fraction. Legume fibres have good water-binding and oil-binding capacities and can therefore be used as fat replacers in bakery products.

5.3.5 Chitin and chitosan

Chitin is the main component of the exoskeleton of insects and shells of crustaceans, for example shrimp, lobster and crab. It is also a structural polysaccharide widely distributed in fungi, yeasts and algae (Muzzarelli, 2009). Chitin is insoluble in water. The structure is similar to cellulose except that the hydroxyl groups at O-2 of the β-D-Glc*p* are substituted with *N*-acetylamino groups. Chitin forms a highly ordered crystalline structure by intermolecular hydrogen bonds, and its isolates are different from each other in many respects (e.g. degree of acetylation, nitrogen content, molecular size and polydispersity). When treated with strong alkali, the *N*-acetal groups of chitin are substituted by amino groups, thereby forming the water-soluble polysaccharide chitosan. The linkage of chitosan is 1,4-linked 2-amino-2-deoxy-β-D-glucopyranosyl (Izydorczyk *et al.*, 2005). It is the only polysaccharide carrying a positive charge. Therefore, chitosan is widely used as a multi-layer emulsifier and encapsulating agent.

5.4 Soluble high molecular weight dietary fibre ingredients

5.4.1 Pectins

Pectins are the major components of cell walls in plants. They are composed of both oligosaccharides and polysaccharides (Ridley *et al.*, 2001). Three major pectic polysaccharides are recognized: homogalacturonan, rhamnogalacturonan-I and rhamnogalacturonan-II. Homogalacturonan is a linear polymer consisting of 1,4-linked a-D-GalA; rhamnogalacturonan-I consists of the repeating disaccharide 4-α-D-GalA-(1,2)-α-L-Rha-1-, among which different glycan chains (arabinan and galactan) are attached to the Rha residues; rhamnogalacturonan-II has a backbone of homogalacturonan chain with complex side chains attached to the rhamnosyl residues (Ridley *et al.*, 2001). The carboxylic acid groups can be methyl esterified in galacturonans, and the degree of esterification was observed to have key impacts on the conformation and solution properties (Axelos and Branger, 1993; Morris *et al.*, 2000).

Based on the degree of esterification, pectins are classified into two categories: low methyl pectins (LMP) with less than 50% methyl esters, and high methyl pectins (HMP) with more than 50% methyl esters (Izydorczyk *et al.*, 2005). If the degree of esterification is lower than 5%, the pectin is in its insoluble form, that is, pectic acid. On the other hand, pectic acid can be converted into monovalent forms (sodium or potassium pectate) to become soluble. In solution, pectins display a random coil conformation with some degree of rigidity. The solution viscosity decreases with increased temperature, decreased concentration and molecular weight. Both HMP and LMP can form gels at concentrations above 0.5 ~ 1%. HMP form thermally irreversible gels in the presence of sugars or other co-solutes at relatively high concentration (>50%) in an acid environment (pH<3.6). However, LM pectin gels formed at low pH are thermally reversible (Izydorczyk *et al.*, 2005). LMP can also form gels in the presence of divalent cations such as Ca^{2+}. The required amount of co-solute increases with increasing degree of polymerization. Meanwhile, gelation is favoured by increased soluble solids and decreased pH.

5.4.2 β-Glucans

β-Glucans are polysaccharides that occur in the subaleurone and endosperm cell walls of the seeds of cereals, including oats, barley, rye and wheat. The level of β-glucan in cereals varies from as low as 0.5–1% in whole wheat to 3–11% in barley (Cui and Roberts, 2009). β-Glucans are homopolysaccharides which only have a single sugar unit, β-D-glucopyranose. The β-D-glucopyranose residues are arranged as blocks of two or three consecutive (1,4)-linked units separated by a single (1,3) linkage, which form the two building blocks of cereal β-glucan: a cellotriosyl unit and a cellotetraosyl unit. The tri/tetrasaccharide ratios for β-glucan from wheat, barley and oats are 4.5, 3.0 and 2.3, respectively. This ratio is an important factor controlling the solution property of the polysaccharides. In aqueous solution, β-glucans adopt a disordered random coil conformation. The gelation capacity of cereal β-glucans is in the order of wheat>barley>oat, which is the same as the order of the tri/tetrasaccharides ratio of wheat, barley and oat. Molecular weight is another important factor influencing solution properties. The gelation rate of β-glucan solutions usually decreases with increased molecular weight (Cui, 2001; Izydorczyk *et al.*, 2005). β-Glucans have been widely used in bakery products, yogurts, processed meats, sausages and beverages as stabilizers, bulking agents and/or fat replacers.

Galactoglucomannans

Galactoglucomannans are cell wall polysaccharides in the seeds of legumes such as carob tree, guar plant, tara shrub and fenugreek plant. Galactoglucomannan consists of a glucomannan backbone composed of β-(1,4)-D-mannosyl units with an α-D-galactose side chain at O-6. The mannose to galactose (M/G) ratio is dependent on the source of the galactoglucomannan. Typically, the M/G ratios for fenugreek gum (FG), guar gum (GG), tara gum (TG) and locust bean gum (LBG) are close to 1, 2, 3 and 4, respectively. M/G ratio may vary even in the same species, which can be caused by varietal or environmental differences (Dea and Morrison, 1975). Because of their high water-binding capacity, galactoglucomannans can form highly viscous solutions at low concentrations without forming gels, except for LBG, which can form a gel at high concentrations under specific conditions (Dea *et al.*, 1977; Richardson *et al.*, 1999). The high water-binding capacity and highly viscous solutions make galactoglucomannans effective thickeners and stabilizers in the food industry. In addition, LBG, TG, GG and FG are all found to exhibit some surface, interfacial and emulsifying activities (Garti *et al.*, 1997). The solubility and hydration rate are influenced by the degree and pattern of substitution of the galactosyl unit, particle size, pH, ionic strength, temperature, co-solute and agitation method (Wang *et al.*, 2003, 2006, 2008; Izydorczyk *et al.*, 2005). The presence of the galactosyl units improves solubility. Molecular weight, M/G ratio and galactose substitution pattern play vital roles in the emulsification and rheological properties of galactoglucomannans. At low concentrations, all galactoglucomannans show Newtonian flow behaviour in that the viscosity is independent of shear rate. At higher concentrations and higher shear rate, the solutions are pseudoplastic, whereby the viscosity decreases with increasing shear rate (Wu *et al.*, 2009b, 2012).

Xyloglucan

Xyloglucan is a major structural polysaccharide of higher plants (or vascular plants). Xyloglucans have linear backbones of (1,4)-linked β-D-glucopyranose with xylopyranosyl units attached. Some xylose residues may carry additional galactosyl and fucosyl units. Xyloglucan can be obtained from cotyledons of tamarind seed, and is commercially available as a thickener, stabilizer, gelling agent, ice-crystal stabilizer and starch modifier. The molecular weight of tamarind seed xyloglucan was reported to be from 115 kDa to 1160 kDa (Nishinari and Takemasa, 2009). Xyloglucans are soluble in cold water, and the solution is stable against heat, pH and shear. The solution exhibits Newtonian flow behaviour at low concentrations and shear-thinning flow behaviour at high concentrations, which is similar to the behaviour of galactoglucomannans. Gels can be formed in the presence of alcohol, a substantial amount of sugar (40–70% w/w) or polyphenolic compounds. Sugar-induced gels are elastic and have good water-holding properties, while a freeze-thaw process can make the gel harder and more elastic (Nishinari and Takemasa, 2009; Izydorczyk *et al.*, 2005).

Arabinoxylan

Arabinoxylans have been found in all major cereal grains, including rye, wheat, barley, oats, sorghum, maize, millet, psyllium, flaxseed, pangola grass, bamboo shoot and rye grass. The highest content of arabinoxylan is found in rye, followed by wheat, barley, oats, rice and sorghum. Arabinoxylans form a major dietary fibre source in the diet. They consist of a linear backbone chain of β-D-xylopyranosyl residues linked through (1,4) glycosidic linkages. An α-L-arabinofuranosyl residue is attached to some of the Xyl*p* residues at O-2, O-3, and/or at both O-2,3 positions. The majority of Ara*f* residues are present as monomeric substituents, while a small portion are oligomeric side chains consisting of two or more Ara*f* residues linked via 1,2, 1,3 and 1,5 linkages. The amount of arabinose and glucuronic acids in glucuronoarabinoxylans may range from substitution at almost all Xyl*p* to polymers having more than 90% unsubstituted β-Xyl*p* units (Izydorczyk *et al.*, 2005). Many cereal (wheat, barley, rye, oats) arabinoxylans do not carry glucuronic acid units.

Arabinoxylans can form a random coil conformation in aqueous solutions. Wheat arabinoxylans can form thermally irreversible gels upon oxidation or cross-linking with ferulic acid residues. According to the extraction procedures and material sources, the molecular weight of arabinoxylans ranges from 300 kDa to 2 MDa, covering soluble and insoluble fractions. The solubility of arabinoxylans in aqueous solutions is related to the degree and pattern of substitutions along the xylan backbone. The flow behaviour of arabinoxylan is concentration- and shear rate-dependent, similarly to galactoglucomannans and xyloglucan. Arabinoxylans with high molecular weights may form weak pseudo-gels. Cereal arabinoxylans containing ferulic acid residues can form gel networks by covalent crosslinks between feruloyl groups of neighbouring chains. Higher gel strength is related to higher content of ferulic acid, higher molecular weight and lower degree of substitution. In aqueous solution, arabinoxylans form random coil structures (Izydorczyk and Dexter, 2008). As a food ingredient, arabinoxylan can affect water-holding capacity, dough rheology or starch retrogradation. Arabinoxylans have important effects on cereal processes such as milling, brewing, and breadmaking quality (Vinkx and Delcour, 1996; Izydorczyk and Dexter, 2008). They can also be used as film-forming agents, cryostabilizers and surface active agents in various food products.

5.4.3 Mucilages

Flaxseed gum

Flaxseed gum can be easily extracted from the whole seeds or flaxseed hulls by soaking them in warm water. Upon hydration of the seeds, the mucilage will be exuded on the surface of the seeds. Flaxseed gum contains a mixture of neutral and acidic polysaccharides. The neutral fraction has a (1,4)-linked β-D-xylopyranosyl backbone chain together with 16.2% (w/w) terminal D-xylose. The acidic fraction has a rhamnogalacturonan backbone composed of 1,2-linked (15.4%) (w/w), 1,2,3-linked (13.1%) (w/w) L-rhamnosyl residues and (1,4)-linked D-galacturonic acid (10.2%) (w/w) (Cui, 2001). Flaxseed gum is soluble in cold water. The solution exhibits Newtonian flow behaviour at low concentrations, and shear thinning flow behaviour at high concentrations. It can form a viscous solution and the viscosity is markedly influenced by the pH. Higher viscosity can be obtained at neutral pH (6–8) (Izydorczyk *et al.*, 2005). Flaxseed gum shows surface activity and can stabilize oil/water emulsions and foams, and is therefore used as a thickener, stabilizer, and water-holding agent.

Mustard mucilage

Yellow or white mustard seeds are used as condiments. Previous research has shown that the neutral fraction of white mustard mucilage is composed primarily of glucose (39.3%), arabinose (25.4%), galactose (17.9%), mannose (5.4%), rhamnose (4.0%) and xylose (7.0%) (w/w) (Vose, 1974). Current research is mainly focused on yellow mustard mucilage (Cui *et al.*, 1993; Sehgal *et al.*, 2002; Wu *et al.*, 2009a). The water-soluble part of yellow mustard mucilage includes glucose (22.3%), galactose (15.2%), mannose (6.3%), rhamnose (3.9%), arabinose (3.2%), xylose (1.8%) and uronic acid (18.7%) (w/w). It contains two fractions, pectic and non-pectic polysaccharides. The pectic polysaccharides are mainly of the rhamnogalacturonan-II type of structure, composed of (1,4)-linked α-D-galacturonopyranosyl and (1,2)-linked α-L-rhamnopyranosyl residues (Cui *et al.*, 1993). The non-pectic polysaccharides are composed of a β-(1,4)-linked D-glucosidic backbone with occasional branches at the O-2, O-3 and O-6 positions. The non-pectic fraction is responsible for synergistic interactions with galactoglucomannans (Wu *et al.*, 2009). Water-soluble yellow mustard mucilage forms either viscous solutions or weak gels depending on the concentration. It shows high surface activity, and also can be used as a thickener and stabilizer.

Psyllium gum

Psyllium gum can be extracted from the seed coat (husk or hull) of *ispaghula* or psyllium seeds of the *Plantago* genus. The hull can be mechanically separated from the rest of the seed, and the gum can be extracted with hot water or mild alkaline solutions. Psyllium husk is commercially available as particles or in powder form. Psyllium gum is composed mainly of arabinose (22%), xylose (57%) and uronic acids (10–15%) (w/w) with small amounts of galactose, rhamnose, glucose and mannose. It is a highly branched acidic arabinoxylan with a high molecular weight (~1500 kDa). The xylan backbone has both β-1,4 and β-1,3 linkages, and the majority of the side chains are connected to the backbone through O-2 or O-3 positions with single L-Ara*f* and D-Xyl*p* residues or disaccharides containing L-Rha*p* and D-Gal*p*A (Guo *et al.*, 2007; Yin *et al.*, 2012). Psyllium gum does not completely dissolve in water due to its high molecular weight. It forms a gel-like paste or dispersion when hydrated. Freshly prepared psyllium gum dispersion (1%) showed Newtonian flow behaviour at low shear rates. Shear thinning flow behaviour was observed at higher shear rates (Izydorczyk *et al.*, 2005). Psyllium gel is thermally stable, with G′ and G″ decreasing with increased temperature. No melting is observed unless the temperature exceeds 80°C (Guo *et al.*, 2008). When Ca^{2+} is added to the gel, the gel becomes more resistant to temperature; meanwhile, its bioavailability is reduced (Cho and Clark, 2001). Psyllium has been used in beverages, confectionery and bakery products as a stabilizer and a gel filling.

5.4.4 Gum arabic

Gum arabic is exuded from the bark of *Acacia* trees that grow primarily in Africa. The main chain is built from (1,3)-linked β-D-galactopyranosyl units with α-L-rhamnopyranose, β-D-glucuronic acid, β-D-galactopyranose and α-L-arabinofuranosyl units as side chains (Williams and Phillips, 2009). Compared with other exuded gums, gum arabic has higher water solubility (up to 50% w/v), and its solution exhibits Newtonian flow behaviour even at high concentrations. The highly branched molecular structure is responsible for the high solubility. Gum arabic is also associated with a protein moiety, which is responsible for the emulsifying and foaming properties of the gum. The protein-rich high molecular weight fraction of gum arabic can be adsorbed onto the surface of oil droplets, whereas the polysaccharide main chain inhibits coalescence by electrostatic and steric repulsion forces (Al-Assaf *et al.*, 2007). Gum arabic is usually used as a food emulsifier and stabilizer in the food industry. Gum arabic can be easily incorporated into beverages and processed foods without changing the original taste or texture due to its high solubility and relatively low viscosity, thus becoming an ideal functional dietary fibre ingredient in food.

5.4.5 Konjac glucomannan

Konjac glucomannan exists in the tubers of konjac (*Lasioideae amorphophallus*), which is distributed in the Far East and southeast Asia. The raw tuber of konjac contains 8–10% of Konjac glucomannan (Takigami, 2009). As a type of glucomannan, it is a heteropolysaccharide consisting of β-D-glucose and β-D-mannose, with a glucose to mannose ratio of 1 to 3. It is reported that konjac glucomannan has side chains and the branches are at the O-3 position of the mannose residue or both glucose and mannose residues. It also contains acetyl groups along the main chain. Konjac glucomannan is water-soluble; however, constant stirring is required to completely dissolve it in water at room temperature. Hot water is not effective at dissolving it. The viscosity of konjac glucomannan solutions increases with concentration. After the concentration reaches 1%, the viscosity increases remarkably. The viscosity is not affected by salt concentration but by the pH of a solution. The viscosity decreases with decreasing pH value, while the solution changes to a gel at higher pH values. Konjac glucomannan can interact with many other polysaccharides, such as xanthan, carrageenan and agar, and forms thermally reversible gels. Adding sugar can enhance the strength of the synergistic gel, while adding salt can inhibit the formation of the synergistic gel; this can be used to control its gel-forming capacity in food. Konjac glucomannan is also suitable as a fat replacer in meat and dairy products.

5.4.6 Seaweed polysaccharides

Alginate

Alginates are structural polysaccharides in marine brown algae (*Phaeophyceae*), and they can also be synthesized by the bacteria *Pseudomonas aeruginosa* and *Azobacter vinelandii* (Draget, 2009). Alginates are composed of (1,4)-linked β-D-mannuronic acid and α-L-guluronic acid residues. There are homomeric blocks of contiguously linked mannuronic acid or guluronic acid and mixed blocks containing both residues. If the uronic acids are in the acid form, the polysaccharide is called alginic acid, which is water-insoluble. The ratio of mannuronic acid and guluronic acid residues is usually 2:1. The ratio may vary with the algae species, age of the plant and the type of the tissues. In bacterial alginates, the content of guluronic acid may range from 15 to 90%. Alginates form thermally stable gels in the presence of ions, and the gels' strength depends on the type of ions and the method of introduction of ions. The effect of ions on the gelation potential of alginates generally follows the order of $Mg^{2+} \ll Ca^{2+} < Sr^{2+} < Ba^{2+}$. High guluronic alginates produce strong but brittle gels with good heat stability, whereas high mannuronic acid alginates produce weaker but more elastic gels with good freeze-thaw stability (Onsøyen, 2001).

Carrageenan

Carrageenans are structural polysaccharides of marine red algae (*Rhodophyceae*) (Imeson, 2009). They are high molecular weight linear polysaccharides including three different types: κ-, ι- and λ-carrageenan. Their structures differ in 3,6-anhydro-α-D-galactose and sulphate group contents. The repeating disaccharide units in the backbone of κ- and ι-carrageenans are sulphate esters of (1,3)-linked β-D-galactose and (1,4)-linked 3,6-anhydro-α-D-galactose. λ-Carrageenans consist of β-D-galactopyranosyl residues sulphated at C-2 (instead of C-4 as in ι- and κ-carrageenans) and 2,6-di-O-sulfato-α-D-galactopyranosyl units (instead of 3,6-anhydro-α-D-galactopyranosyl residues) (Izydorczyk *et al.*, 2005). κ-Carrageenan has one sulphate group per repeating disaccharide unit; ι-carrageenan has two sulphate groups; and λ-carrageenan carries three sulphated groups (Imeson, 2009).

In solution, κ- and ι-carrageenans form a double helix conformation which is stabilized by hydrogen bonds. κ-Carrageenan exhibits firm but brittle gels with poor freeze-thaw stability. It has been used widely in dairy products as a stabilizer to prevent whey separation. ι-Carrageenan forms soft elastic gels with good freeze-thaw stability. κ- and ι-Carrageenans can be used as thickeners, gelling and suspending agents. λ-Carrageenan cannot form gels because of the sulphate groups, and it exhibits a flat and ribbon-like conformation in aqueous solution. λ-Carrageenan can be used as a cryoprotectant to improve the freeze-thaw stability of frozen products (Izydorczyk *et al.*, 2005).

Agar

Agar is a linear structural polysaccharide from red-purple algae (agarophytes) (Armisén and Galatas, 2009). The repeating disaccharide unit in the backbone of agar is (1,3)-linked β-D-galactose and (1,4)-linked 3,6-anhydro-α-L-galactose (instead of the D-enantiomer as in ι- and κ-carrageenans). The double helices of agar are more compact than those of carrageenans due to the lightly sulphated structure. Agar can form a stiff gel at low concentrations, and it is the best gelling agent among all commercial gums. Agar forms cold-set gels at around 38°C, with the melting temperature higher than 85°C (Izydorczyk *et al.*, 2005). Thus, agar is widely used in bakery products because of its heat-resistant characteristics and large gelling/melting hysteresis. Its thermo-reversible gelling property helps to prevent chipping, cracking or sweating of icings, toppings and glazes in baked food products.

5.4.7 Microbial polysaccharides

Xanthan gum

Xanthan gum, produced by the microorganism *Xanthomonas campestris*, is an extracellular polysaccharide (Sworn, 2009). The primary structure of xanthan gum consists of the cellulose-like backbone of (1,4)-linked β-D-Glc*p* residues substituted at O-3 of alternate glucose residues, with a trisaccharide side chain. The trisaccharide side chain consists of a β-D-Man*p*-(1,4)-β-D-Glc*p*A-(1,2)-α-D-Man*p*-(1→) unit. Non-carbohydrate substituents include an acetyl group at O-6 of the inner Man*p* residue and a pyruvate group at O-4,6 of the terminal Man*p*. The pyruvic acid content of xanthan can vary according to the producing bacterial strain. The molecular weight of xanthan gum ranges from 300 kDa to 8 MDa. Xanthan gum is soluble in cold water, and it exhibits very high viscosity at low shear rate range and relatively low viscosity at high shear rate range. Strong synergism is observed between xanthan gum and some mannan-containing polysaccharides, such as galactomannans and glucomannans (Izydorczyk *et al.*, 2005).

Gellan gum

Gellan gum, produced by the bacterium *Auromonas elodea*, is a deacetylated form of the extracellular polysaccharide. Gellan gum consists of a linear tetrasaccharide repeating unit: (1,3)-β-D-Glc*p*-(1,4)-β-D-Glc*p*A-(1,4)-β-D-Glc-(1,4)-α-L-Rha-(1→). Two acyl substituents, L-glyceryl and acetyl, are present at the O-3-linked glucose at the O-2 and O-6 positions, respectively (Sworn, 2009). During commercial processing, these substituents are easily lost. According to the degree of acyl substitution, gellan gums can be categorized as high acyl (HA) gellan gum and low acyl (LA) gellan gum. Both forms are insoluble in cold water, but readily dispersed in water by stirring and adding the gum powder slowly. As ion concentration in water increases, the dispersion becomes easier. Both forms of gellan gum are readily dispersible in milk and reconstituted milk systems. The polysaccharide chains of gellan can form double helices in aqueous solution after cooling, leading to the formation of weak gel structures (Izydorczyk *et al.*, 2005). In the presence of appropriate cations, the double helices form cation-mediated aggregates, which can lead to strong gel networks. Acyl substituents in gellan interfere with the aggregation process; the gel characteristics mainly depend on the degree of acylation and presence of counter-ions.

Gellan gum is commonly used as a gelling agent. HA gellan gum gives soft, elastic and transparent gels at concentrations higher than 0.2%. HA gels set and melt at 70 to 80°C with no thermal hysteresis. However, LA gellan gum can form hard, non-elastic and brittle gels in the presence of cations; the gel strength of LA gellan gum increases with increasing ion concentration. The LA gellan gels also exhibit significant thermal hysteresis (Valli and Miskiel, 2001). It is important to note that the gelling property of gellans restricts their use as dietary fibre ingredients in food, because high concentrations cannot be used in order to maintain the original food texture.

Curdlan

Curdlan is an extracellular microbial polysaccharide produced from the mutant strain of bacteria *Agrobacterium biovar I* (Nishinari, 2009). Curdlan is known as a 1,3-β-D-glucan, which is solely composed of 1,3-β-D-glycosidic linkages. The molecular weight of curdlan normally ranges from 66 to 680 kDa, and it can be higher than 2 MDa for commercial uses. Curdlan is not soluble in water at room temperature but can be dissolved in alkaline solution. The water insolubility may be due to the intramolecularly and intermolecularly hydrogen bonded crystalline structure. The viscosity of curdlan in alkaline solution depends on the concentration of sodium hydroxide. In the range of 0.05–0.10 M sodium hydroxide, curdlan can form triple helices. When the concentration of sodium hydroxide increases to 0.25 M, the triple helices can be dissociated into single chains of lower molecular weight; this will result in a reduction of viscosity.

Concentrated curdlan solution shows almost Newtonian flow behaviour in strongly alkaline solution. Curdlan aqueous solutions can form gels upon heating. When it is heated up to 55°C then cooled, curdlan in aqueous solution can form a thermally reversible gel (Izydorczyk *et al.*, 2005). When the heating temperature is above 80°C, the gel is thermo-irreversible. The gel strength is related to gelling temperature. The gel strength stays stable at 60–80°C, and increases with heating temperature until 100°C. The gel strength also increases with increased concentration. Between pH 3 and 10, the gel strength does not change. Curdlan is a neutral polysaccharide, which is tasteless, odourless and colourless (Yotsuzuka, 2001). Therefore, it has been used widely in the food industry as a gelling agent and fat replacer.

5.5 Soluble low molecular weight dietary fibre ingredients

5.5.1 Non-digestible oligosaccharides

According to the International Union of Pure and Applied Chemistry (IUPAC), oligosaccharides are compounds containing three to ten monomeric sugar residues. Only the non-digestible oligosaccharides are of interest in this section.

Some oligosaccharides occur naturally as free compounds in milk, honey, fruits, vegetables and cereals. Examples are raffinose oligosaccharides in legume seeds, xylooligosaccharides in bamboo shoots, fructooligosaccharides in asparagus, galactooligosaccharides in milk, and so on. Commercial production of oligosaccharides may involve extraction from plant materials using water or aqueous methanol or ethanol solutions, hydrolysing polysaccharides, or enzymatic or chemical synthesis from disaccharide substrates.

There is a wide variety of non-digestible oligosaccharides, all of which exert beneficial physiological effects on humans by affecting the intestinal microflora as dietary fibres; these works have been described and discussed in the literature (Meyer and Tungland, 2008; Playne and Crittenden, 1996; Mussatto and Mancilha, 2007). Due to their relatively low sweetness (0.3–0.6 times as sweet as sucrose) and high water solubility, resistant oligosaccharides have been widely used as dietary fibre ingredients or prebiotics in various foods, for example yoghurt drinks, desserts, ice cream, cheese products, and so on (Meyer, 2009). Compared with monosaccharides and disaccharides, oligosaccharides can provide increased viscosity to improve mouthfeel. Oligosaccharides can also be used to alter the freezing temperature of frozen foods, as well as to provide moisture-retaining capacity and to lower water activity, thus controlling the stability and shelf-life of food products.

5.5.2 Inulin

Inulin occurs in many plants, and can also be synthesized in microbes. It can be found in banana, chicory, barley, onion and wheat, among others (Meyer and Tungland, 2008; Meyer, 2009). Inulin is built up of 2–60 fructose units with one glucosyl terminal unit. When the degree of polymerization is lower than 20, it is considered an oligosaccharide. The main structure of inulin is β-(2,1) fructan, and the solubility mostly depends on the chain length. It is harder to dissolve inulin with longer chain length. At high temperature (80°C), a concentration of up to 20% inulin can be prepared. It is very stable at temperatures up to 140°C.

Inulin is susceptible to acid hydrolysis. The hydrolysis may occur at a pH lower than 4. Inulin solution is very low in viscosity. However, when combined with other ingredients, inulin can compete with other polysaccharides for binding with water molecules, thus changing their rheological behaviour. Therefore, inulin can be used for modifying the rheology and texture of food products. When concentration exceeds 15%, inulin can form a gel or cream (Coussement and Franck, 2001). The strength of the gel can be affected by many factors, such as chain length, concentration and temperature. Long chain inulin molecules can form firmer gels. When inulin is added to beverages with a thickener such as xanthan, guar gum or pectin, the system will become more homogeneous. It can also provide a fat-like flow and satisfactory spreadability when applied in gum-based fat-free dressings and sauces. A creamy mouthfeel can be obtained when inulin is added to dairy products due to interactions with the dairy components. This effect could be enhanced when combined with κ-carrageenan. As summarized by Meyer (2009), inulin has been widely used in dairy, bakery and meat products as a fat replacer, bulking agent and foam stabilizer.

5.6 Resistant starch

Resistant starches (RS) are a variety of starch that can resist digestion and pass through the gastrointestinal tract (Taggart, 2009). According to its physical and chemical characteristics, resistant starch is divided into four types: types I, II, III and IV resistant starch. Type I resistant starch is the physically protected starch in whole or partially ground grains. Type II resistant starch is in raw starch granules. The intact granules cannot be gelatinized due to the compact structure and thus cannot be digested by enzymes. Type III resistant starch is retrograded starch. It generally results from food processing applications. After gelatinization, the retrogradation process can lead to recrystallization of some single chains to form double helices via hydrogen bonds. Many new approaches have been developed for producing type III resistant starch. Type IV resistant starch includes chemically modified starch such as that produced by etherification, oxidation or cross-linking.

Resistant starches have a low water-binding capacity. They can be added to food products at high concentration (up to 30%) by controlling the processing conditions, such as moisture content, pH, temperature, and so on. Recently, resistant starches have been considered as new ingredients for creating fibre-rich food. Resistant starches have small particle size, white appearance and bland taste. They can be used to replace flour on a one-for-one basis without significantly affecting dough handling or rheology (Ranhotra, 2008). Resistant starches can also increase swelling, viscosity and gel-forming capacity. Compared with traditional high-fibre products, resistant starches can form low-bulk high-fibre products with improved texture, appearance and mouthfeel.

5.7 Conclusion

This chapter has presented various kinds of dietary fibres, which are commonly used in food for techno-functional and/or biofunctional (nutrition) purposes. They can be widely used as thickeners, emulsifiers, stabilizers, fat replacers, and suspending and gelling agents, as well as providing beneficial physiological effects. The preparation of dietary fibres and their techno-functionalities and applications in food are summarized in Table 5.1.

There are still challenges in adding dietary fibres to food products in reasonable quantities to achieve their biofunctional effects while maintaining good organoleptic properties. Many dietary fibres or gums are unsuitable for applications in particular foods in large amounts. Therefore, developing purified, colourless dietary fibres with bland taste and low viscosity is of particular interest to related food companies in preparing novel high dietary fibre food products.

Table 5.1 The origin, source and major techno-functionalities of dietary fibres and their applications in food

Dietary fibres (DF)	Origin and source	Major techno-functionalities	Applications in food	Reference
Insoluble DF				
Cellulose and lignin	Cell walls of higher plants.	Bulking capacity.	Improve the loaf volume in bakery products.	Izydorczyk *et al*., 2005
Oat bran	Outer layer of oat groats.	Bulking capacity, fat replacement.	Bulking agent in cereal products; fat replacer in ground beef and pork sausage products.	Mälkki, 2001; Verma and Banerjee, 2010
Wheat bran	Outer coat of wheat grain, by-products of milling wheat into white flour.	Bulking capacity, laxative effect.	Functional DF ingredients.	Cho and Clark, 2001
Legume fibres	Legume seeds including soys, peas, beans, peanuts and lupins, etc.	Water-binding and oil-binding capacity.	Fat replacer in bakery products.	Pfoertner and Fischer, 2008
Chitin	Cell walls of lower plants, exoskeleton of insects, and shells of crustaceans.	Bulking capacity; as raw material for chitosan.	Functional DF ingredients for weight control.	Muzzarelli, 2009; Izydorczyk *et al*., 2005
Soluble high molecular weight (HMw) DF				
Pectin	Middle lamellae of plant cell walls.	Water-binding, emulsifying, gel-forming and thickening capacity.	Stabilizer, thickener and emulsifier in beverages; fat replacer in cheese; low sugar jams and jellies.	Fernandez, 2001; Dhingra *et al*., 2012
β-Glucan	Cell wall components of cereal grains, higher concentration in oats and barley.	Very good fat replacement capacity; water-holding, emulsifying, and film-forming capacity.	Functional DF ingredients showing bioactivity; fat replacer in meat, dairy and bakery products; to improve freeze-thaw stability.	Izydorczyk *et al*., 2005; Wood, 1994; Brennan and Tudorica, 2008; Izydorczyk and Dexter, 2008

Galactoglucomannan	Albuminous and endospermic seeds, such as carob, guar, tara and fenugreek, etc.	Very good emulsifying capacity; thickening properties; interacting with other DF components.	Emulsifier and stabilizer in beverages; fat replacer in cheese and yogurt; to improve shelf-life and freeze-thaw stability.	Wielinga, 2009; Brennan and Tudorica, 2008; Dhingra *et al*., 2012
Xyloglucan	Primary cell wall of higher plants.	Water-binding capacity; thickening properties; stabilizing, gelling and emulsifying capacity; fat replacement capacity.	Effective stabilizer in frozen desserts; thickener in beverages; fat replacer and gelling agent.	Nishinari and Takemasa, 2009; Izydorczyk *et al*., 2005
Arabinoxylan	Tissue cells of terrestrial plants and algae.	Very good water-binding capacity; film-forming, emulsifying and cryostabilizing properties.	Film-forming agent, cryostabilizer and surface active agent; to moderate dough behaviour and loaf volume.	Izydorczyk, 2009
Flaxseed gum	Outer layer of flaxseed hull.	Emulsifying, stabilizing and texture-modifying capacity; fat replacement.	Emulsifier, stabilizer, texture modifier and moisturizer; can be largely added into food as functional DF.	Cui, 2001; Izydorczyk *et al*., 2005
Mustard mucilage	Outer layer of mustard seed.	Emulsifying and stabilizing capacity; interacting with other DF components.	Emulsifier, stabilizer and moisturizer; to prepare different gums by synergistic interactions.	Cui *et al*., 1993; Wu *et al*., 2009a
Psyllium gum	Seed coat of ispaghula or psyllium seeds.	Very good laxative capacity; gel-forming, stabilizing and thickening capacity.	Stabilizer and thickener in beverages and ice cream; gel filling agent in confectionery products.	Cho and Clark, 2001; Izydorczyk *et al*., 2005
Gum arabic	Exuded gum from Acacia trees.	Emulsifying, stabilizing and flavour-encapsulating capacity.	Emulsifier, stabilizer and flavour encapsulator; can be largely added into food as functional DF.	Williams and Phillips, 2009; Izydorczyk *et al*., 2005

(*Continued overleaf.*)

Table 5.1 (Continued)

Dietary fibres (DF)	Origin and source	Major techno-functionalities	Applications in food	Reference
Konjac glucomannan	Tubers of konjac.	Thickening, gel-forming, water-binding capacity.	Film- and gel-forming agent; thickener and fat replacer	Takigami, 2009
Alginate	Brown algae (*Phaeophyceae*).	Thickening, gel-forming, film-forming and stabilizing capacity.	Thickener and stabilizer; gel-forming and film-forming agent.	Draget, 2009; Onsøyen, 2001
Carrageenan	Red algae (*Rhodophyceae*).	Thickening and water-binding capacity; gel-forming capacity (κ-, and ι-carrageenan); interacting with other DF components.	Very good stabilizer in dairy products, thickener, gel-forming agent.	Imeson, 2009
Agar	Red-purple algae (agarophytes).	Very good gel-forming capacity.	Gel-forming agent with large gelling/melting hysteresis; texture modifier.	Armisén and Galatas, 2009
Xanthan gum	Produced by the microorganism *Xanthomonas campestris.*	Stabilizing and texture-modifying capacity; interacting with other DF components; fat replacement.	Stabilizer and texture modifier, thickener and gel-forming agent; interacted with carrageenan gel, avoiding shrinkage and syneresis.	Sworn, 2009; Izydorczyk *et al.*, 2005
Gellan gum	Produced by the microorganism *Auromonas elodea.*	Stabilizing, texture-modifying, gel-forming and film-forming capacity; fat replacement.	Stabilizer and texture modifier, gel-forming agent, fat replacer.	Sworn, 2009; Valli and Miskiel, 2001
Curdlan	Produced by the microorganism *Agrobacterium biovar I.*	Very good gel-forming capacity even with high amount of oil; water-binding and oil-binding capacity.	Gel-forming agent, fat replacer, texture modifier.	Nishinari and Zhang, 2009; Yotsuzuka, 2001

Chitosan	N-acetal groups of chitin are replaced by amino groups in strong alkali.	Very good emulsifying and film-forming capacity.	Multi-layer emulsifier, edible films and coatings.	Muzzarelli; 2009 Izydorczyk *et al*., 2005
Soluble low molecular weight (LMw) DF				
Non-digestible oligosaccharides	DF containing 3 to 10 monomeric sugar residues.	Moisture-retaining capacity, low viscosity.	Functional DF ingredients in low calorie food; to improve the flavour, mouthfeel, and shelf life of food products.	Meyer and Tungland, 2008
Inulin	Widely distributed in higher plants, including banana, chicory, barley, onion and wheat.	Gel-forming capacity; low viscosity, heat and acid stability; interacting with other DF components.	Functional DF ingredient; fat replacer in cheese and muffin; gel-forming agent and foam stabilizer.	Dhingra *et al*., 2012; Zahn *et al*., 2010
Resistant starch (RS)	Degradation and/or modification of starch.	Water- and oil-binding, and flavor-encapsulating capacity; interacting with other DF components.	Fat replacer and flavour encapsulator; can be largely added into food as functional DF.	Brown *et al*., 2008; Ranhotra, 2008; Taggart, 2009

5.8 References

AGOUB A.A., SMITH A.M., GIANNOULI P., RICHARDSON R.K. and MORRIS E.R. (2007). 'Melt-in-the-mouth' Gels from Mixtures of Xanthan and Konjac Glucomannan under Acidic Conditions: A Rheological and Calorimetric Study of the Mechanism of Synergistic Gelation, *Carbohydrate Polymers*. **69**(4), 713–24.

AL-ASSAF S., PHILLIPS G. O., AOKI H. and SASAKI Y. (2007). Characterization and Properties of Acacia Senegal (L.)Willd. var. Senegal with Enhanced Properties (Acacia (sen) SUPER GUM™): Part 1—Controlled Maturation of Acacia Senegal var. Senegal to Increase Viscoelasticity, Produce a Hydrogel Form and Convert a Poor into a Good Emulsifier. *Food Hydrocolloids*. **21**(3), 319–28.

ARMISÉN R. and GALATAS F. (2009). In: *Handbook of hydrocolloids*. PHILLIPS G. O. and WILLIAMS P. A., eds. FL: CRC Press. 82–107.

AXELOS M. A. V. and BRANGER M. (1993). The Effect of the Degree of Esterification on the Thermal-Stability and Chain Conformation of Pectins. *Food Hydrocolloids*. **7**(2), 91–102.

BERTRAND D., BRILLOUET J. M., RASPER V. F., BOUCHET B. and MERCIER C. (1981). Effects of Rat Digestion upon Native, Enzymically Or Chemically Modified Wheat Brans and Native Oat Bran. *Cereal Chemistry*. **58**(5), 375–80.

BRENNAN C. S. and TUDORICA C. M. (2008). Carbohydrate-based fat replacers in the modification of the rheological, textural and sensory quality of yoghurt: comparative study of the utilisation of barley beta-glucan, guar gum and inulin. *International Journal of Food Science and Technology*. **43**(5), 824–33.

BREWER M. S. (2012). Reducing the Fat Content in Ground Beef without Sacrificing Quality: A review. *Meat Science*, **91**(4), 385–95.

BROOKS M., CAMPBELL R. and MCCLEARY B. V. (2008). In: *Advanced dietary fibre technology*. MCCLEARY B. V. and PROSKY L., eds. FL: Blackwell Science Ltd. 331–44.

BROWN I. L., MCNAUGHT K. J., ANDREWS D., MORITA T. (2008). In: *Advance dietary fibre technology*. MCCLEARY B. V. and PROSKY L., eds. FL: Blackwell Science Ltd. 401–412.

CAPREZ A., ARRIGONI E., AMADO R. and NEUKOM H. (1986). Influence of Different Types of Thermal-Treatment on the Chemical-Composition and Physical-Properties of Wheat Bran. *Journal of Cereal Science*. **4**(3), 233–9.

CARRE B. and BRILLOUET J. M. (1986). Yield and Composition of Cell-Wall Residues Isolated from various Feedstuffs used for Non-Ruminant Farm-Animals. *Journal of the Science of Food and Agriculture*. **37**(4), 341–51.

CHO S. S. and CLARK C. (2001). In: *Handbook of dietary fiber*. CHO S. S. and DREHER M., eds. FL: Marcel Dekker, Inc. 473–96.

COUSSEMENT P. and FRANCK A. (2001). In: *Handbook of dietary fiber*. CHO S. S. and DREHER M., eds. FL: Marcel Dekker, Inc. 721–36.

CUI S.W. (2001). In: *Handbook of dietary fiber. Polysaccharide gums from agricultural products*. CUI S.W., ed. FL: Technomic Publishing Company, Inc. 59–102,103–66, 229–38.

CUI S. W. and ROBERTS K. (2009). In: *Modern biopolymer science: bridging the divide between fundamental treatise and industrial application*. KASAPIS S., NORTON I. T., and UBBINK J. B., eds. London: Academic Press. 399–449.

CUI S.W., ESKIN N. A. M. and BILIADERIS C. G. (1993).Chemical and Physical-Properties of Yellow Mustard (Sinapis-Alba L) Mucilage. *Food Chemistry*. **46**(2), 169–76.

CUI Y., WANG X., XU Q. and XIA Z. (2011). Research on Moisture Absorption Behavior of Recycled Polypropylene Matrix Wood Plastic Composites. *Journal of Thermoplastic Composite Materials*. **24**(1), 65–82.

DEA I. C. M., MORRIS E. R., REES D. A., WELSH E. J., BARNES H. A. and PRICE J. (1977). Associations of Like and Unlike Polysaccharides – Mechanism and Specificity in Galactomannans, Interacting Bacterial Polysaccharides, and Related Systems. *Carbohydrate Research*. **57**, 249–72.

DEA I. C. M. AND MORRISON A. (1975). Chemistry and interactions of seed galactomannans. *Advances in Carbohydrate Chemistry and Biochemistry*. **31**, 241–312.

DHINGRA D., MICHAEL M., RAJPUT H. and PATIL R. T. (2012). Dietary Fibre in Foods: A Review. *Journal of Food Science and Technology*. **49**, 255–66.

DICKINSON E. (2009). Hydrocolloids as Emulsifiers and Emulsion Stabilizers. *Food Hydrocolloids*. **23**(6), 1473–82.

DOUBLIER J. L. and WOOD P. J. (1995). Rheological Properties of Aqueous Solutions of (1–3) (1–4)-beta-D-glucan from Oats (*Avena sativa* L.). *Cereal Chemistry*. **72**(4), 335–40.

DRAGET K. I. (2009). In: *Handbook of hydrocolloids*. PHILLIPS G. O. and WILLIAMS P. A., eds. FL: CRC Press. 807–28.

ELLEUCH M., BEDIGIAN D., ROISEUX O., BESBES S., BLECKER C. and ATTIA H. (2011). Dietary Fibre and Fibre-Rich By-Products of Food Processing: Characterisation, Technological Functionality and Commercial Applications: A Review. *Food Chemistry*. **124**(2), 411–21.

FERNANDEZ M. L. (2001). In: *Handbook of dietary fiber*. CHO S. S. and DREHER M., eds. FL: Marcel Dekker, Inc. 583–602.

GARTI N., MADAR Z., ASERIN A. and STERNHEIM B. (1997). Fenugreek Galactomannans as Food Emulsifiers. *Food Science and Technology – Lebensmittel-Wissenschaft & Technologie*. **30**(3), 305–11.

GUO Q., CUI S. W., WANG Q. and YOUNG J.C. (2007). Fractionation and Physicochemical Characterization of Psyllium Gum. *Carbohydrate Polymers*. **73**(1), 35–43.

GUO Q., CUI S. W., WANG Q., GOFF H.D. AND SMITH A. (2008). Microstructure and Rheological Properties of Psyllium Polysaccharide Gel. *Food Hydrocolloids*. **23**(6), 1542–7.

IMESON A. P. (2009). In: *Handbook of hydrocolloids*. PHILLIPS G. O. and WILLIAMS P. A., eds. FL: CRC Press. 164–85.

IZYDORCZYK M. and DEXTER J. E. (2008). Barley β-Glucans and Arabinoxylans: Molecular Structure, Physicochemical Properties, and Uses in Food Products–A Review. *Food Research International*. **41**(9), 850–68.

IZYDORCZYK M., CUI S.W. and WANG Q. (2005). In: *Food carbohydrates; chemistry, physical properties, and applications*. CUI S., ed. FL: Oxford: CRC Press.

MÄLKKI Y. (2001). In: *Handbook of dietary fiber*. CHO S. S. and DREHER M., eds. FL: Marcel Dekker, Inc. 497–518.

MÄLKKI Y. and VIRTANEN E. (2001). Gastrointestinal Effects of Oat Bran and Oat Gum – A Review. *Lebensmittel-Wissenschaft Und Technologie – Food Science and Technology*. **34**(6), 337–47.

MEYER D. (2009). In: *Handbook of hydrocolloids*. PHILLIPS G. O. and WILLIAMS P. A., eds. FL: CRC Press. 829–48.

MEYER D. and TUNGLAND B. (2008). In: *Advanced dietary fibre technology*. MCCLEARY B. V. and PROSKY L., eds. FL: Blackwell Science Ltd. 455–70.

MORRIS G. A., FOSTER T. J. and HARDING S. E. (2000). The Effect of the Degree of Esterification on the Hydrodynamic Properties of Citrus Pectin. *Food Hydrocolloids*. **14**(3), 227–35.

MURRAY J. C. F. (2009). In: *Handbook of hydrocolloids*. PHILLIPS G. O. and WILLIAMS P. A., eds. FL: CRC Press. 710–23.

MUSSATTO S. I. and MANCILHA I. M. (2007). Non-Digestible Oligosaccharides: A Review. *Carbohydrate Polymers*. **68**(3), 587–97.

MUZZARELLI R. A. A. (2009). In: *Handbook of hydrocolloids*. PHILLIPS G. O. and WILLIAMS P. A., eds. FL: CRC Press. 849–87.

NISHINARI K. and TAKEMASA M. (2009). In: *Handbook of hydrocolloids*. PHILLIPS G. O. and WILLIAMS P. A., eds. FL: CRC Press. 535–66, 567–91.

NISHINARI K. and ZHANG H. (2009). In: *Handbook of hydrocolloids*. PHILLIPS G. O. and WILLIAMS P. A., eds. FL: CRC Press. 567–591.

NOORT M. W. J., VAN HAASTER D., HEMERY Y., SCHOLS H. A. and HAMER R. J. (2010). The Effect of Particle Size of Wheat Bran Fractions on Bread Quality – Evidence for Fibre Protein Interactions. *Journal of Cereal Science*. **52**(1), 59–64.

ONSØYEN E. (2001). In: *Handbook of dietary fiber*. CHO S. S. and DREHER M., eds. FL: Marcel Dekker, Inc. 659–74.

OZBOY-OZBAS O., SEKER I. T. and GOKBULUT I. (2010). Effects of Resistant Starch, Apricot Kernel Flour, and Fiber-rich Fruit Powders on Low-fat Cookie Quality. *Food Science and Biotechnology*. **19**(4), 979–86.

PFOERTNER H. P. and FISCHER J. (2008). In: *Advanced dietary fibre technology*. MCCLEARY B. V. and PROSKY L., eds. FL: Blackwell Science Ltd. 361–6.

PHILLIPS G. O. and CUI S. W. (2011). An Introduction: Evolution and Finalisation of the Regulatory Definition of Dietary Fibre. *Food Hydrocolloid*, **25**(2), 139–43.

PLAYNE M. J. and CRITTENDEN R. (1996). Commercially Available Oligosaccharides. *Bulletin of the International Dairy Federation*. **313**, 10–22.

RALET M. C., DELLAVALLE G. and THIBAULT J. F. (1993). Raw and Extruded Fiber from Pea Hulls .1. Composition and Physicochemical Properties. *Carbohydrate Polymers*. **20**(1), 17–23.

RANHOTRA G. (2008). In: *Advanced dietary fibre technology*. MCCLEARY B. V. and PROSKY L., eds. FL: Blackwell Science Ltd. 424–9.

RICHARDSON P. H., CLARK A. H., RUSSELL A. L., AYMARD P. and NORTON I. T. (1999). Galactomannan Gelation: A Thermal and Rheological Investigation Analyzed Using the Cascade Model. *Macromolecules*. **32**(5), 1519–27.

RIDLEY B. L., O'NEILL M. A. and MOHNEN D. A. (2001). Pectins: Structure, Biosynthesis, and Oligogalacturonide-Related Signaling. *Phytochemistry*. **57**(6), 929–67.

SEHGAL G., CHAUHAN G. S., and KUMBHAR B. K. (2002). Physical and Functional Properties of Mucilages from Yellow Mustard (*Sinapis alba* L.) and Different Varieties of Fenugreek (*Trigonella foenum-graecum* L.) Seeds. *Journal of Food Science and Technology-Mysore*. **39**(4), 367–70.

SWORN G. (2009). In: *Handbook of hydrocolloids*. PHILLIPS G. O. and WILLIAMS P. A., eds. FL: CRC Press. 186–227.

TAGGART P. (2009). In: *Handbook of hydrocolloids*. PHILLIPS G. O. and WILLIAMS P. A., eds. FL: CRC Press. 123–25.

TAKIGAMI S. (2009). In: *Handbook of hydrocolloids*. PHILLIPS G. O. and WILLIAMS P. A., eds. FL: CRC Press. 889–901.

TOSH S. M. and YADA S. (2010). Dietary Fibres in Pulse Seeds and Fractions: Characterization, Functional Attributes, and Applications. *Food Research International*. **43**(2), 450–60.

VALLI R. C. and MISKIEL F. J. (2001). In: *Handbook of dietary fiber*. CHO S. S. and DREHER M., eds. FL: Marcel Dekker, Inc. 695–720.

VERMA A. K. and BANERJEE R. (2010). Dietary fibre as Functional Ingredient in Meat Products: A Novel Approach for Healthy Living — a review. *Journal of Food Science and Technology*. **47**(3), 247–57.

VINKX C. J. A. and DELCOUR J. A. (1996). Rye (*Secale cereale* L.) Arabinoxylans: A Critical Review. *Journal of Cereal Science*. **24**(1), 1–14.

VOSE J. R. (1974). Chemical and Physical Studies of Mustard and Rapeseed Coats. *Cereal Chemistry*. **51**, 658–9.

WANG Q. and CUI S. (2005). In: *Food carbohydrates; chemistry, physical properties, and applications*. CUI S., ed. FL: Oxford: CRC Press.

WANG Q., ELLIS P. R. and ROSS-MURPHY S. B. (2003). Dissolution Kinetics of Guar Gum Powders—II. Effects of Concentration and Molecular Weight. *Carbohydrate Polymers*. **53**(1), 75–83.

WANG Q., ELLIS P. R. and ROSS-MURPHY S. B. (2006). Dissolution Kinetics of Guar Gum Powders—III. Effect of Particle Size. *Carbohydrate Polymers*. **64**(2), 239–46.

WANG Q., ELLIS P. R. and ROSS-MURPHY S. B. (2008). Dissolution Kinetics of Water-Soluble Polymers: The Guar Gum Paradigm. *Carbohydrate Polymers*. **74**(3), 519–26.

WIELINGA W. C. (2009) In: *Handbook of hydrocolloids*. PHILLIPS G. O. and WILLIAMS P. A., eds. FL: CRC Press. 228–51.

WILLIAMS P. A. and PHILLIPS G. O. (2009) In: *Handbook of hydrocolloids*. PHILLIPS G. O. and WILLIAMS P. A., eds. FL: CRC Press. 252–273.

WOOD P. J. (1994). Evaluation of Oat Bran as a Soluble Fibre Source. Characterization of Oat, β-Glucan and its Effects on Glycaemic Response. *Carbohydrate Polymers*. **25**(4), 331–6.

WU Y., CUI S. W., ESKIN N. A. M. & GOFF H. D. (2009a). Rheological Investigation of Synergistic Interactions between Galactomannans and Non-Pectic Polysaccharide Fraction from Water Soluble Yellow Mustard Mucilage. *Carbohydrate Polymers*. **78**(1), 112–16.

WU Y., CUI S. W., ESKIN N. A. M. & GOFF H. D. (2009b). An Investigation of Four Commercial Galactomannans on Their Emulsion and Rheological Properties. *Food Research International*. **42**(8), 1141–6.

WU Y., CUI S. W., ESKIN N. A. M. and GOFF H. D. (2012). A Molecular Modeling Approach to Understand Conformation–Functionality Relationships of Galactomannans with Different Mannose/Galactose Ratios. *Food Hydrocolloids*. **26**(2), 359–64.

YIN J., LIN H., LI J., WANG Y., CUI S. W., NIE S. and XIE M. (2012). Structural Characterization of a Highly Branched Polysaccharide from the Seeds of *Plantago asiatica* L. *Carbohydrate Polymers*. **87**(4), 2416–24.

YOTSUZUKA F. (2001). In: *Handbook of dietary fiber*. CHO S. S. and DREHER M., eds. FL: Marcel Dekker, Inc. 737–58.

ZAHN S., PEPKE F. and ROHM H. (2010). Effect of Inulin as a Fat Replacer on Texture and Sensory Properties of Muffins. *International Journal of Food Science and Technology*. **45**(12), 2531–7.

6

Consumption and consumer challenges of wholegrain foods

K. W. Dammann, Cargill, Incorporated, USA, D. Hauge, Grains for Health Foundation, USA, R. A. Rosen, Independent Consultant, USA, N. Schroeder, Johns Hopkins University, USA, and L. Marquart, Grains for Health Foundation and University of Minnesota, USA

DOI: 10.1533/9780857095787.1.120

Abstract: Whole grain intake is associated with health benefits such as reduced risk of cardiovascular disease. However, lack of a global definition of what constitutes a wholegrain food complicates interpretation and communication of research findings. Many populations underconsume wholegrain foods due to both internal factors (difficulty in identifying wholegrain foods and their unique sensory characteristics) and external factors (availability, cost, and the convenience of refined grains). Approaches to introducing wholegrain foods include promoting them early in life, employing the repeated exposures technique, and minimizing sensory differences. Emerging trends include improving the nutritional quality of the final product. Future research may focus on outcomes that improve the healthfulness and availability of grain-based foods, while collaboration will be necessary to ensure that pivotal findings reach industry in a timely manner. Whole grains offer a unique opportunity to enhance diets globally.

Key words: whole grain, fiber, consumption, consumer behavior.

6.1 Introduction

Despite accumulating evidence of the benefits of whole grain and dietary fiber intake for human health, the majority of the population's consumption continues to lag behind recommendations proposed by the scientific community and authoritative health agencies. International surveillance of whole grain intake and analysis of consumer trends have proven difficult, as the definitions of 'whole grain' and related serving sizes vary among experts (Lang and Jebb, 2003; Jones, 2010). Furthermore, whole grain intervention studies have produced mixed results, also complicating the communication of consistent messages around whole grains and health (Seal and Brownlee, 2010). This chapter examines whole grain consumption trends, along with dietary fiber intake, in various countries in the context of health-based recommendations. Internal and external factors that pose challenges to the consumption of wholegrain foods, such as taste and availability, are presented in greater depth in the subsequent sections. Future trends and opportunities for introducing more whole grain and fiber into the food supply are also discussed.

6.2 Whole grain and fiber consumption

6.2.1 Definitions

Wholegrain foods are defined as containing all the essential parts and naturally occurring nutrients of the entire grain seed. If the grain has been processed (e.g. cracked, crushed, rolled, extruded, and/or cooked), the food product should deliver approximately the same balance of nutrients that is found in the original grain seed (AACC, 2000; Whole Grains Council, 2007).

Dietary fiber is usually found in whole grains, fruits, vegetables, legumes, and nuts with various sub-components including cellulose, hemicellulose, pectins, beta-glucans, fructans, gums, mucilages, and non-polysaccharide lignins. Functional fiber is defined as the isolated components of non-digestible carbohydrates that produce positive physiological effects in humans (Slavin, 2005). Total fiber is the sum of dietary fiber and functional fiber (Slavin, 2005). The different fiber components may function in a variety of ways *via* viscosity, fermentability, bulking, volume, water-holding capacity, and binding, which help contribute to the beneficial physiological responses (Burton-Freeman, 2000). High-fiber foods are generally less energy-dense and palatable and are greater in volume than low-fiber foods, providing greater satiety (Porikos and Hagamen, 1986; Holt *et al.*, 1995; Rolls *et al.*, 1999; Saris, 2003).

6.2.2 Consumption data

In the US, the 2005 Dietary Guidelines for Americans for the first time recommended that at least half of grains consumed should be whole grains, with at least three or more 1-ounce equivalents coming from wholegrain products daily (USDA and USDHHS, 2005). Healthy People 2010 objectives, the latest iteration of national benchmarks designed for monitoring US progress towards health promotion and disease prevention, included an evaluation of the proportion of Americans who meet the Dietary Guidelines' recommended intake of six servings of grain products per day with at least three servings of whole grains. While the target for this Healthy People 2010 objective was set at 50%, a recent progress report indicated that the percentage of Americans meeting this recommendation dropped from 4% to 3% between 1994–6 and 2003–4, with approximately 7% of children's and 10% of adults' total grain intake in 2003–4 coming from whole grains (USDHHS, 2008). Healthy People 2020 objectives released late in

December 2010 also continue to monitor the adequacy of whole grain intake (USDHHS, 2010). Shortly thereafter, the 2010 Dietary Guidelines were released, echoing the previous whole grain recommendations and also putting into perspective the imbalance of the American diet with respect to overall grain intake. The new guidelines emphasize that Americans typically exceed recommendations for total grain intake, yet whole grain (and dietary fiber) intake is indeed insufficient, and, thus, dietary guidance should be directed more specifically at increasing whole grain intake by substituting whole grains for refined grains. However, lack of standards for quantifying the wholegrain content of foods can make such recommendations difficult to put into practice (USDA and USDHHS, 2010).

Mean whole grain intake among most age groups in the US generally equates to less than one serving per day. O'Neil *et al.* (2010) recently examined Americans' dietary quality using 1998–2004 National Health and Nutrition Examination (NHANES) data and defined whole grain servings in terms of one-ounce equivalents from the United States Department of Agriculture's (USDA) Pyramid database. For adults aged 19 to 50 years, mean intake of whole grains was 0.63 servings per day, and for adults aged 51 years or more, mean intake was slightly higher at 0.77 servings. Results also showed that a mere 4.8% and 6.6% of individuals in the two respective age groups met the recommendations of at least three servings of whole grains per day (O'Neil *et al.*, 2010). Children's whole grain intake was reportedly similar at 0.59 servings per day for 6–12-year-olds and 0.63 servings per day for 13–18-year-olds (Zanovec *et al.*, 2010). The most recent estimate of dietary fiber intake for Americans aged 2 years and older is 15.2 g/day, in comparison to the Daily Value for dietary fiber of 25 g/day (USDA ARS, 2010).

The majority of Americans consume whole grains in the form of ready-to-eat cereals, followed by yeast breads, hot cereal, and popcorn, according to data from the 2001–2 NHANES (Bachman *et al.*, 2008). Other food products such as crackers, grain-based desserts, pancakes, and rice make smaller contributions to total whole grain intake. On the other hand, major sources of non-whole grains are yeast breads, grain-based desserts, and pizza, suggesting that, with increased functionality and palatability of whole grains as food ingredients, substitution of refined grains for whole grains in such products is certainly a potential avenue for gradually increasing the American population's whole grain intake (Bachman *et al.*, 2008).

It is noteworthy that US dietary surveillance data reflect whole grain intake estimates up until 2004, while specific whole grain intake recommendations made *via* the Dietary Guidelines were introduced in 2005 (Mancino *et al.*, 2008). Thus, ascertaining the true impact of such dietary guidance on consumer behavior has posed a challenge. Publication of NHANES 2007–8 will likely shed light on more current trends in whole grain consumption in the near future. Other organizations such as the American Dietetic Association (ADA) and the Whole Grains Council have presented results of surveys commissioned to help further understand consumer behavior, including that related to whole grain intake. According to the

ADA's 'Nutrition and You: Trends 2008' survey of 783 adults aged 18-years-old and up, 56% reported increasing their intake of wholegrain foods, a trend particularly more prevalent among the 18–34-year-old age group. However, 36% reported no change over the past five years (ADA, 2008). A consumer survey conducted by the NPD Group and presented by the Whole Grains Council at the 2009 'Make Half Your Grains Whole Conference' provided data from 1998 to 2008. The NPD Group sampled 2000 US households with the intent of capturing a nationally representative sample of Americans. Fourteen days' worth of dietary intake data, including at-home and away-from-home foods consumed, were collected. Key findings showed an estimated 20% increase in whole grain consumption among Americans since 2005, with the largest increase among 18–34-year-olds, similar to the results of the ADA's findings (Whole Grains Council, 2009a). Yet, despite reported increases in consumption, mean intake of whole grains was still less than one serving per day. Only 11% of total grains consumed were whole grains in 2008, not much of an improvement since the 2003–4 NHANES data were published. Findings from the International Food Information Council (IFIC) '2010 Food and Health Survey' of 1024 individuals also indicated that, of those who have heard of 'fiber' and 'whole grains,' more than 70% are trying to increase their intakes (IFIC, 2010). While these trends appear to be moving in a positive direction, consumer behavior evolves at a slow pace (Rowe *et al.*, 2011a).

The inclusion of a whole grain message in dietary recommendations throughout Europe varies widely, but, for the most part, bodies disseminating such authoritative guidance encourage intake of wholegrain foods. For example, in the UK, Germany, Austria, Switzerland, and Greece, whole grains are specifically noted as preferable in the context of choosing bread, cereal, starches, and other grains (UK Food Standards Agency, n.d.; Health Grain, 2006; Supreme Scientific Health Council, 1999). In Denmark, four servings of whole grain per day are recommended for citizens (National Food Institute, 2008).

Similarly to US adults and children, whole grain intake in the UK is low. Results from the Dietary and Nutritional Survey of British Adults, which included participants aged 16–64 years, indicated that whole grain intake has declined throughout Great Britain from surveys conducted between 1986–7 and 2000–1 (Thane *et al.*, 2007). In this study, intake of foods containing ≥10% whole grain was assessed. Mean whole grain intake decreased from 29 g/day to 23 g/day over this time period, while the median intake fell from 16 g/day to 14 g/day. Key sources of whole grains were bread and breakfast cereals in 1986–7. By 2000–1, breakfast cereal became the top contributor, with bread following closely behind. The most common type of whole grain consumed was wheat in comparison to other whole grains such as oats, rye, and barley. Among older British adults (aged 65 years or more), median weekly intake of whole grains was five servings, with approximately one-third of the sample not consuming any whole grains on a daily basis (Lang *et al.*, 2003). National data have also demonstrated sub-optimal whole grain intake among British youth aged 4–18 years. Mean intake in 1997 was 13 g/day, with a median intake of 7 g/day. As for British adults, breakfast cereals and breads were the top two types of food contributing most to whole grain intake (Thane *et al.*, 2005).

In contrast to UK dietary patterns, estimated whole grain intake among Finnish adults is much higher, at 218 g/day for men and 150 g/day for women, in which a major source of whole grain in the diet is rye bread (Montonen *et al.*, 2003). Relatively higher whole grain intakes have also been observed among German youth participating in the Dortmund Nutritional and Anthropometric Longitudinally Designed (DONALD) Study, during which nutrition and health data were collected at various time points between 1988 and 2007. Whole grains were categorized based on the US Food and Drug Administration (FDA) definition and absolute intake was calculated (g/day) (Alexy *et al.*, 2010). Mean intake among age groups in the sample ranged from 20 to 33 g/day, with the highest intakes reported for 13–18-year-olds. However, whole grain intake expressed as a percent of total grain intake decreased with age (Alexy *et al.*, 2010).

In Canada, the Food Guide was revised in 2007 to include recommendations for whole grain intake similar to those of the US, encouraging consumption of whole grains as half of total grains consumed (Health Canada, 2007a). However, whole grain intake data are also lacking for this geography. Results from the Quebec Nutrition Survey conducted in 1990 showed that just 44% of the dietary recalls conducted among 2104 adults surveyed included whole grains, and the mean intake of wholegrain breads and cereal was 35 g/day, although how whole grains were defined in this study was not specified (Beaudry *et al.*, 1998). It is important to note that the definition of whole grain in Canada is remarkably different from that in the US: '100% whole wheat' does not ensure the product is wholegrain, because food regulations allow much of the germ to be removed in 'wholewheat' flour (Health Canada, 2007b). Other research has shown that since the mid-1970s carbohydrate intake has increased by 18% in Canadian diets, and fiber intake has also risen from 11 g to almost 14 g (Peng, 2004). Results from a recent consumer survey showed that 10% of Canadian adults meet the recommendation for whole grain intake, but this proportion decreased with age (Canadian Grocer, 2011).

Dietary guidance in Australia also recommends intake of plenty of grain-based foods (at least four) with an emphasis on whole grains (NHMRC, 2003). Australians' whole grain intake has been estimated at 1.45 servings per day or about one-third of their total grain intake (Go Grains Health and Nutrition Ltd, 2010). Yet, interest in whole grains, likely because of their touted health benefits, appears to be growing among this population. Nearly 44% of Australians have reported increasing their whole grain consumption in the past two years, while about three-quarters have expressed desire to learn more about the benefits of whole grains (Griffiths, 2010).

Strong epidemiological data from other regions of the world, such as South America, Asia, and Africa, are lacking with regard to evaluating whole grain and fiber intake. With the nutrition transition, processed and refined grains are increasingly making their way into the diet, in effect reducing overall intake of dietary fiber and other nutritional aspects of whole grains. For example, since the

1970s, obesity rates in the Middle East and across North Africa have dramatically risen (Mehio *et al.*, 2010). Per capita per day total energy supply has also risen, with dietary patterns exhibiting a shift away from traditional food habits, including decreased consumption of wholegrain cereals (Mehio *et al.*, 2010). In Mexico, results of the 2006 National Health and Nutrition Survey demonstrated that dietary patterns departing from the traditional maize-based diet (i.e. characterized by either more refined foods and sweets or overall greater dietary diversity, including animal products, non-maize carbohydrates, saturated fat, fruits, and vegetables) were associated with increased risk of overweight and obesity (Flores *et al.*, 2010). In sum, inadequate whole grain consumption is a global issue, and the health of many would benefit from a diet rich in whole grains.

6.2.3 Socio-demographic differences

Socio-demographic factors such as gender, age, race, ethnicity, income, and education have been associated with whole grain consumption. In the US, older survey data (from the 1990s) indicated that, while males typically consumed more whole grains than females, females consumed a higher proportion of their total grain intake as whole grains (Lin and Yen, 2007). The US Hispanic population demonstrated relatively higher whole grain consumption than white, black, and Asian sub-groups, and greater intakes have also been reported among individuals with higher levels of income and education (Adams and Engstrom, 2000; Lin and Yen, 2007). Thane *et al.* (2007) reported no significant gender differences in whole grain intake for British adults, though whole grain intake increased with age. Additionally, in Britain (Thane *et al.*, 2007) and in France (Touvier *et al.*, 2010), lower education levels and manual labor occupations were also linked to lower whole grain intakes compared with those with higher education and in different (non-manual) occupations. Whole grain consumption may be lower for those with lower incomes and those of different racial/ethnic identities due to a lack of resources (including money and availability in their food environment) and cultural dietary habits that exclude or have begun to exclude whole grains as eating patterns become more Westernized. Nonetheless, whole grain consumption remains low regardless of socio-demographic characteristics. Therefore, understanding the magnitude of the influence of these inherent differences across various socio-demographic groups may inform strategies for increasing whole grain intake among these populations.

6.3 Wholegrain foods and consumer challenges: internal (personal) factors

6.3.1 Identification of whole grains and high fiber foods

One factor that may contribute to lower consumption of whole grains relative to dietary guidance may be consumers' inability to correctly identify whole grains and high fiber foods. One governmental initiative to assist consumers in the identification of healthier foods was the use of health claims on package labels. In the early 1990s, the initial dietary health claims were developed and implemented as a strategy to guide consumer food choices *via* food labeling by helping consumers to identify whole grains and sources of dietary fiber and helping to increase their understanding of diet–disease relationships (US Congress, 1990). In July 1999, the US FDA approved the first whole grain health claim, stating: 'Diets rich in wholegrain foods and other plant foods and low in total fat, saturated fat, and cholesterol, may help reduce the risk of heart disease and certain cancers.' In 2003, the whole grain health claim was modified to state: 'Diets rich in whole grain foods and other plant foods, and low in saturated fat and cholesterol, may help reduce the risk of heart disease' (US FDA CFSAN, 2003). The FDA mandates that foods labeled with the whole grain health claim must contain 51% or more wholegrain ingredients by weight per reference amount and be low or moderate in fat (up to 6.5 g fat per reference amount) (US FDA CFSAN, 2003). Additionally, in 2006, the Whole Grains Council modified their wholegrain stamps to help consumers identify legitimate wholegrain products (Whole Grains Council, 2006). A wholegrain stamp that reads '8 g or more per serving' can be used on products that offer half a serving or more of whole grain. A 100% wholegrain stamp that reads '16 g or more per serving' can be used on products made with all of the grain (e.g. flour, crushed grain, intact kernel) as whole grain. See Table 6.1 for other US whole grain and fiber health claims.

In other industrialized countries, the whole grain requirement and acceptance of whole grain health claims differ per country. In the UK, the Joint Health Claims Initiative agreed that foods containing 51% or more wholegrain ingredients by weight per serving constituted a whole grain. In addition, the whole grain contains the germ, bran, and endosperm, and the term whole grain includes major cereal grains like wheat, rice, maize, and oats (Binns, 2010). The allowed health claim from 2002 stated: 'People with a healthy heart tend to eat more whole grain foods as part of a healthy lifestyle' (JHCI, 2002). In 2003, the Swedish Nutrition Foundation provided whole grain guidelines stating the product should contain at least 50% whole grain on a dry matter basis. The 'Keyhole' criteria should be fulfilled when applicable, meaning the food should also meet certain requirements for at least one of the following: fat, sugar, salt, or dietary fiber. Further, flour, flakes, and grains of cereals should be 100% whole grain; two-thirds whole grain and a maximum of 13% sugar for breakfast cereals (and less than 10% fat), gruels, and porridges; and two-thirds whole grain and a maximum of 10% fat for bread biscuits, rusks, and pasta products. The accepted Swedish health claim reads: 'A healthy lifestyle and a well balanced diet rich in whole grain products reduces the risk for (coronary) heart disease. The product X is rich in whole grains (contains Y% of whole grain)' (SNF, 2004). Similarly to Sweden, the whole grain requirement in Denmark is ≥50 % wholegrain ingredients on a dry matter basis (EFSA Panel on Dietetic Products, Nutrition and Allergies, 2010). In contrast, wholegrain bread must be 90% whole grain according to standards set in Germany (EFSA Panel on Dietetic Products, Nutrition and Allergies, 2010). Although health-related interest in whole grains continues to increase in Australia, the

Table 6.1 Other US whole grain and fiber related health claims

Ingredient/ Source	Year authorized	Soluble fiber per reference amount customarily consumed of the food product	Model claim wording
Whole oat products	1997	≥ 0.75 g	3 grams or more per day of beta-glucan soluble fiber from whole oats, in a diet low in saturated fat and cholesterol, may reduce the risk of heart disease.
Psyllium	1998	≥ 1.7 g	Diets low in saturated fat and cholesterol that include 7 grams of soluble fiber per day from psyllium may reduce the risk of heart disease by lowering cholesterol.
Oatrim	2003	≥ 0.75 g	Diets low in saturated fat and cholesterol that include 3 grams of soluble fiber per day from Oatrim may reduce the risk of heart disease. One serving of [name of food] provides [x] grams of this soluble fiber.
Wholegrain and dry milled barley products	2006	≥ 0.75 g	Soluble fiber from foods such as [name of food], as part of a diet low in saturated fat and cholesterol, may reduce the risk of heart disease. A serving of [name of food] supplies [x] grams of the soluble fiber necessary per day to have this effect.
Barley betafiber (concentrated beta-glucan soluble fiber)	2008	≥ 0.75 g	Diets low in saturated fat and cholesterol that include 3 grams of beta-glucan soluble fiber per day from barley betafiber may reduce the risk of heart disease. A serving of [name of food] supplies [x] grams of this soluble fiber.

Source: Code of Federal Regulations, 2011.

proposed health claim was rejected as Food Standards Australia/New Zealand stated that the whole grain intake and coronary heart disease relationship does not reach a convincing level of evidence (FSANZ, 2006). The rejected claim was as follows: 'A healthy lifestyle and a well balanced diet rich in whole grain products reduces the risk for (coronary) heart disease. The product X is rich in whole grains (contains Y% of whole grain)' (FSANZ, 2006).

Identification of a wholegrain food is extremely difficult because a universal definition for a wholegrain ingredient and/or wholegrain food does not exist, and, as a result, labeling of wholegrain foods is inconsistent and confusing

(Kantor *et al.*, 2001; Britten *et al.*, 2006). One may carefully read labels and purchase high-fiber foods or multi-grain products, but remain unaware as to whether the product is wholegrain. Consumers appear to have a limited understanding regarding the differences between whole grains, high fiber foods, and fiber supplements. This ultimately limits the consumer's ability to identify, select, and purchase wholegrain foods to incorporate into their diet. Furthermore, it is likely that if parents cannot identify whole grains, then wholegrain foods will not be made available to children in the home.

Whole grains are broadly recognized as a food or a component of a food group in the US (Marquart *et al.*, 2006). In addition to consumers, even food service personnel and nutrition professionals appear to have limited knowledge regarding specific application of the whole grain concept (Warber *et al.*, 1996; Adams and Engstrom, 2000; Kennedy and Davis, 2000; Kantor *et al.*, 2001; Chase *et al.*, 2003a; Chase *et al.*, 2003b; Lang *et al.*, 2003; Chase *et al.*, 2004; Britten *et al.*, 2006; Burgess-Champoux *et al.*, 2006; Marquart *et al.*, 2006; Chan *et al.*, 2009; Hesse *et al.*, 2009). Studies have reported that consumers said they look for the words 'whole grain' when finding wholegrain products (Burgess-Champoux *et al.*, 2006; Britten *et al.*, 2006). Burgess-Champoux *et al.* (2006) also found that adults generalized whole grains as 'wheat' or 'having more fiber' and lacked confidence in correctly identifying wholegrain foods. Nutrition professionals and food service personnel may also lack knowledge in identifying wholegrain foods (Warber *et al.*, 1996; Chase *et al.*, 2003a; Marquart *et al.*, 2006). One study examined the beliefs about wholegrain foods among food and nutrition professionals, health club members, participants in the Special Supplemental Nutrition Program for Women, Infants, and Children (WIC), and state fair attendees (Marquart *et al.*, 2006). Interestingly, the largest percentage of food and nutrition professionals reported wholewheat bread as a wholegrain food, while only a few reported wholegrain bread and even fewer reported wholegrain cereal as wholegrain foods. Hesse *et al.* (2009) found that some school food service personnel do not have the necessary resources and skills to identify, purchase, serve, and promote wholegrain foods in school food services. Their lack of understanding of whole grain definitions may be attributed to confusion regarding the use of grams, percentages, or ingredients as a means to identify the amount of whole grain in a food item (Hesse *et al.*, 2009). Chan *et al.* (2009) also reported limited knowledge of wholegrain foods, ingredient definitions, and use of product label information in ordering and purchasing among school food service personnel. Three general categories were used to identify a wholegrain food: 'descriptors,' 'percent whole grain,' and 'label ingredients.' For the wholegrain food 'descriptors,' 'fiber' was the most frequently mentioned. For 'percent whole grain,' most participants knew that wholegrain foods contain at least 50% whole grain. However, most did not know the definition for the US whole grain health claim. Additionally, only a few school food service personnel could identify the three components of a whole grain: bran, germ, and endosperm.

Although whole grains are widely considered an integral part of a healthy diet, one study with Canadian consumers showed that they consistently identified fruits and vegetables as part of a healthy diet, whereas grains they generally did not (Paquette, 2005). Results from a recent TNS Canadian Facts Survey of 1015 adults, reported by the Baking Association of Canada, may shed some light on why whole grain intake appears to be low in Canada. Approximately 46% of respondents agreed with the statement: 'Carbohydrates, including those found in whole grains, are fattening' (Pasut, 2005). Thus, understanding how consumers perceive public health messages and debunking diet-related myths, which may vary by geography, will be critical to the success of improving their dietary habits.

Encouragingly, appropriate curricula for targeted demographics may improve consumers' ability to identify wholegrain foods. In schools, educational interventions may improve both parents' and children's ability to identify whole grains. A school-based pilot study involving older elementary children found the combination of a classroom curriculum on whole grains, greater availability of whole grains at school, and family-oriented activities like interactive newsletters and grocery tours increased whole grain consumption by one serving and decreased refined grain consumption by one serving (Burgess-Champoux *et al.*, 2008). These children also improved their ability to identify wholegrain foods. In another intervention, two versions of a supermarket tour for parents and children were developed to improve parents' skills in identifying whole grains and children's ability to define whole and refined grain terms and identify wholegrain foods (Lafferty *et al.*, 2006). The intervention was successful in increasing both parents' and children's ability to identify whole grains with either one field trip or one evening session, and it also enhanced their ability to confidently select wholegrain foods at the point-of-purchase in the supermarket. Therefore, even basic education programs designed to improve children's skills in identifying whole grains could help to increase consumption of these foods. However, it is important to emphasize that the educational components should be hands-on and age-appropriate for the targeted demographic. On the other end of the age spectrum, in a senior-based curriculum intervention, individuals attending congregate meals at senior centers were provided education on how to identify a wholegrain food. After completing the curriculum, their ability to identify whole grains significantly improved from 45% to 62% (Ellis *et al.*, 2005).

Additional work is necessary to facilitate communication between industry, academia, and consumers to clearly delineate definitions of whole grains and dietary fiber and their beneficial effects. Developing a definition with common ground for both the consumer and industry will not only help consumers better identify whole grains, but also help capture more accurately whole grain consumption patterns and their relationship to chronic disease risks.

6.3.2 Lack of knowledge about whole grains and fiber in relation to disease prevention

Although many consumers associate whole grains with more fiber in helping to maintain regularity, being generally good for you, and being less processed than refined grains, they appear to lack a deeper level of understanding that links whole grain consumption with reduced risk of specific chronic diseases (Chase *et al.*, 2003b; Burgess-Champoux *et al.*, 2006; Marquart *et al.*, 2006). Many consumers do not understand that their risk of heart disease, diabetes, and cancer may be lowered when whole grains are included as part of a healthy eating pattern (Adams and Engstrom, 2000; Kantor *et al.*, 2001; Lang *et al.*, 2003; Smith *et al.*, 2003; Marquart *et al.*, 2006). Therefore, increasing general awareness of the substantial health benefits of wholegrain foods may be one approach to motivate consumers to increase their consumption. Ujszaszy *et al.* (2004) reported that a majority (77%) among school food service personnel agreed that the inclusion of wholegrain foods in school meals would provide health benefits for their students. Although school food service personnel attributed a wide array of health benefits to whole grains, such as reducing the risk of heart disease, diabetes, and cancer, and aiding in weight management, little specificity was noted for any one chronic disease. More recent studies also indicate that school food service personnel associate wholegrain foods with non-specific health benefits (Hesse *et al.*, 2009; Chan *et al.*, 2009).

The average consumer is becoming more aware of whole grains and health. Approximately 81% of US consumers recognize the term 'whole grains' (IFIC, 2009), yet there is a disconnect when translating this knowledge into action. When consumers were asked open-ended questions in an IFIC survey ($n = 1064$), only 33% reported attempting to consume specific foods for health reasons, with 3.5% seeking out whole grains (IFIC, 2009). In Australia, approximately 400 adults were assessed as to their readiness to switch to a plant-based diet, which included whole grains (Lea *et al.*, 2006). Most respondents were in the precontemplation stage with very few in the maintenance stage. Those in the precontemplation stage lacked awareness regarding the health benefits of a plant-based diet, whereas those in the action or maintenance stages recognized the health benefits of the plant-based diet. In a survey of first-year college students, those who consumed the recommended number of whole grain servings displayed greater knowledge of dietary guidelines for major food categories than those not meeting the recommended servings (Kolodinsky *et al.*, 2007). In another study, college nutrition students were introduced to a variety of whole grains (Lacey, 2007). Results from an evaluation showed that nutrition students had only ever cooked two whole grains before the experiment and had only tasted four whole grains in total. From this project, the nutrition students gained greater understanding of how to appropriately educate future clients about wholegrain foods. Thus, more in-depth knowledge, training, and effective communication skills for future dietitians related to whole grains would likely improve the public's knowledge on whole grains and help to further increase consumption levels.

6.3.3 Lack of familiarity and sensory attributes

In addition to consumers being unfamiliar with different whole grains and their health benefits, the distinct sensory qualities of whole grains may also contribute to an overall lower intake. Several studies have shown that consumers tend not to like the taste (dryness), palatability (bland), appearance, texture or color of wholegrain foods (Chang and Chambers, 1992; Adams and Engstrom, 2000; Murray *et al.*, 2002; Bakke *et al.*, 2007). Of these sensory qualities, the increased bitter taste and possibly the coarser, rougher, and harsher texture associated with wheat bran are the most innately disliked. Because people differ in their perceptions of taste and texture, these perceptions lead to variable preferences. Some people perceive bitter compounds more strongly than others. These people have functional receptors that create a perceived bitterness of certain compounds like 6-*n*-propylthiouracil (PROP) (Dinehart *et al.*, 2006). Further, PROP tasters tend to experience a higher intensity of oral stimuli than non-tasters (Duffy *et al.*, 2004). If some consumers have an increased sensitivity to bitterness or other sensations, then a wholegrain product may be less preferred to a refined grain product. However, even if whole grains are preferred by one family member within a household, a household preference for more familiar products will have greater influence on grain purchases to appease preferences for most family members (Burgess-Champoux *et al.*, 2006) and not waste money on uneaten foods (Chase *et al.*, 2003b).

Wholegrain foods have remained unfamiliar to consumers, who have often not associated brand-name foods with whole grains (Marquart *et al.*, 2006). Since consumers think of whole grains as part of a food group, strategies to help them become more familiar with whole grains may work similarly to strategies used in fruit and vegetable promotion. Once whole grains become a more familiar food product, identifying them should be less of a barrier to consumption. According to Ujszaszy *et al.* (2004), school food service personnel were familiar with wholegrain foods, somewhat or very motivated to serve wholegrain foods in their school cafeterias, and somewhat or very motivated to look for wholegrain alternatives to include in school meals. More recent studies indicate that school food service personnel are serving wholegrain foods in school meals on a regular basis (Chan *et al.*, 2009; Hesse *et al.*, 2009).

Unfamiliarity appears to be a major barrier to children's consumption of wholegrain foods. Burgess-Champoux *et al.* (2006) found that most children preferred white, mild, soft breads without particles, nuts, or crusts. After children tried 50% wholegrain cheesebreads, they reported liking the taste and texture, but more than half did not like the appearance. Additionally, children liked the specific characteristics of the wholegrain cereal and 50% wholegrain cheesebread tested, but they were less likely to choose these test foods if served in the school lunch program (Burgess-Champoux *et al.*, 2006). These findings led the authors to believe that, if children are given a choice between whole grains and refined grains, it is not certain that they will choose the wholegrain product. Similarly to most adults, children are unable to clearly identify wholegrain foods (Burgess-Champoux *et al.*, 2006). In another study examining whole grain acceptability, children readily accepted common wholegrain foods such as corn bread and brown rice, whereas less common whole grains such as barley were not as well accepted (Gellar *et al.*, 2009). Thus, familiarity plays a major role in whole grain selection, and children need to be exposed to 'friendly' wholegrain foods and taught how to identify wholegrain products for these foods to become more familiar and to further enhance selection of whole grains outside the home.

Additional factors that influence the overall quality and acceptability of baked wholegrain products include: 1) the stability, storage, and handling of the grain ingredients; 2) the product formula (including levels of sugar, salt, and other ingredients that influence product flavor, texture, and appearance) and processing methods (including mixing and baking); 3) the storage and handling of the baked products (including packaging, shelf life, and storage conditions); and 4) the time period the products sit in the open air before consumed (freshness). As measured by flavor, texture, and appearance, these attributes are important factors for successful introduction of wholegrain products in the home, school cafeterias, and other venues.

6.4 Wholegrain foods and consumer challenges: external factors

6.4.1 Availability in food supply and in specific food environments

In the past, limited availability was indicated as a significant barrier to whole grain consumption (Kantor *et al.*, 2001). Over the last decade, an increasing stream of wholegrain products has emerged in the marketplace. In 2000, 168 wholegrain products were launched (Whole Grains Council, 2008). Mintel 'New Product Launch History' data reported by the Whole Grains Council indicate that over 12 000 new wholegrain products have been introduced since then, with most items in the breakfast cereals category, followed by the bakery and snacks category, and fewer items in the meals and side dishes category (Mintel Global New Products Database, 2010).

The availability of wholegrain foods in the retail marketplace hinges on consumer demand along with cost and industry's ability to produce wholegrain products and maintain an adequate return on investment. Recent reports indicate that the production of wholegrain ingredients and wholegrain foods continues to increase due to consumer demand (Gelski, 2007). Therefore, driving forces behind whole grain availability and consumption may be less associated with consumer demand and more an issue of manufacturers offering new wholegrain products or reformulated grain products that include whole grains (Mancino *et al.*, 2008).

While the average number of new wholegrain product introductions by food manufacturers quadrupled between 2001 and 2006 (Golan *et al.*, 2009), the question remains: in order to facilitate adhering to the Dietary Guidelines, are half of the grain products available to consumers whole grains? A small-scaled study of a US northeastern supermarket chain showed that the numbers were close, with wholegrain foods making up almost 35% of all the grain food products on shelf (Whole Grains Council, 2009a). Whole grains from hot cereal, cold cereal, bread, dry pasta, crackers, and cookies contributed 80%, 68%, 39%, 22%, 20%, and 6%, respectively, to total grain products available within that food category (Whole

Grains Council, 2009a). This study focused on the availability of wholegrain products in a large supermarket chain, but what about availability of whole grains in other food establishments?

'Food deserts' is a fairly new term that was first coined in 1990 by a Nutrition Task Team to describe neighborhoods with few or no food outlets (Beaumont *et al.*, 1995). Since that time, research suggests that food deserts exist and are more prevalent in disadvantaged areas; however, the definition and subsequent identification of food deserts have been inconsistent (Cummins and Macintyre, 2002; USDA, 2009; Walker *et al.*, 2010; Gordon *et al.*, 2011). Whole grain availability in food deserts has not historically been reported in the literature. However, research has indicated that foods available in both urban and rural food deserts were of inferior quality to foods found in non-food deserts (Henderickson *et al.*, 2006); grocery stores were found to have more healthier foods available than convenience stores (Glanz *et al.*, 2007). Jetter and Cassady (2005) found that 100% wholewheat bread and grain products were less likely to be available in low-income neighborhood grocery stores, with 100% wholewheat bread being less available at the end of the month in small independent grocery stores. Kantor *et al.* (2001) also found that wholegrain breads, breakfast cereals, and brown rice and tortilla chips were widely available at conventional supermarkets, but other products like bulgur or quinoa may only be available at health food stores, specialty stores, or ethnic stores, and through the Internet (Kantor *et al.*, 2001), making these products less available to people with lower incomes. Although many food deserts have less healthier options, changes in the WIC food packages being implemented in the US may impact the likelihood of an increased presence of nutritious food options in small grocery stores and corner stores. The new food packages include allocations for the purchase of whole grains, low-fat milk, fruits, and vegetables, and may help to increase (and maintain) demand for these foods in stores in neighborhoods that are home to high concentrations of WIC participants (USDA, 2009).

The limited availability of healthier food options like whole grains is not exclusive to food deserts and low-income neighborhoods. Much of the commercial food business, including school food service programs, has not experienced an increased demand for whole grains as observed for foods consumed at home. The Whole Grains Council (2009b) assessed attitudes towards and implementation of wholegrain foods in schools. Results indicated that more than half of the schools served whole grains at every meal, with breads (e.g. rolls, hamburger and hot dog buns), pizza, and chips topping the list of lunch items, while breakfast commonly included wholegrain cold cereals, granola bars, and breakfast bars. Although these schools exhibited successful incorporation of whole grains into their menus, barriers cited were cost, taste, appearance, and availability of the actual products. Resistant staff, confusion in identifying wholegrain products, and more time and labor needed for preparation of whole grains were environmental barriers (Whole Grains Council, 2009b). Chan *et al.* (2009) reported similar barriers to introducing more wholegrain foods into schools, including sensory characteristics, availability, and cost. Availability of wholegrain products in schools may also be related to the schools' location and size, as well as distance from distribution hubs, which may have an effect on the service, quality, and demand for wholegrain products (Hesse *et al.*, 2009; Rosen *et al.*, 2011). Moreover, few wholegrain products have been made available to schools through the USDA Schools/Child Nutrition Commodity Program. In 2007, only nine out of the 45 grain products available to school food programs contained whole grains (Whole Grains Council, 2010a). Wholegrain pasta, rather common on supermarket shelves, was not available until the 2008–9 school year (USDA FNS, 2010).

The availability of whole grains in smaller business settings, such as childcare centers, is also limited. It is recommended that childcare facilities provide half to two-thirds of the Recommended Dietary Allowances for children who attend for the full day (ADA, 2005). For children's daily intake from the grains category, five ounces are recommended, of which 2.5 ounces should be whole grain. In a recent study that investigated whether these recommendations were being met by childcare centers in North Carolina, Ball *et al.* (2008) found that all children were served a grain product during meals. However, the ratio of refined grains to whole grains fell far below 2:1, with 2.09 ounces of total grains served, including just 0.39 ounces of whole grain (Ball *et al.*, 2008).

Due to the demand for whole grains originating from a policy perspective rather than from consumer demand, retail and commercial food chains have not been as quick to implement changes in their grain offerings. Some retail stores, such as Great Harvest Bread Company and Whole Foods, have been serving whole grains since they opened, and several other independent and chain restaurants, including California Pizza Kitchen and Jack in the Box, have been gradually incorporating more whole grains into menu items to meet their customers' requests for whole grains (Whole Grains Council, 2010b). Whole grains do appear to be gaining some traction on restaurant menus, as a recent survey of 76 national chain restaurant headquarters showed that 41 chains offered at least one whole grain choice on the daily menu (Whole Grains Council, 2009b).

6.4.2 Cost

Some may argue that eating healthily costs more money. Bernstein *et al.* (2010) evaluated the cost of dietary patterns of US women as related to prevention of cardiovascular disease. In this study, a healthier diet was more costly; however, large improvements in the diet could be achieved without spending significantly more money. The authors recommended increasing spending on healthier, nutrient-dense items such as nuts, soy, other beans, and whole grains, while decreasing spending on red and processed meats and high-fat dairy products (Bernstein *et al.*, 2010). With respect to whole grains, it is well known that the cost difference associated with switching to whole grains is a commonly cited barrier to their purchase. Historically, various wholegrain products have been considered specialty items and, thus, were produced in smaller quantities (Buzby *et al.*, 2005). Therefore, the higher cost of manufacturing and marketing whole grains relative to the cost of refined grains, which benefit from economies of scale, could stifle the demand for whole grains. If the price differential is due solely to economies of scale, then an expanding whole grain market, fueled by demand, would ease existing price differentials and further increase the demand for whole grains. However, this may not be the whole picture. According to the most recent Consumer Pricing Index Detailed Report, wholewheat bread in the US costs on average $0.40 more than a loaf of refined bread ($1.76 versus $1.36) (Crawford *et al.*, 2010). Similar price gaps have been reported elsewhere, indicating about a 25% increase in the cost of wholegrain products over their refined counterparts (Kantor *et al.*, 2001; Buzby *et al.*, 2005). Some products, such as cookies, crackers, and chips, may be close to or equal to the cost of the refined equivalent (Whole Grains Council, 2009a). Added cost in the same food category may dissuade consumers from purchasing some wholegrain products for their household.

Although the added cost of whole grains may seem relatively minor for individuals to incur, especially given the increased health benefits, the monetary impact becomes more difficult for schools and other institutions to face. As previously mentioned, the cost of wholegrain items for schools has been reported as an issue in the attainment of wholegrain products for their menus (Chan *et al.*, 2009; Hesse *et al.*, 2009; Rosen *et al.*, submitted), rendering it an unrealistic change. The cost for schools to purchase wholegrain items compared with their refined counterparts may be as little as a penny per serving, but this penny per serving times the thousands of lunches served daily can turn into a substantial amount for a district to incur. The hardship of increased cost for wholegrain products and other healthy, nutrient-dense foods in American schools was recently acknowledged in the report *Solving the Problem of Childhood Obesity within a Generation*, which recommends the provision of 'economic incentives for healthy foods such as fruits, vegetables and whole grains' to schools as part of a concerted effort to fight the epidemic of childhood obesity (White House Task Force on Childhood Obesity, 2010). Despite the incurred cost, school districts will have to make these changes due to the new requirements of the updated nutrition standards for school lunches, which mandate that by 2014, all grains offered be wholegrain-rich (FNS, 2012).

6.4.3 Convenience

Along with cost as a major factor influencing food purchasing behavior, many consumers, whether individuals or at the commercial level, value convenience. In the US, consumption patterns have shifted towards more away-from-home foods with less time spent on at-home food preparation. Grain-based foods are low cost, energy-dense items that are typically less expensive than fruits and vegetables (Drewnowski, 2010). Therefore, when families, food service directors, or retail businesses are looking for foods that are convenient and inexpensive, they often purchase grain-based foods. However, many of these foods, including snack foods, can contain significant amounts of added fat, sugar, and sodium to enhance palatability and, in some cases, extend shelf life. In recent years, this notion of added sugar has been recognized by various food manufacturers, who have since pledged to decrease sugar in various products such as ready-to-eat cereals. Additionally, manufacturers have begun to incorporate whole grains into many convenience foods to meet various nutrition standards set by schools. Some of these products, such as graham crackers, have been tested with schoolchildren and were as well liked as their refined counterparts (Sadeghi and Marquart, 2009; Sadeghi and Marquart, 2010).

Preparation time is often an important aspect of convenience, and it can present a barrier to whole grain consumption, depending on the grain product; some take considerably more time to cook than their refined counterparts. For example, brown rice takes almost twice as long to cook as white rice. On the other hand, wholewheat pasta typically takes less time to cook than conventional pasta, and overcooking and holding can lead to undesirable changes in texture, posing a challenge in food service settings where timing is crucial when serving mass quantities. In general, the time that people have to spend on cooking has decreased over the past 30 years (Rose, 2007; Zick and Stevens, 2009). The Thrifty Food Plan (TFP) has a unique role in US nutrition policy, integrating both dietary guidance and anti-hunger policies and providing the basis for the Supplemental Nutrition Assistance Program. To be economical, the TFP logically assumes that most dishes are prepared from raw ingredients, yet research has indicated that meal time preparation has decreased by about 25% for both working and non-working women, and that this plan may be somewhat unrealistic (Rose, 2007). Davis and You (2010) further investigated the aspect of time and also examined the cost of labor in addition to the cost of food. Results indicated the TFP falls well below the Dietary Guidelines when factoring in labor costs. The trade-offs between time and money used in the preparation of meals for low-income families may be a contradiction of policy, warranting further acknowledgement.

6.5 Approaches to introducing wholegrain foods

Eating habits become engrained in an individual's lifestyle and can be hard to change. Therefore, starting healthy eating habits when one is young may contribute to a healthy lifestyle later in life. Introducing acceptable wholegrain foods for children remains a challenge. Children's food preferences and dietary choices are primarily driven by taste, and they tend to prefer foods that are familiar in taste, texture, flavor, and appearance (Burgess-Champoux *et al.*, 2006). It may be important to consider food preferences when selecting popular grain-based foods or other appropriate foods to deliver wholegrain ingredients. Additionally, research suggests that children's preferences for most foods are shaped by repeated experience (Birch, 1999; Koivisto Hursti, 1999). Thus, one approach to enhance children's preference for whole grains might be to frequently introduce different types of high quality wholegrain foods at home and in the school cafeteria. This approach gives children the opportunity for repeated exposures to wholegrain foods. The incorporation of white wholewheat flour versus traditional red whole wheat into grain-based foods can help minimize changes to the appearance, flavor, and texture of the product. Preliminary sensory research suggested that white whole wheat might provide more acceptable products as judged by children.

Lukow *et al.* (2004) found that children preferred the appearance of pan bread made with lighter colored white wholewheat flour two and half times more than the darker traditional red wholewheat flour. Further, children preferred the taste of bread made with white whole wheat twice as much as red whole wheat. If children are frequently exposed to a 'friendly' or more familiar looking food that contains whole grains, they may gradually become accustomed to wholegrain foods. Alternatively, introducing traditional wholegrain foods with the distinct taste, texture, and flavor profiles that children may find offensive has the possibility of lessening children's enthusiasm for trying wholegrain foods in the future.

The introduction of wholegrain flour into familiar grain products such as pizza, bread, and hamburger buns may potentially increase whole grain and dietary fiber consumption at home and in food service settings. Table 6.2 provides an overview of consumption patterns of partial and 100% wholegrain foods by elementary school children. When a wholegrain ingredient was introduced gradually, children

Table 6.2 Consumption of partial and 100% wholegrain foods by elementary school children

Grain products served (per serving)	Average number of children (*n*)	Percentage of grain ingredients as WG	Amount of WG (g/serving)	Consumption average	Source
Hamburger bun (2 oz)	320	0–91	0–25	63%	Rosen *et al.*, 2008
Pizza (1 slice)[a]	290	0–50	0–16	74%	Chan *et al.*, 2008 Schroeder *et al.*, in press
Pasta (1/2 cup)	340	23–100	6–25	73%	Unpublished data, University of Minnesota
Rolls (1.5 oz)	360	0–91	0–19	68%	Rosen *et al.*, 2008
French bread (1 oz)	345	50	6	45%	Schroeder *et al.*, in press
Crackers (30 g)	115	0–100	0–26	71%	Sadeghi and Marquart, 2009; 2010
Cookie (30 g)	275	75–100	5–10	74%	Unpublished data, University of Minnesota

Source: Adapted from Rosen *et al.*, 2009.

Notes: WG, whole grain.

[a] Pizza slices were 129–144 g per serving.

were found to accept red wholewheat and white wholewheat buns and rolls at consumption levels comparable to refined grain versions in a school food service setting (Rosen *et al.*, 2008). Children accepted whole grains made from red and white wheat products at 12.9 grams and 10.7 grams, respectively. Preliminary studies by Chan *et al.* (2008) found that school children consumed pizza crust made with a 50:50 blend of white wholewheat flour and refined wheat flour at levels similar to pizza crust made with 100% refined grain flour. However, there is limited research on children's acceptance of various types of wholewheat flour in traditional grain foods in a school cafeteria setting. More research on incorporating whole grains into school meals is needed to increase the acceptability and consumption of wholegrain foods.

Few studies have examined varied approaches to introducing wholegrain foods. Approaches have mainly focused on increasing children's consumption of wholegrain foods. In a recent intervention, WIC participants in California were provided with a two-month curriculum on whole grains (Ritchie *et al.*, 2010). Consumption of whole grains increased among English speakers, but not Spanish speakers. Additionally, even though there was an increase in intent to use whole grains, there was no change in label reading after the intervention. In a 12-week program aimed at improving physical activity and nutrition in children with parental involvement, more than 75% of children increased their intake of whole grains (Slawta *et al.*, 2008). Another intervention focused on improving the content of sack lunches brought to childcare centers (Sweitzer *et al.*, 2010). Parents and teachers were educated on increasing fruits, vegetables, and whole grains. At the end of the study, whole grain servings in sack lunches increased to one serving. However, actual consumption of sack lunch contents by children was not documented. In a YMCA after-school program intervention, researchers aimed to improve the snack and beverage choices (Mozaffarian *et al.*, 2010). YMCA staff members were educated on healthy eating standards and advised to incorporate these standards into their after-school programs. Although improvements were seen in fruit and vegetable consumption, an increase in whole grain servings did not occur. YMCA staff reported whole grains based on higher fiber grains versus as a whole grain; thus, it remains unclear how whole grain consumption was affected by the intervention. Wholegrain foods are complex to understand when trying to integrate into a meal plan, and this reiterates the need for a clear definition for whole grains and increased effort in identifying these products for the public. Additionally, nutrition education on whole grains should be designed for the targeted demographic, and parental involvement appears to improve desired outcomes related to whole grain awareness and consumption by children.

In a recent dietary modeling study, whole grain intake was modeled by replacing varying proportions of refined flour in common grain products; thus, the impact of substituting whole grain for <51% of the refined grain in 100% refined grain products was examined (Keast *et al.*, 2011). Post-modeling whole grain intake increased by 1.7 ounce equivalents per day. Further, whole grain intake did not differ by poverty level post-modeling.

While a few studies have examined the inclusion of whole grains into grain-based foods, mainly in school settings, others have explored the addition of dietary fiber to the regular diets of nursing home or long-term care residents. In a 12-week study, seniors were provided an oat bran fiber supplement (18 g fiber/100 g) in the form of a cake (Sturtzel and Elmadfa, 2008). Laxative use was significantly reduced by 59%, body weight was maintained, and the seniors' quality of life improved, while in the control group laxative use increased by 8% and body weight significantly decreased. Because the oat bran was adapted into a product the seniors were familiar with and enjoyed, adequate dietary fiber was incorporated into their diet, providing significant targeted health benefits. In another study, residents in a long-term care facility received 1–3 g/serving of pea hull fiber integrated into three to four foods each day (Dahl *et al.*, 2003). After six weeks, bowel frequency significantly increased and laxative use decreased. Thus, careful thought when integrating dietary fiber into the regular diet creates an inexpensive, acceptable higher fiber food product that helps one to meet the fiber recommendations.

Various approaches focused on the grain (versus educational interventions) have been suggested as means to introduce wholegrain foods into the marketplace for consumers in general: 1) use a gradual approach (slowly add more whole grain into the product formulation over time) (Rosen *et al.*, 2009); 2) use white whole wheat and other light-colored wholegrain ingredients instead of red whole wheat (minimize perceptible change in color); 3) use finer particle size wholegrain flours (minimize perceptible change in texture and appearance); 4) make more 100% wholegrain breads, breakfast cereals, and other products available; and 5) develop innovative/novel products containing whole grains in beverages, extenders in protein items, and soups (Marquart *et al.*, 2006). These approaches may be valuable to introduce acceptable and palatable wholegrain foods into school menus, as well as restaurants, and in the retail market for home purchase.

6.6 Future trends

6.6.1 Wholegrain foods and consumer demand

Although consumption of whole grains and fiber remains below dietary recommendations worldwide, consumer purchasing trends are currently shifting towards increased whole grain purchases, at least in the US marketplace (Arndt, 2010). This gradual shift in consumer preferences may be due to several factors previously discussed, including the health benefits of whole grains, increased consumer awareness, evolving taste preferences, and also the increased availability of whole grain options in a variety of settings. Even while progress is being made towards increasing availability of whole grain and fiber, significant barriers still exist in establishing whole grains and fiber as the societal or cultural norm worldwide. Several of these barriers have been discussed, including taste, familiarity, availability, cost, and convenience. Overall, industry has responded to the mounting scientific evidence of the health benefits of whole grains and fiber, as well as to consumer demand, with a dramatic increase in the introduction of wholegrain and higher fiber products into the marketplace. In some cases, these were modifications to existing products, while others came from innovative new product solutions. In addition to maintaining the growth of wholegrain and higher fiber products, a next step in product innovation aimed at improving public health will include addressing issues of caloric and nutrient density, overall nutrition, and modifying the fats, sugars, and sodium added to grain-based foods.

Consumers currently eat far more calories than recommended through dietary guidance for health and weight maintenance. Children obtain most of these excess calories through grain-based dishes, including grain desserts and pizza (Reedy and Krebs-Smith, 2010). Both a push from the food industry and increasing demand from consumers will be needed to improve the availability of wholegrain foods for all consumers everywhere. It is unlikely that consumer demand alone will be sufficient to sustain a healthy food supply, given the logistics and economics of the current distribution of food (Krebs-Smith *et al.*, 2010). However, several key groups informing consumers about healthy food choices, such as physicians and registered dietitians, will be essential in growing a sustained demand for healthy foods (Rowe *et al.*, 2011a). Policy-makers and industry must also make a concerted effort to advance a healthy, sustainable food supply, while consumers must take more responsibility and seek education through various public health programs and initiatives (DGAC, 2010). Changes to the USDA's WIC food package that require program participants to purchase wholegrain foods are a recent example of policy modifications that may help to facilitate increased consumer demand for a healthy food supply, including wholegrain and fiber foods (Committee to Review the WIC Food Packages, 2005). Industry's role in the development and delivery of a healthy food supply may include innovative product development, marketing healthy products, and providing easy access for delivery of healthy foods to all (Porter and Kramer, 2011; Rowe *et al.*, 2011b).

Several product formulation strategies may be considered for reducing overall calorie intake through grain-based foods. Each strategy should be carefully evaluated for effectiveness of calorie reduction in the specific end audience. For example, if a calorie-reduction strategy is to introduce more fiber and reduced saturated fat in a cookie served at schools, the cookie should be tested through school food service channels in the natural setting to assure quality and acceptability with students. Other segments of the value chain may play key roles in creating a healthier food supply. For example, Wal-mart, the world's largest retailer, has recently announced an initiative to make healthier foods more widely available and less costly by reformulating many of their owned brand products (Scott-Thomas, 2011).

In addition to evaluating added calories in grain-based foods, opportunities still exist in specific product categories for increasing consumer acceptance of wholegrain and higher fiber food options. For example, breads and cereals have enjoyed a relatively smooth transition to more wholegrain, higher fiber options in the marketplace with increasing consumer acceptance in these categories. Pasta, however, presents unique challenges to consumer acceptance of wholegrain texture and flavor. Addition of the bran to pasta dough leads to challenges such as less acceptable taste and texture, as well as potential storage and shelf life issues. Thus, research should be performed in a coordinated manner that will lead all stakeholders to improve wholegrain pasta and develop and deliver a quality product that is highly accepted by consumers.

6.6.2 Wholegrain foods stakeholder collaboration

Pasta is one example of a grain-based product in the food supply that will benefit from a coordinated research and development effort of the grains community working together. Coordination, collaboration, and working toward collective solutions will be necessary to continue to effectively address consumer challenges to accepting healthy wholegrain and higher fiber foods. Including government, industry, academia, and other organizations when formulating research agendas and work plans will be necessary to delineate the health benefits of wholegrain and fiber components. Coordination of efforts will also be necessary to develop and deliver the most healthful grain-based foods possible to the consumer while maintaining favorable taste profiles and a competitive cost compared with refined grain products. In short, improving the health of the grain food supply will require everyone working together. Australia's Go Grain initiative is an example of a specific work plan that crosses sectors to benefit all. Go Grains specifically recommends aiming for an intake of 48 g of whole grains per day and is working with food manufacturers and organizations to communicate this message, such as on food packaging and in promotional materials, in an effort to increase whole grain consumption and promote the health of the Australian population (Griffiths, 2010).

The execution of a comprehensive effort to increase consumer intake of wholegrain and higher fiber foods will require contributions from all sectors, segments and disciplines within the food system. This interdisciplinary work calls for different sets of skills from those used to accomplish individual work or even collaboration within a defined discipline. One approach is not superior to the other, and both interdisciplinary work and individual work will be necessary to improve the availability, cost, taste, and acceptability of healthy wholegrain, higher fiber products. Leaders of an interdisciplinary effort will need the ability to actively listen with intent, suspend judgment and individual agendas, and frame issues through a systemic approach in order to work successfully across sectors and disciplines. Thus, networking, relationship-building, and negotiating skills are all essential to produce expected outcomes from interdisciplinary groups that move complex societal issues towards desired outcomes rather than creating conflict. Training for young professionals who will enter the food industry should include opportunities to learn collaborative skills through multi-sector, interdisciplinary experiences that prepare them to work through real issues in the food supply. Both training for young professionals and coaching for seasoned professionals in the grain community to operate from a base of core values, rather than focusing only on the bottom line, will drive innovation by allowing corporate responsibility efforts to shape healthier product development, marketing, and business models. In some cases, grain companies are already successfully maintaining healthy economics by selling healthy grain-based foods. These successful models should be understood and replicated through interdisciplinary efforts to work towards the challenge of making the healthy choice the easy choice for consumers (DGAC, 2010).

6.7 Sources of further information and advice

There are a number of different organizations that specialize through various segments of the grain supply chain. The collaboration of these organizations will benefit industry, policy-makers, and consumers alike as they collectively work to deliver healthier grain-based foods to the consumer.

- American Bakers Association: www.americanbakers.org
- Go Grains: www.gograins.com.au
- Grain Foods Foundation: www.gowiththegrain.org
- Grains for Health Foundation: www.grainsforhealth.org
- HEALTHGRAIN Forum: www.healthgrain.org
- IFIC: www.foodinsight.org
- Wheat Foods Council: www.wheatfoods.org
- Whole Grains Council: www.wholegrainscouncil.org

6.8 References

AACC (2000), 'AACC whole grain ingredient definition', *Cereal Foods World*, **45**, 79.

ADA (2005), 'Position of the American Dietetic Association: benchmarks for nutrition programs in child care settings', *J Am Diet Assoc*, **105**, 979–86.

ADA (2008), *Nutrition and you: trends 2008 summary of findings, ADA*. Available from: http://www.eatright.org/Media/content.aspx?id=7639 (Accessed 25 November 2010).

ADAMS JF and ENGSTROM A (2000), 'Helping consumers achieve recommended intakes of whole grain foods', *J Am Coll Nutr*, **19**(3 Suppl), 339S–344S.

ALEXY U, ZORN C and KERSTING M (2010), 'Whole grain in children's diet: intake, food sources and trends', *Eur J Clin Nutr*, **64**, 745–751.

ARNDT E (2010), 'Functionality and health aspects of whole grains for product development', Institute of Food Technologists Annual Meeting, Chicago, IL.

BACHMAN JL, REEDY J, SUBAR AF and KREBS-SMITH SM (2008), 'Sources of food group intakes among the US population, 2001-2002', *J Am Diet Assoc*, **108**(5), 804–14.

BAKKE A, VICKERS Z, MARQUART L and SJOBERG S (2007), 'Consumer acceptance of refined and whole-wheat breads', in MARQUART L, JACOBS D, MCINTOSH G, POUTANEN K and REICKS M, *Whole grains and health*, Ames, Iowa, Blackwell Publishing, 255–61.

BALL SC, BENJAMIN SE and WARD DS (2008), 'Dietary intakes in North Carolina child-care centers: are children meeting current recommendations?', *J Am Diet Assoc*, **108**(4), 718–21.

BEAUDRY M, GALIBOIS I and CHAUMETTE P (1998), 'Dietary patterns of adults in Quebec and their nutritional adequacy', *Can J Public Health*, **89**(5), 347–51.

BEAUMONT J, LANG T, LEATHER S and MUCKLOW C (1995), *Report from the policy sub-group to the Nutrition Task Force Low Income Project Team of the Department of Health*, Hertfordshire, Radlett Institute of Grocery Distribution.

BERNSTEIN AM, BLOOM DE, ROSNER BA, FRANZ M and WILLETT WC (2010), 'Relation of food cost to healthfulness of diet among US women', *Am J Clin Nutr*, **92**(5), 1197–203.

BINNS NM (2010), 'Regulatory aspects for whole grain and whole grain food: an EU perspective', *Cereal Chem*, **87**(2), 162–6.

BIRCH L (1999), 'Development of food preferences', *Ann Rev Nutr*, **19**, 41.

BRITTEN P, LYON J, WEAVER CM, et al. (2006), 'MyPyramid food intake pattern modeling for the Dietary Guidelines Advisory Committee', *J Nutr Educ Behav*, **38**(6 Suppl), S143–152.

BURGESS-CHAMPOUX T, MARQUART L, VICKERS Z and REICKS M (2006), 'Perceptions of children, parents, and teachers regarding whole-grain foods, and implications for a school-based intervention', *J Nutr Educ Behav*, **38**(4), 230–7.

BURGESS-CHAMPOUX TL, CHAN HW, ROSEN R, MARQUART L and REICKS M (2008), 'Healthy whole-grain choices for children and parents: a multi-component school-based pilot intervention', *Public Health Nutr*, **11**(8), 849–59.

BURTON-FREEMAN B (2000), 'Dietary fiber and energy regulation', *J Nutr*, **130**(2S Suppl), 272S–275S.

BUZBY J, FARAH H and VOCKE G (2005), 'Will 2005 be the year of the whole grain?', *Amber Waves*, **3**(3).

CANADIAN GROCER (2011), *Canadians misjudging grain intake*, Ontario, Rogers Publishing Limited. Available from: http://www.canadiangrocer.com/research/canadians-misjudging-grain-intake-2876 (Accessed 22 January 2011).

CHAN HW, BURGESS-CHAMPOUX TL, VICKERS Z, REICKS M and MARQUART L (2008), 'White whole grain flour can be substituted for red in pizza crust for school children', *J of Nutr Manag*, **32**(1).

CHAN H, HESSE D, REICKS M and MARQUART L (2009), 'Group interviews with school foodservice personnel regarding whole grain foods in foodservice operations', *J of Foodservice*, **20**(3), 109–16.

CHANG C and CHAMBERS EI (1992), 'Flavor characterization of breads made from hard red winter wheat and hard white winter wheat', *Cereal Chem*, **69**, 556–9.

CHASE K, REICKS M, SRINVASAN P and MARQUART L (2004), 'Factors influencing production of whole grain foods: perceptions of members of the American Association of Cereal Chemists', *J Food Distr Res*, **35**, 53–9.

CHASE K, REICKS M and JONES JM (2003a), 'Applying the theory of planned behavior to promotion of whole-grain foods by dietitians', *J Am Diet Assoc*, **103**(12), 1639–42.

CHASE K, REICKS M, SMITH C, HENRY H and REIMER K (2003b), 'Use of the think-aloud method to identify factors influencing purchase of bread and cereals by low-income African American women and implications for whole-grain education', *J Am Diet Assoc*, **103**(4), 501–4.

CODE OF FEDERAL REGULATIONS (2011), 'Health claims: Soluble fiber from certain foods and risk of coronary heart disease (CHD)', 21 CFR 101.81 (current through 27 May 2011). Available from: http://ecfr.gpoaccess.gov/cgi/t/text/text-idx?c=ecfr;sid=866c04a76b3e9aa5174a45ed5f95b1a7;rgn=div8;view=text;node=21%3A2.0.1.1.2.5.1.12;idno=21;cc=ecfr (Accessed 29 May 2011).

COMMITTEE TO REVIEW THE WIC FOOD PACKAGES (2005), *WIC food packages: time for a change*, The National Academies Press, Washington, DC. Available from: http://www.nap.edu (Accessed 3 January 2011).

CRAWFORD M, KATZ S and MAURO A (2010), 'CPI detailed report data for January 2010', Bureau of Labor Statistics. Available from: www.bls.gov/cpi/cpid1001.pdf (Accessed 10 May 2011).

CUMMINS S and MACINTYRE S (2002), 'Food deserts': evidence and assumption in health policy making, BMJ, **325**(7361), 436–8.

DAHL WJ, WHITING SJ, HEALEY A, ZELLO GA and HILDEBRANDT SL (2003), 'Increased stool frequency occurs when finely processed pea hull fiber is added to usual foods consumed by elderly residents in long-term care', *J Am Diet Assoc*, **103**, 1199–202.

DAVIS GC and YOU W (2010), 'The Thrifty Food Plan is not thrifty when labor cost is considered', *J Nutr*, **140**(4), 854–7.

DGAC (2010), *Report of the Dietary Guidelines Advisory Committee (DGAC) on the Dietary Guidelines for Americans, 2010: Part A: Executive Summary*. ARS and USDA, Washington, DC. Available from: http://www.cnpp.usda.gov/Publications/DietaryGuidelines/2010/DGAC/Report/A-ExecSummary.pdf (Accessed 22 November 2010).

DINEHART M, HAYES JE, BARTOSHUK LM, LANIER SL and DUFFY VB (2006), 'Bitter taste markers explain variability in vegetable sweetness, bitterness, and intake', *Physiol Behav*, **87**, 304–13.

DREWNOWSKI A (2010), 'The cost of US foods as related to their nutritive value', *Am J Clin Nutr*, **92**(5), 1181–8.

DUFFY VB, PETERSON JM and BARTOSHUK LM (2004), 'Associations between taste genetics, oral sensation and alcohol intake', *Physiol Behav*, **82**(2–3), 435–45.

EFSA PANEL ON DIETETIC PRODUCTS, NUTRITION AND ALLERGIES (2010), 'Scientific opinion on the substantiation of health claims related to whole grain (ID 831, 832, 833, 1126, 1268, 1269, 1270, 1271, 1431) pursuant to Article 13(1) of Regulation (EC) No 1924/2006', *EFSA Journal*, **8**(10), 1766.

ELLIS J, JOHNSON MA, FISCHER JG and HARGROVE JL (2005), 'Nutrition and health education intervention for whole grain foods in the Georgia older Americans nutrition programs', *J Nutr Elderly*, **24**(3), 67–83.

FLORES M, MACIAS N, RIVERA M, et al. (2010), 'Dietary patterns in Mexican adults are associated with risk of being overweight or obese', *J Nutr*, **140**(10), 1869–73.

FNS (2012), *Nutrition Standards in the National School Lunch and School Breakfast Programs; Final Rule*, Federal Register 77:17 (January 26, 2012) p. 4088.

FSANZ (2006), 'Review of high level health claim on wholegrains and coronary heart disease, FSANZ'. Available from: http://www.foodstandards.gov.au/foodmatters/healthnutritionandrelatedclaims/reviewsforhighlevelc3090.cfm (Accessed 23 January 2011).

GELLAR L, ROVNER AJ and NANSEL TR (2009), 'Whole grain and legume acceptability among youths with type 1 diabetes', *Diabetes Educ*, **35**(3), 422–7.

GELSKI J (2007), 'Let them eat whole grain cake: formulators begin to explore adding more whole grains to indulgent items', *Milling and Baking News*, **86**(4), 23–30.

GLANZ K, SALLIA JF, SAELENS BE and FRANK LD (2007), 'Nutrition Environment Measures Survey in Stores (NEMS-S): development and evaluation', *Am J Prev Med*, **32**(4), 282–9.

GO GRAINS HEALTH AND NUTRITION LTD (2010), *The grains and legumes health report: a review of the science*, New South Wales, Go Grains Health and Nutrition Ltd. Available at: http://www.gograins.com.au/pdfs/Go+Grains+Report+22.04.10.pdf (Accessed 27 November 2010).

GOLAN E, MANCINO L and UNNEVEHR L (2009), 'Food policy: check the list of ingredients', *Amber Waves*, **7**(2).

GORDON C, PURCIEL-HILL M, GHAI NR, KAUFMAN L, GRAHAM R and VAN WYE G (2011), 'Measuring food deserts in New York City's low-income neighborhoods', *Health Place*, **17**(2), 696–700.

GRIFFITHS T (2010), 'Promoting cereal grain and whole grain consumption: an Australian perspective', *Cereal Chem*, **87**(2), 159–61.

HEALTH CANADA (2007a), *Canada's food guide*, Health Canada. Available from: http://www.hc-sc.gc.ca/fn-an/food-guide-aliment/index-eng.php (Accessed 15 December 2010).

HEALTH CANADA (2007b), *Whole grains – get the facts*, Health Canada. Available from: http://www.hc-sc.gc.ca/fn-an/nutrition/whole-grain-entiers-eng.php (Accessed 22 January 2011).

HEALTH GRAIN (2006), *How much whole grain is good for you?*, Health Grain. Available from: http://www.healthgrain.eu/pub/chapter-five.php#DACH (Accessed 7 May 2011).

HENDERICKSON D, SMITH C and EIKENBERRY N (2006), 'Fruit and vegetable access in four low-income food deserts communities in Minnesota', *Agr Human Values*, **23**, 371–83.

HESSE D, BRAUN C, DOSTAL A, JEFFERY R and MARQUART L (2009), 'Barriers and opportunities related to whole grain foods in Minnesota school foodservice', *J Child Nutr Manag*, **33**(1).

HOLT SH, MILLER JC, PETOCZ P and FARMAKALIDIS E (1995), 'A satiety index of common foods', *Eur J Clin Nutr*, **49**(9), 675–90.

IFIC (2009), *2009 Food and health survey: consumer attitudes toward food safety, nutrition and Health*, Washington, DC, IFIC. Available from: http://www.foodinsight.org/Resources/Detail.aspx?topic=2009_Food_Health_Survey_Consumer_Attitudes_toward_Food_Nutrition_and_Health (Accessed 25 February 2010).

IFIC (2010), *2010 Food and health survey: consumer attitudes toward food safety, nutrition and health*, Washington, DC, IFIC. Available from: http://www.foodinsight.org/Content/3651/2010FinalFullReport.pdf (Accessed 25 November 2010).

JETTER KM and CASSADY DL (2005), 'The availability and cost of healthier food', *AIC Issue Brief No. 29*, University of California, Davis Agricultural Issues Center.

JHCI (2002), *Joint Health Claims Initiative approved generic health claim*, JHCI. Available from: http://www.jhci.org.uk/approv/wgrainh.htm (Accessed 23 January 2011).

JONES JM (2010), 'Regulatory aspects of whole grain and whole grain foods: definitions and labeling', *Cereal Chem*, **87**(2), 150–4.

KANTOR LS, VARIYAM JN, ALLSHOUSE JE, PUTNAM JJ and LIN BH (2001), 'Choose a variety of grains daily, especially whole grains: a challenge for consumers', *J Nutr*, **131**(2S-1), 473S–486S.

KEAST DR, ROSEN RA, ARNDT EA and MARQUART LF (2011), 'Dietary modeling shows that substitution of whole grain for refined grain ingredients of foods commonly consumed by US children and teens can increase intake of whole grains', *J Am Diet Assoc*, **111**(9), 1322–8.

KENNEDY E and DAVIS CA (2000), 'Dietary guidelines 2000 – the opportunity and challenges for reaching the consumer', *J Am Diet Assoc*, **100**(12), 1462–5.

KOIVISTO HURSTI UK (1999), 'Factors influencing children's food choice', *Annals of Med*, **31**(1), 26–32.

KOLODINSKY J, HARVEY-BERINO JR, BERLIN L, JOHNSON RK and REYNOLDS TW (2007), 'Knowledge of current dietary guidelines and food choice by college students: better eaters have higher knowledge of dietary guidance', *J Am Diet Assoc*, **107**(8), 1409–13.

KREBS-SMITH SM, REEDY J and BOSIRE C (2010), 'Healthfulness of the US food supply: little improvement despite decades of dietary guidance', *Am J Prev Med*, **38**(5), 472–7.

LACEY JM (2007), 'Enhancing students' understanding of whole cereal grains in a university experimental foods course', *J Nutr Edu Behav*, **39**(4), 235–6.

LAFFERTY A, MARQUART L and REICKS M (2006), 'Hunting for whole grains: a supermarket tour', *J Nutr Educ Behav*, **38**(3), 197–8.

LANG R and JEBB SA (2003), 'Who consumes whole grains, and how much?', *Proc Nutr Soc*, **62**, 123–7.

LANG R, THANE CW, BOLTON-SMITH C and JEBB SA (2003), 'Consumption of whole-grain foods by British adults: findings from further analysis of two national dietary surveys', *Public Health Nutr*, **6**(5), 479–84.

LEA EJ, CRAWFORD D and WORSLEY A (2006), 'Consumers' readiness to eat a plant-based diet', *Eur J Clin Nutr*, **60**(3), 342–51.

LIN BW and YEN ST (2007), *The US grain consumption landscape: who eats grain, in what form, where, and how much? Report No. 50*, Washington, DC, USDA Economic Research Service.

LUKOW OM, GUINARD JX and ADAMS KM (2004), 'Whole wheat bread preference of children', AACC Annual Meeting, San Diego, CA.

MANCINO L, KUCHLER F and LEIBTAG E (2008), 'Getting consumers to eat more whole grains: the role of policy, information, and food manufacturers', *Food Policy*, **33**, 489–96.

MARQUART L, PHAM AT, LAUTENSCHLAGER L, CROY M and SOBAL J (2006), 'Beliefs about whole-grain foods by food and nutrition professionals, health club members, and special supplemental nutrition program for women, infants, and children participants/state fair attendees', *J Am Diet Assoc*, **106**(11), 1856–60.

MEHIO SA, NASREDDINE L, MOKDAD AH, ADRA N, TABET M and HWALLA N (2010), 'Nutrition transition and cardiovascular disease risk factors in the Middle East and North Africa Countries: reviewing the evidence', *Ann Nutr Metab*, **57**(3–4), 193–203.

MINTEL GLOBAL NEW PRODUCTS DATABASE (2010), 'Whole grain growth worldwide, 2000-2010'. Available from: http://www.wholegrainscouncil.org/newsroom/whole-grain-statistics (Accessed 10 December 2010).

MONTONEN J, KNEKT P, JARVINEN R, AROMAA A and REUNANEN A (2003), 'Whole-grain and fiber intake and the incidence of type 2 diabetes', *Am J Clin Nutr*, **77**, 622–9.

MOZAFFARIAN RS, WIECHA JL, ROTH BA, NELSON TF, LEE RM and GORTMAKER SL (2010), 'Impact of an organizational intervention designed to improve snack and beverage quality in YMCA after-school programs', *Am J Public Health*, **100**(5), 925–32.

MURRAY JM, COX D, EASTON K and MIALON VS (2002), 'Descriptive sensory analysis of Australian breads', *Food Australia*, **54**, 247–52.

NATIONAL FOOD INSTITUTE (2008), *Wholegrain – definition and scientific background for recommendations of wholegrain intake in Denmark*, Technical University of Denmark. Available from: http://www.food.dtu.dk/ (Accessed 27 November 2010).

NHMRC (2003), *Guidelines for all Australians*, Australian Government. Available from: www.nhmrc.gov.au/publications/synopses/dietsyn.htm (Accessed 13 May 2011).

O'NEIL CE, NICKLAS TA, ZANOVEC M and CHO S (2010), 'Whole-grain consumption is associated with diet quality and nutrient intake in adults: the National Health and Nutrition Examination Survey, 1999-2004', *J Am Diet Assoc*, **110**(10), 1461–8.

PAQUETTE M (2005), 'Perceptions of healthy eating: state of knowledge and research gaps', *Can J Public Health*, **96**(3), S15–S19.

PASUT L (2005), *Grains: essential for healthy eating*, Ontario, Baking Association of Canada. Available from: http://www.bakingassoccanada.com (Accessed 14 December 2010).

PENG Y (2004), *Canadian consumer trends in obesity and food consumption*, Alberta, Alberta Agriculture, Food and Rural Development. Available from: http://www1.agric.gov.ab.ca/$department/deptdocs.nsf/all/sis8438 (Accessed 22 January 2011).

PORIKOS K and HAGAMEN S (1986), 'Is fiber satiating? Effects of a high fiber preload on subsequent food intake of normal-weight and obese young men', *Appetite*, **7**(2), 153–62.

PORTER ME and KRAMER MR (2011), 'Creating shared value', *Harvard Business Review*, January–February, 64–77.

REEDY J and KREBS-SMITH SM (2010), 'Dietary sources of energy, solid fats, and added sugars among children and adolescents in the United States', *J Am Diet Assoc*, **110**(10), 1477–84.

RITCHIE LD, WHALEY SE, SPECTOR P, GOMEZ J and CRAWFORD PB (2010), 'Favorable impact of nutrition education on California WIC families', *J Nutr Educ Behav*, **42**(3), S2–10.

ROLLS BJ, BELL EA, CASTELLANOS VH, CHOW M, PELKMAN CL and THORWART ML (1999), 'Energy density but not fat content of foods affected energy intake in lean and obese women', *Am J Clin Nutr*, **69**(5), 863–71.

ROSE D (2007), 'Food Stamps, the Thrifty Food Plan, and meal preparation: the importance of the time dimension for US nutrition policy', *J Nutr Educ Behav*, **39**(4), 226–32.

ROSEN RA, SADEGHI L, SCHROEDER N, REICKS MM and MARQUART L (2008), 'Gradual incorporation of whole wheat flour into bread products for elementary school children improves whole grain intake', *J Child Nutr Manag*, **32**(2). http://www.schoolnutrition.org/content.aspx?id=10584

ROSEN RA, SCHMITZ K, COHEN EA, ARNDT EA, REICKS M and MARQUART L (2009), 'A gradual approach to increasing whole grain consumption in children', *Cereal Foods World*, **54**(3), 113–17.

ROSEN R, HAUGE D, ARNDT E, VEAL M and MARQUART L (submitted), 'Exploring the use of whole grain pasta in school lunches', *J Child Nutr Manag*, **35**(2).

ROSEN R, ARNDT E and MARQUART L (submitted), 'Pasta dishes as a vehicle for meeting whole grain requirements in school meals: Challenges, opportunities and benefits', *Journal of Foodservice Management and Education.*

ROWE S, ALEXANDER N, ALMEIDA NG, et al. (2011a), 'Translating the Dietary Guidelines for Americans 2010 to bring about real behavior change', *J Am Diet Assoc*, **111**, 28–39.

ROWE S, ALEXANDER N, ALMEIDA N, et al. (2011b), 'Food science challenge: translating the Dietary Guidelines for Americans to bring about real behavior change', *J Food Sci*, **76**(1), R29–R37.

SADEGHI L and MARQUART L (2009), 'Whole grain snack intake in an after-school snack program: a pilot study', *Journal of Foodservice*, **20**(2), 71–80.

SADEGHI L and MARQUART L (2010), 'Consumption of graham snacks in after-school snack programs based on whole grain flour content', *Br Food J*, **112**(7), 723–36.

SARIS WH (2003), 'Glycemic carbohydrate and body weight regulation', *Nutr Rev*, **61**(5 Pt 2), S10-6.

SCHROEDER N, RONNEI J, ARNDT B and MARQUART L (in press), 'Perspectives on the incorporation of whole grain foods into school meals', *J Cul Sci and Tech.*

SCOTT-THOMAS C (2011), 'Wal-Mart pledges to promote healthy foods', Food Navigator. Available from: http://www.foodnavigator-usa.com/Financial-Industry/Walmart-pledges-to-promote-healthy-foods/?c=92q9RxsjRfWosUbIrivi5l9juuJwNQjz&utm_source=newsletter_daily&utm_medium=email&utm_campaign–Newsletter%2BDaily (Accessed 11 February 2011).

SEAL CJ and BROWNLEE IA (2010), 'Whole grains and health, evidence from observational and intervention studies', *Cereal Chem*, **87**(2), 167–74.

SLAVIN JL (2005), 'Dietary fiber and body weight', *Nutr*, **21**(3), 411–18.

SLAWTA J, BENTLEY J, SMITH J, KELLY J and SYMAN-DEGLER L (2008), 'Promoting healthy lifestyles in children: a pilot program of be a fit kid', *Health Promot Pract*, **9**(3), 305–12.

SMITH AT, KUZNESOF S, RICHARDSON DP and SEAL CJ (2003), 'Behavioural, attitudinal and dietary responses to the consumption of wholegrain foods', *Proc Nutr Soc*, **62**(2), 455–67.

SNF (2004), Health claims in the labelling and marketing of food products. The food sector's code of practice.

STURTZEL B and ELMADFA I (2008), 'Intervention with dietary fiber to treat constipation and reduce laxative use in residents of nursing homes', *Ann Nutr Metab*, **52**(1), 54–6.

SUPREME SCIENTIFIC HEALTH COUNCIL (1999), *Dietary guidelines for adults in Greece*, Athens, Ministry of Health and Welfare. Available from: http://www.mednet.gr/archives/1999-5/pdf/516.pdf (Accessed 27 November 2010).

SWEITZER SJ, BRILEY ME, ROBERTS-GRAY C, et al. (2010), 'Lunch is in the bag: increasing fruits, vegetables, and whole grains in sack lunches of preschool-aged children', *J Am Diet Assoc*, **110**(7), 1058–64.

THANE CW, JONES AR, STEPHEN AM, SEAL CJ and JEBB SA (2005), 'Whole-grain intake of British young people aged 4-18 years', *Br J Nutr*, **94**, 825–31.

THANE CW, JONES AR, STEPHEN AM, SEAL CJ and JEBB SA (2007), 'Comparative whole-grain intake of British adults in 1986-7 and 2000-1', *Br J Nutr*, **97**(5), 987–92.

TOUVIER M, MÉJEAN C, KESSE-GUYOT E, et al. (2010), 'Variations in compliance with starchy food recommendations and consumption of types of starchy foods according to sociodemographic and socioeconomic characteristics', *Br J Nutr*, **103**(10), 1485–92.

UJSZASZY B, BURGESS-CHAMPOUX TL, REICKS M, LAZARUS W and MARQUART L (2004), 'It's time for whole grain products in school meals', *J Child Nutr Manag*, 2.

UK FOOD STANDARDS AGENCY (n.d.), *Healthy eating nutrition essentials*, Food Standards Agency. Available from: http://www.eatwell.gov.uk/healthydiet/nutritionessentials (Accessed 27 November 2010).

US CONGRESS (1990), *Nutrition Labeling and Education Act*. Washington, DC: US Government Printing Office.

USDA (2009), *Access to affordable and nutritious food: measuring and understanding food deserts and their consequences*, USDA. Available from: http://www.ers.usda.gov/Publications/AP/AP036/ (Accessed 10 February 2011).

USDA ARS (2010), *Nutrient intakes from food: mean amounts consumed per individual by gender and age, in the United States, 2007-2008*, USDA ARS. Available from: http://www.ars.usda.gov/SP2UserFiles/Place/12355000/pdf/0708/Table_1_NIN_GEN_07.pdf (Accessed 22 January 2011).

USDA FNS (2010), *USDA white paper on USDA foods in the National School Lunch Program*, USDA FNS. Available from: http://www.fns.usda.gov/fdd/foods/healthy/WhitePaper.pdf (Accessed 19 April 2010).

USDA AND USDHHS (2005), *Dietary Guidelines for Americans, 2005* (6th Edition), Washington, DC, US Government Printing Office. Available from: http://www.health.gov/dietaryguidelines/dga2005/document/pdf/DGA2005.pdf (Accessed 7 May 2011).

USDA AND USDHHS (2010), *Dietary Guidelines for Americans, 2010* (7th Edition), Washington, DC, US Government Printing Office. Available from: http://www.cnpp.usda.gov/Publications/DietaryGuidelines/2010/PolicyDoc/PolicyDoc.pdf (Accessed 12 February 2011).

USDHHS (2008), *Healthy People 2010 progress review: nutrition and overweight*, Washington, DC, USDHHS. Available from: http://www.healthypeople.gov/Data/2010prog/focus19/2008Focus19.pdf (Accessed 25 November 2010).

USDHHS (2010), *Healthy People 2020 summary of objectives: nutrition and weight status*, USDHHS. Available from: http://www.healthypeople.gov/2020/topicsobjectives2020/pdfs/NutritionandWeight.pdf (Accessed 22 January 2011).

US FDA CFSAN (2003), 'Health claim notification for whole grain foods with moderate fat content', Docket No. 03Q-0547.

WALKER RE, KEANE CR and BURKE JG (2010), 'Disparities and access to healthy food in the United States: a review of food deserts literature', *Health Place*, **16**(5), 876–84.

WARBER JP, HADDAD EH, HODGKIN GE and LEE JW (1996), 'Foodservice specialists exhibit lack of knowledge in identifying whole-grain products', *J Am Diet Assoc*, **96**(8), 796–8.

WHITE HOUSE TASK FORCE ON CHILDHOOD OBESITY (2010), *Solving the problem of childhood obesity within a generation*. Available from: http://www.letsmove.gov/white-house-task-force-childhood-obesity-report-president (Accessed 10 May 2011).

WHOLE GRAINS COUNCIL (2006), *The whole grain stamp*, Whole Grains Council. Available from: http://wholegrainscouncil.org/whole-grain-stamp (Accessed 30 July 2007).

WHOLE GRAINS COUNCIL (2007), *A consumer definition of whole grains*, Whole Grains Council. Available from: http://wholegrainscouncil.org/whole-grains-101/definition-of-whole-grains (Accessed 30 July 2007).

WHOLE GRAINS COUNCIL (2008), *Whole grain statistics*, Whole Grains Council. Available from: http://www.wholegrainscouncil.org/newsroom/whole-grain-statistics (Accessed 19 May 2008).

WHOLE GRAINS COUNCIL (2009a), 'Are we there yet? Measuring progress on making at least half our grains whole', Make Half Your Grains Whole Conference, Alexandria, VA. Available from: http://www.wholegrainscouncil.org/files/3.AreWeThereYet.pdf (Accessed 25 November 2010).

WHOLE GRAINS COUNCIL (2009b), 'Schools and whole grains', Make Half Your Grains Whole Conference, Alexandria, VA. Available from: http://www.wholegrainscouncil.org/files/5.Schools+WG.pdf (Accessed 25 November 2010).

WHOLE GRAINS COUNCIL (2010a), *Barriers to whole grains in schools*, Whole Grains Council. Available from: http://www.wholegrainscouncil.org/resources/barriers-to-whole-grains-in-schools (Accessed 10 April 2011).

WHOLE GRAINS COUNCIL (2010b), *Eating away from home*, Whole Grains Council. Available from: http://www.wholegrainscouncil.org/find-whole-grains/eating-away-from-home (Accessed 10 May 2011).

ZANOVEC M, O'NEIL CE, CHO SS, KLEINMAN RE and NICKLAS TA (2010), 'Relationship between whole grain and fiber consumption and body weight measures among 6- to 18-year-olds', *J Pediatr*, **157**(4), 578–83.

ZICK CD and STEVENS RB (2009), 'Trends in Americans' food-related time use: 1975-2006', *Public Health Nutr*, **13**(7), 1064–72.

Part II

Dietary fibre sources

7

Improving the content and composition of dietary fibre in wheat

P. R. Shewry, Rothamsted Research, UK, and University of Reading, UK

DOI: 10.1533/9780857095787.2.153

Abstract: The major dietary fibre (DF) components in wheat grain are the cell wall polysaccharides arabinoxylan (AX) and (1→3,1→4)-β-D-glucans (β-glucan). Extensive variation exists between wheat genotypes in the amounts and structures of AX in bran and flour and in the amount of total β-glucan in wholemeal. A high proportion of this variation is heritable and chromosomal regions that determine the amount and properties of AX are being identified by genetic analyses. The variation in DF can be exploited by plant breeders, facilitated by the development of molecular markers, near infrared calibrations and antibody-based kits.

Key words: wheat, dietary fibre, arabinoxylan, β-glucan, genetic variation.

7.1 Introduction

Wheat is the most important staple food in temperate zones, including the UK and North America. It contributes calories (mainly from starch), protein, minerals and vitamins to the diet. It is also a major source of dietary fibre (DF), which mainly comprises non-starch polysaccharides (NSP) derived from the cell walls. For example, in the UK the NSP from wheat contributes about 20% of the total daily intake of DF (Steer *et al.* 2008).

A recent study reported that NSP accounted for between 7.7% and 11.4% of the grain dry weight (average 9.5% dry weight), based on analyses of 26 lines grown in six environments. The total DF content of the same material, including lignin, was 9.6–14.4% (average 11.7%) (Gebruers *et al.* 2010a).

Wheat grain comprises several tissues which are partially separated by milling (Fig. 7.1).The major storage tissue of the grain is the endosperm, accounting for about 90% of the grain dry weight (Barron *et al.* 2007).This comprises two tissues: the starchy endosperm, which accounts for about 83–84% and forms the white

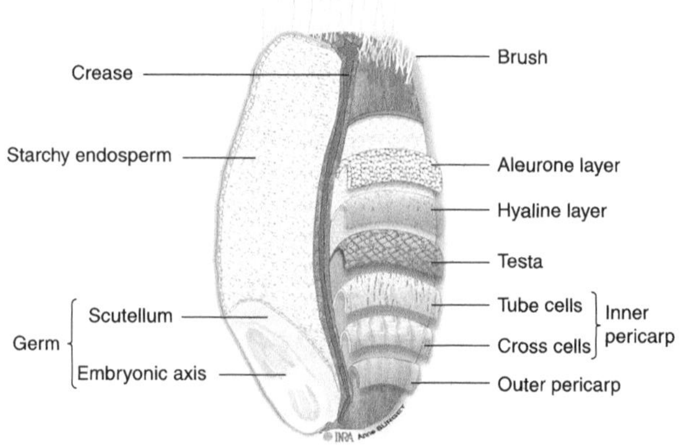

Fig. 7.1 Structure of the mature wheat grain showing the major tissues. Reproduced with permission from Surget and Barron (2005).

flour on milling, and a single layer of thick walled outer cells, the aleurone, which accounts for about 6.5% and is recovered in the bran fraction on milling. The bran fraction also contains the outer layers of the grain (pericarp, hyaline layer and testa; about 7–8% dry weight). Finally, the embryo (germ) is about 3% of the dry weight and is also recovered in the bran on milling.

7.2 Fibre content and composition of wheat fractions

The different organs and milling fractions of wheat differ widely in their content and composition of DF, and hence the dietary intake will vary depending on the fractions that are consumed.

7.2.1 White flour (starchy endosperm cells)

The cell walls of the wheat starchy endosperm (i.e. white flour) account for about 2–3% of the dry weight and consist of two major components, arabinoxylan (AX) and (1→3,1→4)-β-D-glucan (β-glucan), with small amounts of cellulose ((1→4)-β-D-glucan) and glucomannan. The classic and widely quoted study of Mares and Stone (1973) reported that these four types of polysaccharide accounted for about 70%, 20%, 2% and 7%, respectively, of wheat starchy endosperm cell walls. AX is also often divided into two tractions, depending on whether it is extractable (WE-AX) or unextractable (WU-AX) with water. These tractions may differ in their health benefits (as discussed elsewhere in this volume).

AX comprises a backbone of β-D-xylopyranosyl residues linked through (1→4) glycosidic linkages, with some residues being substituted with α-L-arabinofuranosyl residues at either position 3 or positions 2 and 3. Substitution at

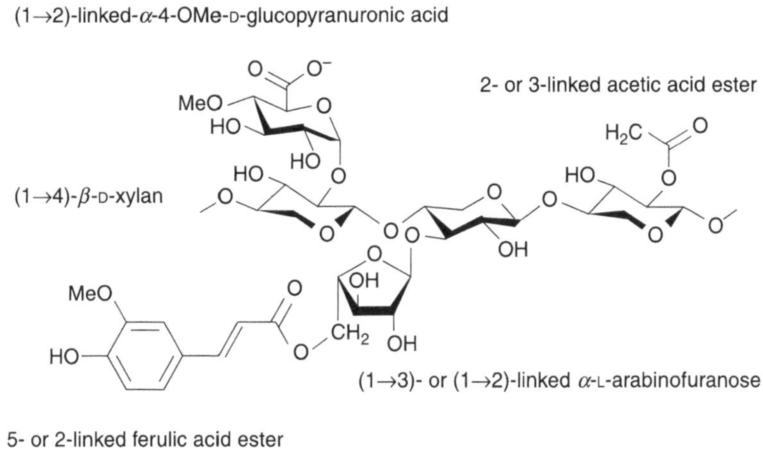

Fig. 7.2 Structure of arabinoxylan showing major substituents identified in fractions from flour, aleurone and pericarp. Reproduced from Stone and Morell (2009) with permission.

position 2 only has also been reported, but occurs rarely (Stone and Morell 2009). Some arabinofuranosyl residues at position 3 of the xylan residues may themselves be substituted with ferulic acid at the 5 position (Fig. 7.2). This substitution with ferulic acid allows the formation of cross-links by oxidation of ferulate present on adjacent AX chains to give dehydrodimers (diferulates). The extent of AX cross-linking is important as it affects the physio-chemical properties (notably solubility and viscosity) of AX, and hence its behaviour in food processing, and the health benefits. Starchy endosperm AX contain only low levels of ferulic acid, which has been estimated to account for 0.2–0.4% (w/w) of WE-AX and 0.6–0.9% (w/w) of WU-AX of wheat flour (Bonnin *et al.* 1998).

β-glucan has a simpler structure than AX, comprising only glucose residues joined by (1→3) and (1→4) linkages (Fig. 7.3(a)). Single (1→3) linkages are usually separated by two or three (1→4) linkages, resulting in the release of

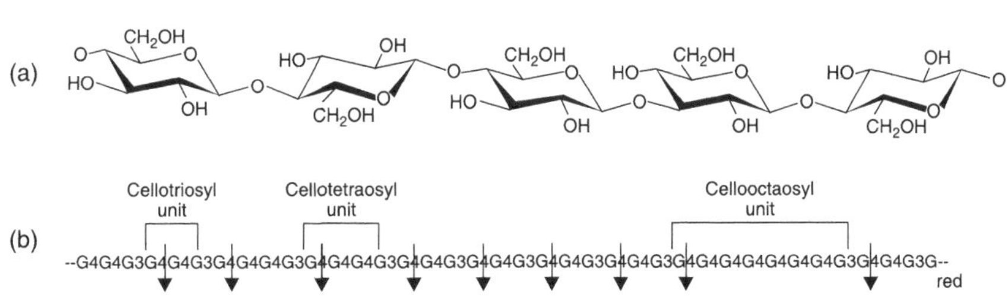

Fig. 7.3 (a) Structure of a (1→3, 1→4)-*β*-D-glucan molecule. (b) Distribution of 1→3 and 1→4 linkages in a (1→3, 1→4)-*β*-D-glucan molecule, showing sites of cleavage by lichenase ((1→3, 1→4)-*β*-D-glucan endohydrolase) to release glucans of three, four and more units. Reproduced from Stone and Morell (2009) with permission.

trisaccharide (G3) and tetrasaccharide (G4) units on digestion with a specific lichenase ((1→3, 1→4) endohydrolase) enzyme (Fig. 7.3(b)). However, longer stretches of (1→4) β-D-glucan linked glucan of up to 14 units have been reported for wheat bran β-glucan (Li *et al.* 2006). Such regions are sometimes referred to as 'cellulose-like', as cellulose is (1→4)-β-D-glucan without any (1→3) linkages.

7.2.2 Aleurone cells

The aleurone cells have thick cell walls and cell wall sugars account for about 35–40% of the dry weight (Barron *et al.* 2007). The cell wall composition is similar to that of the starchy endosperm cell walls, with 29% β-glucan, 65% arabinoxylan and only 2% each of cellulose and glucomannan (Bacic and Stone 1981). However, the ratio of arabinose to xylose is lower than that of starchy endosperm AX: 0.41 and 0.47 for two cultivars compared with 0.81 and 0.87, respectively (Barron *et al.* 2007). The aleurone AX are also highly esterified and cross-linked, with about 3.2% of the AX dry weight being ferulic acid and 0.45% being diferulic acid (Antoine *et al.* 2003; Parker *et al.* 2005). Additional esterification with *p*-coumaric acid and acetyl groups also occurs (Rhodes *et al.* 2002; Antoine *et al.* 2004).

7.2.3 Outer layers of the grain

The outer layers of the mature wheat grain comprise about 45–50% cell wall material (Barron *et al.* 2007). The major tissue is the pericarp, which is more similar in cell wall composition to wheat straw than to the seed tissues: about 30% cellulose, 60% arabinoxylan and 12% lignin (reviewed by Stone and Morell 2009).

The pericarp AX also has a more complex and highly branched structure than the endosperm AX, with galactose and glucuronic acid residues, and is hence often termed glucuronoarabinoxylan (GAX). It also has high contents of ferulic acid and diferulic acid (Saulnier and Thibault 1999; Antoine *et al.* 2003; Parker *et al.* 2005) and acetylation (Mandalari *et al.* 2005) and significant amounts of ferulic acid trimer (Barron *et al.* 2007).

7.2.4 Embryo (germ)

Little information is available on the content and composition of fibre in wheat germ, although commercial wheat germ fractions have been analysed in detail for many other components. Also, because the germ is difficult to separate from bran contamination, except by painstaking hand dissection, those values which have been published vary widely. The recent study of Barron *et al.* (2007) probably provides the most reliable data, based on neutral sugar analysis of hydrolysates. The scutellum (cotyledon) and embryonic axis contained about 12% and 25% of neutral carbohydrate, respectively, with arabinose and xylose (presumably derived from AX) accounting for about 65% of the total. Other sugars released were glucose (presumably from β-glucan), galactose and, for the embryonic axis only, mannose (possibly from mannans or glucomannans).

7.3 Genetic variation in arabinoxylan (AX) amount, structure and composition

7.3.1 Variation in amount and composition

A number of studies have reported the contents of β-glucan and AX fractions in wheat, analysing collections of lines, lines grown on different sites, and lines grown with different levels of nitrogen fertiliser and irrigation. The results of some of these studies are summarised in Table 7.1. Despite the analyses having been carried out in different laboratories with different methods over a period of 20 years, there is remarkably good agreement between the mean contents of β-glucan and AX that have been reported.

The content of β-glucan in wholegrain varies from about 0.5 to 1.1% dry weight, with the content in the endosperm being about half of this. Total arabinoxylan (TOT-AX) generally accounts for about 6% of the whole grain, with only a tenth of this being water-extractable. The content of total AX is much higher in bran fractions, 17–18% dry weight, but WE-AX is only about 0.4% (i.e. about 2% of the TOT-AX in this fraction). By contrast, the content of TOT-AX in flour is lower (about 2% dry weight) but the water-extractable fraction accounts for about 25% of the total. However, there is also significant variation in the contents of β-glucan and AX between genotypes and environments. For example, Ordaz-Ortiz *et al.* (2005) reported that the contents of WE-AX in 20 wheat varieties varied from 0.26 to 0.75% dry weight (mean 0.51%) and of WU-AX from 0.88 to 1.52% dry weight (mean 1.15%).

A more extensive study of 151 wheat lines (131 winter type and 20 spring type) grown on a single site in Hungary showed substantial variation in the contents of WE-AX and TOT-AX in both flour and bran fractions and in the content of β-glucan in wholemeal (see Table 7.1).The data for the AX fractions are shown graphically in Fig. 7.4. Particularly noteworthy is the variation in the WE-AX content of flour, with one line (the Chinese breadmaking wheat Yumai 34) having about 1.4% dry weight of WE-AX compared with between 0.3% and 0.9% dry weight in the other 150 lines.

A more recent study reported by Gebruers *et al.* (2010b) compared 26 wheat lines, of which 23 had been grown for three years on the same site in Hungary and for the third year on three additional sites (in the UK, France and Poland), and three had been grown on the same four sites except for year 1. This showed substantial variation in the contents of AX (in the flour and bran) and β-glucan (in wholemeal) in the grain from the different years and sites, as well as variation between genotypes (Fig. 7.5).The content of WE-AX in flour was particularly variable, with high contents in the samples grown in the UK in 2007 (Gebruers *et al.* 2010b). Nevertheless, the amount was highly heritable (see below).

Table 7.1 Contents of arabinoxylan (AX) and β-glucan reported for wholegrain, flour and bran fractions of wheat. Results are expressed on a % dry weight basis

Lines	Tissue	Soluble β-glucan			Insoluble β-glucan			Total β-glucan			WE-AX			WU-AX			TOT-AX			Notes	Ref
		min	max	mean	min	max	mean	min	max	mean	min	max	mean	min	max	mean	min	max	mean		
2	Endosperm							0.24	0.36								2.26	2.33			1
2	Whole grain							0.60	0.65								6.25	6.93			1
18	Whole grain										0.31	0.75					4.07	6.06		Values for pentosans, on FW basis.	2
49	Flour	0.09	0.41	0.24				0.25	0.63	0.44	0.48	1.23	0.81	0.88	1.66	1.24				Based on sugar analysis.	3
20	Flour										0.36	0.78	0.56								4
22	Wholemeal										0.36	0.83	0.56				5.53	7.79	6.36		5
1	Whole grain										5.7	7.0	6.4							One cultivar, two seasons, 12 treatments.	6
22	White flour										0.26	0.91	0.49							22 lines grown at three locations for two years.	7
3	Whole grain							0.21	1.08											Based on analyses of three cultivars grown with three levels of N and three of irrigation.	8

20	Flour				0.26	0.75	0.51	1.21	2.31	1.67	1.66	2.87	2.18		9
20	Whole grain										4.79	6.92	5.76	Same samples as above.	10
6	Whole grain				0.42	0.86	0.63				5.81	7.19	6.62	Based on data for three years.	11
131	Flour				0.30	1.40	0.50				1.35	2.75	1.90	131 winter wheats on one site.	
	Bran														
	Whole grain				0.30	0.85	0.40				13.2	22.1	18.0		
		0.50	0.95	0.75											12
20	Flour				0.30	0.75	0.50				1.65	2.75	2.00	20 spring wheats on one site.	
	Bran														
	Whole grain				0.30	0.55	0.40				12.7	19.2	16.8		
		0.50	0.65	0.60											
26	Flour				0.24	1.03	0.54				1.31	2.73	1.99	23 wheats on six sites + three wheats on five sites only.	13
	Bran				0.27	0.92	0.44				12.1	22.6	17.3		
	Whole grain	0.46	0.95	0.66											

Notes: FW, fresh weight; WE-AX, water-extractable AX; WU-AX, water-unextractable AX; TOT-AX, total AX.

1. Henry, 1987; 2. Hong *et al.*, 1989; 3. Andersson *et al.*, 1992; 4. Andersson *et al.*, 1994; 5. Saulnier *et al.*, 1995; 6. Coles *et al.*, 1997; 7. Martinant *et al.*, 1999; 8. Güler, 2003; 9. Ordaz-Ortiz and Saulnier, 2005; 10. Ordaz-Ortiz *et al.*, 2005; 11. Dornez *et al.*, 2008a; 12. Gebruers *et al.*, 2008; 13. Gebruers *et al.*, 2010b.

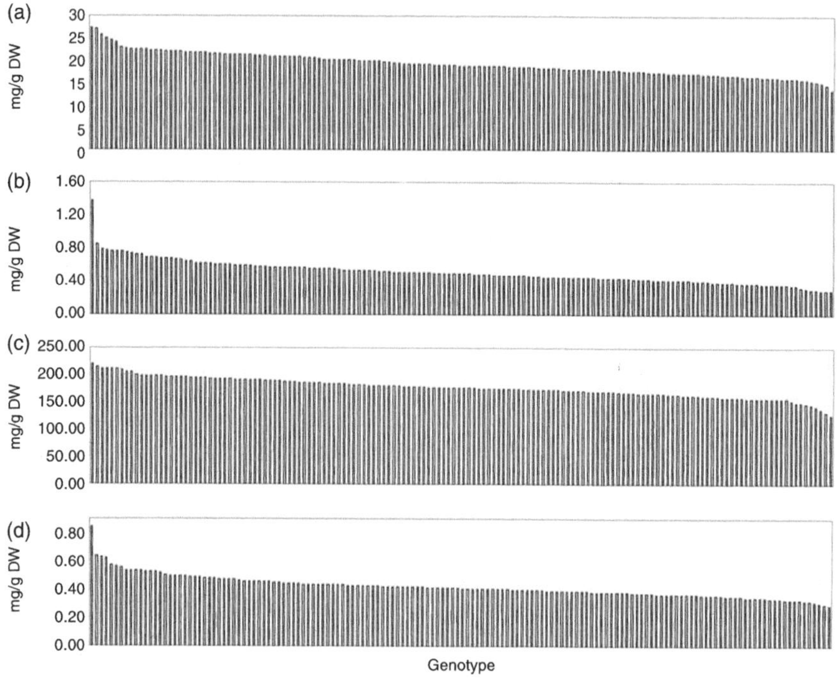

Fig. 7.4 Contents of arabinoxylan (AX) fibre in flour and bran of 150 wheat cultivars grown on a single site as part of the EU FP6 HEALTHGRAIN project.
(a) Total AX in flour; (b) water-extractable AX in flour; (c) total AX in bran; (d) water-extractable AX in bran. Taken from Shewry *et al.* (2010b) and based on data reported by Gebruers *et al.* (2008).

7.3.2 Variation in AX structure

Wheat AX is a complex mixture of polymers which may vary significantly in their structure, including the extent of substitution of the xylan backbone with arabinose and the substitution of monosubstituted arabinose with ferulic acid.

A frequently used measure of diversity in AX structure is the ratio of arabinose to xylose residues on hydrolysis (A:X ratio). The HEALTHGRAIN study reported by Gebruers *et al.* (2008) and Ward *et al.* (2008) showed significant variation in this ratio in flour and bran samples from 150 wheat lines grown on a single site, from 0.39 to 0.57 for flour WE-AX, from 0.49 to 0.71 for flour TOT-AX, from 0.71 to 1.63 for bran WE-AX and from 0.53 to 0.71 for bran TOT-AX (Fig. 7.4). Similarly, Saulnier *et al.* (2007) reported that the A:X ratio of WE-AX varied from 0.39 to 0.57 in a population of 90 lines from the cross W7984 (synthetic) x Oparta.

These differences imply the existence of variation in the ratio of xylose residues with arabinose at the 3 position (monosubstituted) and with arabinose at the 2 and 3 positions (disubstituted), which is sometimes also called the 'branching ratio'.

Further information on the fine structure of AX can be provided by a number of spectroscopic and biochemical approaches, with the most accessible of these being enzyme fingerprinting. This method is based on the digestion of the AX

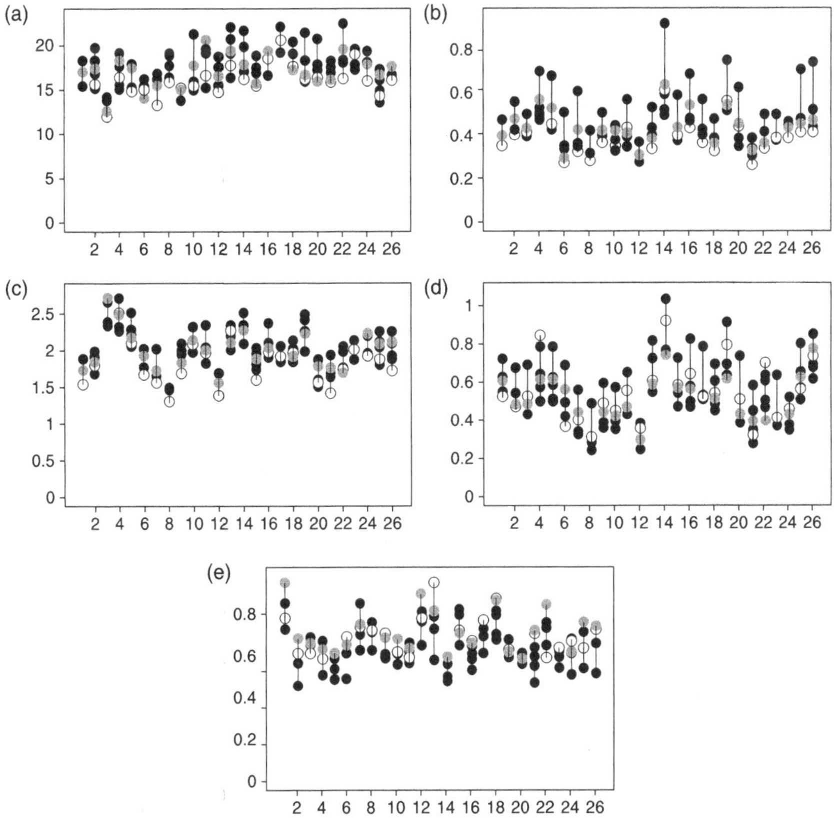

Fig. 7.5 Contents of dietary fibre components in the 26 wheat lines from six site × year combinations. Vertical axis = % dry weight, Horizontal axis = cultivar number. Samples are coloured by year of growth (light grey circles – 2005, open circles – 2006, dark grey circles – 2007). (a) Bran TOT-AX; (b) bran WE-AX; (c) flour TOT-AX; (d) flour WE-AX; (e) wholemeal β-glucan. Units are % dry weight. Taken from Shewry *et al.* (2010a), based on data reported by Gebruers *et al.* (2010b).

with a specific endoxylanase enzyme followed by separation of the released AX oligosaccharides (AXOS) by High Performance Liquid Chromatography (HPLC) (Ordaz-Ortiz *et al.* 2005) or gel electrophoresis (Goubet *et al.* 2002). The individual AXOS fragments can be further analysed to determine their structures while the patterns of AXOS released from different lines can be used as fingerprints to determine the range of structural diversity.

Saulnier and colleagues have applied this approach in a range of studies, including the wheat lines grown in Hungary in 2007 as part of the HEALTHGRAIN project and 128 lines from the cross Valoris x Isengrain (discussed below). Principal component analysis of the AXOS fingerprints showed that the major separation in PC1, accounting for 78.6% and 66.7% of the variation, respectively, in the two populations, related to differences in the proportions of monosubstituted and disubstituted xylose residues (see Shewry *et al.* 2010b).

7.4 Specific effects of agronomy and environment on arabinoxylan (AX) and β-glucan content and composition

A number of studies have shown that the agronomic conditions and climate can substantially affect the content and composition of AX and β-glucan. A limited number of studies have also related these effects to specific conditions (temperature, water availability and nitrogen nutrition).

The best documented effect is that of pre-harvest sprouting (PHS), due to wet conditions during the later stages of grain development and harvesting. PHS is premature germination and associated with the production of hydrolytic enzymes, including endoxylanases. This effect has been reported by Dornez *et al.* (2008a), who determined the levels of AX, endoxylanase activity and endoxylanase inhibitors in grain of 14 cultivars grown over three years (2002, 2003, 2004). They reported that 2002 was an exceptionally wet summer and that the grain had high levels of WE-AX and endoxylanase activity. By contrast, no significant variation in the content of TOT-AX was found.

A similar association between high endoxylanase activity and high content of WE-AX was reported by Gebruers *et al.* (2010a, b) for 26 wheat lines grown in the UK in 2007, another wet summer. In this study, the availability of meteorological data allowed correlations to be calculated, based on analyses of six sets of samples (grown in Hungary in 2005, 2006 and 2007 and in France, Poland and the UK in 2007 only). This showed strong negative correlations of both bran WE-AX and flour WE-AX with the average daily temperature and positive correlations with the total precipitation, both measured during the period between heading and harvest. However, no significant correlations between TOT-AX or wholemeal β-glucan and weather conditions were found (Table 7.2).

By contrast, Coles *et al.* (1997) compared grain from irrigated and non-irrigated plots of wheat cv Batten and showed a positive relationship between TOT-AX

Table 7.2 Correlations between the contents of DF in 26 wheat lines grown in six environments and the total precipitation and average temperature between heading and harvest

	Average temperature		Precipitation heading to harvest	
	R	*p* value	*R*	*p* value
Bran TOT-AX	0.060	0.911	0.138	0.795
Bran WE-AX	**−0.889**	**0.018**	**0.737**	0.095
Flour TOT-AX	−0.516	0.295	0.259	0.620
Flour WE-AX	**−0.868**	**0.025**	**0.692**	0.128
Wholemeal β-glucan	0.306	0.555	−0.684	0.134

Taken from Shewry *et al.* (2010b) with permission. Based on DF data reported by Gebruers *et al.* (2010b).
Notes: numbers in bold are statistically significant.

content and drought, while Güler (2003) reported that the total β-glucan content also increased under drought conditions.

The effect of N fertilisation on grain fibre content is less clear. Güler (2003) reported a positive effect of N on grain β-glucan in one year only out of a three-year study of three cultivars, while Dornez *et al.* (2008b) reported no effect on AX content in a three-year study of two cultivars. Coles *et al.* (1997) also showed that N fertilisation had no effect on the proportion of AX, with the total content per grain (but not the proportion) increasing with grain weight when late N fertilisation was combined with irrigation.

It is clear, therefore, that the major impact of environmental factors on dietary fibre content is that of endoxylanase on the proportion of WE-AX, due to the initiation of premature germination under wet climatic conditions.

7.5 Heritability and genetic analysis of arabinoxylan (AX) and β-glucan content

7.5.1 Heritability

The availability of compositional data for wheat lines grown under different environmental and agronomic conditions allows the variation to be partitioned between the effects of environment and genotype.

Hong *et al.* (1989) analysed wholemeals from 18 wheat lines (seven hard red winter, seven hard white winter and four club wheats) grown on two sites in Washington State, USA, and calculated that the genotypic variance was 1.6 times the environmental variance for water-soluble pentosans (i.e. WE-AX) and 2.4 times for total pentosans (i.e. TOT-AX).

Martinant *et al.* (1999) compared 19 cultivars grown at three locations in France and calculated the broad sense heritability (genotypic variance/phenotypic variance) as 0.75 for WE-AX of flour and 0.80 for the viscosity (which is largely determined by WE-AX) of flour water extracts. Dornez *et al.* (2008a) similarly analysed 14 cultivars grown in Belgium for three years and calculated broad sense heritabilities of 0.53 for TOT-AX and 0.96 for WE-AX, both in wholemeal. Similar studies of wholemeal samples of five durum wheat cultivars grown under four agronomic regimes gave genotype/environment ratios of 4.5 for TOT-AX and 4.9 for WE-AX (Lempereur *et al.* 1997).

Similarly high heritabilities of WE-AX and TOT-AX in flour were reported by Finnie *et al.* (2006), who analysed seven spring wheat lines grown in 10 environments and 20 winter wheat lines grown in 12 environments.

The analyses reported by Gebruers *et al.* (2010b) are typical of most studies and are summarised in Fig. 7.6 (taken from Shewry *et al.* 2010a).These show that the AX content of flour is highly heritable, with genotype accounting for about 60% of the variation in WE-AX and 70% of the variation in TOT-AX. Wholemeal β-glucan and bran WE-AX also show about 50% heritability. Thus, WE-AX in flour is a particularly attractive target for selection in plant breeding programmes. This study, and several others discussed above, also showed some interaction

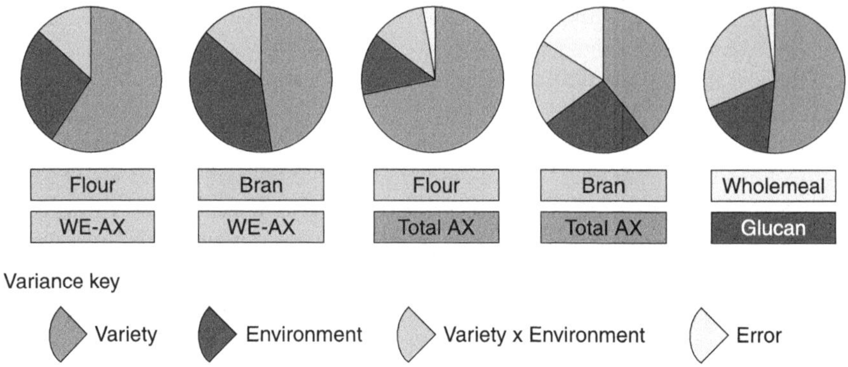

Fig. 7.6 Variance components of dietary fibre (AX and β-glucan) components of wheat grain. Taken from Shewry *et al.* (2010a) and based on data reported by Gebruers *et al.* (2010b).

between the genotype and environment, but this aspect has not been explored in detail.

However, a note of caution must be introduced based on the study of Li *et al.* (2009). They analysed wholemeals of 25 hard winter wheats and 25 hard spring wheats, with the two sets each being grown at three locations (although the locations differed for the two sets). They showed that environment had a much greater effect than genotype on WE-AX and TOT-AX in the winter lines, by more than an order of magnitude. Environment also had a greater impact than genotype on WE-AX in spring wheats, but had no significant effect on TOT-AX in these lines. The authors concluded that the relative effects of genotype and environment depended on the genotypes and environments which were sampled.

7.5.2 Genetic analysis

Martinant *et al.* (1998) used two mapping populations; 91 doubled haploid (DH) lines from the cross Courtot x Chinese Spring and 115 F_7 single seed descent lines from the cross W7984 (synthetic) x Oparta. They measured WE-AX, extract viscosity (which is largely determined by WE-AX) and the ratio of arabinose:xylose in WE-AX. A major quantitative trait locus (QTL) for all three traits was identified on chromosome 1B, which explained 32–37% of the variation in extract viscosity and 35–42% of the variation in the A:X ratio.

Further studies of five additional crosses were reported by Quraishi *et al.* (2010). These were populations of 187 recombinant inbred lines (RILs) from the cross Courtot x Chinese Spring (Perretant *et al.* 2000), 241 DH lines from the cross Arche x Recital (Laperche *et al.* 2007), 194 RILs from the cross Renan x Recital (Quraishi *et al.* 2009), 124 DH lines from Valoris x Isengrain and 280 lines from RE006 x CF007 (Charmet *et al.* 2009), with the latter two populations being constructed between parents with contrasting levels of WE-AX viscosity. Several of these crosses had been characterised for AX viscosity in previous studies and these data were therefore collated with new analyses to identify 'meta-QTL'. In this way the 12 QTL identified in the five populations were reduced to three meta-QTL for WE-AX viscosity located on chromosomes 1B, 3D and 6B.The 1B QTL corresponded to that identified by Martinant *et al.* (1998), while Charmet *et al.* (2009) reported that the QTL on 6B accounted for up to 59% of the variation in WE-AX viscosity in the Valoris x Isengrain and RE006 x CF007 populations.

Quraishi *et al.* (2010) complemented their meta-QTL analysis with association genetic analysis of the HEALTHGRAIN diversity collection of 156 wheat lines (131 winter and 20 spring bread wheats and five *Triticum spelta* lines grown in Hungary in 2005) (Ward *et al.* 2008). This identified seven loci involved in WE-AX viscosity: three co-located with the meta-QTL located on chromosomes 1B, 3D and 6B with four additional loci on chromosomes 3A, 5B, 7A and 7B.

The most significant locus identified by both these approaches was that on chromosome 1B, and Quraishi and co-workers (2010) have shown that this region of the chromosome contains four genes which may contribute to the trait. They have established molecular markers which are linked to the loci determining WE-AX viscosity and hence may be appropriate for use in plant breeding programmes.

7.6 Exploitation of genetic variation in grain dietary fibre in plant breeding

It is clear from the studies discussed above that extensive variation exists in the amount, properties and structure of AX in different wheat lines and samples, and that a substantial proportion of this variation is genetically controlled. It should therefore be feasible for plant breeders to select for increased, or decreased, contents of TOT-AX and/or WE-AX in their programmes. However, to do this it is necessary to establish screening methods which are robust but also sufficiently cheap and simple to be applied to large numbers of samples in breeding programmes. The viscosity of water extracts has been used as a measure of WE-AX in genetic studies, but viscosity may also be affected by other grain components (notably β-glucan) and no comparably simple methods are available for TOT-AX. Work is therefore in progress in several laboratories to develop rapid methods to quantify TOT-AX and determine specific structural characteristics, focusing on three approaches.

Near infrared (NIR) spectroscopy is widely used in plant breeding programmes, including the determination of moisture, protein, hardness (particle size index), colour, flour yield and flour water absorption on whole grain and milled samples of wheat (Osborne, 2006). Salgó *et al.* (2009) have developed NIR calibrations for TOT-AX, using the grain samples (wheat and other cereals) analysed for fibre components in the HEALTHGRAIN programme (Gebruers *et al.* 2008, 2010b; Ward *et al.* 2008; Shewry *et al.* 2010a) and based on analysing wholegrain, wholemeal, bran and white flour fractions. Using the data for wheat samples only, the correlation coefficients (R^2) between the predicted and determined values for TOT-AX were 0.7883 in bran and 0.5701 in flour, but these increased to 0.9354 and 0.8569, respectively, when the non-wheat samples were included in the datasets. These calibrations provide a good basis for the development of NIR systems which are appropriate for use in commercial plant breeding programmes.

The second promising approach is the development of antibodies which are specific for TOT-AX and for structural features of AX (such as diferulate cross-links). Toole *et al.* (2009) have discussed progress in the development of antibodies to AX and their use as probes in the spatial mapping of cell wall components in cereal grain. The challenge is to incorporate such antibodies into kit formats which enable them to be used in high throughput automated analyses.

Finally, the identification of QTL and candidate genes for AX synthesis is allowing the development of molecular markers (Charmet *et al.* 2009; Quraishi *et al.* 2010) which could be exploited in marker-assisted selection (MAS).The latter is perhaps the most promising, as MAS is being increasingly used to select for traits that are not readily selected at the phenotypic level in breeding programmes for wheat and other crops (Koebner and Summers 2003; Collard and Mackill 2008).

7.7 Conclusion

There is wide variation in the amount and composition of dietary fibre components between commercial wheat lines, particularly AX in white flour. Furthermore, a high proportion of the variation in amount is heritable; about 70% of the total variation for TOT-AX in white flour, 60% of the variation in WE-AX in white flour and about 50% of the variation in TOT-AX and WE-AX in bran. Genetic studies are leading to the identification of chromosomal regions and genes that determine this variation, which will facilitate the development of molecular markers to allow plant breeders to select for AX amount and composition in their breeding programmes. These markers will be complemented by other screening tools, with NIR calibrations allowing selection for total amount and antibody-based kits allowing identification of specific structural features. This should lead to the development of a new generation of wheat cultivars in which improved health benefits are combined with high yields, good agronomic properties and good quality for traditional end uses.

7.8 Acknowledgements

Part of the work described in this publication was financially supported by the European Commission in the Communities 6th Framework Programme, Project HEALTHGRAIN (FOOD-CT-2005-514008). It reflects the authors' views and the Community is not liable for any use that may be made of the information contained in this publication. I have quoted extensively from analyses carried out during the HEALTHGRAIN project and wish to thank my colleagues who contributed to these studies, notably Gilles Charmet, Catherine Ravel, Luc Saulnier, Jerome Salse, Umar Masood Quraishi (INRA, France), Kurt Gebruers, Christophe Courtin, Jan Delcour (Katholieke Universiteit Leuven, Belgium), Zoltan Bedő, Mariann Rakszegi (Agricultural Research Institute of the Hungarian Academy of Sciences, Martonvásár, Hungary) and Jane L. Ward (Rothamsted, UK). Rothamsted Research receives grant-aided support from the Biotechnology and Biological Sciences Research Council of the UK.

7.9 References

ANDERSSON R, WESTERLUND E, TILLY A-C and ÅMAN P (1992), 'Natural variations in the chemical composition of white flour', *J Cereal Sci*, **17**, 183–99.

ANDERSSON R, WESTERLUND E and ÅMAN P (1994), 'Natural variations in the contents of structural elements of water-extractable non-starch polysaccharides in white flour', *J Cereal Sci*, **19**, 77–82.

ANTOINE C, PEYRON S, MABILLE F, LAPIERRE C, BOUCHET B, *et al.* (2003), 'Individual contribution of grain outer layers and their cell wall structure to the mechanical properties of wheat bran', *J Agric Food Chem*, **51**, 2026–33.

ANTOINE C, PEYRON S, LULLIEN-PELLERIN V, ABECASSIS J and ROUAU X (2004), 'Wheat bran tissue fractionation using biochemical markers', *J Cereal Sci*, **39**, 387–93.

BACIC A and STONE BA (1981), 'Chemistry and organisation of aleurone cell wall components from wheat and barley', *Australian Journal of Plant Physiology*, **8**, 475–95.

BARRON C, SURGET A and ROUAU X (2007), 'Relative amounts of tissues in mature wheat (*Triticum aestivum* L.) grain and their carbohydrate and phenolic acid composition', *J Cereal Sci*, **45**, 88–96.

BONNIN E, LE GOFF A, SAULNIER L, CHAURAND M and THIBAULT JF (1998), 'Preliminary characterisation of endogenous wheat arabinoxylan-degrading enzymic extracts', *J Cereal Sci*, **28**, 53–62.

CHARMET G, MASOOD-QURAISHI U, RAVEL C, ROMEUF I, BALFOURIER F, *et al.* (2009), 'Genetics of dietary fibre in bread wheat', *Euphytica* **170**, 155–68.

COLES GD, HARTUNIAN-SOWA SM, JAMIESON PD, HAY AJ, ATWELL WA and FULCHER RG (1997), 'Environmentally-induced variation in starch and non-starch polysaccharide content in wheat', *J Cereal Sci*, **26**, 47–54.

COLLARD BCY and MACKILL DJ (2008), 'Marker-assisted selection: an approach for precision plant breeding in the twenty-first century', *Phil Trans Royal Soc B*, **363**, 557–72.

DORNEZ E, GEBRUERS K, JOYE IJ, DE KETELAERE B, LENARTZ J, *et al.* (2008a), 'Effects of genotype, harvest year and genotype-by-harvest year interactions on arabinoxylan, endoxylanase activity and endoxylanase inhibitor levels in wheat kernels', *J Cereal Sci*, **47**, 180–9.

DORNEZ E, GEBRUERS K, JOYE IJ, DE KETELAERE B, LENARTZ J, *et al.* (2008b), 'Effects of fungicide treatment, N-fertilisation and harvest date on arabinoxylan, endoxylanase activity and endoxylanase inhibitor levels in wheat kernels', *J Cereal Sci*, **47**, 190–200.

FINNIE SM, BETTGE AD and MORRIS CF (2006), 'Influence of cultivar and environment on water-soluble and water-insoluble arabinoxylans in soft wheat', *Cereal Chem*, **83**, 617–23.

GEBRUERS K, DORNEZ E, BOROS D, FRAS A, DYNKOWSKA W, *et al.* (2008), 'Variation in the content of dietary fiber and components thereof in wheats in the HEALTHGRAIN diversity screen', *J Agric Food Chem*, **56**, 9740–9.

GEBRUERS K, DORNEZ E, BEDO Z, RAKSZEGI M, COURTIN CM and DELCOUR JA (2010a), 'Variability in xylanase and xylanase inhibition activities in different cereals in the HEALTHGRAIN diversity screen and contribution of environment and genotype to this variability in common wheat', *J Agric Food Chem*, **58**, 9362–71.

GEBRUERS K, DORNEZ E, BEDO Z, RAKSZEGI M, FRAS A, *et al.* (2010b), 'Environment and genotype effects on the content of dietary fiber and its components in wheat in the HEALTHGRAIN diversity screen', *J Agric Food Chem*, **58**, 9353–61.

GOUBET F, JACKSON P, DEERY MJ and DUPREE P (2002), 'Polysaccharide analysis using carbohydrate gel electrophoresis: a method to study plant cell wall polysaccharides and polysaccharide hydrolases', *Anal Biochem*, **300**, 53–68.

GÜLER M (2003), 'Nitrogen and irrigation effects on β-glucan content of wheat grain', *Acta Agric Scand B*, **53**, 156–60.

HENRY RJ (1987), 'Pentosan and (1→3),(1→4)-β-glucan concentrations in endosperm and wholegrain of wheat, barley, oats and rye', *J Cereal Sci*, **6**, 253–8.

HONG BH, RUBENTHALER GL and ALLAN RE (1989), 'Wheat pentosans. I. Cultivar variation and relationship to kernel hardness', *Cereal Chem*, **66**, 369–73.

KOEBNER RMD and SUMMERS RW (2003), '21st century wheat breeding: plot selection or plate detection?' *Trends Biotechnol*, **21**, 59–63.

LAPERCHE A, BRANCOURT-HULMEL M, HEUMEZ E, GARDET O, HANOCQ E, *et al.* (2007) 'Using genotype x nitrogen interaction variables to evaluate the QTL involved in wheat tolerance to nitrogen constraints', *Theor Appl Genet*, **115**, 399–415.

LEMPEREUR I, ROUAU X and ABECASSIS J (1997), 'Genetic and agronomic variation in arabinoxylan and ferulic acid contents of durum wheat (*Triticum durum* L.) grain and its milling fractions', *J Cereal Sci*, **25**, 103–10.

LI S, MORRIS CF and BETTGE AD (2009), 'Genotype and environment variation for arabinoxylans in hard winter and spring wheats of the US Pacific Northwest', *Cereal Chem*, **86**, 88–95.

LI W, CUI SW and KAKUDA Y (2006), 'Extraction, fractionation, structural and physical characterization of wheat β-D-glucans', *Carbohyd Polym*, **63**, 408–16.

MANDALARI G, FAULDS CB, SANCHO AI, SAIJA A, BISIGNANO G, *et al.* (2005), 'Fractionation and characterisation of arabinoxylans from brewers' spent grain and wheat bran', *J Cereal Sci*, **42**, 205–12.

MARES DJ and STONE BA (1973), 'Studies on wheat endosperm. I. Chemical composition and ultrastructure of the cell walls', *Aus J Biol Sci*, **26**, 793–812.

MARTINANT JP, CADELEN T, BILLOT A and CHARTIER S (1998), 'Genetic analysis of water-extractable arabinoxylans in bread wheat endosperm', *Theor Appl Genet*, **97**, 1069–75.

MARTINANT JP, BILLOT A, BOUGUENNEC A, CHARMET G, SAULNIER L and BRANLARD G (1999), 'Genetic and environmental variations in water-extractable arabinoxylans content and flour extract viscosity', *J Cereal Sci*, **30**, 45–8.

ORDAZ-ORTIZ JJ and SAULNIER L (2005), 'Structural variability of arabinoxylans from wheat flour. Comparison of water-extractable and xylanase-extractable arabinoxylans', *J Cereal Sci*, **42**, 119–25.

ORDAZ-ORTIZ JJ, DEVAUX M-F and SAULNIER L (2005), 'Classification of wheat varieties based on structural features of arabinoxylans as revealed by endoxylanase treatment of flour and grain', *J Agric Food Chem*, **53**, 8349–56.

OSBORNE BG (2006), 'Applications of near infrared spectroscopy in quality screening of early-generation material in cereal breading programmes', *J Near Infrared Spec*, **14**, 93–101.

PARKER ML, NG A and WALDRON KW (2005), 'The phenolic acid and polysaccharide composition of cell walls of bran layers of mature wheat (*Triticum aestivum* L. cv. Avalon) grains', *J Sci Agric Food Chem*, **85**, 2539–47.

PERRETANT MR, CADALEN T, CHARMET G, SOURDILLE P, NICOLAS P, *et al.* (2000), 'QTL analysis of bread-making quality in wheat using a doubled haploid population', *Theor Appl Genet*, **100**, 1167–75.

QURAISHI U-M, ABROUK M, BOLOT S, PONT C, THROUDE M, *et al.* (2009), 'Genomics in cereals: from genome-wide conserved orthologous set (COS) sequences to candidate genes for trait dissection', *Funct Integ Genom*, **9**, 473–84.

QURAISHI U-M, MURAT F, ABROUK M, PONT C, CONFOLENT C, *et al.* (2010), 'Combined meta-genomics analyses unravel candidate genes for the grain dietary fibre content in bread wheat (*Triticum aestivum* L.)', *Funct Integ Genom*, **11**, 71–83. (doi 10.1007/s10142-010-0183-2).

RHODES DI, SADEK M and STONE BA (2002), 'Hydroxycinnamic acids in walls of wheat aleurone cells', *J Cereal Sci*, **36**, 67–81.

SALGÓ A, GERGELY S and GEBRUERS K (2009), 'Screening for dietary fibre constituents in cereals by near infrared spectroscopy', in SHEWRY PR and WARD JL, *HEALTHGRAIN methods. Analysis of bioactive components in small grain cereals*, St Paul, MN, AACC, 247–72.

SAULNIER L and THIBAULT JF (1999), 'Ferulic acid and diferulic acids as components of sugar-beet pectins and maize bran heteroxylans', *J Sci Food Agric*, **79**, 396–402.

SAULNIER L, PENEAU N and THIBAULT J-F (1995), 'Variability in grain extract viscosity and water-soluble arabinoxylan content in wheat', *J Cereal Sci*, **22**, 259–64.

SAULNIER L, SADO P-E, BRANLARD G, CHARMET G and GUILLON F (2007), 'Wheat arabinoxylans: exploiting variation in amount and composition to develop enhanced varieties', *J Cereal Sci*, **46**, 261–81.

SHEWRY PR, PIIRONEN V, LAMPI A-M, EDELMANN M, KARILUOTO S, *et al.* (2010a), 'The HEALTHGRAIN wheat diversity screen: effects of genotype and environment on phytochemicals and dietary fiber components', *J Agric Food Chem*, **58**, 9291–8.

SHEWRY PR, SAULNIER L, GUILLON F, GEBRUERS K, COURTIN C, *et al.* (2010b), 'Improving the benefits of wheat as a source of dietary fibre', in VAN DER KAMP JW, JONES J, MCCLEARY B and TOPPING D, *Dietary fibre: new frontiers for food and health*, Wageningen, Wageningen Academic Publishers, 65–78.

STEER T, THANE C, STEPHEN A and JEBB S (2008), 'Bread in the diet: consumption and contribution to nutrient intakes of British adults', *Proc Nutr Soc*, **67**, E363.

STONE B and MORELL MK (2009), 'Carbohydrates', in KHAN K and SHEWRY PR, *Wheat: Chemistry and Technology*, 4th ed., St Paul, MN, AACC, 299–362.

SURGET A and BARRON C (2005), 'Histologie du grain de blé', *Industrie des Céréales*, **145**, 3–7.

TOOLE GA, WELLNER N, FAULDS CB, MILLS ENC, BARRON C, *et al.* (2009), 'Spatial mapping of cell wall components in the cereal endosperm using spectroscopic, fluorescent and immunochemical methods', in SHEWRY P R and WARD J L, *HEALTHGRAIN methods. Analysis of bioactive components in small grain cereals*, St Paul, MN, AACC, 217–46.

WARD J, POUTANEN K, GEBRUERS K, PIIRONEN V, LAMPI A-M, *et al.* (2008), 'The HEALTHGRAIN cereal diversity screen: concept, results and prospects', *J Agric Food Chem*, **56**, 9699–709.

8

Cereal brans as dietary fibre ingredients

J. Sibakov, P. Lehtinen and K. Poutanen, VTT Technical Research Centre of Finland, Finland

DOI: 10.1533/9780857095787.2.170

Abstract: This chapter reviews the technologies for production and use of wheat, rye, oat, barley and rice bran. These important ingredients increase the grain fibre content of cereal-based foods in particular. Wheat bran, a co-product of milling wheat into flour, is a commodity with a long history of use as an ingredient. Even though the commercial use pattern of oats, rye and barley is different from that of wheat in the sense that they are more often consumed as wholegrain products, their brans, as well as rice bran, are also commercially available as milling side streams. All brans have their specific composition, functional properties and flavour, and, in addition to providing fibre, assist in diversifying the grain based product portfolio.

Key words: wheat, rye, oats, barley, rice, bran, fibre, ingredient, milling.

8.1 Introduction

From a quantitative point of view, wheat, rice, maize, rye, oats, barley, sorghum and various millets are the most important cereal grains and have a variety of food uses. Cereal products are an essential part of the diet for the majority of the world's population, providing 30–60% of daily energy worldwide. At the same time, they are an important source of all major nutrients. For example, in Finland around 48% of carbohydrate, 3% of lipid and 20% of protein intake is through cereal products (Pietinen *et al.*, 2010). Cereal products are also a major source of dietary minerals and vitamins, especially B vitamins. However, cereal processing typically involves refining steps so that in the majority of commercial food products the outer parts of the grains, and concomitantly a large part of dietary fibre, minerals, vitamins and phytochemicals, are removed. Thus, the majority of breads and other cereal foods have lower density of these nutrients than the original grain raw material. It has been estimated that in 2005 around 90% of the intake of cereal foods in the USA was based on refined products (Wells and Buzby, 2008). Processing also has a large impact on cereal food structure, which is important for food digestibility and nutrient absorption.

Recent epidemiological studies show an increasing body of evidence for a protective role of wholegrain foods and grain fibre against chronic diseases, such as type 2 diabetes (de Munter *et al.*, 2007) and cardiovascular disease (Jensen *et al.*, 2004; Mellen *et al.*, 2007). This has raised awareness of the importance of cereal food quality in health maintenance. The importance of dietary fibre as a health protective component has long been recognised. It is concentrated in the outer layers of the grains, which also contain phytochemicals, vitamins and minerals. Evidently, a high proportion of the potentially bioactive components are present in bran, making it an excellent source for nutritional enrichment of refined foods. It is hence an important dietary strategy to change the consumption of cereal products from refined to healthier products. Here, new tools are needed to increase the use of products enriched with wholegrain, bran or germ.

8.2 Cereal cell walls as dietary fibre

The non-starch polysaccharides building up the cell walls of cereal grains are one of the most important dietary fibre sources in the human diet. The main dietary fibre components are similar in all major cereals, consisting of cellulose, arabinoxylan (AX), (1→3)(1→4) mixed linked β-D-glucans and lignin. The proportions of these components vary between different cereals and grain layers. Outer pericarp layers of grains are enriched with cellulose, AX and lignin, whereas aleurone and endosperm cell walls contain mainly AX and β-glucans (Fincher and Stone, 1986; Mandalari *et al.*, 2005; Schwarz *et al.*, 1988). Rye and wheat also contain fructan, which contributes to the dietary fibre content in these grains (Karppinen *et al.*, 2003; Haskå *et al.*, 2008).

The composition of cereal cell walls, in relation to their suggested health relevance, was recently reviewed by Collins *et al.* (2010). The insoluble nature of the cereal fibre complex has been suggested to be a reason for its protective role against type 2 diabetes (Weickert and Pfeiffer, 2008). Antioxidative properties in the gastrointestinal tract (Vitaglione *et al.*, 2008; Saura-Calixto, 2011) and bifidogenic properties (Neyrinck *et al.*, 2011) have been suggested as some of the mechanisms important for the health effects of cereal fibre.

Oat and barley bran are well-known sources of β-glucan. The health effects of viscous β-glucan dietary fibre are well documented with respect to both cholesterol-lowering properties (Wood, 2007; Othman *et al.*, 2011) and attenuation of glycaemic and insulin responses (Butt *et al.*, 2008; Kim *et al.*, 2009; Panahi *et al.*, 2007; Wood *et al.*, 2000). Especially with respect to the latter, retaining the highly viscous character of β-glucan in food systems is important. Health claims referring to the reduction of cholesterol levels can be connected to oat bran both in the USA (FDA, 1997; 2003) and in the EU (EFSA, 2009).

AX, the major constituent of the wheat, rye and rice bran fibre complex, has recently gained much interest as dietary fibre, as reviewed by Bach Knudsen and Laerke (2010), Broekaert *et al.* (2011) and Saeed *et al.* (2011). AXs are heteropolysaccharides consisting of a backbone of β-1,4-linked D-xylopyranoside units, the major substituents of which are L-arabinofuranose residues, attached by α-1,2 and/or α-1,3-glycosidic linkages. Hydroxycinnamic acids, mainly ferulic acid, but also dehydrodiferulic, *p*-coumaric and sinapic acids, may be linked to the C-(*O*)-5 position of some terminal arabinose units. The heterogeneous structure of the polysaccharide, in terms of contents of unsubstituted, mono- and disubsituted xylopyranose units, as well as in terms of molecular weight distribution and water extractability, makes AX a blend of materials with a range of physiological responses. AX and AX-oligosaccharides have recently been studied for their prebiotic and bifidogenic properties (Broekaert *et al.*, 2011; Neyrinck *et al.*, 2011).

In some studies, the cholesterol lowering effect of full-fat rice bran has been shown to be almost equal to that of oat bran (Gerhardt and Gallo, 1998). According to Most *et al.* (2005), defatted rice bran does not lower the plasma lipid concentrations. However, rice bran oil can lower the serum cholesterol levels in healthy, moderately hypercholesterolaemic adults (Cicero and Derosa, 2005).

In addition to dietary fibre, brans contain different types of small molecular weight components with known and potential nutritional significance, such as vitamins, minerals and various phenolic compounds. They will be introduced below for each bran.

8.3 Cereal bran production technology

The term 'cereal bran' is relatively vague and refers to various types of milling products comprising outer layers of kernels enriched with dietary fibre. Typically, cereal bran products contain cellulose- and lignin-rich outer pericarp layers of grain, aleurone and subaleurone layers rich in hemicelluloses, and cell wall material from the endosperm part of the grain. Often, the germ of the grain is recovered with the bran fraction. Rye and oat brans typically contain a much larger proportion of subaleurone and endosperm tissues than wheat bran (Fig. 8.1).

The bran fraction is traditionally collected as a leftover from the production of flour (Delcour and Hoseney, 2010). However, with increased knowledge of the nutritional importance of dietary fibre, there has been an increasing interest in producing high quality bran fractions as a primary product, or isolating and further functionalising specific bran components, such as β-glucan-rich cell walls from oats and barley (Lehtinen *et al.*, 2009; Morgan, 1998; Redmond and Fielder, 2004; Sibakov *et al.*, 2011; Wu and Doehlert, 2002), phytochemical-rich aleurone layers of wheat (Harris *et al.*, 2005; Hemery *et al.*, 2007) and AX-oligosaccharides (Broekaert *et al.*, 2011), into value added products.

Prior to the separation of grain into bran and endosperm fractions, grains can be pre-treated to modify their mechanical properties (tissue dissociation and

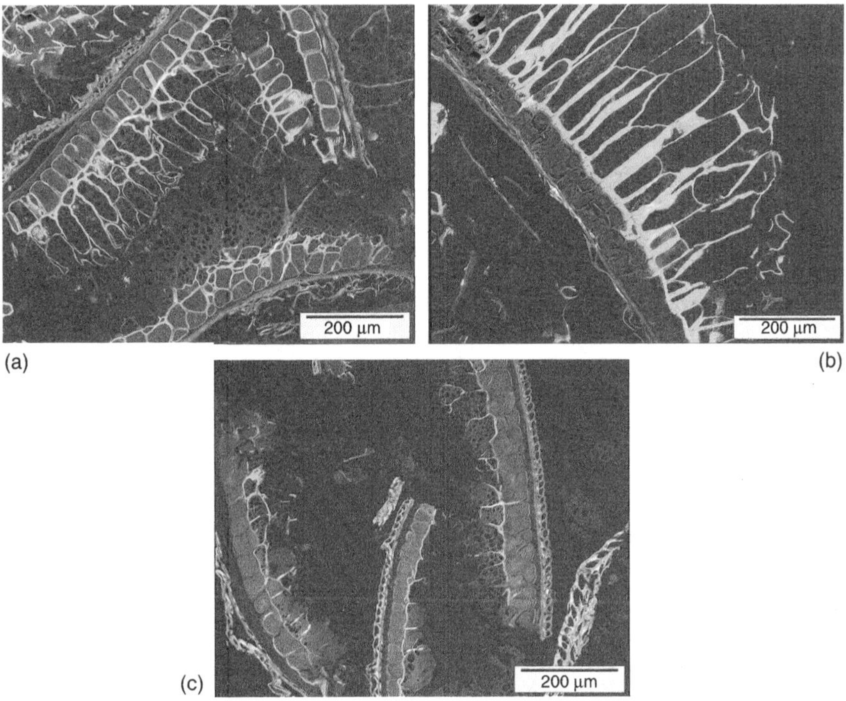

Fig. 8.1 Micrographs of (a) rye bran, (b) oat bran and (c) wheat bran produced from non-peeled grains. *β*-Glucan in cell walls is stained with Calcofluor (blue) and protein with Acid Fuchsin (red) in the sections cut of resin embedded samples. Starch granules are not stained and are seen as black spaces in the protein matrix (courtesy of Ulla Holopainen, VTT Technical Research Centre, Finland).

fragmentation) or to influence the tissue composition. Pre-treatment techniques include grain moistening, changing grain temperature, and ultra-violet radiation. The actual fractionation process is generally performed in several steps, including fragmentation steps in which bran tissues are disintegrated and dissociated by grinding and separation.

Debranning, degerming, peeling or pearling can be used before milling to remove the outer pericarp layers and/or the embryo to improve the quality of end products. Wholegrain cereals contain not only nutritionally valuable compounds, but also detrimental microorganisms, heavy metals, sand and pesticide residues. However, the contamination is not uniformly distributed in the grain. For example, Fleurat-Lessard *et al.* (2007) showed that about 80% of pesticide residues are present in the outer layers of wheat grain. The outer pericarp usually contains most of the contaminating bacteria and moulds. According to Laca *et al.* (2006), 87% of the total microbial contamination is eliminated by removing only 4% of the total grain weight using debranning.

In the separation steps, the bran particles can be fractionated according to size, shape, mass, density or dielectric properties. Several separation methods can be combined to obtain efficient tissue separation (Hemery *et al.*, 2007). For example, the wheat aleurone layer, which contains most of the antioxidant potential of the grain, is recovered by efficient dry fractionation with grinding, air classification and electrostatic separation (Mateo Anson *et al.*, 2009).

8.3.1 Wheat bran

Wheat bran is produced as a side product of milling of wheat into white flour. Wheat is usually milled by roller milling, which delivers multiple product streams that the miller can combine into flour or bran fractions. Thus, the composition of wheat bran from different mills varies significantly. The worldwide consumption of wheat was around 693 million tons in 2011 (WASDE, 2012). Milling of one million tons of wheat can yield up to 0.25 million tons of wheat bran (Javed *et al.*, 2012). The composition and quantity of wheat bran depend on the extraction rate of milling, that is, how much of the kernel is recovered in flour. Wheat bran contains the outer layers of the wheat kernel and is composed mainly of insoluble AX, cellulose, starch, protein, β-glucan and lignin (Hemery *et al.*, 2007). It is well known for its effects in increasing faecal bulk and reducing intestinal transit time. EFSA has accepted health claims related to these effects, provided that either a food is 'high in fibre' or 10 g of wheat bran are consumed daily, respectively (EFSA, 2010).

According to Gebruers *et al.* (2008; 2010), the dietary fibre content in different wheats varies between 11.5 and 18.3%. The total AX concentration varies between 6.1 and 22.1% and between 1.4 and 2.8% in the bran and flour fractions, respectively. On average, bran AX makes up about 29% of the total dietary fibre content of wheat. Bran yield is inversely related to the AX content in bran and positively related to the dietary fibre content in wholemeal. During milling, around 80–85% of the dietary fibre is usually recovered in the bran fraction.

Kamal-Eldin *et al.* (2009) characterised two commercial wheat bran samples from the Nordic countries. The dietary fibre content in these wheat bran products varied from 40 to 53% of dry matter and starch content from 9 to 25%. The ash content of wheat bran samples was 5.5–6.5%. Around 55% of the dietary fibre in wheat bran is AX; the rest is cellulose (9–12%), lignin (3–5%), fructan (3–4%) and mixed linked β-glucan (2.2–2.6%). About 95% of the dietary fibre in wheat bran is insoluble (Cornell and Hoveling, 1998; Pomeranz, 1988).

Wheat bran consists of several layers: outer pericarp, inner pericarp, testa/seed coat, hyaline layer and aleurone layer (Fig. 8.2). The pericarp is composed of intermediate cells, cross cells and tube cells. The total pericarp comprises about 5% of the grain. It consists mainly of insoluble AX, cellulose and lignin. The outermost layer of the pericarp is called the outer epidermis. It is 15–20 μm thick, and is composed of long, narrow cells that are arranged alternately (Hemery *et al.*, 2007; Khan and Shewry, 2009). The testa layer comprises about 1% of the grain and is composed of mainly AX and lignin. The proportion of cellulose is lower

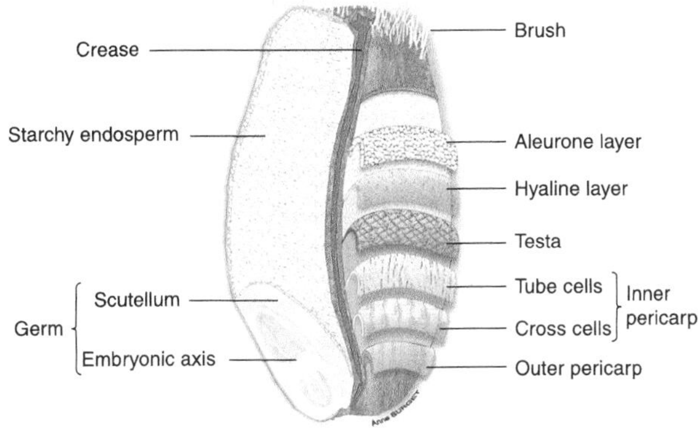

Fig. 8.2 The different layers of wheat bran illustrated from aleurone to outer pericarp. (Surget and Barron, 2005).

than in the pericarp (Hemery *et al.*, 2007). The testa contains almost all of the grain alkylresorcinols (Landberg *et al.*, 2008), a class of phenolic lipids reported to exhibit antioxidant properties and anti-cancer activity (Kozubek and Tyman, 1999).

Wheat bran, especially aleurone, is an interesting layer, as it contains most of the antioxidant potential of wheat grain (Mateo Anson *et al.*, 2009; Verma *et al.*, 2008; Adom *et al.*, 2005) due to its high content of lignans and phenolic acids (Buri *et al.*, 2004; Esposito *et al.*, 2005; Zhou *et al.*, 2004). Aleurone represents about 7% of the wheat grain dry mass but contains the major part of the B vitamins and about half of the total mineral content (Antoine *et al.*, 2003; Pomeranz, 1988). Compared to the other peripheral layers, the aleurone layer has high protein content, with a better balance of amino acids (particularly higher levels of lysine) than the proteins of endosperm (Buri *et al.*, 2004; Rhodes and Stone, 2002).

Recently, electric separation of wheat bran was developed to separate mixtures of aleurone and other outer layer particles. The charged particles are separated from one another due to their distinct dielectric properties and/or their different electrical polarisation (Behrens and Bohm, 2004; Bohm and Kratzer, 2005; Hemery *et al.*, 2011a, b). In addition, the aleurone fraction can be separated by enzymatic approaches (Bohm *et al.*, 2003).

Depending on the milling process, wheat bran fraction may also contain the germ. The wheat germ comprises 2.5 to 3.5% of the kernel. It is composed of the embryonic axis and the scutellum, which functions as a storage organ for wheat. The germ contains about 25% protein, 18% sugars and 16% lipids. Sugars are mainly sucrose and raffinose. The germ does not contain starch, but is rich in B vitamins (Delcour and Hoseney, 2010). Plant sterols are also concentrated in the germ (Nyström *et al.*, 2007).

8.3.2 Rye bran

Rye bran is a commercial milling product that contains grain outer layers and cell walls from endosperm. Similarly to wheat, rye is often milled by roller milling, which delivers multiple product streams that can be combined into flour or bran fractions. This results in various compositions of rye bran depending on the manufacturer, and it is not always clear whether the product should be described as rye bran or rye flour. A relatively large part (in Finland, for example, 90% of the rye consumption of 14 kg/capita/year) is used as wholegrain flour (Finnish Bread Information, 2012). EFSA has recently accepted a health claim about consumption of rye fibre and changes in bowel function (EFSA, 2011).

The content of dietary fibre in different rye varieties is between 20.4 and 25.2%, whereas total AX concentrations vary between 12.1 and 14.8% and between 3.1 and 4.3% in the bran and flour fractions, respectively (Nyström *et al.*, 2008). In rye, the aleurone, pericarp and testa are not as easily separated from endosperm as in wheat. Kamal-Eldin *et al.* (2009) characterised eight commercial rye bran samples from the Nordic countries. The dietary fibre content in these rye bran products varied from 41 to 48% of dry matter and starch content from 13 to 28%. Around 50% of the dietary fibre in rye bran is AX; the rest is a mixture of linked β-glucan, lignin, cellulose and fructan. All of the rye bran samples had ash contents higher than 2.8%. Also, rye bran fractions are enriched in protein, and Kamal-Eldin *et al.* (2009) reported a protein content of 14 to 18% in rye bran, whereas in rye flour the protein content is much lower at 5 to 16% (Gómez *et al.*, 2009).

Glitsø and Bach Knudsen (1999) showed that pericarp and testa have different dietary fibre composition and solubility from aleurone, and thus different functionality. In addition, Härkönen *et al.* (1997) showed that the AX in the outermost milling fractions of rye is less substituted (A:X 0.6–0.8) than in the endosperm (A:X 1.1–1.2). Rye AX, with a molecular weight of 1.38×10^6 g/mol in rye bran, is more resistant than rye β-glucan to depolymerisation in food processing (Rakha *et al.*, 2010).

Rye bran is relatively rich in low molecular weight phenolic compounds such as lignans and phenolic acids (Nilsson *et al.*, 1997; Liukkonen *et al.*, 2003). The contents and physiological effects of these compounds in rye bran and other rye products have been reviewed by Bondia-Pons *et al.* (2009). Rye bran is also a good source of plant sterols (Nyström *et al.*, 2007).

8.3.3 Oat bran

Oat grain contains a highly insoluble cellulose-rich outer shell or hull. Dehulling yields two products: hull material and the inner kernel, the oat groat. Only a few food ingredients are derived from hull, and the majority of the hull fraction, the main component of which is cellulose, is used as ruminant feed. The chemical composition and properties of the hull-based dietary fibre ingredients are very different from the bran obtained by milling of groats.

Unlike wheat and rye, oats are normally thermally treated prior to processing to ensure adequate shelf life. The thermal treatment, kilning, renders the majority of oat ingredients enzymatically inactive (NAMA, 2010). In further processing, kilned oat groats are milled into flour, usually in hammer mills or rollstands. The product is either whole oat flour (hammer mill) or a combination of starchy oat flour and oat bran (rollstands). Roller milling takes the oat groats through several rollstands to flatten and separate the bran from the endosperm flour (Paton and Lenz, 1993).

The effects of roller and impact milling on differently conditioned oat groats have been compared by Doehlert and Moore (1997). Tempering oats to 12% moisture improved bran yield from roller milling nearly twofold, but had little effect on bran composition. Bran yield from the impact-type mill was significantly affected by grinding screen size. Bran generated with 2.0 and 3.0 mm grinding screens on the mill had significantly higher starch concentration and significantly lower protein, β-glucan and ash concentrations than brans produced with 0.5 and 1.0 mm grinding screen sizes. Wang *et al.* (2007) combined dry milling with a pearling process, which efficiently removed trichomes and surface-borne aluminium and microbial contamination.

Oat bran consists of the outer layers of the grain, mainly aleurone, subaleurone and pericarp. Oat bran contains substantially more starchy endosperm and soluble dietary fibre components and less cellulose than wheat bran (Fulcher and Miller, 1993). In the definition of the American Association of Cereal Chemists (AACC), the oat bran fraction is not more than 50% of the dehulled oat kernel, and has a total β-glucan content of at least 5.5% (dry weight basis) and a total dietary fibre content of at least 16.0% (dry weight basis). In addition, at least one-third of the total dietary fibre should be soluble (AACC, 1989).

A review by Marlett (1993) lists published ranges of oat bran composition of 6.6–7.4% β-glucan, 12–26% protein, 47–53% starch, 2–11% fat and 2–9% ash. According to Shewry *et al.* (2008), the bran fractions of different oat varieties contain 6.2–8.4% β-glucan and 3.8–13.2% total AX, respectively. Only a minor part of the AX (0.2%) is water-extractable. Quantitative scanning microspectrofluorometry has been used to examine the distribution of β-glucan in the oat groat by Fulcher and Miller (1993). They concluded that oat cultivars with lower total β-glucan concentration have a higher proportion of the β-glucan in the subaleurone layers, whereas cultivars with higher total β-glucan concentration have a more uniform β-glucan distribution.

Air classification (Stevenson *et al.*, 2008; Vasanthan and Temelli, 2008; Wu and Doehlert, 2002) or extensive sieving procedures (Knuckles *et al.*, 1992) provide a way to enrich oat β-glucan to a much higher degree than in regular oat bran obtained by a rollstand process. Thus far, the highest β-glucan concentration obtained by air classification from regular, heat-treated and non-defatted oats has been 20–23%, with a mass yield of 33–39% (Lehtomäki and Myllymäki, 2010). With the non-heat-treated and defatted oats as the starting material, β-glucan concentration as high as 34% with a mass yield of 8–9% has been obtained by dry fractionation (Sibakov *et al.*, 2011). In addition to β-glucan, bran fractions are also usually enriched with protein and AX.

The viscosity of β-glucan solutions increases with both molecular weight and concentration of β-glucan in solutions, but decreases with increase in temperature

(Autio *et al.*, 1987; Dawkins and Nnanna, 1995). β-Glucan can be depolymerised during food processing due to the action of endogenous or exogenous enzymes, or because of thermo-mechanical treatment. According to Åman *et al.* (2004), intact oats and oat brans have β-glucan of high average molecular weight ($M_w = 2.0–2.3 \times 10^6$ g/mol). Most dry processed foods, such as extruded flakes, macaroni and muffins, retain the high molecular weight β-glucan. Large bran particle size and short fermentation time limit β-glucan degradation during baking. On the other hand, β-glucan in pasteurised juice, fresh pasta and teacake is degraded into smaller molecules ($M_w = 4.5–5.8 \times 10^5$ g/mol).

Compared with other cereals, oats contain unique polyphenols called avenanthramides, which have strong *in vitro* and *in vivo* antioxidant activity. Avenanthramides exhibit anti-inflammatory, antiproliferative and anti-itching activity. They may provide protection against coronary heart disease, colon cancer and skin irritation (Guo *et al.*, 2010; Meydani, 2009). Together with β-glucan, avenanthramides can be concentrated into cell wall-enriched fractions (Sibakov *et al.*, 2010). Based on pearling experiments, Peterson *et al.* (2001) showed that antioxidant activity is highest in the short-pearling-time fractions and decreases as more endosperm tissue is included. In contrast, concentrations of avenanthramides were not correlated with pearling time, indicating that they were more uniformly distributed in the groats.

8.3.4 Barley bran

The majority of the barley crop is used as a feed or for malting and brewing. Barley is surrounded by a husk that is usually not separated from the kernel during threshing, except in the case of hull-less or naked barleys. The husk is usually removed from the barley that is used for food by blocking or pearling until the pericarp, the testa, and in some cases also the aleurone layer have been removed (Slavin *et al.*, 2001). The barley kernel has a shallow crease, which makes it more attractive to start the milling process with a decortication step for removing the outer parts of the kernel instead of initially breaking up the kernel with roller mills to extract the endosperm as fine flour.

The total dietary fibre and starch contents in barley can vary significantly with the variety. For example, Andersson *et al.* (2008) reported 15.0–23.8% and 51.1–58.5% for dietary fibre and starch, respectively. The β-glucan concentration of barley is usually 3.7–6.5%, and the average molecular weight of β-glucan $1.5–1.8 \times 10^6$ g/mol (Andersson *et al.*, 2008; Yalçin *et al.*, 2007; Zhang *et al.*, 2002). The total AX content in barley flour and bran has been reported to be 1.4–2.2% and 4.8–9.8%, respectively. Only a minor part of the AX (0.2–0.4%) is water-extractable (Andersson *et al.*, 2008).

Pearling of barley produces groats with higher β-glucan content than in grains with cellulose-rich husk and protein-rich aleurone (Holopainen *et al.*, 2012; Klamczynski *et al.*, 1998; Marconi *et al.*, 2000). Barley groat can subsequently be flaked or milled into different kinds of flour. Barley flour can be fractionated into β-glucan-enriched products by air classification process or by roller milling and sieving. Ferrari *et al.* (2009) studied the air classification of pin disc milled barley flour and produced a fraction with 15.6% β-glucan with 28.4% yield, whereas Vasanthan and Bhatty (1995) produced a fraction with 23.8% β-glucan with a yield of 7.6%. Roller milling and sieving yield fractions relatively similar to air classification. Izydorczyk *et al.* (2003) were able to produce a fraction with over 15% β-glucan content and over 20% yield.

Soluble dietary fibre components from barley have also been recovered using aqueous processes. Benito-Román *et al.* (2011) used a systematic study design to identify critical parameters for β-glucan extraction. They found 55°C to be an optimal temperature for β-glucan extraction and also pointed out the importance of particle size and pH in extraction. A more complex protocol for β-glucan recovery was presented by Ghotra *et al.* (2008). In this process, patented by Vasanthan and Temelli (2002), the β-glucan is initially concentrated by removing other grain constituents in aqueous ethanol. In addition, a soluble barley β-glucan product has been developed using a proprietary hot water extraction method (Zheng *et al.*, 2004).

8.3.5 Rice bran

Commercial rice milling consists of cleaning, hull removal and subsequent milling processes. In brown rice, only the hull is removed (Slavin *et al.*, 2001). Usually, a part or all of the bran and germ is removed by abrasive scouring or pearling. Regular milled rice is brown rice from which practically all of the germ and pericarp, and most of the aleurone, have been removed, leaving mostly the starchy endosperm. This is usually called polished or white rice. Brown rice and white rice have similar levels of calories, carbohydrates and protein. The main differences between the two forms of rice lie in processing and nutritional content. Several vitamins (vitamins B_1 and B_3) and minerals (such as iron), as well as small amounts of fatty acids and dietary fibre, are lost in bran removal and subsequent polishing. The average level of dietary fibre in brown rice is usually 3–4% (Kahlon, 2009).

Rice bran has a light, slightly sweet taste. The bran layers of the rice kernel contain the highest concentration of some nutrients and the bran is a good source of protein and iron. The bran is traditionally used as feed for animals, because of a rapid tendency to become rancid and because of the microbial activity generally associated with raw rice bran. Highly active lipase enzymes begin to hydrolyse the neutral fat into free fatty acids and glycerol right after the milling. For example, the amount of free fatty acids can be increased by up to 16% within four days and up to 30% or more within two weeks (Babcock, 1987). To avoid the problems related to rancidity, Randall *et al.* (1985) inactivated the lipase enzymes by heating the bran in an extrusion cooker at 125–135°C for 1–3 s at 11–15% moisture. Extrusion cooking also reduces the microbial activity. This procedure prevents the increase in free fatty acid concentration for at least four weeks even under warm and humid storage conditions. According to Babcock (1987), the storage life can be as long as six months if the bran material is stored at or below 20°C.

Abdul-Hamid *et al.* (2007) collected samples of freshly milled raw rice bran from each of four different milling fractions produced during the multi-pass whitening process for brown rice. During commercial milling, brown rice is processed by polishing the kernels four times. For this study, the bran was collected after each rubbing. The first fraction had the highest concentration of dietary fibre (about 30%) and the fourth had the lowest (about 18%).

Abdul-Hamid and Luan (2000) showed that rice bran originally contains about 27% dietary fibre. When the oil of the rice bran is removed (e.g. by extraction with n-hexane), the bran can have an even higher content of dietary fibre, in the 35–48% range (Babcock, 1987). Saunders (1990) investigated the dietary fibre content of both non-defatted and defatted bran fractions. According to this study, the stabilised bran contains 20–25% total dietary fibre (of which 1.8–2.6% is soluble), bran from parboiled rice 31–33% (2.0–2.5%), defatted stabilised bran 24–28% (2.0–2.4%) and defatted bran from parboiled rice 44–51% (2.4–2.9%), respectively. The stabilised bran typically consists of 7.0–8.3% pentosans, 9.5–16.9% hemicelluloses, 5.9–9.0% cellulose and 2.8–3.9% lignin. The extraction of soluble fibres from rice has been studied by Aoe *et al.* (1993). β-Glucans are present at less than 1% in rice bran (Kahlon *et al.*, 1984).

8.4 Technologies to improve the properties of cereal brans as source of dietary fibre

Technological, nutritional and safety properties of cereal brans can be improved by different processing techniques. These techniques can be targeted at more specific fractionation, modification of structural properties, introduction of new functionalities or improving the sensory quality. An obvious parameter important for the functionality of bran as an ingredient is the particle size. It plays a significant role when adding the bran in baking (see Chapter 10, e.g. Zhang and Moore, 1999 and Noort *et al.*, 2010) and also in extrusion (see Chapter 15, e.g. Robin *et al.*, 2011). Current milling technologies allow ultra-fine milling (Hemery *et al.*, 2011a; Paltakari *et al.*, 2012; Zhu *et al.*, 2010), which itself creates possibilities for bran modification.

Removal of 1–3% of the wheat kernel by peeling prior to grain breakage and subsequent bran separation improves the sensory properties of bran (Hemery *et al.*, 2010). In the case of wheat bran, this improvement is also attributed to a removal of microbes, mycotoxins, heavy metals and pesticides. Simultaneously, the sensory and technological properties of the wheat bran are greatly improved. The subsequent limited grinding and bran separation enable an aleurone fraction to be produced in which the majority of the whole grain's beneficial properties are concentrated (Behrens and Bohm, 2004; Bohm *et al.*, 2003; Bohm and Kratzer, 2005; Hemery *et al.*, 2007; 2011b).

In the case of rye, the effective peeling rate of the kernel is much higher than in the case of wheat. For example, Heiniö *et al.* (2012) reported peeling rates of 10–20%. The improved properties of rye bran from peeled kernels were attributed to the lower content of certain phenolic compounds, while the dietary fibre content of bran remained the same as for rye bran without peeling. Fermentation of rye bran from peeled kernels with lactic acid bacteria prior to use in baking improved the bread making process (Katina *et al.* 2007). The fermentation lowers the pH, which in turn activates endogenous cell wall-degrading enzymes in rye. Bioprocessing with yeast and lactic acid starters and cell wall-degrading enzymes is an efficient technology for improving wheat bran as a bread baking ingredient (Salmenkallio-Marttila *et al.*, 2001; Katina *et al.*, 2012). The performance of bran in baking applications can also be improved by using enzymes such as xylanases (Laurikainen *et al.*, 1998) and oxidative enzymes (Gül *et al.*, 2009). Hydrothermal processing of bran has also been suggested (Amirkaveei *et al.*, 2009).

The particle properties and/or viscosity of soluble dietary fibre components have limited the use of bran in beverage applications. However, viscous properties of fibres can be effectively controlled by tailoring the molecular weight of soluble cell wall components. Tailoring of molecular weight is indeed an important tool in producing cereal dietary fibre components, especially in applications with high water content. Zheng *et al.* (2004) described an enzymatic method to produce a low molecular weight β-glucan composition with lower viscosity. Later, Kaukovirta-Norja *et al.* (2009) described a process for producing low molecular weight β-glucan by acid-catalysed hydrolysis at low water content, and Lehtomäki and Myllymäki (2009) developed a process based on enzymatic hydrolysis of β-glucan at low water content. Similarly, Broekaert *et al.* (2010) have described a process for producing soluble low molecular weight AX from distiller wet grains via enzymatic hydrolysis. Depolymerisation obviously influences both technological functionality and nutritional properties.

8.5 Food applications of cereal fibre ingredients

Cereal brans have been investigated as sources of dietary fibre in many different food applications. They are especially suited for use in cereal foods, where they are usually used in combination with refined flour. The most common products studied for bran fibre enrichment are presented in Table 8.1.

Bran, especially wheat bran, is the most common source of added dietary fibre in baking (Sanz Penella *et al.*, 2008), and rye bran has also been used to increase the dietary fibre content of bread (Katina *et al.*, 2007). The use of barley bran derived from naked or dehusked barley or oat bran derived from husked oat kernels is also becoming more widespread due to their high soluble fibre content, in particular their content of mixed-linked β-glucan. The challenges of high fibre and wholegrain baking are dealt with in Chapter 10, and those of adding fibre to extruded products in Chapter 12, pasta in Chapter 13 and noodles in Chapter 14. The specific feature of cereal brans as dietary fibre ingredients is their insolubility, as well as the presence of other grain components as part of the bran tissue.

Oat bran has been successfully incorporated into bread, extruded snack products, noodles, muffins and pancakes. However, its usability is limited because

Table 8.1 Examples of studies on effects of bran addition to food products

Food application	Wheat bran	Rye bran	Oat bran	Barley bran/Spent grains	Rice bran
Bread	Damen *et al.*, 2012; Hemery *et al.*, 2010; Katina *et al.*, 2006; Katina *et al.*, 2012; Lai *et al.*, 1989; Noort *et al.*, 2010; Salmenkallio-Marttila *et al.*, 2001; Sanz Penella *et al.*, 2008; Seyer and Gélinas, 2009; Zhang and Moore, 1999	Katina *et al.*, 2007; Larsson and Sandberg, 1991; Laurikainen *et al.*, 1998	Åman *et al.*, 2004; Kerckhoffs *et al.*, 2003; Larsson and Sandberg, 1991	Knuckles *et al.*, 1997; Moriartey *et al.*, 2011; Rasco *et al.*, 1990	Sairam *et al.*, 2011; Hu *et al.*, 2009
Extruded snack-products	Brennan *et al.*, 2008; Singh *et al.*, 2000; Robin *et al.*, 2011	Gambuś *et al.*, 2012; Myllymäki and Saapunki, 2010	Lobato *et al.*, 2011; Myllymäki *et al.*, 2002; Rzedzicki *et al.*, 2000	Ainsworth *et al.*, 2007; Stojceska *et al.*, 2008	Sekhon *et al.*, 1997
Muffins and cookies	Gujral *et al.*, 2003; Sloan and James, 1988	Kristensen *et al.*, 2005	Tosh *et al.*, 2008; Hudson *et al.*, 1992	Hudson *et al.*, 1992; Rasco *et al.*, 1990	Hudson *et al.*, 1992; Sloan and James, 1988; Sharif *et al.*, 2009
Noddles and pasta	Chen *et al.*, 2011; Sudha *et al.*, 2011; Wójtowicz and Mościcki, 2011	–	Reungmaneepaitoon *et al.*, 2006	Marconi *et al.*, 2000; Knuckles *et al.*, 1997	Kim *et al.*, 1998
Breakfast cereals	Baublis *et al.*, 2000; Brennan *et al.*, 2008; Kahlon and Woodruff, 2003; Kamran *et al.*, 2008; Monro, 2002	Lorenz and Al-Ruqaie, 1992	Bartram *et al.*, 1992; Kahlon and Woodruff, 2003; Tappy *et al.*, 1996; Tosh *et al.*, 2010	–	–
Pancakes, crepes, blinis, pie crust and pizza crust	Hebden *et al.*, 1998; Moore *et al.*, 2009	–	Dukan, 2009	–	Sharma *et al.*, 2004; De Delahaye *et al.*, 2005
Ice cream	–	–	Soukoulis *et al.*, 2009	–	–

of its high lipid content. In bread, the highest amount of oat bran that can be used without deterioration of the texture of the bread is usually around 20%. However, higher concentrations, up to 55–60%, have been studied in clinical trials and model products (Kerckhoffs *et al.*, 2003; Åman *et al.*, 2004). Addition of barley bran decreases bread loaf volume, increases firmness and gives darker and redder bread (Moriartey *et al.*, 2011). Breads with 20% β-glucan rich barley bran contain 4.2 times more total dietary fibre and 7.6 times more β-glucan than control bread. Such breads are still acceptable in laboratory acceptance tests (Knuckles *et al.*, 1997).

Defatted rice bran can be incorporated into breads at a level of up to 10–15%, as such or with bread improvers (Sairam *et al.*, 2011). Sharif *et al.* (2009) concluded that up to 10–20% of wheat flour can be substituted with defatted rice bran to prepare rice bran supplemented cookies without adversely affecting the sensory and structural quality.

8.6 Conclusion and future trends

Cereal brans are increasingly important dietary fibre ingredients, as the body of evidence about their health-protective effects is increasing, and new ways of tailoring their properties are emerging. Wheat bran has long been a common ingredient, but in recent years new milling technologies as well as bioprocessing methods have opened the door to an array of new ingredients with improved technological functionality. Interest in wheat bran is expected to increase. Rye bran is mainly used in the Northern and Eastern parts of Europe. It has distinct properties with high nutritional potential, and due to its high starch content, may serve in slightly different applications from wheat bran.

Oat and barley brans have attracted interest especially due to their soluble fibre content and cholesterol-lowering properties. Several specialty products with elevated β-glucan content are available, facilitating the formulation of a range of foods high in soluble fibre. The rheological properties of these brans also offer technological benefits in product formulations. Due to established health claims, the use of these fibre sources is expected to continue. Rice bran also has its established uses, and offers an interesting raw material for further modification.

The separation of brans in the milling process was originally developed because of the greater palatability of products made from refined flour. Now that the health relevance of the bran fraction has been established and realised, new technologies will enable production of cereal fibre-enriched foods with palatable taste and high sensorial quality.

8.7 References

AACC (1989), 'AACC committee adopts oat bran definition', *Cereal Food World*, **34**, 1033.
ABDUL-HAMID A and LUAN YS (2000), 'Functional properties of dietary fibre prepared from defatted rice bran', *Food Chem*, **68**, 15–19.

ABDUL-HAMID A, RAJA SULAIMAN RR, OSMAN A and SAARI N (2007), 'Preliminary study of the chemical composition of rice milling fractions stabilized by microwave heating', *J Food Comp Anal*, **20**, 627–37.

ADOM KK, SORRELLS M and LIU RH (2005), 'Phytochemicals and antioxidant activity of milled fractions of different wheat varieties', *J Agric Food Chem*, **53**, 2297–306.

AINSWORTH P, IBANOĞLU S, PLUNKETT A, IBANOĞLU E and STOJCESKA V (2007), 'Effect of brewers spent grain addition and screw speed on the selected physical and nutritional properties of an extruded snack', *J Food Eng*, **81**, 702–9.

ÅMAN P, RIMSTEN, L and ANDERSSON, R (2004), 'Molecular weight distribution of β-glucan in oat-based foods', *Cereal Chem*, **81**, 356–60.

AMIRKAVEEI SH, SHAHEDI M, KABIR GH and KADIVAR M (2009), 'Effects of treated and untreated bran in dough dynamic rheology', *Int J Food Sci Nutr*, **60**, 90–198.

ANDERSSON AAM, LAMPI A-M, NYSTRÖM L, PIIRONEN V, LI L, *et al.* (2008), 'Phytochemical and dietary fiber components in barley varieties in the HEALTHGRAIN diversity screen', *J Agric Food Chem*, **56**, 9767–76.

ANTOINE C, PEYRON S, MABILLE F, LAPIERRE C, BOUCHET B, *et al.* (2003), 'Individual contribution of grain outer layers and their cell wall structure to the mechanical properties of wheat bran', *J Agric Food Chem*, **51**, 2026–33.

AOE S, ODA T, TATSUMI K, YAMAUCHI M and AYANO Y (1993), 'Extraction of soluble dietary fibres from defatted rice bran', *Cereal Chem*, **70**, 423–5.

AUTIO K, MYLLYMÄKI O and MÄLKKI Y (1987), 'Flow properties of solutions of oat β-glucans', *J Food Sci*, **52**, 1364–6.

BABCOCK D (1987), 'Rice bran as a source of dietary fibre', *Cereal Foods World*, **32**, 538–40.

BACH KNUDSEN KE and LAERKE HN (2010), 'Rye arabinoxylans: Molecular structure, physicochemical properties and physiological effects in the gastrointestinal tract', *Cereal Chem*, **87**, 353–62.

BARTRAM P, GERLACH S, SCHEPPACH W, KELLER F and KASPER H (1992), 'Effect of a single oat bran cereal breakfast on serum cholesterol, lipoproteins, and apolipoproteins in patients with hyperlipoproteinemia type IIa', *J Parent Ent Nutr*, **16**, 533–7.

BAUBLIS AJ, LU C, CLYDESDALE FM and DECKER EA (2000), 'Potential of wheat-based breakfast cereals as a source of dietary antioxidants', *J Am Coll Nutr*, **19**, 308S–311S.

BEHRENS R and BOHM A (BÜHLER AG) (2004), *Method for the electric contact charging of a mixture containing aleurone and shell particles*. PCT application WO 2004/016354, 2004-Feb-26.

BENITO-ROMÁN O, ALONSO E and LUCAS S (2011), 'Optimization of the β–glucan extraction conditions from different waxy barley cultivars', *J Cereal Sci*, **53**, 271–6.

BOHM A and KRATZER A (2005), 'Method for isolating aleurone particles', US patent application US 2005/0103907 A1, 2005-May-19.

BOHM A, BOGONI C, BEHRENS R and OTTO T (2003), 'Method for the extraction of aleurone from bran', US patent application US 2003/0175384 A1, 2003-Sep-18.

BONDIA-PONS I, AURA A-M, VUORELA S, KOLEHMAINEN M, MYKKÄNEN H and POUTANEN K (2009), 'Rye phenolics in nutrition and health', *J Cereal Sci*, **49**, 323–36.

BRENNAN MA, MERTS I, MONRO J, WOOLNOUGH J and BRENNAN CS (2008), 'Impact of guar gum and wheat bran on the physical and nutritional quality of extruded breakfast cereals', *Starch/Staerke*, **60**, 248–56.

BROEKAERT W, COURTIN C and DELCOUR J (FUGEIA NV) (2010), 'Method for making soluble arabinoxylans as co-product of fermentation of whole-grain cereals', US patent application US2010/0035302 A1, 2010-Feb-11.

BROEKAERT WF, COURTIN CM, VERBEKE K, VAN DE WIELE T, VERSTRAETE W and DELCOUR JA (2011), 'Prebiotic and other health-related effects of cereal-derived arabinoxylans, arabinoxylan-oligosaccharides, and xylooligosaccharides', *Crit Rev Food Sci Nutr*, **51**, 178–94.

BURI RC, VON REDING W and GAVIN MH (2004), 'Description and characterization of wheat aleurone', *Cereal Food World*, **49**, 274–82.

BUTT MS, TAHIR-NADEEM M, KHAN MKI, SHABIR R and BUTT MS (2008), 'Oat: unique among the cereals', *Eur J Nutr*, **47**, 68–79.

CHEN JS, FEI MJ, SHI CL, TIAN JC, SUN CL, ZHANG H, MA Z and DONG HX (2011), 'Effect of particle size and addition level of wheat bran on quality of dry white Chinese noodles', *J Cereal Sci*, **53**, 217–224.

CICERO AFG and DEROSA G (2005), 'Rice bran and its main components: Potential role in the management of coronary risk factors', *Curr Top Nutraceut Res*, **3**, 29–46.

COLLINS HM, BURTON RA, TOPPING DL, LIAO M-L, BACIC A and FINCHER GB (2010), 'Variability in fine structures of noncellulosic cell wall polysaccharides from cereal grains: potential importance in human health and nutrition', *Cereal Chem*, **87**, 272–82.

CORNELL HJ and HOVELING AW (1998), *Wheat: Chemistry and utilization*, Pensylvania USA, Technomic Publishing Company Ltd, 426 p.

DAMEN B, POLLET A, DORNEZ E, BROEKAERT WF, HAESENDONCK IV, TROGH I, ARNAUT F, DELCOUR, JA and COURTIN, CM (2012), 'Xylanase-mediated in situ production of arabinoxylan oligosaccharides with prebiotic potential in whole meal breads and breads enriched with arabinoxylan rich materials', *Food Chem*, **131**, 111–118.

DAWKINS N and NNANNA IA (1995), 'Studies on oat gum [(1→3, 1→4)-β-D-glucan]: Composition, molecular weight estimation and rheological properties', *Food Hydrocoll*, **9**, 1–7.

DE DELAHAYE EP, JIMÉNEZ P and PÉREZ E (2005), 'Effect of enrichment with high content dietary fiber stabilized rice bran flour on chemical and functional properties of storage frozen pizzas', *J Food Eng*, **68**, 1–7.

DELCOUR, JA and HOSENEY RC (2010), *Principles of Cereal Science and Technology*, AACC-I, St Paul, MN, USA, 280 p.

DE MUNTER JSL, HU FB, SPIEGELMAN D, FRANZ M and VAN DAM RM (2007), 'Whole grain, bran, and germ intake and risk of type 2 diabetes: A prospective cohort study and systematic review', *PLoS Medicine*, **4**, 1385–95.

DUKAN P (APPLICANT) (2009), 'Cereal-base food preparation, consisting mainly of oat bran, for the industrial manufacture of food products', US patent application US2009297682 A1, 2009-Dec-03.

DOEHLERT DC and MOORE WR (1997), 'Composition of oat bran and flour prepared by three different mechanisms of dry milling', *Cereal Chem*, **74**, 403–6.

EFSA (2009), 'Scientific Opinion on the substantiation of health claims related to beta-glucans and maintenance of normal blood cholesterol concentrations (ID 754, 755, 757, 801, 1465, 2934) and maintenance or achievement of a normal body weight (ID 820, 823) pursuant to Article 13(1) of Regulation (EC) No 1924/2006', *EFSA Journal*, **7**, 1254.

EFSA (2010), 'Scientific Opinion on the substantiation of health claims related to wheat bran fibre and increase in faecal bulk (ID 3066), reduction in intestinal transit time (ID 828, 839, 3067, 4699) and contribution to the maintenance or achievement of a normal body weight (ID 829) pursuant to Article 13(1) of Regulation (EC) No 1924/2006', *EFSA Journal*, **8**, 1817.

EFSA (2011), 'Scientific Opinion on the substantiation of health claims related to rye fibre and changes in bowel function (ID 825), reduction of post-prandial glycaemic responses (ID 826) and maintenance of normal blood LDL-cholesterol concentrations (ID 827) pursuant to Article 13(1) of Regulation (EC) No 1924/2006', *EFSA Journal*, **9**, 2258.

ESPOSITO F, ARLOTTI G, BONIFATI AM, NAPOLITANO A, VITALE D and FOGLIANO V (2005), 'Antioxidant activity and dietary fibre in durum wheat bran by-products', *Food Res Int*, **38**, 1167–73.

FDA (1997), 'Food labeling: Health claims; oats and coronary heart disease', *Federal Register*, **62**, 3584–601.

FDA (2003), 'Food labeling: Health claims; Soluble dietary fiber from certain foods and coronary heart disease', *Federal Register*, **68**, 44207–9.

FERRARI B, FINOCCHIARO F, STANCA AM and GIANINETTI A (2009), 'Optimization of air classification for the production of β-glucan-enriched barley flours', *J Cereal Sci*, **50**, 152–8.

FINCHER GB and STONE BA (1986), 'Cell walls and their components in cereal grain technology', *Adv Cereal Sci Technol*, **8**, 207–95.

FINNISH BREAD INFORMATION (2012), Available from: http://www.leipatiedotus.fi/tietoa_leivasta/ravitsemussuositukset_ja_niiden_toteutuminen/viljan_kulutus_suomessa

FLEURAT-LESSARD F, CHAURAND M, MARCHEGAY G and ABECASSIS J (2007), 'Effects of processing on the distribution of pirimiphos-methyl residues in milling fractions of durum wheat', *J Stor Prod Res*, **43**, 384–95.

FULCHER GR and MILLER SS (1993), 'Structure of oat bran and distribution of dietary fiber components', in Wood PJ, *Oat bran*, St Paul, MN, USA, AACC-I, 1–24.

GAMBUŚ H, MATUSZ-MIRLAK A, DULIŃSKI R, ZIOBRO R and GOLACHOWSKI A (2012), 'The influence of extrusion process on myo-inositol phosphate content and profile in snacks containing rye bran', *Int J Food Sci Nutr*, **63**, 41–4.

GEBRUERS K, DORNEZ E, BOROS D, FRAŚ A, DYNKOWSKA W, *et al.* (2008), 'Variation in the content of dietary fiber and components thereof in wheats in the HEALTHGRAIN diversity screen', *J Agric Food Chem*, **56**, 9740–9.

GEBRUERS K, DORNEZ E, BEDÕ Z, RAKSZEGI M, FRÁS A, *et al.* (2010), 'Environment and genotype effects on the content of dietary fiber and its components in wheat in the HEALTHGRAIN diversity screen', *J Agric Food Chem*, **58**, 9353–61.

GERHARDT AL and GALLO NB (1998), 'Full-fat rice bran and oat bran similarly reduce hypercholesterolemia in humans', *J Nutr*, **128**, 865–9.

GHOTRA BS, VASANTHAN T and TEMELLI F (2008), 'Structural characterization of barley β-glucan extracted using a novel fractionation technique', *Food Res Int*, **41**, 957–63.

GLITSØ LV and BACH KNUDSEN KE (1999), 'Milling of whole grain rye to obtain fractions with different dietary fibre characteristics', *J Cereal Sci*, **29**, 89–97.

GÓMEZ M, PARDO J, OLIETE B and CABALLERO PA (2009), 'Effect of the milling process on quality characteristics of rye flour', *J Sci Food Agric*, **89**, 470–6.

GUJRAL HS, MEHTA S, SAMRA IS and GOYAL P (2003), 'Effect of wheat bran, coarse wheat flour, and rice flour on the instrumental texture of cookies', *Int J Food Prop*, **6**, 329–340.

GÜL H, ÖZER MS and DIZLEK H (2009), 'Improvement of the wheat and corn bran bread quality by using glucose oxidase and hexose oxidase', *J Food Qual*, **32**, 209–22.

GUO W, NIE L, WU D, WISE ML, COLLINS FW, *et al.* (2010), 'Avenanthramides inhibit proliferation of human colon cancer cell lines in vitro', *Nutr Cancer*, **62**, 1007–16.

HÄRKÖNEN H, PESSA E, SUORTTI T and POUTANEN K (1997), 'Distribution and some properties of cell wall polysaccharides in rye milling fractions', *J Cereal Sci*, **26**, 95–104.

HARRIS PJ, CHAVAN RR and FERGUSON LR (2005), 'Production and characterisation of two wheat-bran fractions: An aleurone-rich and a pericarp-rich fraction', *Mol Nutr Food Res*, **49**, 536–45.

HASKÅ L, NYMAN M and ANDERSSON R (2008), 'Distribution and characterisation of fructan in wheat milling fractions', *J Cereal Sci*, **48**, 768–74.

HEBDEN JM, BLACKSHAW PE, PERKINS AC, D'AMATO M and SPILLER RC (1998), 'Small bowel transit of a bran meal residue in humans: Sieving of solids from liquids and response to feeding', *Gut*, **42**, 685–689.

HEINIÖ R-L, NORDLUND E, POUTANEN K and BUCHERT J (2012), 'Use of enzymes to elucidate the factors contributing to bitterness in rye flavor', *Food Res Int*, **45**, 31–8.

HEMERY Y, ROUAU X, LULLIEN-PELLERIN V, BARRON C and ABECASSIS J (2007), 'Dry processes to develop wheat fractions and products with enhanced nutritional quality', *J Cereal Sci*, **46**, 327–47.

HEMERY YM, MATEO ANSON N, HAVENAAR R, HAENEN GRMM, NOORT MWJ and ROUAU X (2010), 'Dry-fractionation of wheat bran increases the bioaccessibility of phenolic acids in breads made from processed bran fractions', *Food Res Int*, **43**, 1429–38.

HEMERY Y, CHAURAND M, HOLOPAINEN U, LAMPI A-M, LEHTINEN P, *et al.* (2011a), 'Potential of dry fractionation of wheat bran for the development of food ingredients, part I: Influence of ultra-fine grinding', *J Cereal Sci*, **53**, 1–8.

HEMERY Y, HOLOPAINEN U, LAMPI A-M, LEHTINEN P, NURMI T, *et al.* (2011b), 'Potential of dry fractionation of wheat bran for the development of food ingredients, part II: Electrostatic separation of particles', *J Cereal Sci*, **53**, 9–18.

HOLOPAINEN URM, PIHLAVA J-M, HIETANIEMI V, WILHELMSON A, POUTANEN K and LEHTINEN P (2012), 'Evaluating milling and water uptake properties of different barley (*Hordeum vulgare* L.) cultivars in relation to their grain composition and structure', *J Food Sci*, Paper currently under review.

HU G, HUANG S, CAO S and MA Z (2009), 'Effect of enrichment with hemicellulose from rice bran on chemical and functional properties of bread', *Food Chem*, **115**, 839–42.

HUDSON CA, CHIU MM and KNUCKLES BE (1992), 'Development and characteristics of high-fiber muffins with oat bran, rice bran or barley fiber fractions', *Cereal Food World*, **37**, 373–8.

IZYDORCZYK MS, JACOBS M and DEXTER JE (2003), 'Distribution and structural variation of nonstarch polysaccharides in milling fractions of hull-less barley with variable amylose content', *Cereal Chem*, **80**, 645–53.

JAVED MM, ZAHOOR S, SHAFAAT S, MEHMOODA I, GUL A, *et al.* (2012), 'Wheat bran as a brown gold: Nutritious value and its biotechnological applications', *Afr J Microbiol Res*, **6**, 724–33.

JENSEN MK, KOH-BANERJEE P, HU FB, FRANZ M, SAMPSON L, *et al.* (2004), 'Intakes of whole grains, bran, and germ and the risk of coronary heart disease in men', *Am J Clin Nutr*, **80**, 1492–9.

KAHLON TS (2009), 'Rice Bran: Production, composition, functionality and food application, physiological benefits', in CHO SS and SAMUEL P, *Fiber Ingredients: Food Applications and Health Benefits*, CRC Press, 305–18.

KAHLON TS and WOODRUFF CL (2003), 'In vitro binding of bile acids by ready-to-eat breakfast cereals', *Cereal Food World*, **48**, 73–5.

KAHLON TS, SAUNDERS RM, CHOW FI, CHIU MC and BETCHART AA (1984), 'Effect of rice bran and oat bran on plasma cholesterol in hamsters', *Cereal Foods World*, **34**, 768.

KAMAL-ELDIN A, LÆRKE HN, KNUDSEN K-EB, LAMPI A-M, PIIRONEN V, *et al.* (2009), 'Physical, microscopic and chemical characterisation of industrial rye and wheat brans from the Nordic countries', *Food Nutr Res*, **53**, 1–11.

KAMRAN M, SALEEM N and UMER ZN (2008), 'Ready-to-eat (RTE) wheat bran breakfast cereal as a high-fiber diet', *J Food Process Pres*, **32**(5), 853–67.

KARPPINEN S, MYLLYMÄKI O, FORSSELL P and POUTANEN K (2003), 'Fructan content of rye and rye products', *Cereal Chem*, **80**, 168–71.

KATINA K, SALMENKALLIO-MARTTILA M, PARTANEN R, FORSSELL P and AUTIO K (2006), 'Effects of sourdough and enzymes on staling of high-fibre wheat bread', *LWT – Food Sci Technol*, **39**, 479–91.

KATINA K, LAITILA A, JUVONEN R, LIUKKONEN K-H, KARILUOTO S, *et al.* (2007), 'Bran fermentation as a means to enhance technological properties and bioactivity of rye', *Food Microbiol*, **24**, 175–86.

KATINA K, JUVONEN R, LAITILA A, FLANDER L, NORDLUND E, *et al.* (2012), 'Fermented wheat bran as a functional ingredient in baking', *Cereal Chem*, **89**, 126–34.

KAUKOVIRTA-NORJA A, LEHTINEN P, VIRKAJÄRVI I, SUORTTI M, MYLLYMÄKI O, *et al.* (VTT TECHNICAL RESEARCH CENTRE OF FINLAND) (2009), 'Method of processing beta-glucan', PCT application WO 2009/077659 A1, 2009-Jun-25.

KERCKHOFFS DAJM, HORNSTRA G and MENSINK RP (2003), 'Cholesterol-lowering effect of β-glucan from oat bran in mildly hypercholesterolemic subjects may decrease when β-glucan is incorporated into bread and cookies', *Am J Clin Nutr*, **78**, 221–7.

KHAN K and SHEWRY P (2009), *Wheat: Chemistry and technology*, St Paul, Minnesota, USA, AACC, 480 p.

KIM H, STOTE KH, BEHALL KM, SPEARS K, VINYARD B and CONWAY JM (2009), 'Glucose and insulin responses to whole grain breakfasts varying in soluble fiber, β-glucan – A dose response study in obese women with increased risk for insulin resistance', *Eur J Nutr*, **48**, 170–5.

KIM YS, HA TY, LEE SH and LEE HY (1998), 'Effect of rice bran dietary fiber on flour rheology and quality of wet noodles', *Korean J Food Sci Technol*, **29**, 90–5.

KLAMCZYNSKI A, BAIK B-K and CZUCHAJOWSKA Z (1998), 'Composition, microstructure, water imbibition, and thermal properties of abraded barley', *Cereal Chem*, **75**, 677–85.

KNUCKLES BE, CHIU MM and BETSCHART AA (1992), 'Beta-glucan-enriched fractions from laboratory-scale dry milling and sieving of barley and oats', *Cereal Chem*, **69**, 198–202.

KNUCKLES BE, HUDSON CA, CHIU MM and SAYRE RN (1997), 'Effect of β-glucan barley fractions in high-fiber bread and pasta', *Cereal Food World*, **42**, 94–9.

KOZUBEK A and TYMAN JHP (1999), 'Resorcinolic lipids, the natural non-isoprenoid phenolic amphiphiles and their biological activity', *Chem Rev*, **99**, 1–26.

KRISTENSEN MB, HELS O and TETENS I (2005), 'No changes in serum enterolactone levels after eight weeks' intake of rye bran products in healthy young men', *Scand J Nutr*, **49**, 62–7.

LACA A, MOUSIA Z, DIAZ M, WEBB C and PANDIELLA SS (2006), 'Distribution of microbial contamination within cereal grains', *J Food Eng*, **72**, 332–8.

LAI CS, HOSENEY RC and DAVIS AB (1989), 'Effects of wheat bran in breadmaking', *Cereal Chem*, **66**, 217–19.

LANDBERG R, KAMAL-ELDIN A, SALMENKALLIO-MARTTILA M, ROUSSET M and ÅMAN P (2008), 'Localization of alkylresorcinols in barley, wheat and rye kernels', *J Cereal Sci*, **48**, 401–6.

LARSSON M and SANDBERG A-S (1991), 'Phytate reduction in bread containing oat flour, oat bran or rye bran', *J Cereal Sci*, **14**, 141–9.

LAURIKAINEN T, HÄRKÖNEN H, AUTIO K and POUTANEN K (1998), 'Effects of enzymes in fibre–enriched baking', *J Sci Food Agric*, **76**, 239–49.

LEHTINEN P, KAUKOVIRTA-NORJA A, SIBAKOV J, MYLLYMÄKI O, POUTANEN K and PIHLAVA J-M (2009), 'Functional oat ingredients – Opportunities and challenges for food technology', *Cereal Food World*, **54**, 267–71.

LEHTOMÄKI I and MYLLYMÄKI O (POLAR GLUCAN OY) (2009), 'Method of producing a bran product', PCT application WO 2009/109703 A1, 2009-Sep-11.

LEHTOMÄKI I and MYLLYMÄKI O (APPLICANTS) (2010), 'New dry-milling method for preparing bran', PCT application WO 2010/000935 A1, 2010-Jan-07.

LIUKKONEN K-H, KATINA K, WILHELMSON A, MYLLYMÄKI O, LAMPI A-M, *et al.* (2003), 'Process-induced changes on bioactive compounds in whole grain rye', *Proc Nutr Soc*, **62**, 117–22.

LOBATO LP, ANIBAL D, LAZARETTI MM and GROSSMANN MVE (2011), 'Extruded puffed functional ingredients with oat bran and soy flour', *LWT– Food Sci Technol*, **44**, 933-9.

LORENZ K and AL-RUQAIE A (1992), 'Alkylresorcinols in commercial and experimental extruded high fiber breakfast cereals', *LWT – Food Sci Technol*, **25**, 248–52.

MANDALARI G, FAULDS CB, SANCHO AI, SAIJA A, BISIGNANO G, *et al.* (2005), 'Fractionation and characterisation of arabinoxylans from brewers' spent grain and wheat bran', *J Cereal Sci*, **42**, 205–12.

MARCONI E, GRAZIANO M and CUBADDA R (2000),'Composition and utilization of barley pearling by-products for making functional pastas rich in dietary fiber and β-glucans', *Cereal Chem*, **77**, 133–9.

MARLETT JA (1993), 'Comparisons of dietary fiber and selected nutrient compositions of oat and other bran fractions', in WOOD PJ, *Oat Bran*, St Paul, MN, AACC, 49–82.

MATEO ANSON N, VAN DEN BERG R, HAVENAAR R, BAST A and HAENEN GRMM (2009), 'Bioavailability of ferulic acid is determined by its bioaccessibility', *J Cereal Sci*, **49**, 296–300.

MELLEN PB, LIESE AD, TOOZE JA, VITOLINS MZ, WAGENKNECHT LE and HERRINGTON DM (2007), 'Whole-grain intake and carotid artery atherosclerosis in a multiethnic cohort: The insulin resistance atherosclerosis study', *Am J Clin Nutr*, **85**, 1495–502.

MEYDANI M (2009), 'Potential health benefits of avenanthramides of oats', *Nutr Rev*, **67**, 731–5.

MONRO JA (2002), 'Dietary fibre content and nutrient claims relative to the faecal bulking efficacy of breakfast cereals', *Asia Pac J Clin Nutr*, **11**, 274–84.

MOORE J, LUTHER M, CHENG Z and YU L (2009), 'Effects of baking conditions, dough fermentation, and bran particle size on antioxidant properties of whole-wheat pizza crusts', *J Agric Food Chem*, **57**, 832–839.

MORGAN KR (IND RES LTD) (1998), 'Beta-glucan products and extraction processes from cereals', PCT application WO 98/13056 A1, 1998-Apr-2.

MORIARTEY S, TEMELLI F, VASANTHAN T and GÄNZLE M (2011), 'Viscosity and solubility of β-glucan extracted under *in vitro* conditions from barley β-glucan-fortified bread and evaluation of loaf characteristics', *Cereal Chem*, **88**, 421–8.

MOST MM, TULLEY R, MORALES S and LEFEVRE M (2005), 'Rice bran oil, not fiber, lowers cholesterol in humans', *Am J Clin Nutr*, **81**, 64–8.

MYLLYMÄKI O, POUTANEN K, OKSMAN-CALDENTEY K-M, LAITILA A and HEINIÖ, R-L (VTT TECHNICAL RESEARCH CENTRE OF FINLAND) (2002), 'Method for producing an oat product and an oat cereal and a snack product produced with said method', PCT application WO/0228201 A1, 2002-Apr-11.

MYLLYMÄKI O and SAAPUNKI M (MUNCH OY) (2010), 'Food product having high dietary fiber content', PCT application WO 2010/124922 A1, 2010-Nov-4.

NAMA – NORTH AMERICAN MILLERS' ASSOCIATION (2010), 'Oat milling', Available from: http://www.namamillers.org/oldsite/ci_products_oats_mill.html (accessed 2 November 2012).

NEYRINCK AM, POSSEMIERS S, DRUART C, VAN DE WIELE T, DE BACKER F, *et al.* (2011), 'Prebiotic effects of wheat arabinoxylan related to the increase in bifidobacteria, roseburia and bacteroides/prevotella in diet-induced obese mice', *PLoS ONE*, 6, e20944.

NILSSON M, ÅMAN P, HÄRKÖNEN H, HALLMANS G, BACH KNUDSEN KE, *et al.* (1997), 'Content of nutrients and lignans in roller milled fractions of rye', *J Sci Food Agric*, **73**, 143–8.

NOORT MWJ, VAN HAASTER D, HEMERY Y, SCHOLS HA and HAMER RJ (2010), 'The effect of particle size of wheat bran fractions on bread quality – Evidence for fibre-protein interactions', *J Cereal Sci*, **52**, 59–64.

NYSTRÖM L, PAASONEN A, LAMPI, A-M and PIIRONEN V (2007), 'Total plant sterols, steryl ferulates and steryl glycosides in milling fractions of wheat and rye', *J Cereal Sci*, **45**, 106–15.

NYSTRÖM L, LAMPI A-M, ANDERSSON AAM, KAMAL-ELDIN A, GEBRUERS K, *et al.* (2008), 'Phytochemicals and dietary fiber components in rye varieties in the HEALTHGRAIN diversity screen', *J Agric Food Chem*, **56**, 9758–66.

OTHMAN RA, MOGHADASIAN MH and JONES PJ (2011), 'Cholesterol-lowering effects of oat beta-glucan', *Nutr Rev*, **69**, 299–309.

PALTAKARI J, LAINE J, ÖSTERBERG M, SUBRAMANIAN R and TERIFOLK J-E (UPM KYMMENE OYJ) (2012), 'Method for producing modified cellulose', US patent application 2012/0043039 A1, 2012-Feb-23.

PANAHI S, EZATAGHA A, TEMELLI F, VASANTHAN T and VUKSAN V (2007), 'β-Glucan from two sources of oat concentrates affect postprandial glycemia in relation to the level of viscosity', *J Am Coll Nutr*, **26**, 639–44.

PATON D and LENZ MK (1993), 'Processing: Current practice and novel processes', in WOOD PJ, *Oat Bran*, St Paul, MN, USA, AACC-I, 25–47.

PETERSON DM, EMMONS CL and HIBBS AH (2001), 'Phenolic antioxidants and antioxidant activity in pearling fractions of oat groats', *J Cereal Sci*, **33**, 97–103.

PIETINEN P, PATURI M, REINIVUO H, TAPANAINEN H and VALSTA LM (2010), 'FINDIET 2007 Survey: energy and nutrient intakes', *Public Health Nutr*, **13**, 920–4.

POMERANZ Y (1988), 'Chemical composition of kernel structures', in POMERANZ Y, *Wheat: Chemistry and Technology*, St Paul, MN, USA, AACC-I, 97–158.

RAKHA A, ÅMAN P and ANDERSSON R (2010), 'Characterisation of dietary fibre components in rye products', *Food Chem*, **119**, 859–67.

RANDALL JM, SAYRE RN, SCHULTZ WG, FONG RY, MOSSMAN AP, *et al.* (1985), 'Rice bran stabilization by extrusion cooking for extraction of edible oil', *J Food Sci*, **50**, 361–4.

RASCO BA, RUBENTHALER G, BORHAN M and DONG FM (1990), 'Baking properties of bread and cookies incorporating distiller's or brewer's grain from wheat and barley', *J Food Sci*, **55**, 424–9.

REDMOND MJ and FIELDER DA (CEAPRO INC) (2004), 'Improved extraction and purification method for cereal beta-glucan', PCT application WO 2004/096862 A2, 2004-Nov-11.

REUNGMANEEPAITOON S, SIKKHAMONDHOL C and TIANGPOOK C (2006), 'Nutritive improvement of instant fried noodles with oat bran', *Songklanakarin J Sci Technol*, **28**, 89–97.

RHODES DI and STONE BA (2002), 'Proteins in walls of wheat aleurone cells', *J Cereal Sci*, **36**, 83–101.

ROBIN F, DUBOIS C, PINEAU N, SCHUCHMANN HP and PALZER S (2011), 'Expansion mechanism of extruded foams supplemented with wheat bran', *J Food Eng*, **107**, 80–9.

RZEDZICKI Z, SZPRYNGIEL B and SOBOTA A (2000), 'Estimation of some chosen physical properties of extrudates obtained from corn semolina and oat bran mixtures', *Int Agrophysics*, **14**, 233–9.

SAEED F, PASHA I, ANJUM FM and SULTAN MT (2011), 'Arabinoxylans and arabinogalactans: a comprehensive treatise', *Crit Rev Food Sci Nutr*, **51**, 467–76.

SAIRAM S, GOPALA KRISHNA AG and UROOJ A (2011), 'Physico-chemical characteristics of defatted rice bran and its utilization in a bakery product', *J Food Sci Technol*, **48**, 478–83.

SALMENKALLIO-MARTTILA M, KATINA K and AUTIO K (2001), 'Effects of bran fermentation on quality and microstructure of high-fiber wheat bread', *Cereal Chem*, **78**, 429–35.

SANZ PENELLA JM, COLLAR C and HAROS M (2008), 'Effect of wheat bran and enzyme addition on dough functional performance and phytic acid levels in bread', *J Cereal Sci*, **48**, 715–21.

SAUNDERS RM (1990), 'The properties of rice bran as a foodstuff', *Cereal Foods World*, **35**, 632–4.

SAURA-CALIXTO F (2011), 'Dietary fiber as a carrier of dietary antioxidants: an essential physiological function', *J Agric Food Chem*, **59**, 43–9.

SCHWARZ PB, KUNERTH WH and YOUNGS VL (1988), 'The distribution of lignin and other fiber components within hard red spring wheat bran', *Cereal Chem*, **65**, 59–64.

SEKHON KS, DHILLON SS, SINGH N and SINGH B (1997), 'Functional suitability of commercially milled rice bran in India for use in different food products', *Plant Foods Human Nutr*, **50**, 127–40.

SEYER M-È and GÉLINAS P (2009), 'Bran characteristics and wheat performance in whole wheat bread', *Int J Food Sci Technol*, **44**, 688–693.

SHARIF M, BUTT MS, ANJUM FM and NAWAZ H (2009), 'Preparation of fiber and mineral enriched defatted rice bran supplemented cookies', *Pakistan J Nutr*, **8**, 571–7.

SHARMA HR, CHAUHAN GS and AGRAWAL K (2004), 'Physico-chemical characteristics of rice bran processed by dry heating and extrusion cooking', *Int J Food Propert*, **7**, 603–14.

SHEWRY PR, PIIRONEN V, LAMPI A-M, NYSTRÖM L, LI L, *et al.* (2008), 'Phytochemical and fiber components in oat varieties in the HEALTHGRAIN diversity screen', *J Agric Food Chem*, **56**, 9777–84.

SIBAKOV J, MYLLYMÄKI O, HIETANIEMI V, PIHLAVA J-M, KAUKOVIRTA-NORJA A, *et al.* (2010), 'Combination of defatting and dry fractionation technologies to produce oat ingredients with high β-glucan concentration' in VAN DER KAMP J, MCCLEARY B and TOPPING D, *Dietary Fibre: New frontiers for food and health*, Amsterdam, Wageningen Academic Publishers, 79–89.

SIBAKOV J, MYLLYMÄKI O, HOLOPAINEN U, KAUKOVIRTA-NORJA A, HIETANIEMI V, *et al.* (2011), 'Lipid removal enhances separation of oat grain cell wall material from starch and protein', *J Cereal Sci*, **54**, 104–9.

SINGH D, CHAUHAN GS, SURESH I and TYAGI SM (2000), 'Nutritional quality of extruded snacks developed from composite of rice brokens and wheat bran', *Int J Food Prop*, **3**, 421–431.

SLAVIN JL, JACOBS D and MARQUART L (2001), 'Grain processing and nutrition', *Crit Rev Biotechnol*, **21**, 49–66.

SLOAN S and JAMES C (1988), 'Extruded full-fat rice bran in muffins', *LWT – Food Sci Technol*, **21**, 245–7.

SOUKOULIS C, LEBESI D and TZIA C (2009), 'Enrichment of ice cream with dietary fibre: Effects on rheological properties, ice crystallisation and glass transition phenomena', *Food Chem*, **115**, 665–71.

STEVENSON DG, ELLER FJ, JANE J-L and INGLETT GE (2008), 'Structure and physicochemical properties of defatted and pin-milled oat bran concentrate fractions separated by air-classification', *Int J Food Sci Technol*, **43**, 995–1003.

STOJCESKA V, AINSWORTH P, PLUNKETT A and IBANOĞLU S (2008), 'The recycling of brewer's processing by-product into ready-to-eat snacks using extrusion technology', *J Cereal Sci*, **47**, 469–79.

SUDHA ML, RAMASARMA PR and RAO GV (2011), 'Wheat bran stabilization and its use in the preparation of high-fiber pasta', *Food Sci Technol Int*, **17**, 47–53.

SURGET A and BARRON C (2005), 'Histologie du grain de blé', *Industrie des Céréales*, **145**, 3–7.

TAPPY L, GÜGOLZ E and WÜRSCH P (1996), 'Effects of breakfast cereals containing various amounts of β-glucan fibers on plasma glucose and insulin responses in NIDDM subjects', *Diabetes Care*, **19**, 831–4.

TOSH SM, BRUMMER Y, WOLEVER TMS and WOOD PJ (2008), 'Glycemic response to oat bran muffins treated to vary molecular weight of β-glucan', *Cereal Chem*, **85**, 211–17.

TOSH SM, BRUMMER Y, MILLER SS, REGAND A, DEFELICE C, *et al.* (2010), 'Processing affects the physicochemical properties of β-glucan in oat bran cereal', *J Agric Food Chem*, **58**, 7723–30.

VASANTHAN T and BHATTY RS (1995), 'Starch purification after pin milling and air classification of waxy, normal, and high amylose barleys', *Cereal Chem*, **72**, 379–84.

VASANTHAN T and TEMELLI F (UNIV ALBERTA) (2002), 'Grain fractionation methods and products', PCT application WO 02/27011A2, 2002-Apr-04.

VASANTHAN T and TEMELLI F (2008), 'Grain fractionation technologies for cereal beta-glucan concentration', *Food Res Int*, **41**, 876–81.

VERMA B, HUCL P and CHIBBAR RN (2008), 'Phenolic content and antioxidant properties of bran in 51 wheat cultivars', *Cereal Chem*, **85**, 544–9.

VITAGLIONE P, NAPOLITANO A and FOGLIANO V (2008), 'Cereal dietary fibre: a natural functional ingredient to deliver phenolic compounds into the gut', *Trends Food Sci Technol*, **19**, 451–63.

WANG R, KOUTINAS AA and CAMPBELL GM (2007), 'Effect of pearling on dry processing of oats', *J Food Eng*, **82**, 369–76.

WASDE (2012), 'World Agricultural Supply and Demand Estimates, World Agricultural outlook board: March, 2012'. Available from: http://www.usda.gov/oce/commodity/wasde/latest.pdf

WEICKERT MO and PFEIFFER AF (2008), 'Metabolic effects of dietary fiber consumption and prevention of diabetes', *J Nutr*, **138**, 439–42.

WELLS HF and BUZBY JC (2008), 'Dietary assessment of major trends in U.S. food consumption 1970–2005', *Economic Information Bulletin*, **33**, 1–27. Available from: www.ers.usda.gov/Publications/EIB33/

WÓJTOWICZ A and MOŚCICKI L (2011), 'Effect of wheat bran addition and screw speed on microstructure and textural characteristics of common wheat precooked pasta-like products', *Pol J Food Nutr Sci*, **61**, 101–107.

WOOD PJ (2007), 'Cereal β–glucans in diet and health', *J Cereal Sci*, **46**, 230–8.

WOOD PJ, BEER MU and BUTLER G (2000), 'Evaluation of role of concentration and molecular weight of oat beta-glucan in determining effect of viscosity on plasma glucose and insulin following an oral glucose load', *Br J Nutr*, **84**, 19–23.

WU YV and DOEHLERT DC (2002), 'Enrichment of β-glucan in oat bran by fine grinding and air classification', *LWT – Food Sci Technol*, **35**(1), 30–3.

YALÇIN E, ÇELIK S, AKARC T, SAYIM I and KÖKSEL H (2007), 'Effects of genotype and environment on β-glucan and dietary fiber contents of hull-less barleys grown in Turkey', *Food Chem*, **101**, 171–6.

ZHANG D and MOORE W (1999), 'Wheat bran particle size effects on bread baking performance and quality', *J Sci Food Agric*, **79**, 805–9.

ZHANG G, JUNMEI W and JINXIN C (2002), 'Analysis of β-glucan content in barley cultivars from different locations of China', *Food Chem*, **79**, 251–4.

ZHENG G-H, HESS R, KHARE A, HILBERT B, DEGUISE M (CARGILL INC.) (2004), 'Improved dietary fiber containing materials comprising low molecular weight glucan', PCT application WO 2004/086878 A3, 2004-Oct-14.

ZHOU K, LAUX JJ and YU L (2004), 'Comparison of Swiss red wheat grain and fractions for their antioxidant properties', *J Agric Food Chem*, **52**, 1118–23.

ZHU KX, HUANG S, PENG W, QIAN HF and ZHOU HM (2010), 'Effect of ultrafine grinding on hydration and antioxidant properties of wheat bran dietary fiber', *Food Res Int*, **43**, 943–8.

9

Vegetable, fruit and potato fibres

M. Nyman and L. Haskå, Lund University, Sweden

DOI: 10.1533/9780857095787.2.193

Abstract: As much as one-third of the dietary fibre intake in a normal Western diet originates from fruits and vegetables. Nutritional effects of dietary fibre can to a great extent be related to the physicochemical properties of the fibre, such as composition, solubility, viscosity, water-holding capacity and molecular weight. In fruits and vegetables the structure of the cell wall matrix (tertiary structure) is also extremely important for nutritional characteristics and texture of the product. Fruits and vegetables are often processed in some way prior to consumption. During this processing the cell wall composition and also the physicochemical properties of the plant material may be changed considerably. The effects of mechanical, chemical, enzymatic and thermal processing will be discussed in this chapter.

Key words: vegetables, fruits, dietary fibre, processing, physicochemical properties, solubility, viscosity, water-holding capacity, molecular weight, cross-links.

9.1 Introduction

Diet has been suggested to be a common denominator of many chronic disorders of the Western world, such as cardiovascular diseases, type 2 diabetes mellitus and some types of colonic diseases. In this respect dietary fibre could play an interesting role (Galland 2010). A number of studies regarding physiological properties of dietary fibre have been performed on cereals, while vegetables and berries are often overlooked as a fibre source due to their low fibre content. However, considering that at least one-third of the dietary fibre intake in a normal diet originates from fruits and vegetables, the intake of these types of fibre is extremely important. During the period 1986–2009 the total consumption of vegetables (not including potatoes) in Sweden increased by 85% to 76 kg per capita and year, and fruits by 10% to 92 kg per capita and year, while the intake of potatoes decreased by 20% to 56 kg per capita and year (Swedish Board of Agriculture 2011). Further, these dietary sources do not only differ in the composition of the dietary fibre but are often delivered fresh and are very sensitive to storage. Of the total consumption, nearly 30% of the vegetables (not including potatoes) and approximately 35% of the fruits are industrially processed (Swedish Board of Agriculture 2011). Unknown quantities of the fresh products are also prepared at home. Another source of dietary fibre from fruits and vegetables is side streams from industrial processing, such as the production of juice, wine and sugar (Schieber *et al.* 2001). It is of great interest to find food applications for these types of products, from both an economic and a functional and nutritional point of view. Pectin is a well-known example in this respect, and it is already widely used as a gelling agent in various food items such as yogurt, ketchup and fruit jellies. It is found in high amounts in apples and citrus fruits but can also be extracted from orange peel, for example.

Functional and nutritional effects of dietary fibre can to a great extent be related to the physicochemical properties of the dietary fibre, such as composition, solubility, viscosity and molecular weight. The structure of the cell wall matrix (tertiary structure) is also of great importance for the properties of the product, and the architecture may, for example, influence the porosity and the surface area of the plant material (Guillon and Champ 2000). However, during processing the cell wall composition may be modified, and as a result also its physicochemical properties. This may be especially important for vegetable foods, since they are often processed or cooked in some way before consumption, not least to prolong the storage period. A number of things can happen during both heat-related activities and other intense treatments. For example, glycosidic linkages in the dietary fibre polysaccharides may be hydrolysed, resulting in a decrease in molecular weight and viscosity of the soluble dietary fibres (Svanberg *et al.* 1995, Selvendran and Robertson 1994). Also the amount of insoluble dietary fibre can be affected when cross-linkages between cell wall components are broken (Wennberg *et al.* 2003). Different types of plant materials, but also different genotypes within the same plant species, may be influenced variously by processing, depending on factors such as the number of cross-linkings between cell wall components and the esterification of the pectic compounds in the original product. Furthermore, the degree of maturity at harvest and storage conditions may alter the properties of the starting material, and perhaps even the final product (Wennberg *et al.* 2003).

9.2 Fruits and vegetables as sources of dietary fibre

9.2.1 Definitions and dietary fibre recommendations

Fruits and vegetables are a diverse group of plants consumed by humans. There is no strict botanical or chemical definition of what is meant by fruits and vegetables. These plant materials are therefore often classified according to how they are prepared or consumed, that is, vegetables as plants or plant parts generally eaten as a component of the main course of the meal, and fruits as parts of an appetiser or a dessert. From a botanical point of view, vegetables are derived from most families of flowering plants and also from some algae and fungi (Brouk 1975), while fruits are defined as the ripened ovary with or without the adjoining parts (Haard and Chism 1996). The main component of fresh fruits and vegetables is water (80–90%), while the solid matter is mainly constituted of carbohydrates, including dietary fibre (2–20% of the fresh weight), and some protein (5–7% of the fresh weight). Most fruits and vegetables contain very low amounts of lipids (<0.5%), while they are rich sources of vitamins, minerals and antioxidants. In fact, most vitamin C (~63%) and a great part of the dietary fibre (~30%), folacin (~32%), β-carotene (16%) and potassium (~30%) originate from this type of plant materials in a mixed Western diet, while plants only contribute 8% of the energy and 5% of the fat intake (Swedish Board of Agriculture 2011; Becker 1994). The contribution may be even higher, since the level of domestic production is unknown. The recommended dietary fibre intake for adults according to the Nordic Nutrition Recommendations is 3 g/MJ, which corresponds to an intake of between 25 and 35 g dietary fibre per day. A similar intake is recommended for many other Western countries (Galvin *et al.* 2001). No exact amounts of dietary fibre have been recommended by the WHO/FAO Expert Consultation group (Mann *et al.* 2007). Instead it was considered that the intake of fruit, vegetables and wholegrain cereals should provide at least 25 g of dietary fibre per day, until dietary fibre has been defined correctly.

9.2.2 Chemistry of cell wall components in fruits and vegetables

The cell wall components in fruits and vegetables consist of cellulose (~35%), hemicelluloses (~15%), pectins (~40%), proteins (~5%) and some lignin/polyphenols (~5%) (Selvendran and Robertson 1990). A model of the primary cell wall in flowering plants and the interaction between its components has been presented by Carpita and Gibeaut (1993). In contrast to cereals, the dietary fibre in fruits and vegetables contains high proportions of pectic substances. Pectin is a highly branched polysaccharide consisting of α-(1,4) galacturonic acid units in the backbone, sometimes interspersed with rhamnose. Two main types of pectin exist: linear homogalacturonans and rhamnogalacturonans with neutral sugar side chains attached to the rhamnosyl residue. Arabinose, galactose, xylose and glucuronic acid may be present in the side chain (Kays 1997). The galacturonic acid in the backbone may be esterified with carboxyl groups, and the solubility of pectin depends partly on this esterification. The cellulose in vegetables and fruits has been reported to be less crystalline than cellulose in cereals (Hsu and Penner 1989), partly because the cellulose is less lignified. The crystallinity index of cellulose in banana and sugar cane bagasse has been reported to be 39 and 48%, respectively (Guimaraes *et al.* 2009), while it was 81% in microcrystalline cellulose from wood (Hsu and Penner 1989). Xyloglucan is an important hemicellulosic substance in some vegetables, whereas high amounts of arabinans are present in sugar beet fibre and galactans in potatoes (Zykwinska *et al.* 2006). However, the composition of the cell wall polysaccharides varies considerably between different species, as can be seen in Table 9.1, and also between different cultivars of specific species (Wennberg *et al.* 2002).

Table 9.1 Plant family of different fruits and vegetables and total content of dietary fibre polysaccharides (g/100g dry weight basis), soluble fraction (% of total dietary fibre polysaccharides), monomeric composition (arabinose, xylose, galactose, glucose, uronic acids, other sugars, i.e. rhamnose + mannose and resistant starch in % of total dietary fibre polysacharides), Klason lignin (g/100g dry weight basis registered in the first column within parentheses) and fructo-oligosaccharides (FOS, g/100g dry weight basis, registered in the last column) of some selected plants

Latin name	Examples[1]	Dietary fibre polysaccharides (Klason lignin)	Soluble fraction	Arabinose	Xylose	Galactose	Glucose	Uronic acids	Other sugars	Resistant starch	FOS
Apiaceae	*Carrot*, celery, parsnip	28.4[2](0)	49	7	4	12	58	15	4	0	–
Asteraceae	Lettuce, endive, artichoke										
Brassicaceae	*Cabbage*, radish, turnip,	24.1[3](0)	26	10	1	16	30	39	4	0	–
	swedes, cauliflower, broccoli,	34.6[4](0)	20–43	7	8	7	42	30	6	0	–
	Brussels sprouts	33.5[4](0)	35	20	5	13	33	27	4	0	–
Chenopodiaceae	*Spinach*,	51.7[5](0)	30	9	3	8	35	42	3	0	–
	beetroot, *sugar beet*, chard	66.0[6](3)	31	26	2	6	28	35	3	–	–
Cucurbitaceae	Cucumber, squash, melon										
Ericaceae	*Bilberry*, cranberry, lingonberries	26.4[7] (14.0)	9	5	20	7	39	25	4	0	–

Liliaceae	*Onion*, garlic, leek, asparagus	24.7[8](0.2)	50	2	2	15	17	16	1	0	47[9]
Rosaceae	*Apple*, pear, cherry, plum, peach,	71.4[10](1.3)	39	14	6	9	36	27	6	2	0
	raspberry, *apricot* and strawberry	24.6[6](1.0)	35–45	10	6	8	33	40	3	0	0
Rutaceae	Orange, grapefruit, lemon, lime										
Solanaceae	*Potato*, tomato, sweet pepper	70.0[10](0.2–0.7)	24	4	1	25	22	14	2	32	–

Notes: 0 means <0.5%. – Not analysed.

1 Dietary fibre content/composition is given in each case for the fruit/vegetable in italics.
2 Carrots from Nyman and Nilsson (1994).
3 Cabbage from Wennberg *et al.* (2002).
4 Swedes from Nyman *et al.* (1987).
5 Spinach from Gustafsson *et al.* (1993).
6 Sugar beet fibre, onions and apricots from Marlett and Vollendorf (1994), Nyman and Asp (1982) and Prosky *et al.* (1994).
7 Bilberries from Bränning *et al.* (2008).
8 Onions from Marlett and Vollendorf (1993).
9 Onions from Muir *et al.* (2007).
10 Potato powder and apples from Henningsson *et al.* (2002).

9.3 Effects of processing on fruit and vegetable dietary fibre

9.3.1 Mechanical processing

Grinding of dietary fibre-rich raw materials not only decreases the particle size but may also change the shape of the particles and the physical structure; intense mechanical treatment may open up the cell wall structure (Lario *et al.* 2004). Swelling, water-binding capacity and water-holding capacity of sugar beet fibre and citrus fibre preparations have been observed to decrease when the particle size was decreased, which was attributed to a collapse of the pore structure (Auffret *et al.* 1994; Lario *et al.* 2004). In contrast, hydration properties of coconut fibre increased when the particle size was reduced, although they decreased after reduction beyond a certain point (Raghavendra *et al.* 2006). Micronisation (milling to extremely fine particles (~100 microns)), and especially high-pressure micronisation, of fractions high in insoluble fibre from carrot pomace and carambola pomace increased swelling, water-holding, oil-holding, cation-exchange and glucose adsorption capacities and increased the inhibitory effect on lipase and α-amylase activities (Chau *et al.* 2006; Chau *et al.* 2007). These effects were proposed to be caused by a larger surface area and more water-binding sites available after the decrease in particle size. Fibre components were also redistributed from insoluble to soluble fractions in the micronisation process. Thus, different results after reduction in particle size may be explained by two competing effects. Although a decreased particle size is related to an increased theoretical surface area, that is, an increased capacity to hold water, the water-holding capacity may also decrease due to a destruction of the pore structure (Cadden 1987; Guillon and Champ 2000).

Mechanical fractionation processing is often used when extracting different types of juices. The end products typically contain less dietary fibre than the raw material, while the side stream contains a lot of dietary fibre. The side streams represent an unexploited source of dietary fibre, which is currently used for animal feed or is discarded, but has great potential to be a part of tomorrow's food with health benefits.

9.3.2 Chemical processing

Chemical treatments may be used to change the properties of dietary fibre. The use of acidic or basic solutions affects the texture of cooked vegetables, which have been reported to be firmer when prepared at a pH of 4 than at pH 10 (Brandt *et al.* 1984). This may be explained by the promotion of the β-elimination reaction of pectin at pH > 4.5 at elevated temperatures (Sila *et al.* 2005), which in turn is dependent on the degree of esterification of the pectin and the presence of anions and cations. Heat treatment at low pH may instead lead to acidic hydrolysis of the pectic polysaccharides (Sila *et al.* 2009). Commercially produced pectin is usually extracted at a pH of 1–3, and the exact extraction conditions determine the degree of esterification and thus the functionality (gelling properties) of the final product (Harris and Smith 2006). The use of oxalate, acidic and basic solutions has also been shown to increase swelling of sugar beet fibre (Bertin *et al.* 1988; Elleuch *et al.* 2011). Improved water-holding and oil-holding capacities, bleaching and reduced lignin content may be obtained by treatment with hydrogen peroxide (Sangnark and Noomhorm 2003). The dietary fibre content and the distribution between soluble and insoluble fibre are also affected by the presence of salts. Thus, when salt was present in the cooking water of carrots an increased degradation of pectic substances occurred (Sajjaanantakul *et al.* 1993; Nyman and Svanberg 2002). Since the increased loss was mostly due to insoluble dietary fibre, it was suggested that the breakage of weak bonds was catalysed by monovalent cations during the heat treatment. Similar results have been seen in potatoes, in which the strong associations between cellulosic and pectic substances were damaged after boiling (Ryden and Selvendran 1990). When divalent ions were added at low concentrations (100 mM) to the cooking water of carrots there was instead an increased cross-linking between pectic polysaccharides, an increased amount of insoluble dietary fibre and a denser plant structure (Nyman and Svanberg 2002). A more stable plant structure may also decrease the loss of low molecular weight material into the boiling water. However, a higher concentration (400 mM) led to an extensive degradation of the dietary fibre polysaccharides in carrots, which was also reflected in the viscosity.

9.3.3 Enzymatic processing

Dietary fibre may be degraded by enzymes present in the raw material or added during processing. Both endogenous and exogenous enzymes are able to degrade pectin and thus change structure and properties (Sila *et al.* 2009). Depending on the application, it may be desirable to inactivate or to maintain, or even increase, the enzymatic activity (Duvetter *et al.* 2009). The enzyme pectin methylesterase (PME) (Van Buren 1979), usually reported to be rather inactive in plant tissues, was suggested to be activated during long-term storage of white cabbage (Wennberg *et al.* 2002). During storage for 24 weeks there was a redistribution of soluble to insoluble fibre, while no such effect could be seen after 7 weeks of storage. PME demethoxylates pectic substances, and Ca^{2+} ions can then cross-link the pectin molecules and in this way increase the amount of insoluble dietary fibre.

In the study by Wennberg *et al.* (2002) there was a considerable loss of polymers containing arabinose and galactose, suggesting that other endogenous enzymes, such as arabinases, galactosidases and endoglucanases, are also activated during storage (Brummell and Harpster 2001). Another endogenous enzyme that instead may degrade pectic substances, increasing the amount of soluble dietary fibre, is polygalacturanase. This enzyme only acts on de-esterified pectin, but may explain the increased proportion of soluble fibre after storage found in a specific cultivar of carrots (Svanberg *et al.* 1997). Dietary fibre may also be formed through the action of enzymes, such as the creation of callose (β-1,3-linked glucose) as protection against leakage of water and nutrients when plant materials are wounded during cutting and peeling (Shea *et al.* 1989).

Dietary fibre from waste fractions and side streams may also be exposed to exogenous enzymes that have been added to facilitate processing, such as in the production of juice and wine. Furthermore, the use of enzymes to specifically improve the properties of dietary fibre preparations is an important area within the food industry today. Several pectinolytic enzymes with tailored properties are available on the market to optimise functional characteristics, for example, giving different gelling capacities. This important and huge field is summarised by Schols *et al.* (2009) and will not be further discussed in detail here. Oligosaccharides with potentially prebiotic and other physiological effects can also be produced from dietary fibre polysaccharides by enzymatic means (Martínez *et al.* 2009; Martínez *et al.* 2010).

Fermentation (anaerobic preservation of the raw material, usually by lactic acid bacteria) is another type of enzymatic processing that may affect the dietary fibre. The changes depend on the enzymatic activity during the fermentation process, that is, the amount and the activity of the bacteria added and the length of the fermentation period. However, such a process would be expected to result mainly in degradation of glycosidic linkages, and as a consequence solubilisation of different cell wall polysaccharides. Several dietary fibre-degrading enzymes (polygalacturonase, cellulase and β-galactosidase) have been found in fermentation liquids (Rodríguez *et al.* 2006). These enzymes may increase the solubility of the dietary fibre or, if the degradation is extensive, cause a loss of dietary fibre into the fermentation liquid, as is seen in green olives (Jiménez *et al.* 1998). However, there may also be a loss of insoluble fibre, as is seen in fermentation of white cabbage with *Lactobacillus plantarum* 299v (Nyman and Wennberg, unpublished results). The considerable loss of insoluble fibre in that study indicates that weak bonds between polysaccharide chains are mostly affected by the low pH obtained during fermentation and not by bacterial enzymes. Similar findings were seen in a study of white cabbage soured with acetic acid (Wennberg *et al.* 2006).

Functional properties may also be affected by enzymatic treatment. A degradation of attached side chains by exogenous or endogenous enzymes may reduce the viscosity. A lower viscosity was seen with fermented cabbage products compared with raw cabbage (Nyman and Wennberg, unpublished results), most probably due to splitting of glycosidic linkages during processing. Such changes in functional properties may also have nutritional implications and reduce positive metabolic effects of the fibre. On the other hand, the low pH that is formed during fermentation may counteract such an effect. For example, the effects on glucose and insulin response were augmented in healthy subjects consuming carrots steeped in lactic acid compared with untreated carrots (Gustafsson *et al.* 1994).

9.3.4 Thermal processing

Heat treatment of vegetables leads to a softening of the texture, due to loss of turgor and changes in the cell wall composition (Van Buren 1979). This is mainly due to degradation of heat-labile polysaccharides, mainly pectic polysaccharides, and breakage of cross-links between cell-wall polysaccharides at elevated temperatures. These effects depend on the processing conditions and the dietary fibre material, but the reduction in molecular weight of dietary fibre generally follows the degree of heat treatment (Nyman 2003).

Content and composition

Wet processing of vegetables, such as blanching or boiling, leads to a loss of dry matter of mainly low molecular weight material, for example, sugars, vitamins and minerals. The loss is dependent on the amount of water, temperature and heating time. During this type of treatment the amount of dietary fibre in the cooked material increases (Nyman 2003). In the case of swedes, cauliflower and potatoes a loss of dietary fibre during boiling has also been reported (Brandt *et al.* 1984; Nyman 2003). Cooking losses may further be affected by harvest and storage conditions. During storage the number of cross-links between polysaccharides increases, which may lead to a more dense texture and more insoluble fibre. Long-term storage decreased the cooking loss of pectic substances in cabbage, while short-term storage and an early harvest increased the loss (Wennberg *et al.* 2003). However, the reduction in soluble dietary fibre was higher in stored carrots than in fresh carrots (Nyman *et al.* 2005). Another possible effect of the thermal processing of vegetables with a high starch content, such as potatoes, is the formation of resistant starch. Higher amounts of resistant starch have been found in deep-fried potato products and potato crisps than in boiled potatoes, but storage in a refrigerator increases the amount of resistant starch in boiled potatoes (Åkerberg *et al.* 1998; Liljeberg Elmståhl 2002).

Heat treatment often changes the ratio of soluble to insoluble fibre. An increase in the proportion of soluble dietary fibre was detected in frozen, blanched and canned carrots, swedes and Brussels sprouts (Nyman *et al.* 1987) and in boiled and/or canned carrots (Penner and Kim 1991). Furthermore, a comparison between ordinary cooking, pressure-cooking and microwave treatment of several vegetables showed that all methods reduced the content of insoluble fibre to some extent, but pressure-cooking showed the most pronounced effect (Rehman *et al.* 2003). Solubility of pineapple cell walls increased in canned samples but decreased in air-dried samples (Femenia *et al.* 2007). The decrease in the soluble dietary fibre in the air-dried samples may be explained by the fact that a high proportion of pectic polysaccharides could not be recovered after processing, especially at higher drying temperatures. This was probably due to extensive solubilisation or degradation by β-elimination processes or enzymatic degradation. The degree of esterification of pectins also decreased at higher drying temperatures.

Thermal pasteurisation of pectin also leads to solubilisation and depolymerisation, but by using high-pressure pasteurisation this effect may be reduced (Van Buggenhout *et al.* 2009). Autoclaving (121°C, 15 min) had no significant impact on the content and composition of dietary fibre of beetroots (Villanueva *et al.* 1996) or carrots (Redondo *et al.* 1997), but a small increase in soluble fibre was observed in turnips (Redondo *et al.* 1997), and sterilisation of onion waste (121°C, 17–31 min) decreased the total content of dietary fibre and increased the proportion of soluble fibre (Benítez *et al.* 2011). A formation of resistant starch at a level of 2–8% of the total starch content has also been reported in autoclaved infant purees (Siljeström and Björck 1990).

Extrusion cooking is widely used in the production of snack foods, and also in the treatment of dietary fibre from by-products of the food industry (Wolf 2010). The combination of mechanical and thermal energy used in extrusion cooking generally seems to solubilise the dietary fibre (Arrigoni *et al.* 1986; Camire *et al.* 1997; Hwang *et al.* 1998; Wolf 2010). In contrast, the effect of extrusion on total dietary fibre content is often insignificant, but depends on the conditions and the dietary fibre source. While little effect was observed on total dietary fibre content in apple pomace (Arrigoni *et al.* 1986; Hwang *et al.* 1998), onion waste (Ng *et al.* 1999) and potato peels produced by abrasion peeling (Camire *et al.* 1997), a significant loss of soluble dietary fibre was seen in depectinised apple pomace, probably due to the low pH of the sample (Arrigoni *et al.* 1986). The loss was suggested to be arabinans, arabinogalactans and galactans of lower molecular weight, that is, hemicellulosic substances associated with pectin. An increased dietary fibre content was observed in potato peels produced by steam peeling due to an increase in Klason lignin and a possible formation of resistant starch (Camire *et al.* 1997).

Another high pressure treatment is HHP (high hydrostatic pressure). This quite new low-thermal alternative allows strict control of process conditions and is therefore of interest when producing foods with specific health effects (Knorr *et al.* 2002). A study on white cabbage treated by this method showed little effect on the total dietary fibre content, but the solubility of the dietary fibre decreased when the pressure increased (Wennberg and Nyman 2004).

In addition to variation between different types of dietary fibre and processing conditions used, different results may be caused by different analytical methods, and whether results have been corrected for the loss of low molecular weight material (Redondo *et al.* 1997). The degradation of dietary fibre polysaccharides may also lead to the formation of oligosaccharides that were previously not analysed as dietary fibre but are included in newer definitions of dietary fibre.

Functional properties

Microwaving, blanching, boiling and canning decreased the viscosity of the soluble dietary fibre in carrots and Brussels sprouts, the smallest effect observed from microwaving and blanching and the largest from canning (Nyman *et al.* 1994; Svanberg *et al.* 1995). The decrease in viscosity after processing was generally in accordance with the decrease in molecular weight of the soluble dietary fibre. In contrast, extrusion of citrus peels increased solubility and slightly increased the apparent viscosities, depending on the solvent used (Gourgue *et al.* 1994). While solubility and oil-holding capacity of fibre-rich asparagus powder were higher in freeze-dried fibres than in oven-dried fibres, water-holding capacity was more influenced by thermal treatment (Fuentes-Alventosa *et al.* 2009). Water-holding capacity of extruded apple pomace remained constant when a low mechanical force was used but decreased under more severe conditions, probably due to disintegration of the cell wall (Hwang *et al.* 1998). Similar results have been found for potato peel (Arora *et al.* 1993), while the water-holding capacity of depectinased apple pomace (Arrigoni *et al.* 1986) and the swelling and absorption of water of orange peels were increased after extrusion (Larrea *et al.* 2005). The absorption of water and the water-binding capacity of both untreated and depectinased apple pomace decreased with autoclaving and increased with boiling (Arrigoni *et al.* 1986). Physical properties of a material are thus considerably influenced by thermal processing, although in different ways. It is important to have in mind that results from one material cannot be applied to another one (Chávez-Jáuregui *et al.* 2000). The chemical composition and/or the architecture of the material seem to be of great importance in this respect.

9.4 Conclusion

The effects of processing on dietary fibre in vegetables and fruits are highly dependent on both processing conditions and the structure of the dietary fibre. Physicochemical properties of importance in relation to processing are, for example, the molecular size of the dietary fibre in the raw material, the chemical composition and the degree of esterification of the dietary fibre. Furthermore, these effects have implications for nutritional and functional properties. Although changes regarding molecular weight and viscosity are documented for soluble dietary fibre, it is also important to characterise the insoluble dietary fibre. One way is to document changes in the botanical cell wall structure by microscopy, or to measure hydration properties and the dissolution of cross-links through the analysis of phenolic acids. It is also important to study the effects of modification of the dietary fibre material *in vivo*. A change in viscosity may, for example, influence hypolipidaemic properties of the dietary fibre material.

9.5 References

ÅKERBERG, A. K., LILJEBERG, H. G., GRANFELDT, Y. E., DREWS, A. W. and BJÖRCK, I. M. (1998). An In Vitro Method, Based on Chewing, To Predict Resistant Starch Content in Foods Allows Parallel Determination of Potentially Available Starch and Dietary Fiber. *J. Nutr.* **128**(3): 651–60.

ARORA, A., ZHAO, J. and CAMIRE, M. E. (1993). Extruded Potato Peel Functional Properties Affected by Extrusion Conditions. *J. Food Sci.* **58**(2): 335–7.

ARRIGONI, E., CAPREZ, A., AMADÒ, R. and NEUKOM, H. (1986). Chemical composition and physical properties of modified dietary fibre sources. *Food Hydrocolloid.* **1**(1): 57–64.

AUFFRET, A., RALET, M. C., GUILLON, F., BARRY, J. L. and THIBAULT, J. F. (1994). Effect of Grinding and Experimental Conditions on the Measurement of Hydration Properties of Dietary Fibres. *Lebensmittel-Wissenschaft und-Technologie* **27**:166–72.

BECKER, W. (1994). *Dietary habits and nutrient intake in Sweden 1989.* Swedish National Food Administration, Livsmedelsverkets förlag, Uppsala, Sweden.

BENÍTEZ, V., MOLLÁ, E., MARTÍN-CABREJAS, M. A., AGUILERA, Y., LÓPEZ-ANDRÉU, F. J. and ESTEBAN, R. M. (2011). Effect of sterilisation on dietary fibre and physicochemical properties of onion by-products. *Food Chem.* **127**(2): 501–7.

BERTIN, C., ROUAU, X. and THIBAULT, J.-F. (1988). Structure and properties of sugar beet fibres. *J. Sci. Food Agric.* **44**(1): 15–29.

BRANDT, L. M., JELTEMA, M. A., ZABIK, M. E. and JELTEMA, B. D. (1984). Effects of Cooking in Solutions of Varying pH on the Dietary Fiber Components of Vegetables. *J. Food Sci.* **49**(3): 900–4.

BRÄNNING, C., HÅKANSSON, Å., AHRNÉ, S., MOLIN, G., JEPPSSON, B. and NYMAN M. (2008). Blueberry husk and multi-strain probiotics affect colonic fermentation in rats. *Brit. J. Nutr.* **5**: 1–12.

BROUK, B. (1975). *Plants consumed by man*. London, Academic Press Inc.

BRUMMELL, D. A. and HARPSTER, M. H. (2001). Cell wall metabolism in fruit softening and quality and its manipulation in transgenic plants. *Plant Mol. Biol.* **47**(1): 311–39.

CADDEN, A.-M. (1987). Comparative Effects of Particle Size Reduction on Physical Structure and Water Binding Properties of Several Plant Fibers. *J. Food Sci.* **52**(6): 1595–9.

CAMIRE, M. E., VIOLETTE, D., DOUGHERTY, M. P. and MCLAUGHLIN, M. A. (1997). Potato Peel Dietary Fiber Composition: Effects of Peeling and Extrusion Cooking Processes. *J. Agric. Food Chem.* **45**(4): 1404–8.

CARPITA, N.C. and GIBEAUT, D.M. (1993). Structural models of primary cell walls in flowering plants: consistency of molecular structure with the physical properties of the walls during growth. *Plant Journal* **3**(1): 1–30.

CHAU, C.-F., WEN, Y.-L. and WANG, Y.-T. (2006). Improvement of the functionality of a potential fruit insoluble fibre by micron technology. *Int. J. Food Sci. Tech.* **41**: 1054–60.

CHAU, C.-F., WANG, Y.-T. and WEN, Y.-L. (2007). Different micronization methods significantly improve the functionality of carrot insoluble fibre. *Food Chem.* **100**: 1402–8.

CHÁVEZ-JÁUREGUI, R.N., SILVA, M.E.M.P and ARĚAS, J.A.G. (2000). Extrusion Cooking Process for Amaranth (*Amaranthus caudatus* L.) *J. Food Sci.* **65:** 1009-1015.

DUVETTER, T., SILA, D. N., VAN BUGGENHOUT, S. JOLIE, R., VAN LOEY, A. and HENDRICKX, M. (2009). Pectins in Processed Fruit and Vegetables: Part I—Stability and Catalytic Activity of Pectinases. *Compr. Rev. Food Sci. F.* **8**(2): 75–85.

ELLEUCH, M., BEDIGIAN, D., ROISEUX, O., BESBES, S., BLECKER, C. and ATTIA, H. (2011). Dietary fibre and fibre-rich by-products of food processing: Characterisation, technological functionality and commercial applications: A review. *Food Chem.* **124**(2): 411–21.

FEMENIA, A., SIMAL, S., TABERNER, C. G. and ROSSELLO, C. (2007). Effects of heat treatment and dehydration on pineapple (*Ananas comosus* L. Merr) cell walls. *Int. J. Food Eng.* **3**(2): 1–14.

FUENTES-ALVENTOSA, J. M., RODRÍGUEZ-GUTIÉRREZ, G., JARAMILLO-CARMONA, S., ESPEJO-CALVO, J. A., RODRÍGUEZ-ARCOS, R., *et al.* (2009). Effect of extraction method on chemical composition and functional characteristics of high dietary fibre powders obtained from asparagus by-products. *Food Chem.* **113**(2): 665–71.

GALLAND, L. (2010). Diet and Inflammation. *Nutr. Clin. Pract.* **25**(6): 634–40.

GALVIN, M. A., KIELY, M., HARRINGTON, K. E., ROBSON, P. J., MOORE, R. and FLYNN, A. (2001). The North/South Ireland Food Consumption Survey: the dietary fibre intake of Irish adults. *Public Health Nutr.* **4**(5A):1061–8.

GOURGUE, C., CHAMP, M., GUILLON, F. and DELORT-LAVAL, J. (1994). Effect of extrusion-cooking on the hypoglycemic properties of citrus fiber: an in-vitro study. *J. Sci. Food Agric.* **64**(4): 493–9.

GUILLON, F. and CHAMP, M. (2000). Structural and physical properties of dietary fibres, and consequences of processing on human physiology. *Food Res. Int.* **33**(3–4): 233–45.

GUIMARAES, J. L., FROLLINI, E., DA SILVA, C. G., WYPYCH, F. and SATYANARAYANA, K. G. (2009). Characterization of banana, sugarcane bagasse and sponge gourd fibers of Brazil. *Ind. Crop. Prod.* **30:** 407–15.

GUSTAFSSON, K., ASP, N.-G., HAGANDER, B. and NYMAN, M. (1993) Effects of different vegetables in mixed meals on glucose homeostasis and satiety. *Eur. J. Clin. Nutr.* **47**: 192–200.

GUSTAFSSON, K., ASP, N. G., HAGANDER, B. and NYMAN, M. (1994). Dose-response effects of boiled carrots and effects of carrots in lactic acid in mixed meals on glycaemic response and satiety. *Eur. J. Clin. Nutr.* **48**(6): 386–96.

HAARD, N. F. and CHISM, G. W. (1996). Characteristics of edible plant tissues. In *Food Chemistry*, O. R. FENNEMA. New York, Marcel Dekker Inc.: 943–1011.

HARRIS, P. J. and SMITH, B. G. (2006). Plant cell walls and cell-wall polysaccharides: structures, properties and uses in food products. *Int. J. Food Sci. Tech.* **41**: 129–43.

HENNINGSSON, Å. M., NYMAN, E. M. G. L. and BJÖRCK, I. M. G. (2002). Short-chain fatty acid content in the hind-gut of rats fed various composite foods and commercial dietary fibre fractions from similar sources. *J. Sci. Food Agric.* **82:** 385–93.

HSU, J. C. and PENNER, M. H. (1989). Influence of cellulose structure on its digestibility in the rat. *J. Nutr.* **119**: 872–8.

HWANG, J.-K., CHOI, J.-S., KIM, C.-J. and KIM, C-T. (1998). Solubilization of appled pomace by extrusion. *J. Food Process. Pres.* **22**(6): 477–91.

JIMÉNEZ, A., SÁNCHEZ-ROMERO, C., GUILLÓN, R., FERNÁNDEZ-BOLAÑOS, J. and HEREDIA, A. (1998). Solubilization of Cell Wall Polysaccharides from Olive Fruits into Treatment Liquids during Spanish Green Olive Processing. *J. Agric. Food Chem.* **46**(10): 4376–81.

KAYS, S. J. (1997). *Postharvest physiology of perishable plant products.* Athens, Georgia, USA, Exon Press.

KNORR, D., ADE-OMOWAYE, B. I. O. and HEINZ, V. (2002). Nutritional improvement of plant foods by non-thermal processing. *Proc. Nutr. Soc.* **61**(02): 311–18.

LARIO, Y., SENDRA, E., GARCÍA-PÉREZ, J. FUENTES, C., SAYAS-BARBERÁ, E., *et al.* (2004). Preparation of high dietary fiber powder from lemon juice by-products. *Innov. Food Sci. Emerg. Technol.* **5**(1): 113–17.

LARREA, M. A., CHANG, Y. K. and MARTINEZ-BUSTOS, F. (2005). Some functional properties of extruded orange pulp and its effect on the quality of cookies. *LWT – Food Sci. Technol.* **38**(3): 213–20.

LILJEBERG ELMSTÅHL, H. (2002). Resistant starch content in a selection of starchy foods on the Swedish market. *Eur. J. Clin. Nutr.* **56**(6): 500–5.

MANN, J., CUMMINGS, J. H., ENGLYST, H. N., KEY, T., LIU, S., *et al.* (2007). FAO/WHO Scientific Update on carbohydrates in human nutrition: conclusions. *Eur. J. Clin. Nutr.* **61** (Suppl 1): S132–S137.

MARLETT, J. A. and VOLLENDORF, N. W. (1993). Dietary fiber content and composition of vegetables determined by two methods of analysis. *J. Agric. Food Chem.* **41**: 1608–12.

MARLETT, J. A. and VOLLENDORF, N. W. (1994). Dietary fiber content and composition of fruits. *Food Chem.* **51**: 39–44.

MARTÍNEZ, M., GULLÓN, B., YÁÑEZ, R., ALONSO, J. L. and PARAJÓ, J. C. (2009). Direct Enzymatic Production of Oligosaccharide Mixtures from Sugar Beet Pulp: Experimental Evaluation and Mathematical Modeling. *J. Agric. Food Chem.* **57**(12): 5510–17.

MARTÍNEZ, M., YÁÑEZ, R., ALONSO, J. L. and PARAJÓ, J. C. (2010). Chemical Production of Pectic Oligosaccharides from Orange Peel Wastes. *Ind. Eng. Chem. Res* **49**(18): 8470–6.

MUIR, J.G, SHEPHERD, S.J., ROSELLA, O., ROSE, R., BARRETT, J.S. and GIBSON, P.R. (2007). Fructan and free fructose content of common Australian vegetables and fruits. *J. Agric. Food Chem.* **55:** 6619–27.

NG, A., LECAIN, S., PARKER, M. L., SMITH, A. C. and WALDRON, K. W. (1999). Modification of cell-wall polymers of onion waste: III. Effect of extrusion-cooking on cell-wall material of outer fleshy tissues. *Carbohydr. Polym.* **39**(4): 341–9.

NYMAN, E. M. G. L. (2003). Importance of processing for physico-chemical and physiological properties of dietary fibre. *Proc. Nutr. Soc.* **62**(01): 187–92.

NYMAN, E. M. G. L. and NILSSON, T. (1994). Effect of long-term storage on dietary fibre in different cultivars of carrots. *Acta Agric. Scand. Sect B, Soil and Plant Sci.* **44**, 116–22.

NYMAN, E. M. G. L. and SVANBERG, S. J. M. (2002). Modification of physicochemical properties of dietary fibre in carrots by mono- and divalent cations. *Food Chem.* **76**: 273–80.

NYMAN, E. M. G. L., SVANBERG, S. J. M. and ASP, N.-G. L. (1994). Molecular weight distribution and viscosity of water-soluble dietary fibre isolated from green beans, Brussels sprouts and green peas following different types of processing. *J. Sci. Food Agric.* **66**: 83–91.

NYMAN, E. M. G. L., SVANBERG, S. J. M., ANDERSSON, R. and NILSSON, T. (2005). Effects of cultivar, root weight, storage and boiling on carbohydrate content in carrots (*Daucus carota* L). *J. Sci. Food Agric.* **85**(3): 441–9.

NYMAN, M. and ASP, N.-G. (1982). Fermentation of dietary fibre components in the rat intestinal tract. *Brit. J. Nutr.* **47**: 357–66.

NYMAN, M., PÅLSSON, K.-E. and ASP, N.-G. (1987). Effects of processing on dietary fibre in vegetables. *Lebens-Wiss. Technol.* **20**: 29–36.

PENNER, M. H. and KIM, S. (1991). Nonstarch Polysaccharide Fractions of Raw, Processed and Cooked Carrots. *J. Food Sci.* **56**(6): 1593–6.

PROSKY, L., ASP, N.-G., SCHWEIZER, T. F., DEVRIES, J. W., FURDA, I. and LEE, S. C. (1994) Determination of soluble dietary fiber in foods and food products: collaborative study. *J AOAC Int.* **77**(3): 690–4.

RAGHAVENDRA, S. N., RAMACHANDRA SWAMY, S. R., RASTOGI, N. K., RAGHAVARAO, K. S. M. S., *et al.* (2006). Grinding characteristics and hydration properties of coconut residue: A source of dietary fiber. *J. Food Eng.* **72**(3): 281–6.

REDONDO, A., VILLANUEVA, M. J., RODRIGUEZ, M. D. and SACO, M. D. (1997). Autoclaving effects on the dietary fibre content of carrots (*Daucus carota*) and turnips (*Brassica napus*): an evaluation of different methods. *Z. Lebensm. Unters. Forsch.* **205**(6): 457–63.

REHMAN, Z. U., ISLAM, M. and SHAH, W. H. (2003). Effect of microwave and conventional cooking on insoluble dietary fibre components of vegetables. *Food Chem.* **80**(2): 237–40.

RODRÍGUEZ, R., JIMÉNEZ, A., FERNÁNDEZ-BOLAÑOS, J., GUILLÉN, R. and HEREDIA, A. (2006). Dietary fibre from vegetable products as source of functional ingredients. *Trends Food Sci. Tech.* **17**(1): 3–15.

RYDEN, P. and SELVENDRAN, R. R. (1990). Structural features of cell-wall polysaccharides of potato (*Solanum tuberosum*). *Carbohydr. Res.* **195**(2): 257–72.

SAJJAANANTAKUL, T., VAN BUREN, J. P. and DOWNING, D. L. (1993). Effect of cations on heat degradation of chelator-soluble carrot pectin. *Carbohydr. Polym.* **20**(3): 207–14.

SANGNARK, A. and NOOMHORM, A. (2003). Effect of particle sizes on functional properties of dietary fibre prepared from sugarcane bagasse. *Food Chem.* **80**(2): 221–9.

SCHIEBER, A., STINTZING, F. C. and CARLE, R. (2001). By-products of plant food processing as a source of functional compounds — recent developments. *Trends Food Sci. Technol.* **12**: 401–13.

SCHOLS, H. A., VISSER, R. G. F. and VORAGEN, A. G. J., eds. (2009). *Pectins and pectinases.* Wageningen Academic Publishers.

SELVENDRAN, R. R. and ROBERTSON, J. A. (1990). The chemistry of dietary fibre – an holistic view of the cell wall matrix. In *Dietary fibre: Chemical and biological aspects.* D. A. T. SOUTHGATE, K. WALDRON, I. T. JOHNSON and G. R. FENWICK. Royal Society of Chemistry, Cambridge, UK, pp. 27–43.

SELVENDRAN, R. R. and ROBERTSON, J. A. (1994) Dietary fibre in foods: amount and type. In *Physico-chemical properties of dietary fibre and effect of processing on micronutrients availability.* R. AMADÒ, J.-L. BARRY and W. FRØLICH. Luxembourg, COST 92 Directorate-General XIII: 11–19.

SHEA, E. M., GIBEAUT, D. M. and CARPITA, N. C. (1989). Structural analysis of the cell walls regenerated by carrot protoplasts. *Planta* **179**(3): 293–308.

SILA, D. N., SMOUT, C., VU, S. T., VAN LOEY, A. and HENDRICKX, M. (2005). Influence of Pretreatment Conditions on the Texture and Cell Wall Components of Carrots During Thermal Processing. *J. Food Sci.* **70**(2): E85–E91.

SILA, D. N., VAN BUGGENHOUT, S., DUVETTER, T., FRAEYE, I., DE ROECK, A., *et al.* (2009). Pectins in Processed Fruits and Vegetables: Part II—Structure–Function Relationships. *Compr. Rev. Food Sci. F.* **8**(2): 86–104.

SILJESTRÖM, M. and BJÖRCK, I. (1990). Digestible and undigestible carbohydrates in autoclaved legumes, potatoes and corn. *Food Chem.* **38**(2): 145–52.

SVANBERG, S. J. M., NYMAN, E. M. G. L., ANDERSSON, R. and NILSSON, T. (1997). Effects of Boiling and Storage on Dietary Fibre and Digestible Carbohydrates in Various Cultivars of Carrots. *J. Sci. Food Agric.* **73**(2): 245–54.

SVANBERG, S. J. M., GUSTAFSSON, K. B. H., SUORTTI T. and NYMAN, E. M. G. L. (1995). Molecular weight distribution, measured by HPSEC, and viscosity of water-soluble dietary fiber in carrots following different types of processing. *J. Agric. Food Chem.* **43**(10): 2692–97.

SWEDISH BOARD OF AGRICULTURE (2011). *Livsmedelskonsumtion och näringsinnehåll.* http://www.sjv.se/webdav/files/SJV/Amnesomraden/Statistik,%20fakta/Livsmedel/Statistikrapport2011_2/20112_ikortadrag.htm (accessed 15 June 2011).

VAN BUGGENHOUT, S., SILA, D. N., DUVETTER, T., VAN LOEY, A. and HENDRICKX, M. (2009). Pectins in Processed Fruits and Vegetables: Part III—Texture Engineering. *Compr. Rev. Food Sci. F.* **8**(2): 105–17.

VAN BUREN, J. P. (1979). The chemistry of texture in fruits and vegetables. *J. Texture Stud.* **10**(1): 1–23.

WENNBERG, M. and NYMAN, M. (2004). On the possibility of using high pressure treatment to modify physico-chemical properties of dietary fibre in white cabbage (*Brassica oleracea* var. *capitata*). *Innov. Food Sci. Emerg. Technol.* **5**(2): 171–7.

WENNBERG, M., ENGQVIST, G. and NYMAN, M. (2002). Effects of harvest time and storage on dietary fibre components in various cultivars of white cabbage (*Brassica oleracea* var *capitata*). *J. Sci. Food Agric.* **82**(12): 1405–11.

WENNBERG, M. S., ENGQVIST, G. M. and NYMAN, E. M. G. L. (2003). Effects of Boiling on Dietary Fiber Components in Fresh and Stored White Cabbage (*Brassica oleracea* var. *capitata*). *J. Food Sci.* **68**(5): 1615–21.

WENNBERG, M., EKVALL, J., OLSSON, K. and NYMAN, M. (2006). Changes in carbohydrate and glucosinolate composition in white cabbage (*Brassica oleracea* var. *capitata*) during blanching and treatment with acetic acid. *Food Chem.* **95**(2): 226–36.

VILLANUEVA, M. J., RODRIGUEZ, M. D., REDONDO, A. and SACO, M. D. (1996). Effect of autoclaving on dietary fibre content of beet root (*Beta vulgaris*). Evaluation by different methods. *Z. Lebensm. Unters. Forsch.* **203**(4): 345–50.

WOLF, B. (2010). Polysaccharide functionality through extrusion processing. *Curr. Opin. Colloid In.* **15**(1–2): 50–4.

ZYKWINSKA, A, RONDEAU-MOURO, C., GARNIER, C, THIBAULT, J. F. and RALET, M. C. (2006). Alkaline extractability of pectic arabinan and galactan and their mobility in sugar beet and potato cell walls. *Carbohyd. Polym.* **65:** 510–20.

Part III

Improving the quality of fibre-rich and wholegrain foods: cereal products

10

Fibre-enriched and wholegrain breads

A. Rakha, National Institute of Food Science and Technology, Pakistan, P. Åman and R. Andersson, Swedish University of Agricultural Sciences, Sweden

DOI: 10.1533/9780857095787.3.211

Abstract: Bread is a staple food worldwide. It is a good source of energy, protein, dietary fibre (DF), minerals, vitamins and many other bioactive compounds. Increased intake of DF has been associated with a decreased risk of overweight and obesity, hypertension, cardiovascular diseases, diabetes, certain cancers and constipation. The use of refined flour in bread decreases its content of DF and associated bioactive compounds. Therefore wholemeal flour, composite flour, bran, resistant starch, fructan/fructo-oligosaccharides or fibre concentrates have been added to bread to enrich it with DF. However, these ingredients can modify many properties of the dough and the bread, so the bread-making process has to be adjusted to achieve desirable products. Many processes can result in the loss of functionality and positive health effects of the DF components, an important aspect to consider when creating innovative products.

Key words: bread, dietary fibre enrichment, processing, sensory properties.

10.1 Introduction

Bread is used as a staple food in most countries. In the UK, for instance, the household penetration of bread is about 97.4% with around 66 loaves purchased annually per household (The Federation of Bakers, 2007). White bread is consumed most often and is usually prepared from wheat flour with about 72% extraction rate, thus removing bran and germ. This leads to a bread with a low content of dietary fibre (DF) (<2.5%), minerals and vitamins (Anon, 2003; Bender, 2006).

With rising consumer demand for healthier foods, the incorporation of various fibre-rich ingredients into bread has greatly increased. Dietary fibre has been positively associated with a decreased risk of conditions such as obesity, diabetes, cardiovascular disease, colon cancer and constipation (EFSA, 2010). It also promotes the production of short chain fatty acids in the intestine and may have prebiotic properties. Due to the universal consumption of bread products, enriching bread with DF offers promising potential to increase DF intake. The typical Western diet contains too little DF, 20 g/day compared with the recommended 25–30 g/day (EFSA, 2010).

The most updated definition of DF by Codex is from 2010 (CAC/GL 2-1985) and states that:

> Dietary fibre means carbohydrate polymers[1] with ten or more monomeric units[2], which are not hydrolysed by the endogenous enzymes in the small intestine of humans and belong to the following categories:
>
> - Edible carbohydrate polymers naturally occurring in the food consumed
> - Carbohydrate polymers, which have been obtained from food raw materials by physical, enzymatic or chemical means and which have been shown to have a physiological effect of benefit to health as demonstrated by generally accepted scientific evidence to competent authorities
> - Synthetic carbohydrate polymers which have been shown to have a physiological effect of benefit to health as demonstrated by generally accepted scientific evidence to competent authorities
>
> [1] When derived from a plant origin, dietary fibre may include fractions of lignin and/or other compounds associated with polysaccharides in the plant cell walls. These compounds also may be measured by certain analytical method(s) for dietary fibre. However, such compounds are not included in the definition of dietary fibre if extracted and re-introduced into a food.
>
> [2] Decision on whether to include carbohydrates from 2 to 9 monomeric units should be left to national authorities.

A similar definition has been introduced in the EU by the European Commission (Commission Directive 2008/100/EC). One important difference is that this definition states that all carbohydrates with at least three monomeric units should be included in the definition, so this is not optional for EU member states. At the moment, both Codex and the European Commission are working on a list of approved methods which may be used for the determination of dietary fibre content or content of individual dietary fibre components.

10.1.1 Different types of bread

There is a wide variety of breads differing in morphology, ingredients and method of baking. Breads around the world can be divided into three broad categories (New Zealand Association of Bakers, 2010):

- Those that rise highest and so have to be baked in pans,
- those with a medium volume, like rye and French breads, and
- those that hardly rise at all and consequently are called flatbreads.

Yeast forms an integral part of white bread baking, and white bread baked in pans is the most common type of bread, consumed by large numbers of people around the world. Multigrain and kibbled breads, sourdough bread, wholemeal bread, pumpernickel bread, bagels, hearth breads, French baguettes, and so on belong to the second category. Flatbread is the oldest bread made by humans and its basic ingredients are flour, salt and water. These ingredients are kneaded to workable dough and the bread is shaped by hand and baked. An example of flatbread is chapatti or roti, consumed mostly in South Asia. Flatbread is usually made from wheat flour, but can be supplemented with high fibre ingredients, thus adding nutrient diversity and variety to the bread. It can be made with or without yeast. Other examples of flatbread are tortilla (Mexico), focaccia (Italy), pitta (Middle East) and naan (India). Crispbread is a kind of flat bread consumed in Scandinavia. It was originally made from rye flour, water and salt, but it has since incorporated multiple ingredients, such as yeast, grains from other cereals, and so on, and is made in various shapes.

10.1.2 Major DF components in flour

Arabinoxylan (AX) is a cell wall polysaccharide present in all major cereals. The backbone of the AX molecule consists of (1→4)-linked β-D-xylopyranosyl residues, which are either monosubstituted by an α-L-arabinofuranosyl residue at the O-2 or O-3 position or disubstituted at both these positions (Izydorczyk and Dexter, 2008). Monosubstitution at O-2 is rare in wheat and rye, but occurs more frequently in barley (Saulnier and Quemener, 2009; Viëtor *et al.*, 1992). This substitution pattern also varies depending on cultivar and position in the grain; for example, AX is more highly substituted in outer wheat bran (A/X 0.88) than in the aleurone layer (A/X 0.35) (Bonnand-Ducasse *et al.*, 2010; Izydorczyk and Dexter, 2008; Saulnier *et al.*, 2007). In wheat endosperm the A/X ratio varies from 0.5 to 0.7. Different phenolics, for example, *p*-coumaric acid and ferulic acid, can be esterified at the O-5 position of the arabinose residue and play an important role in oxidative gelation of water-soluble AX (Ishii, 1997). The degree and pattern of substitution control the physicochemical properties (solubility, viscosity, hydration properties) of the polymer (Courtin and Delcour, 2002; Saulnier *et al.*, 2007). Water-unextractable AX is considered to have negative impact on loaf volume, while water-extractable AX, which makes up about 25% of AX in grain endosperm, improves loaf volume (Biliaderis *et al.*, 1995; Courtin and Delcour, 2002). Rye AXs have been classified into four distinct classes based on structure and extractability, which are partly overlapping (Andersson and Åman, 2001; Vinkx *et al.*, 1993). These include a sparsely substituted acidic xylan, a highly branched heteroxylan and two types of soluble AX with different substitution patterns. Enzymatic fingerprinting is a helpful tool to study the structural features of AX (Saulnier and Quemener, 2009). A light scattering detector coupled with refractive index and UV detectors is usually used to characterise AX for molecular mass distribution (Andersson *et al.*, 2009).

Mixed linkage (1→3) (1→4)-β-D-glucan (hereafter referred to as β-glucan) is predominantly composed of (1→4)-linked β-D-glucopyranosyl residues

(~70%) interrupted by (1→3)-linked *β*-D-glucopyranosyl residues (~30%) (Wood, 2001). Most of the (1→4) linkages are present in groups of two or three units, thereby resulting in a structure with predominantly (1→3) linked cellotriosyl and cellotetraosyl units. So far no evidence exists for two or more adjacent (1→3) linkages in the *β*-glucan chain (Izydorczyk and Dexter, 2008). The solution properties of *β*-glucan depend upon amount, molecular weight, solubility/extractability and structure, and therefore changes in these properties will affect the physiological response of the polymer (Autio, 1996; Wood, 2002). The molar ratio of cellotriosyl to cellotetraosyl units differs between cereals and is an important determinant of the physicochemical properties (Autio, 1996). Cellotriosyl and cellotetraosyl units normally constitute 85–90% by weight of cereal *β*-glucan and less than 15% form cellulose-like chains with more than three consecutive (1→4)-linked glucose residues (Izydorczyk and Dexter, 2008; Wood, 2007). *β*-Glucan dominates in the endosperm cell walls of oats and barley, while it is less prominent in rye and wheat endosperm cell walls (Wood, 2007). *β*-Glucan in oats is mainly located in the sub-aleurone layer, while in barley it is more evenly distributed throughout the endosperm (Cui and Wang, 2009). Structural fingerprinting can be carried out by hydrolysing the polymer by lichenase and measuring the oligosaccharides released (Saulnier and Quemener, 2009). Size exclusion chromatography with selective Calcofluor detection is used to measure the molecular mass of the polymer (Rimsten *et al.*, 2003).

Cellulose is the most abundant organic macromolecule present on land (O'Sullivan, 1997). It is a linear polymer of (1→4)-linked *β*-D-glucopyranosyl residues with a wide molecular weight distribution (Franz and Blaschek, 1990). The *β*-configuration forces the chain to rotate, with anhydrocellobiose as the repeating unit. The extended molecules form flat ribbons, which are further stiffened by intramolecular and intermolecular hydrogen bonds. Cellulose provides rigidity to the plant cell wall and protects the interior of the cell. In cereals, bran is usually a rich source of cellulose (Gropper *et al.*, 2009).

Lignin, a polymer of phenyl-propanoids (Vanholme *et al.*, 2010), is present in secondary thickened cell walls in the bran of cereal grains. It is a highly branched and complex polymer with strong intramolecular bonds (Ralph *et al.*, 2004; Vanholme *et al.*, 2010). It is regarded as a structural component of plants and is attached to heteroxylans found in the cell wall (Gropper *et al.*, 2009). Lignin is insoluble in water and is considered to be a poor substrate for the colonic microflora.

Fructans, including fructo-oligosaccharides (FOS) with a degree of polymerisation (DP) 3–9, are soluble dietary fibre components with prebiotic properties (Gibson and Roberfroid, 1995). Among cereals, rye has the highest content of fructans, up to 6.4% (Hansen *et al.*, 2003). Chemically, fructans are polymers of *β*-D-fructofuranosyl residues with a terminal glucose residue (Bornet, 2001; Smeekens *et al.*, 1996). Plant fructans usually have a DP range of 5–60, with only a few species having DP up to 200. The elution profiles of rye (cv. Ottarp) and wheat (cv. Harnesk) fructans are presented in Fig. 10.1.

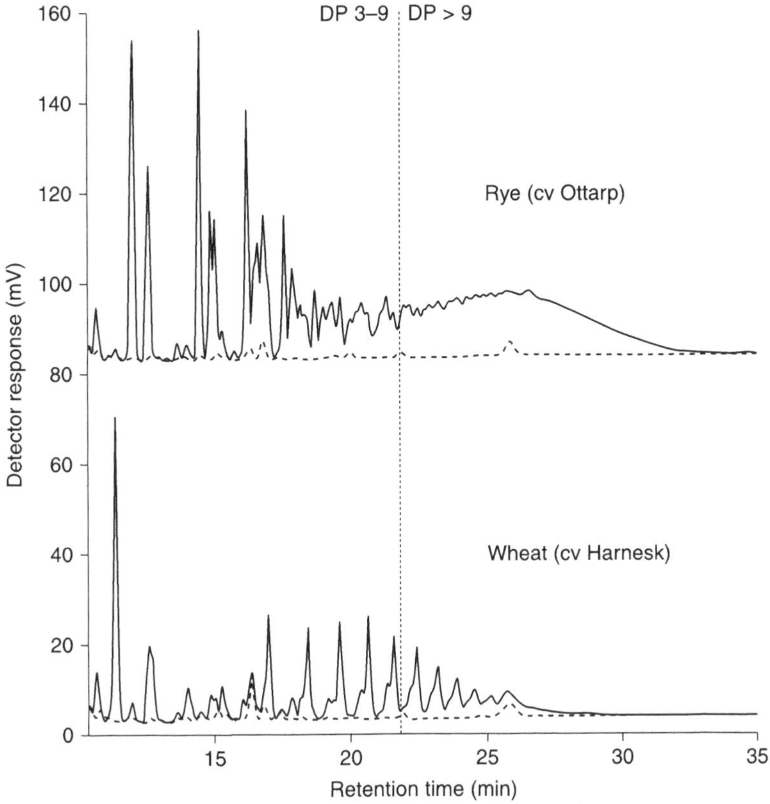

Fig. 10.1 Fructan molecular weight distribution profile of rye (cv. Ottarp) and wheat (cv. Harnesk). The line (—) represents the chromatogram without fructanase treatment and (----) that with fructanase treatment. Unpublished data from the author's laboratory.

In wheat the intermediate DP fructan dominates, while rye has a significant proportion of long chain fructan molecules. Based on the linkage pattern, fructans are divided into three groups: (1) inulin type with (2→1) linkages; (2) levan type with (2→6) linkages; and (3) graminan or mixed type with both (2→1) and (2→6) linkages. Inulin is present, for example, in chicory or Jerusalem artichoke and is the most widely studied fructan, while graminan-type fructans predominate in cereals (Roberfroid, 2005; Smeekens *et al.*, 1996). FOS can be produced from inulin by acid hydrolysis or the action of transferase enzymes. The molecular weight distribution of fructan in cereals and cereal-based foods can be analysed by anion exchange chromatography with pulsed amperometric detection, while enzymatic methods are used for the quantification of fructan (Rakha *et al.*, 2010).

10.2 Fibre enrichment of breads

10.2.1 Wholegrain

Wholegrain bread is considered to be a good source of DF, and the United States Department of Agriculture (USDA) Dietary Guidelines Advisory Committee (2005) recommends a minimum of three servings of whole grains per day. The DF content of wholegrain wheat flour (100% extraction rate) is about 12%, while that of sifted white flour (75% extraction rate) is about 2.5% (Dewettinck *et al.*, 2008), making white flour a poor source of DF. Whole, cracked or crushed kernels can also be incorporated as a topping in crisp or soft breads or as an ingredient in soft bread, adding variety to these breads. The following definition was approved by the Whole Grain Council (WGC) in 2004: 'Whole grains or foods made from them contain all the essential parts and naturally-occurring nutrients of the entire grain seed. If the grain has been processed (e.g., cracked, crushed, rolled, extruded, and/or cooked), the food product should deliver approximately the same rich balance of nutrients that are found in the original grain seed' (Whole Grain Council, 2010). The selected whole grains accepted by WGC and their DF values reported by the USDA National Nutrient Database SR 23 are presented in Fig. 10.2. There is a markedly wide range of DF content, from only 4.6% in brown rice to 15.1% in rye. Other cereal grasses such as canary seed, Job's tears, montina, timothy, fonio, and so on are also included in the definition, but are less common. Legumes and oilseeds are not defined as whole grains by WGC, the American Association of Cereal Chemists (AACC) International or the American Food and Drug Administration (FDA).

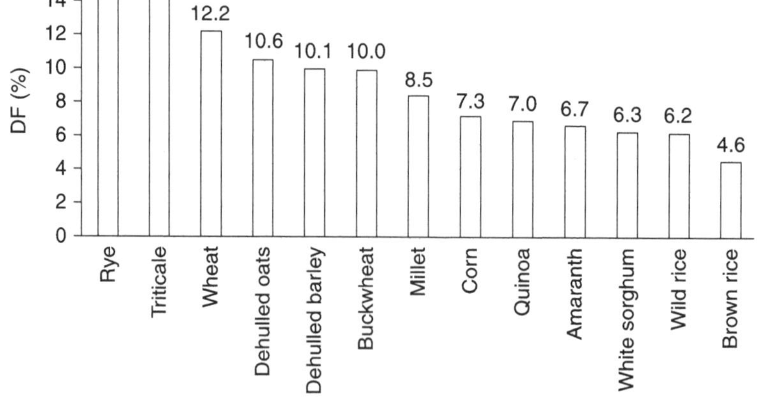

Fig. 10.2 Whole grains and their dietary fibre content (% of fresh weight) as reported in the USDA (SR 23) database.

10.2.2 Bran

Bran obtained from wheat, rye, oat, rice, barley or other cereals offers the most promising prospects of DF fortification in bread. The DF content of bran varies considerably within and between different bran samples; for example, the average content in oat bran is around 15%, while in corn bran it is as high as 79% (Fig. 10.3). Rye bran contains about 38% DF (dry matter basis), but when fructan is included according to the new Codex definition the content increases to about 45% (Kamal-Eldin *et al.*, 2009). Major components of DF in rye bran include AX (25%), fructan (7%), β-glucan (5%), cellulose (6.5%) and Klason lignin (4.5%). Wheat bran contains comparable levels of total DF but varies in relative proportion of DF components. For example, the fructan and β-glucan content is only half that in rye bran. Oat bran is a rich source of β-glucan, with the content generally ranging from 5 to 9% (Luhaloo *et al.*, 1998; Mälkki and Virtanen, 2001). The chemical composition of bran is found to vary with the milling efficiency by which the endosperm is separated from the bran layers. Bran thus offers tremendous potential to raise the DF level in bread. Since bran and outer layers of grain are rich sources of vitamins, minerals and other bioactive components such as phenolics (Dervilly-Pinel *et al.*, 2001; Dewettinck *et al.*, 2008; Kamal-Eldin *et al.*, 2009), addition of bran can result in a significant increase in the nutritive value of bread.

However, the addition of bran can also result in increased content of heavy metals such as cadmium or other toxic substances such as mycotoxins present in the outer layers of the grain (EFSA, 2009: Question No EFSA-Q-2007-138). Furthermore, there is evidence that consumption of bran fibre decreases mineral absorption. Phytic acid, which is present in the aleurone layer of bran, is known to

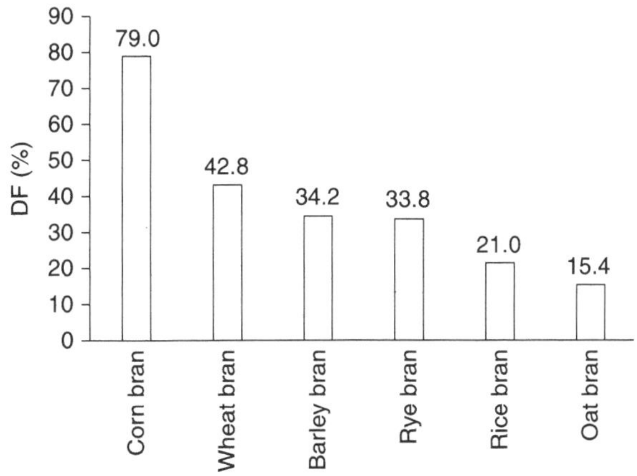

Fig. 10.3 Dietary fibre content (% of fresh weight) of major cereal brans as reported in the USDA (SR 23) database. The DF values (converted to fresh weight basis) for rye and barley bran are from Kamal-Eldin *et al.* (2009) and Sullivan *et al.* (2010), respectively.

bind minerals such as Fe, Ca and Mg, thereby lowering their bioavailability (Ekholm *et al.*, 2003; Idouraine *et al.*, 1996).

10.2.3 Milling fractions

The non-uniform distribution of DF components within cereal grains allows the grain to be fractionated into flour streams enriched in arabinoxylan and β-glucan (Izydorczyk and Dexter, 2008). With modern milling and sieving techniques, it is possible to obtain fractions with as much as 20% β-glucan (Wood, 2002). Pericarp and seed coat, outer layers which are low in β-glucan, can be removed by pearling (Izydorczyk and Dexter, 2008). Air classification is another technique widely used to obtain fractions rich in a particular compound, for example β-glucan. With this technology, a fraction with 40–45% enrichment of β-glucan can be obtained from high β-glucan barley (Andersson *et al.*, 2000). However, it is possible to achieve up to 62% enrichment of β-glucan from barley through air classification if the process is preceded by defatting (Izydorczyk and Dexter, 2008). Izydorczyk *et al.* (2008) reported an increase from 0.2 to 3.0 g in total β-glucan intake and from 2.4 to 4.2 g in AX intake per serving of two-layer wheat flat bread when supplemented with 20% fibre-rich fraction of high amylose pin-milled barley. Such naturally obtained products retain maximum physiological functions and are preferred by the health-conscious consumer. Milling fractions provide a diversity of DF components compared with isolated fibre concentrates.

10.2.4 Composite flour

Composite flour technology is widely used to selectively increase certain DF components in breads. In a study by Trogh *et al.* (2004) on yeast-leavened bread, up to 40% of the wheat flour was replaced with hull-less barley flour. Supplementation of barley flour helped to increase the sum of AX and β-glucan content from 1.7% in wheat flour bread to 3.1% in composite flour bread with acceptable sensory characteristics. The problem of decreased loaf volume was largely overcome by addition of specific xylanase, which preferentially converts the water-unextractable AX into soluble AX, thereby improving the baking performance of the flour. Mariotti *et al.* (2006) produced wheat bread supplemented with 20% oat flour with adjustments in the baking process. The selection of supplemented flour with high falling number (i.e. low enzyme activity) may be important to avoid the endogenous enzyme-related degradation of β-glucan (Andersson *et al.*, 2008).

10.2.5 Bread enriched with fructan and/or fructo-oligosaccharides

In recent years the role of fructan in human health has been widely studied (Roberfroid, 2005). Consumption of fructan has been associated with improving gastrointestinal health and immune functions. The fructan content in various tissues varies depending on the growth stage of the plant. In grains, it is highest during grain filling and the content decreases rapidly thereafter (Nardi *et al.*, 2003). That study found that common wheat contained 18.2% fructan 13 days after anthesis, which decreased to 3.7% 28 days after anthesis. Similarly, rye contained 30% fructan 13 days after anthesis, which decreased to 6.2% 28 days after anthesis. Inulin and its partial hydrolysate are white powders that are easy to incorporate into bread without changing crumb colour, which is the case when using bran or wholegrain flour with dark particles (Meyer and Peters, 2009). Inulin-enriched breads should be baked for a shorter time, however, since inulin accelerates crust colouration via the Maillard reaction (Poinot *et al.*, 2010).

10.2.6 Resistant starch

According to the new Codex definition, resistant starch (RS) is considered part of DF. RS is not digested by the enzymes present in the upper gut of humans, but is fermentable by the colonic microflora. Based on its origin, RS is divided into subclasses 1–4 (Englyst and Macfarlane, 1986). RS1 is physically inaccessible to digestive enzymes because of its presence in intact or partly disintegrated grains with a resistant botanical structure. RS2 is resistant to digestion due to the compact inaccessible structure of the granules, for example potato or green banana starch granules. RS3 is formed naturally from crystallisation of amylose after gelatinisation of starch granules. RS4 is formed during starch derivatisation when the functional properties are modified by substitution or cross-linking of starch (Cummings and Stephen, 2007). The addition of RS as a source of DF in fibre-enriched products offers some promising advantages compared with bran. It does not result in dark colour, which is usually a problem with addition of bran, and it gives better cell structure and loaf volume. Products containing RS also perform physiological functions similar to those of fibre (Sajilata *et al.*, 2006). The fine particle size of RS does not interfere with the dough matrix, a problem that is usually associated with high fibre baking. The relatively low water absorption of RS compared with other fibre sources is advantageous as it does not disrupt bread structure drastically and provides the bread with greater organoleptic appeal (Brown *et al.*, 2001). The incorporation of high amylose maize (starch with more than 80% amylose) produces fibre-enriched bread without compromising loaf volume, crumb colour or texture.

10.2.7 Fortification with fibre concentrate

Commercial fibres from wheat, maize, oats and barley containing high amounts of total DF or individual DF components are available and can be incorporated to produce high fibre bread (Sabanis *et al.*, 2009a). Nutrim® and UltraTrim™ (FutureCeuticals, Inc.), Glucagel® (Polycell Technologies, Crookston, MN), OatWell (CreaNutrition AG, Switzerland) and Viscofibre (Cevena Bioproducts, Inc., Edmonton, AB, Canada) are some examples of isolates/concentrates rich in β-glucan.

Other sources of DF, such as gums, mucilages, pea fibre, pectin, brewer's spent grain, citrus pulp, potato skin, and so on, can also be incorporated into bread. In addition, synthetic fibres such as polydextrose and chemically modified fibres from lignocellulosic non-woody sources are potential sources. Some of these fibre isolates or gums are added for technological purposes to impart favourable characteristics to the bread. Other fibre concentrates carry specific DF components and provide certain health benefits.

10.2.8 Fibre enrichment of gluten-free bread

Gluten-free (GF) products are aimed to target the population suffering from coeliac disease, while retaining the maximum possible sensory and nutritional characteristics. Coeliac disease is an autoimmune genetic disorder that arises by inclusion of gluten in the diet (Hill *et al.*, 2005). It is caused by a prolamin protein sequence specific to wheat (gliadin), rye (secalin) and barley (hordein) and occurs with a mean prevalence of about 1% in the global population (Green and Cellier, 2007). Gluten, being a main structure-forming component in bread-making, is present mostly in wheat and gives elasticity to the dough, helps it to rise and keep its shape during baking, and gives a chewy texture to the bread (Gallagher *et al.*, 2004). Gluten removal therefore poses a tremendous challenge for bakers to produce acceptable GF breads. Since wheat, rye and barley flour are mainly replaced by gluten-free starch in GF bread, the coeliac population generally does not meet the recommended daily intake of DF (Lee *et al.*, 2009).

Rice comprises a major part of the typical GF diet and white rice has a very low DF content (Lee *et al.*, 2009). To rectify this deficiency of fibre in coeliacs, GF breads can be supplemented with commercial fibre made from oat, rice or maize bran. The addition of fibre can impart favourable properties to the bread, as incorporation of 3% maize fibre in GF bread usually produces higher loaf volume and softer crumb compared with non-fibre GF bread (Sabanis *et al.*, 2009a). In an optimised GF bread formulation reported by Sabanis *et al.* (2009b), the addition of 6.5% maize fibre led to 5.2% DF content in bread loaves. The addition of maize fibre to GF bread resulted in a better overall acceptability score compared with non-supplemented GF bread. The incorporation of RS or production of RS during processing offers promising prospects for fibre enrichment of GF bread without impairing the organoleptic properties (Korus *et al.*, 2009). In that study, 20% replacement of maize starch with maize RS resulted in an increase of up to 89% in total DF without impairing the total quality score of GF bread. It is reported that maximum intake of RS should not exceed 30 g/day, as this might have some adverse effects in the form of flatulence and gastric problems (Nugent, 2005).

Other non-cereal fibre sources also offer promising potential to increase the DF level in GF bread. Inulin can be incorporated into GF breads to enhance soluble DF. Incorporation of 8% inulin into wheat starch-based GF bread enhanced the DF content from 1.4% in the control to 7.5% (Gallagher *et al.*, 2004). When incorporated into bread, inulin results in better dough stability and increased loaf volume, with improved crust colour and crumb texture. Pseudo-cereals such as buckwheat and amaranth, which have a high amount of DF, can also help to meet the DF deficiency in GF breads (Alvarez-Jubete *et al.*, 2009). Therefore partial or complete replacement of starch with these cereals can help to alleviate the DF deficit in the diet of coeliacs. Oat is also a GF cereal but is frequently contaminated with wheat during growing, harvesting and processing. New production, handling and processing protocols have been developed by several companies to ensure absolutely pure oats that can be used as a GF ingredient. Different hydrocolloids such as gums (guar gum, xanthan, locust bean gum) and mucilages are also incorporated in GF baking as binding agents and offer a gluten substitute in bread-making (Gallagher *et al.*, 2004). In this way, the DF content of GF bread can be increased with acceptable quality. Therefore the enrichment of GF bread with various fibres not only provides significant amounts of DF, but also offers tremendous technological benefits, resulting in products with better organoleptic properties.

10.3 Processing

Processing is essential to make food palatable, as it adds variety and results in modification of food properties. Some of the process-induced modifications are favourable, while others can have adverse impacts on the nutritional quality of food (Slavin *et al.*, 2000). The importance of judicious processing and the use of whole grain ingredients was already laid down by Hippocrates, who wrote:

> And this I know, moreover, that to the human body it makes a great difference whether the bread be fine, or coarse; of wheat with or without the hull, whether mixed with much or little water, strongly wrought or scarcely at all, baked or raw-and a multitude of similar differences . . . Whoever pays no attention to these things, or, paying attention, does not comprehend them, how can he understand the diseases which befall a man? (Hippocrates, 400 BC)

Different processing parameters, such as mixing, endogenous enzymes, temperature, fermentation, pH, and so on, can result in significant degradation of major DF components during baking (Åman *et al.*, 2004; Andersson *et al.*, 2009; Andersson *et al.*, 2004; Westerlund *et al.*, 1989). Higher temperature is reported to break the glycosidic linkages in DF polysaccharides, resulting in depolymerisation (Selvendran and Robertson, 1994). The extent of this effect is dependent on the intensity of heat treatment.

10.3.1 Total DF

During bread-making, the total content of DF changes depending upon the processing conditions (Andersson *et al.*, 2009; Laurikainen *et al.*, 1998). A varying quantity of RS is formed depending upon processing and ingredients, which accounts for the variation in total DF (Westerlund *et al.*, 1989; Sajilata *et al.*, 2006). Fructans are sensitive to yeast fermentation, which may result in significant loss of soluble DF (Hansen *et al.*, 2002; Praznik *et al.*, 2002). Hansen *et al.* (2002) observed a 4 g/100 g (dry matter basis) decrease in DF in imitated sourdough compared with rye flour, but the baking process did not significantly affect DF content. In contrast to total DF, there is an increase in the content of soluble DF, partly because some insoluble DF is converted to soluble DF (Vasanthan *et al.*, 2002). The relative proportion of water-extractable DF has also been found to increase during baking, to 31% of total DF in bread, compared with 23% water-extractable DF in raw flour (Hansen *et al.*, 2002). In a recent study on the DF content of rye products, the huge variation found was attributed to variations in ingredients and processing conditions (Rakha *et al.*, 2010). In the studied products, the DF content in soft breads ranged from 7.9 to 17.5% (average 12.6%), while that in crispbreads ranged from 13.0 to 19.8% (average 17.8%).

10.3.2 Arabinoxylan

Bread-making results in increased soluble AX content (Trogh *et al.*, 2004) but total content decreases (Andersson *et al.*, 2009). Mixing, fermentation and baking result in the solubilisation of the arabinoxylan molecules (Cleemput *et al.*, 1997). This increased solubilisation can partly be ascribed to physical phenomena that result in disaggregation of the weakly bound AX chains (Rouau, 1993). Endogenous pentosanases also play a role during bread-making (Cleemput *et al.*, 1997). Their action is dependent on processing conditions, pre-treatment of flour and structure of AX, such as extent of AX association with other components and the substitution pattern on the AX chain (Cleemput *et al.*, 1997; Rouau, 1993). After dough kneading in one study, more than 10% of the water-unextractable AX became soluble and at the end of fermentation about 25% became soluble, in the absence of added enzymes (Rouau *et al.*, 1994). In that experiment the ratio of water-extractable AX to water-unextractable AX was 0.4 in flour and 0.9 in fully fermented dough. This increase in solubility was attributed mostly to physical phenomena, that is, temperature increase and mechanical input. The solubility becomes much higher if baking enzymes are added during processing (Cleemput *et al.*, 1997; Rouau *et al.*, 1994; Trogh *et al.*, 2004). The oven baking process itself has been reported to decrease the degree of solubilisation of AX molecules, as the bread crumb has less soluble AX than the corresponding dough (Rouau *et al.*, 1994; Westerlund *et al.*, 1989).

The bread-making process affects the molecular weight distribution of AX by reducing the high molecular weight fraction (Andersson *et al.*, 2009). A comparison of the AX molecular weight distribution profile of rye flour and breads is given in Fig. 10.4. The flour is shown to have a narrower distribution profile. The soft breads and crispbreads exhibit marked degradation, with a shift of the population towards low molecular weight. Cleemput *et al.* (1997) also observed a reduction in molecular weight of water-extractable AX during mixing and fermentation. Since no mechanical input was involved during fermentation, the decrease in molecular weight was attributed to endoxylanases. This decrease was ascribed to either increased solubilisation of lower molecular weight AX or depolymerisation of water-extractable AX. Sourdough bread usually has a lower average molecular weight than other soft breads or crispbreads (Andersson

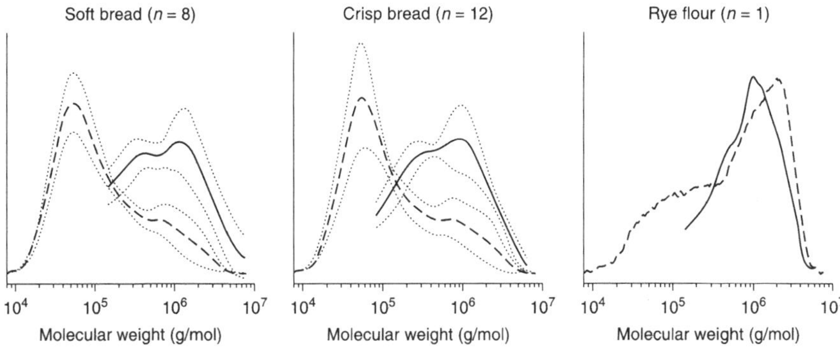

Fig. 10.4 Molecular weight distribution profile of β-glucan (----) and arabinoxylan (—) of rye flour, crispbreads and soft breads. The dotted lines (.......) around the molecular weight distributions of soft breads and crispbreads show the standard deviations. Data adapted from Rakha *et al.* (2010).

et al., 2009). This highlights the role of pH in degradation of AX during the bread-making process.

The role of endogenous enzymes during bread-making was investigated by Debyser *et al.* (1999), who observed that breads containing purified endoxylanase inhibitor had significantly lower volume than those without added inhibitors. Endogenous enzymes are also active during refrigeration of dough and are responsible for the degradation of AX (Gys *et al.*, 2003). This degradation of AX results in decreased water-holding capacity of the polymer and increased dough syruping. The farinograph dough consistency also decreases, for example from 640 BU immediately after mixing to 505 BU after 8 h refrigerated storage (Gys *et al.*, 2003). Initially, during refrigeration of dough the level of water-soluble AX was reported to increase from 0.84% to 1.41% due to solubilisation of water-unextractable AX. It is recommended to use xylanase inhibitors (Courtin *et al.*, 2005; Poulsen and Sørensen, 2001) or competitive inhibition by adding xylan (preferentially degraded by endogenous endoxylanases compared with native AX) to the dough during refrigeration (Atwell, 1998). The unsubstituted xylan from birchwood or oat spelt acts as a competitive inhibitor for endoxylanases native to wheat grain that are responsible for syruping in refrigerated dough. These techniques can be used during the bread-making process to avoid degradation by endogenous enzymes. It can therefore be inferred that degradation of arabinoxylan is associated with both physical and enzymatic factors during bread-making.

10.3.3 β-Glucan

Of the three major DF components, arabinoxylan, β-glucan and fructan, β-glucan is the most sensitive to different processing parameters (Andersson *et al.*, 2009). The viscosity of β-glucan in solution is mainly controlled by concentration, molecular weight distribution and structure (Wood, 2002; Wood, 1991). The effectiveness of oat β-glucan in controlling postprandial glucose and insulin levels in the blood is dependent on its viscosity (Anttila *et al.*, 2004; Cui and Wang, 2009; Tosh *et al.*, 2008; Wood *et al.*, 1994). Similarly, the role of β-glucan in lowering plasma cholesterol is believed to be associated with its viscosity in the human intestine (Wolever *et al.*, 2010). Therefore depolymerisation and degradation of the polymer adversely affect the functional properties of cereal β-glucan.

The endogenous enzymes present in the flour work very rapidly when hydrated and result in a decrease in molecular weight of the polymer (Andersson *et al.*, 2008). Since the endo β-glucanases present in cereals attack randomly, the decrease in molecular weight is very rapid. For example, within 11+6 min of fermentation during the making of rye crispbread with added oat fibre, a 73% decrease in molecular weight of β-glucan was observed (Andersson *et al.*, 2008). Significant effects of endogenous β-glucanases on viscosity development profiles have also been reported in barley samples (Izydorczyk *et al.*, 2000). Along with endogenous enzymes, microbial contamination during grain handling contributes enzymes capable of degrading β-glucan (Mälkki and Virtanen, 2001). The roles of different stages in the bread-making process on the degradation of β-glucan are summarised in Table 10.1. Overall, there is a huge loss of the long chain fraction of β-glucan during bread-making (Fig. 10.4). A comparison of the distribution profiles of rye flour and breads demonstrates the degradation and shift towards low molecular weight of β-glucan during bread-making. The flour has a unimodal distribution profile, while the bread has a bimodal distribution with a shift into a population of low molecular weight chains during processing (Fig. 10.4) (Åman

Table 10.1 Effect of bread making on molecular weight (MW) and extractability of β-glucan

Process in bread-making	β-Glucan MW	Extractability	Reference
Bread-making	↓	↑	Åman *et al.* (2004); Andersson *et al.* (2009); Andersson *et al.* (2008); Andersson *et al.* (2004); Trogh *et al.* (2004)
Mixing	↓	↑	Andersson *et al.* (2004); Trogh *et al.* (2004)
Yeast	–	–	Andersson *et al.* (2004)
Proving/ fermentation	↓	↑	Andersson *et al.* (2004); Trogh *et al.* (2004); Andersson *et al.* (2008)
*Baking	–	– ↑	Andersson *et al.* (2008); Andersson *et al.* (2004); Trogh *et al.* (2004)

Notes: (↑ = increase), (↓ = decrease), (– = no effect).

* Baking may increase the extractability in non-fermented dough or may leave it unchanged in fermented dough. The effects are usually small.

et al., 2004; Rakha *et al.*, 2010). Different soft breads and crispbreads vary in their molecular weight distribution profile of β-glucan.

Dough mixing and fermentation result in a significant decrease in the molecular weight of β-glucan (Andersson *et al.*, 2004). Reducing the β-glucanase activity in dough can help to maintain β-glucan molecular weight and thereby the nutritional value of the bread. The level of β-glucanase activity differs between cultivars (Izydorczyk *et al.*, 2000; Knuckles and Chiu, 1999) and therefore it is important to use cultivars with low endogenous β-glucanase activity. Cultivars with high falling number (low enzyme activity) maintain higher β-glucan molecular weight in bread (Andersson *et al.*, 2008). Grain texture can also play a very important role in determining the fate of β-glucan during processing. Partly milled or crushed grains or bran with coarse particles when included in the bread maintain β-glucan molecular weight and content better than finely milled flour (Åman *et al.*, 2004) (Fig. 10.5). The use of ingredients and processing parameters that minimise the degradation of extractable β-glucan, such as short fermentation and dough mixing time during bread-making and the incorporation of bran with large particle size, is recommended.

The bread-making process also affects the extractability of β-glucan (Table 10.1). The polymer becomes more extractable during processing, probably due to a decrease in molecular mass, and hence the short chain molecules are more easily extractable. The increase in solubility of β-glucan is usually dependent on processing conditions (Vasanthan *et al.*, 2002). Hydrothermal treatment intended to open up the physical barriers to water absorption renders β-glucan more soluble, while drying makes it less extractable (Mälkki and Virtanen, 2001). Hydrothermal treatment also inactivates the endogenous β-glucanase, thus avoiding depolymerisation. Other techniques such as autoclaving followed by

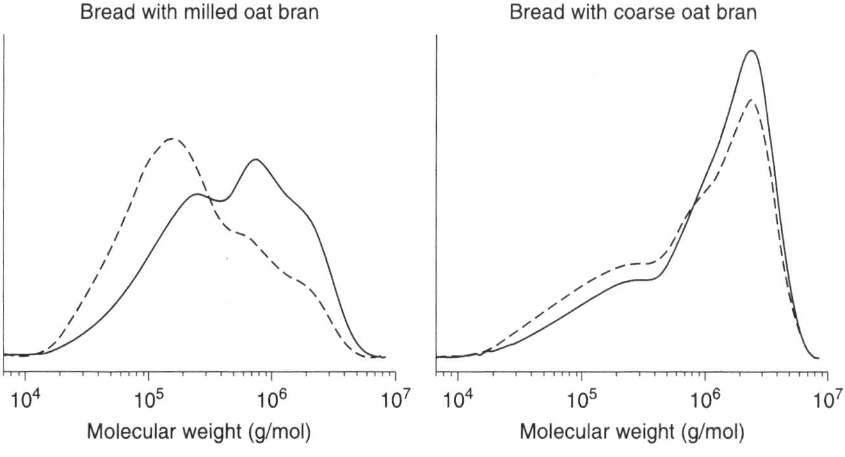

Fig. 10.5 β-Glucan molecular weight distribution profile of coarse and finely milled oat bran fermented for 10 min (—) and 40 min (----). Data adapted from Åman *et al.* (2004).

sonication have been shown to increase the extractable β-glucan content significantly on an experimental scale (Izydorczyk *et al.*, 2000). The use of proteolytic action to disrupt the association of β-glucan with protein molecules also renders it more extractable (Izydorczyk *et al.*, 2000). The increased extractability is generally a positive aspect of processing if degradation can be minimised. While comparing the extractability of β-glucan in crispbreads (29%) and soft breads (35%), it was found that the soft breads usually had a higher amount of extractable β-glucan, but relatively more degradation of β-glucan (Rakha *et al.*, 2010). A sample of extruded crispbread had the highest extractability (47%) and maintained molecular weight better than the other soft breads and crispbreads analysed. The extractability was found to increase with increasing temperature and moisture content during extrusion cooking (Vasanthan *et al.*, 2002). In summary, the extractability and molecular weight of cereal β-glucan are of nutritional importance and can be manipulated by physical, thermal and enzymatic treatment.

10.3.4 Fructan

Degradation of fructan during bread-making has been demonstrated in different studies (Andersson *et al.*, 2009; Hansen *et al.*, 2002). The content of fructan was reported to decrease from 6.2% in rye whole meal to 4.6% in freshly prepared dough, 4.1% after proving and 3.4% in bread crumbs (Hansen *et al.*, 2002). Yeast plays an important role in bread-making. It can degrade fructan, resulting in a significant decrease in the soluble fraction of DF. Soft breads or crispbreads baked with yeast are usually low in fructan compared with those baked without yeast (Rakha *et al.*, 2010). The decrease in fructan content has been found to be higher during sourdough baking (62%) than in yeast-leavened (32%) and air-leavened crispbreads (6%) (Andersson *et al.*, 2009).

Short DP fructan molecules are usually preferred by yeast. The particle size of the incorporated fructan source, also plays an important role in determining the fate of fructan in bread. Coarse particles or whole grains sprinkled on top of the bread retain most of the fructan. A comparison of the fructan distribution profile of breads made from milled and whole rye kernels is given in Fig. 10.6. The relative proportion of short DP fructan is significantly less in bread with finely milled rye kernels, while the longer DP fructans are similar in both types of bread. The preference of yeast for low DP inulin has also been reported by Meyer and Peters (2009), who observed 53% loss of inulin with average DP 8 and only 15.5% loss of inulin with average DP 23 when supplemented in bread. Findings by other authors (Mitterdorfer *et al.*, 2001; Praznik *et al.*, 2002) also corroborate the disposition of yeast for low DP fructans.

10.3.5 Resistant starch

The most relevant form of RS during baking is RS3, which is not present in unprocessed flour but is formed as a result of bread-making due to crystallisation

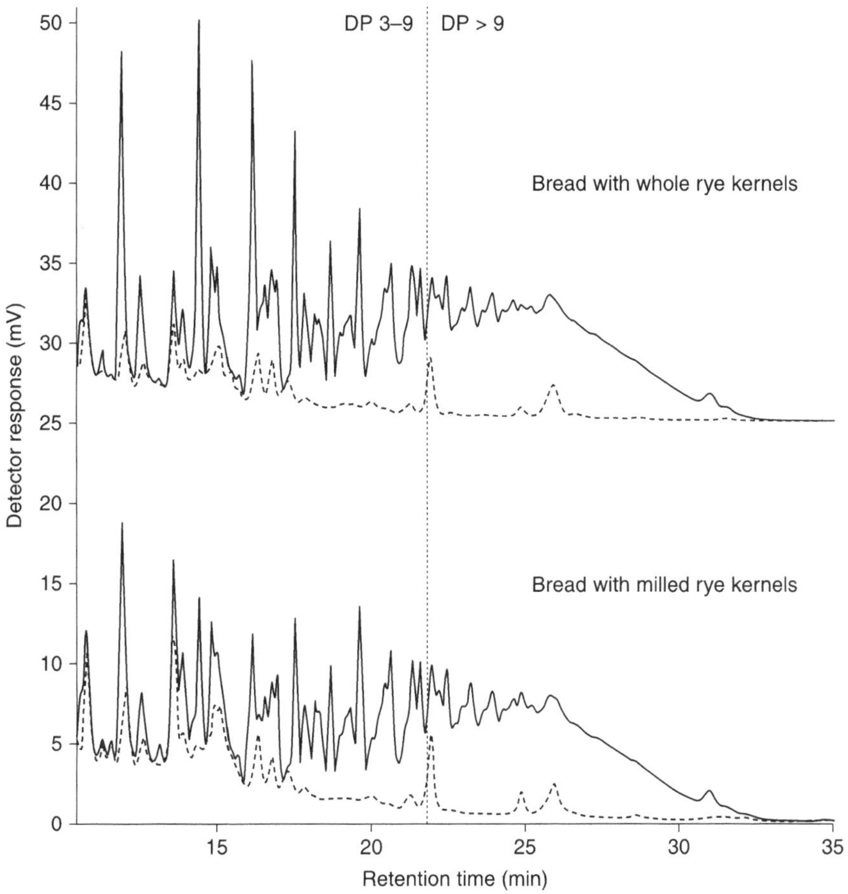

Fig. 10.6 Fructan molecular weight distribution profile of bread made from whole and milled rye kernels. The line (—) represents the chromatogram without fructanase treatment and (----) that with fructanase treatment. Unpublished data from the author's laboratory.

of gelatinised starch during cooling (Englyst and Macfarlane, 1986). Crystallisation of amylopectin (RS3a) is slow and mainly occurs during storage of bread, while crystallisation of amylose (RS3b) is more rapid and forms more stable crystals. Repeated heating and cooling of baked products is reported to increase the content of RS3, since nucleation takes place at the lower temperature and growth of crystals at the higher temperature (Eerlingen *et al.*, 1993; Yadav *et al.*, 2009). Therefore varying processing conditions and ingredients result in different amounts of RS in products and their fractions (Dewettinck *et al.*, 2008; Westerlund *et al.*, 1989). Increasing the baking time and temperature can result in higher RS formation, as reported by Dewettinck *et al.* (2008). The amount of moisture during processing has been found to be critical for the formation of RS3 in extruded barley flour (Vasanthan *et al.*, 2002). In that study, increasing the amount of water from 20% to 50% doubled the RS3 content in the extruded product. However, Dewettinck *et al.* (2008) noted decreased RS formation with increasing amount of water in bread. Furthermore, high amylose starches are more prone to retrogradation and hence can be used to prepare breads with high RS content (Cummings and Stephen, 2007). Sourdough bread is also reported to contain higher amounts of RS due to debranching of amylopectin chains under acidic conditions (Brighenti *et al.*, 1998; Dewettinck *et al.*, 2008). Eerlingen and Delcour (1995) summarised amylose/amylopectin ratio, polymer chain length, lipid content, presence of other constituents and process conditions after starch gelatinisation as possible factors influencing the formation of RS. It is consequently possible to increase the content of RS3 by modifying processing parameters such as moisture, heating time and temperature, pH, number of heating and cooling cycles, freezing and drying (Sajilata *et al.*, 2006).

10.4 Properties of dietary fibre-enriched dough and breads

10.4.1 Dough properties

The physical and rheological properties of fibre-enriched dough vary greatly depending upon the extent of substitution, source of fibre and pre-processing (Rosell *et al.*, 2009). The addition of fibre influences the pasting characteristics of the starch (Santos *et al.*, 2008) and interferes with the starch–gluten matrix (Gan *et al.*, 1992). The high water-holding capacity of DF components results in increased farinographic water absorption, as the added fibre competes for water with gluten, starch and intrinsic DF (Rosell *et al.*, 2010; Skendi *et al.*, 2009). Increased farinographic water absorption was observed when 20% wheat flour was replaced by oat flour (Mariotti *et al.*, 2006). Almeida *et al.* (2010) compared the water absorption of three different fibre sources added to wheat flour and found that locust bean gum presented the highest water absorption index, followed by wheat bran and RS in that order. Skendi *et al.* (2009) investigated the impact of molecular weight of β-glucan on dough water absorption and observed that high molecular weight β-glucan gave higher water absorption values than low molecular weight β-glucan. Dough water absorption also varies with the ratio of soluble DF and insoluble DF in the fibre source (Katina, 2003). The size of fibre particles controls the rate of water absorption, as large particles absorb water more slowly than fine particles. Increased water absorption can decrease the crispness of the crust. The higher water absorption by fibre incorporated into dough can be advantageous for processors, who can get a higher yield of bread units per unit flour on a fresh weight basis (Izydorczyk *et al.*, 2008).

In contrast to other fibres, addition of inulin to dough has been shown to decrease the water absorption (Meyer and Peters, 2009). To solve this problem carboxymethylcellulose (CMC) has been added, particularly in dough with short DP inulin. The extensibility of dough decreases and dough development time increases with increasing level of wheat bran (Sudha *et al.*, 2007). Mariotti *et al.* (2006) observed a sharp decline in dough stability from 15.3 min with 100% wheat flour to 5.9 min with 20% replacement with oat flour. Unlike bran, the non-starch polysaccharides, that is, AX and β-glucan preparations, added in small amounts to wheat dough significantly increase peak dough resistance and mixing stability (Izydorczyk *et al.*, 2001). These polymers also increase the dough strength of weaker flour. However, increased levels of cell wall material result in poor mixing and significant dough weakening (Rosell *et al.*, 2010). Pre-hydration or enzyme treatment of the fibre-rich fraction are reported to improve bread quality (Izydorczyk and Dexter, 2008).

10.4.2 Organoleptic properties of bread

The organoleptic properties of bread play a major role in consumer choice of a particular type of bread. With the addition of DF, certain organoleptic properties of bread may be negatively affected, depending upon the source and content of the DF. The DF enrichment of bread from bran usually results in a darker colour that might not be appealing to the consumer. Polyphenol oxidase can lead to discoloration of, for example, barley-based foods (Quinde-Axtell *et al.*, 2006). However, techniques including steam heating, pearling, enzyme inhibition and exclusion of oxygen may be used to avoid discoloration. Ames *et al.* (2006) describe infrared heat treatment as an effective tool to slow down the darkening of tortilla dough. Taste also plays a very important role in consumer choice of a particular bread. For example, wholemeal breads, particularly those containing bran, may have a slight bitterness (Bakke and Vickers, 2007; Heiniö *et al.*, 2003).

Decreased loaf volume, poor mouth feel and slight off-flavour are other problems associated with breads containing high DF from bran. Addition of defatted rice bran to dough produces bread with significantly less volume and firm crumb (Abdul-Hamid and Luan, 2000). The decreased loaf volume in breads supplemented with DF from different sources has been attributed to dilution of the gluten network, among other factors (Trogh *et al.*, 2004). For example, in a study by Krishnan *et al.* (1987), the volume of bread decreased by 20% with 15% finely milled oat bran replacement. This adverse effect of bran on loaf volume can be overcome to a large extent by a combination of fine grinding and pre-soaking of wheat bran in water (Lai *et al.*, 1989). However, since microorganisms are present on the bran layer of grain, care must be taken during soaking of bran to avoid microbiological hazards (Katina, 2003). Pre-fermentation of bran by yeast or lactic acid bacteria and addition of sourdough are other important tools to compensate for loaf volume in high fibre baking (Salmenkallio-Marttila *et al.*, 2001). Inulin supplementation is also associated with decreased loaf volume. This decrease in bread volume is directly correlated with inulin DP, with the largest decrease occurring with high DP (Meyer and Peters, 2009). Likewise, β-glucan with high molecular weight results in higher loaf volume than β-glucan with low molecular weight (Lazaridou and Biliaderis, 2007). Tenderness of bread is also affected adversely by inulin addition and the effect is more pronounced with long chain molecules, although still acceptable. The addition of inulin can result in crust coloration and crumb hardness (Poinot *et al.*, 2010). However, with slightly decreased baking time (17 min instead of 20 min for normal bread), bread can be produced containing up to 5% inulin with overall acceptability similar to white bread (Poinot *et al.*, 2010). The shorter baking time is also advantageous from an energy point of view.

10.5 Conclusion

Dietary fibre has been shown to provide numerous health benefits in both human and animal models, targeting, for example, maintenance of healthy cholesterol level, gut health, glycaemic index and satiety. It has therefore become imperative in modern food guide pyramids to include a sufficient amount of DF in the daily diet. Bread is considered a staple food across the globe and hence can act as a carrier of DF. However, addition of DF to bread can negatively affect its technological and organoleptic properties, and slight modifications may be required in processing parameters. Processing should be designed on the principle of 'do no harm', that is, care must be taken in the selection of processing methods and conditions such that these do not impair the physiological properties of the DF or compromise bread appeal.

10.6 References

ABDUL-HAMID A and LUAN Y S (2000), 'Functional properties of dietary fibre prepared from defatted rice bran', *Food Chem*, **68**, 15–19.

ALMEIDA E L, CHANG Y K and STEEL C J (2010), 'Effect of adding different dietary fiber sources on farinographic parameters of wheat flour', *Cereal Chem*, **87**, 566–73.

ALVAREZ-JUBETE L, ARENDT E K and GALLAGHER E (2009), 'Nutritive value and chemical composition of pseudo-cereals as gluten-free ingredients', *Int J Food Sci Nutr*, **60**, 240–57.

ÅMAN P, RIMSTEN L and ANDERSSON R (2004), 'Molecular weight distribution of β-glucan in oat-based foods', *Cereal Chem*, **81**, 356–60.

AMES N, RHYMER C, ROSSNAGEL B, THIERRIEN M, RYLAND D, *et al.* (2006), 'Utilization of diverse hull-less barley properties to maximize food product quality', *Cereal Foods World*, **51**, 23–8.

ANDERSSON R and ÅMAN P (2001), 'Cereal arabinoxylan: occurrence, structure and properties', in MCCLEARY B V and PROSKY L, *Advanced dietary fibre technology*, Blackwell Science, Oxford, UK, 315–27.

ANDERSSON A A M, ANDERSSON R and ÅMAN P (2000), 'Air classification of barley flours', *Cereal Chem*, **77**, 463–7.

ANDERSSON A A M, ARMÖ E, GRANGEON E, FREDRIKSSON H, ANDERSSON R and ÅMAN P (2004), 'Molecular weight and structure units of (1→3,1→4)-β-glucans in dough and bread made from hull-less barley milling fractions', *J Cereal Sci*, **40**, 195–204.

ANDERSSON A A M, RÜEGG N and ÅMAN P (2008), 'Molecular weight distribution and content of water-extractable β-glucan in rye crisp bread', *J Cereal Sci*, **47**, 399–406.

ANDERSSON R, FRANSSON G, TIETJEN M and ÅMAN P (2009), 'Content and molecular weight distribution of dietary fibre components in whole-grain rye flour and bread', *J Agric Food Chem*, **57**, 2004–8.

ANON (2003), *Perception and understanding of health components of bread*, The Federation of Bakers, London, UK.

ANTTILA H, SONTAG-STROHM T and SALOVAARA H (2004), 'Viscosity of beta-glucan in oat products', *Agric Food Sci*, **13**, 80–7.

ATWELL W A. (1998), 'Method for reducing syruping in refrigerated doughs', US patent application 5,792,499, 1998-Aug-11.

AUTIO K (1996), 'Functional aspects of cell wall polysaccharides', in ELIASSON A-C, *Carbohydrates in food*, New York, Marcel Dekker, 227–64.

BAKKE A and VICKERS Z (2007), 'Consumer liking of refined and whole wheat breads', *J Food Sci*, **72**, 473–80.

BENDER D A (2006), *Benders' dictionary of nutrition and food technology*, 8th edition, Woodhead Publishing Limited, Abington, England.

BILIADERIS C G, IZYDORCZYK M S and RATTAN O (1995), 'Effect of arabinoxylans on bread-making quality of wheat flours', *Food Chem*, **53**, 165–71.

BONNAND-DUCASSE M, VALLE G D, LEFEBVRE J and SAULNIER L (2010), 'Effect of wheat dietary fibres on bread dough development and rheological properties', *J Cereal Sci*, **52**, 200–6.

BORNET F R J (2001), 'Fructo-oligosaccharides and other fructans: chemistry, structure and nutritional effects', in MCCLEARY B V and PROSKY L, *Advanced dietary fibre technology*, Blackwell Science, Oxford, UK, 480–93.

BRIGHENTI F, CASIRAGHI M C and BAGGIO C (1998), 'Resistant starch in the Italian diet', *Br J Nutr*, **80**, 333–41.

BROWN I L, MCNAUGHT K J, ANDREWS D and MORITA T (2001), 'Resistant starch: plant breeding, applications development and commercial use', in MCCLEARY B V and PROSKY L, *Advanced dietary fibre technology*, Blackwell Science, Oxford, UK, 401–12.

CLEEMPUT G, BOOIJ C, HESSING M, GRUPPEN H and DELCOUR J A (1997), 'Solublisation and changes in molecular weight distribution of arabinoxylans and protein in wheat flours during bread-making, and the effects of endogenous arabinoxylan hydrolysing enzymes', *J Cereal Sci*, **26**, 55–66.

COURTIN C M and DELCOUR J A (2002), 'Arabinoxylans and endoxylanases in wheat flour bread-making', *J Cereal Sci*, **35**, 225–43.

COURTIN C M, GYS W, GEBRUERS K and DELCOUR J A (2005), 'Evidence for the involvement of arabinoxylan and xylanases in refrigerated dough syruping', *J Agric Food Chem*, **53**, 7623–9.

CUI S W and WANG Q (2009), 'Cell wall polysaccharides in cereals: chemical structures and functional properties', *Struct Chem*, **20**, 291–7.

CUMMINGS J H and STEPHEN A M (2007), 'Carbohydrate terminology and classification', *Eur J Clin Nutr*, **61**, 5–18.

DEBYSER W, PEUMANS W J, VAN DAMME E J M and DELCOUR J A (1999), 'Triticum aestivum xylanase inhibitor (TAXI), a new class of enzyme inhibitor affecting bread making performance', *J Cereal Sci*, **30**, 39–43.

DERVILLY-PINEL G, RIMSTEN L, SAULNIER L, ANDERSSON R and ÅMAN P (2001), 'Water-extractable arabinoxylan from pearled flours of wheat, barley, rye and triticale. Evidence for the presence of ferulic acid dimers and their involvement in gel formation', *J Cereal Sci*, **34**, 207–14.

DEWETTINCK K, VAN BOCKSTAEL F, KÜHNE B, VAN DE WALLE D, COURTENS T M and GELLYNCK X (2008), 'Nutritional value of bread: Influence of processing, food interaction and consumer perception', *J Cereal Sci*, **48**, 243–57.

EERLINGEN R C and DELCOUR J A (1995), 'Formation, analysis, structure and properties of type III enzyme resistant starch', *J Cereal Sci*, **22**, 129–38.

EERLINGEN RC, CROMBEZ M and DELCOUR JA (1993), 'Enzyme-resistant starch. I. Quantitative and qualitative influence of incubation time and temperature of autoclaved starch on resistant starch formation', *Cereal Chem*, **70**, 339–44.

EFSA (EUROPEAN FOOD SAFETY AUTHORITY) (2009), 'Scientific opinion: "Cadmium in food" – scientific opinion of the panel on contaminants in the food chain', (Question No EFSA-Q-2007-138). Adopted on 30 January 2009, *EFSA J,* **980**, 1–139. Available from: www.efsa.europa.eu

EFSA PANEL ON DIETETIC PRODUCTS, NUTRITION, AND ALLERGIES (NDA) (2010), 'Scientific opinion on dietary reference values for carbohydrates and dietary fibre', *EFSA J*, **8**, 1462. doi:10.2903/j.efsa.2010.1462. Available from: www.efsa.europa.eu

EKHOLM P, VIRKKI P, YLINEN M and JOHANSSON L (2003), 'The effect of phytic acid and some natural chelating agents on the solubility of mineral elements in oat bran', *Food Chem*, **80**, 165–70.

ENGLYST H N and MACFARLANE G T (1986), 'Breakdown of resistant and readily digestible starch by human gut bacteria', *J Sci Food Agric*, **37**, 699–706.

FEDERATION OF BAKERS (2007), *Our daily bread: the role of bread in the British diet*, Available from: http://www.fabflour.co.uk/download/31/ (Accessed 15 December 2010).

FRANZ G and BLASCHEK W (1990), 'Cellulose, in carbohydrates', in DEY P M and HARBORNE J B, *Methods in plant biochemistry*, Vol. **2**, Academic Press, London.

GALLAGHER E, GORMLEY T R and ARENDT E K (2004), 'Recent advances in the formulation of gluten-free cereal-based products', *Trends Food Sci Technol*, **15**, 143–52.

GAN Z, GALLIARD T, ELLIS P R, ANGOLD R E and VAUGHAN J G (1992), 'Effect of the outer bran layers on the loaf volume of wheat bread', *J Cereal Sci*, **15**, 151–63.

GIBSON G R and ROBERFROID M B (1995), 'Dietary modulation of the human colonic microbiota: introducing the concept of prebiotics', *J Nutr*, **125**, 1401–12.

GREEN P H and CELLIER C (2007), 'Celiac disease', *New Engl J Med*, **357**, 1731–43.

GROPPER S S, SMITH J L and GROFF J L (2009), *Advanced Nutrition and Human metabolism*, 5th Edition, Wadsworth Cengage Learning, Belmont, CA, USA.

GYS W, COURTIN C M and DELCOUR J A (2003), 'Refrigerated dough syruping in relation to the arabinoxylan population', *J Agric Food Chem*, **51**, 4119–25.

HANSEN H B, ANDREASEN M F, NIELSEN M M, LARSEN L M, BACH-KNUDSEN K B, *et al.* (2002), 'Changes in dietary fibre, phenolic acids and activity of endogenous enzymes during rye bread-making', *Eur Food Res Technol*, **214**, 33–42.

HANSEN H B, RASMUSSEN C V, BACH KNUDSEN K E and HANSEN Å (2003), 'Effect of genotype and harvest year on content and composition of dietary fibre in rye (*Secale cereale* L.) grain', *J Sci Food Agric*, **83**, 76–85.

HEINIÖ R-L, LIUKKONEN K-H, KATINA K, MYLLYMÄKI O and POUTANEN K (2003), 'Milling fractionation of rye produces different sensory profiles of both flour and bread', *LWT-Food Sci Technol*, **36**, 577–83.

HILL I D, DIRKS M H, LIPTAK G S, COLLETTI R B, FASANO A and GUANDALINI S (2005), 'Guideline for the diagnosis and treatment of coeliac disease in children: recommendations of the North American Society for pediatric gastroenterology, hepatology and nutrition', *J Pediatr Gastr Nutr*, **40**, 1–19.

IDOURAINE A, KHAN M J and WEBER C W (1996), '*In vitro* binding capacity of wheat bran, rice bran, and oat fiber for Ca, Mg, Cu, and Zn alone and in different combinations', *J Agric Food Chem*, **44**, 2067–72.

ISHII T (1997), 'Structure and functions of feruloylated polysaccharides', *Plant Sci*, **127**, 111–27.

IZYDORCZYK M S and DEXTER J E (2008), 'Barley β-glucans and arabinoxylans: molecular structure, physicochemical properties, and uses in food products—a review', *Food Res Int*, **41**, 850–68.

IZYDORCZYK M S, HUSSAIN A and MACGREGOR A W (2001), 'Effect of barley and barley components on rheological properties of wheat dough', *J Cereal Sci*, **34,** 251–60.

IZYDORCZYK M S, STORSLEY J, LABOSSIERE D, MACGREGOR A W and ROSSNAGEL B G (2000), 'Variation in total and soluble β-glucan content in hulless barley: effects of thermal, physical, and enzymic treatments', *J Agric Food Chem*, **48**, 982–9.

IZYDORCZYK M S, CHORNICK T L, PAULLEY F G, EDWARDS N M and DEXTER J E (2008), 'Physicochemical properties of hull-less barley fibre-rich fractions varying in particle size and their potential as functional ingredients in two-layer flat bread', *Food Chem*, **108**, 561–70.

KAMAL-ELDIN A, LÆRKE H N, BACH-KNUDSEN K E, LAMPI A M, PIIRONEN V, *et al.* (2009), 'Physical, microscopic, and chemical characterisation of industrial rye and wheat brans from the Nordic countries', *Food Nutr* Res, **53**, DOI: 10.3402/fnr.v53i0.1912.

KATINA K (2003), 'High fibre-baking', in CAUVAIN S P, *Bread making: improving quality*, Woodhead Publishing Limited, Cambridge, England, 487–99.

KORUS J, WITCZAK M, ZIOBRO R and JUSZCZAK L (2009), 'The impact of resistant starch on characteristics of gluten-free dough and bread', *Food Hydrocolloids*, **23**, 988–95.

KNUCKLES B E and CHIU M-C M (1999), 'β-Glucanase activity and molecular weight of β-glucans in barley after various treatments', *Cereal Chem*, **76**, 92–5.

KRISHNAN P G, FAUBION J M and HOSENEY R C (1987), 'Effect of commercial oat bran on the characteristics and composition of bread', *Cereal Chem*, **64**, 55–8.

LAI C S, HOSENEY R C and DAVIS A B (1989), 'Effects of wheat bran in bread-making', *Cereal Chem*, **66**, 217–19.

LAURIKAINEN T, HÄRKÖNEN H, AUTIO K and POUTANEN K (1998), 'Effects of enzymes in fibre-enriched baking', *J Sci Food Agric*, **76**, 239–49.

LAZARIDOU A and BILIADERIS C G (2007), 'Molecular aspects of cereal β-glucan functionality: physical properties, technological applications and physiological effects', *J Cereal Sci*, **46**, 101–18.

LEE A R, NG D L, DAVE E, CIACCIO E J and GREEN P H R (2009), 'The effect of substituting alternative grains in the diet on the nutritional profile of the gluten-free diet', *J Hum Nutr Diet*, **22**, 359–63.

LUHALOO M, MÅRTENSSON A-C, ANDERSSON R and ÅMAN P (1998), 'Compositional analysis and viscosity measurements of commercial oat brans', *J Sci Food Agric*, **76**, 142–8.

MÄLKKI Y and VIRTANEN E (2001), 'Gastrointestinal effects of oat bran and oat gum: a review', *LWT – Food Sci Technol*, **34**, 337–47.

MARIOTTI M, LUCISANO M and PAGANI M A (2006), 'Development of a baking procedure for the production of oat-supplemented wheat bread', *Int J Food Sci Technol*, **41**, 151–7.

MEYER D and PETERS B (2009), 'Enhancing the nutritional value of bread with inulin', *AgroFOOD Industry Hi-Tech*, **20**, 48–50.

MITTERDORFER G, KNEIFEL W and VIERNSTEIN H (2001), 'Utilization of prebiotic carbohydrates by yeasts of therapeutic relevance', *Lett Appl Microbiol*, **33**, 251–5.

NARDI S, CALCAGNO C, ZUNIN P, D'EGIDIO M G, CECCHINI C, *et al.* (2003), 'Nutritional benefits of developing cereals for functional foods', *Cereal Res Commun*, **31**, 445–52.

NEW ZEALAND ASSOCIATION OF BAKERS (NZAB) (2010), *Types of bread*, Available from: http://www.bakeinfo.co.nz/school/school_info/types_of_bread.php (Accessed 28 November 2010).

NUGENT A P (2005), 'Health properties of resistant starch', *British Nutrition Foundation: Nutr Bull*, **30**, 27–54.

O'SULLIVAN A C (1997), 'Cellulose: the structure slowly unravels', *Cellulose*, **4**, 173–207.

POINOT P, ARVISENET G, GRUA-PRIOL J, FILLONNEAU C, LE-BAIL A and PROST C (2010), 'Influence of inulin on bread: Kinetics and physico-chemical indicators of the formation of volatile compounds during baking', *Food Chem*, **119**, 1474–84.

POULSEN, C H. and SØRENSEN, J F. (2001), 'Process of forming a refrigerated dough', WIPO patent application WO 01/52657 A1.2001-Jul-26.

PRAZNIK W, CIEŚLIK E and FILIPIAK-FLORKIEWICZ A (2002), 'Soluble dietary fibres in Jerusalem artichoke powders: composition and application in bread', *Nahrung/Food*, **46**, 151–7.

QUINDE-AXTELL Z, POWERS J and BAIK, B-K (2006), 'Retardation of discoloration in barley flour gel and dough', *Cereal Chem*, **83**, 385–90.

RAKHA A, ÅMAN P and ANDERSSON R (2010), 'Characterization of dietary fibre components in rye products', *Food Chem*, **119**, 859–67.

RALPH J, LUNDQUIST K, BRUNOW G, LU F, KIM H, *et al.* (2004), 'Lignins: natural polymers from oxidative coupling of 4-hydroxyphenylpropanoids', *Phytochemistry Rev*, **3**, 29–60.

RIMSTEN L, STENBERG T, ANDERSSON R, ANDERSSON A and ÅMAN P (2003), 'Determination of β-glucan molecular weight using SEC with Calcofluor detection in cereal extracts', *Cereal Chem*, **80**, 485–90.

ROBERFROID M B (2005), 'Introducing inulin-type fructans', *Br J Nutr*, **93**, 13–25.

ROSELL C M, SANTOS E and COLLAR C (2009), 'Physico-chemical properties of commercial fibres from different sources: a comparative approach', *Food Res Int*, **42**, 176–84.

ROSELL C M, SANTOS E and COLLAR C (2010), 'Physical characterization of fiber-enriched bread doughs by dual mixing and temperature constraint using the Mixolab®', *Eur Food Res Technol*, **231**, 535–44.

ROUAU X (1993), 'Investigation into the effect on an enzyme preparation for baking on wheat flour dough pentosans', *J Cereal Sci*, **18**, 145–57.

ROUAU X, EL-HAYEK M-L and MOREAU D (1994), 'Effect of an enzyme preparation containing pentosanases on the bread-making quality of flours in relation to changes in pentosan properties', *J Cereal Sci*, **19**, 259–72.

SABANIS D, LEBESI D and TZIA C (2009a), 'Effect of dietary fibre enrichment on selected properties of gluten-free bread', *LWT – Food Sci Technol*, **42**, 1380–9.

SABANIS D, LEBESI D and TZIA C (2009b), 'Development of fibre-enriched gluten-free bread: a response surface methodology study', *Int J Food Sci Nutr*, **60** (S4), 174–90.

SAJILATA M G, SINGHAL R S and KULKARNI P R (2006), 'Resistant starch—a review', *Compr Rev Food Sci F*, **5**, 1–17.

SALMENKALLIO-MARTTILA M, KATINA K and AUTIO K (2001), 'Effects of bran fermentation on quality and microstructure of high-fiber wheat bread', *Cereal Chem*, **78**, 429–35.

SANTOS E, ROSELL C M and COLLAR C (2008), 'Gelatinization and retrogradation kinetics of high-fiber wheat flour blends: a calorimetric approach', *Cereal Chem*, **85**, 455–63.

SAULNIER L and QUEMENER B (2009), 'Enzymatic mapping of arabinoxylan structure', in SHEWRY P R and WARD J, *HEALTHGRAIN methods: analysis of bioactive components in small grain cereals*, AACC International, St Paul, Minnesota, USA, 191–201.

SAULNIER L, SADO P-E, BRANLARD G, CHARMET G and GUILLON F (2007), 'Wheat arabinoxylans: exploiting variation in amount and composition to develop enhanced varieties', *J Cereal Sci*, **46**, 261–81.

SELVENDRAN R R and ROBERTSON J A (1994), 'Dietary fibre in foods: amount and type', in AMADÒ R, FRØLICH W and BARRY J L, *Physico-chemical properties of dietary fibre and effect of processing on micronutrients availability*, Luxembourg: COST 92 Directorate-general XIII, 11–19.

SKENDI A, PAPAGEORGIOU M and BILIADERIS C G (2009), 'Effect of barley β-glucan molecular size and level on wheat dough rheological properties', *J Food Eng*, **91**, 594–601.

SLAVIN J L, JACOBS D and MARQUART L (2000), 'Grain processing and nutrition', *Crit Rev Food Sci Nutr*, **40**, 309–26.

SMEEKENS S, EBSKAMP M, PILON-SMITS L and WEISBEEK P (1996), 'Fructans', *Ann NY Acad Sci*, **792**, 20–5.

SUDHA M L, VETRIMANI R and LEELAVATHI K (2007), 'Influence of fibre from different cereals on the rheological characteristics of wheat flour dough and on biscuit quality', *Food Chem*, **100**, 1365–70.

SULLIVAN P, O'FLAHERTY J, BRUNTON N, GEE V L, ARENDT E and GALLAGHER E (2010), 'Chemical composition and microstructure of milled barley fractions', *Eur Food Res Technol*, **230**, 579–95.

TOSH S M, BRUMMER Y, WOLEVER T M S and WOOD P J (2008), 'Glycemic response to oat bran muffins treated to vary molecular weight of β-glucan', *Cereal Chem*, **85**, 211–17.

TROGH I, COURTIN C M, ANDERSSON A A M, ÅMAN P, SØRENSEN J F and DELCOUR J A (2004), 'The combined use of hull-less barley flour and xylanase as a strategy for wheat/hull-less barley flour breads with increased arabinoxylan and (1→3,1→4)-β-D-glucan levels', *J Cereal Sci*, **40**, 257–67.

USDA (UNITED STATES DEPARTMENT OF AGRICULTURE) (2010), *National Nutrient Database for Standard Reference*, SR 23, Available from: http://www.nal.usda.gov/fnic/foodcomp/search/ (Accessed 15 December 2010).

USDA (UNITED STATES DEPARTMENT OF AGRICULTURE) CENTER FOR NUTRITION POLICY AND PROMOTION (2005), *Report of the Dietary Guidelines Advisory Committee (DGAC) on the dietary guidelines for Americans*, Available from: http://www.cnpp.usda.gov/DGAs2010-DGACReport.htm (Accessed 15 December 2010).

VANHOLME R, DEMEDTS B, MORREEL K, RALPH J and BOERJAN W (2010), 'Lignin biosynthesis and structure', *Plant Physiol*, **153**, 895–905.

VASANTHAN T, GAOSONG J, YEUNG J and LI J (2002), 'Dietary fiber profile of barley flour as affected by extrusion cooking', *Food Chem*, **77**, 35–40.

VIËTOR R J, ANGELINOT S A G F and VORAGEN A G J (1992), 'Structural features of arabinoxylans from barley and malt cell wall material', *J Cereal Sci*, **15**, 213–22.

VINKX C J A, REYNAERT H R, GROBET P J and DELCOUR J A (1993), 'Physicochemical and functional properties of rye non starch polysaccharides. V. Variability in the structure of water-soluble arabinoxylans', *Cereal Chem*, **70**, 311–17.

WESTERLUND E, THEANDER O, ANDERSSON R and ÅMAN P (1989), 'Effect of baking on polysaccharides in white bread fractions', *J Cereal Sci*, **10**, 149–56.

WHOLE GRAIN COUNCIL (2010), *Definition of whole grains*, Available from: http://www.wholegrainscouncil.org/whole-grains-101/definition-of-whole-grains (Accessed 27 November 2010).

WOLEVER T M S, TOSH M S, GIBBS A L, BRAND-MILLER J, DUNCAN A M, *et al.* (2010), 'Physicochemical properties of oat β-glucan influence its ability to reduce serum LDL cholesterol in humans: a randomized clinical trial', *Am J Clin Nutr*, **92**, 723–32.

WOOD P J (1991), 'Oat β-glucan-physicochemical properties and physiological effects', *Trends Food Sci Technol*, **2**, 311–14.

WOOD P J (2001), 'Cereal β-glucans: structure, properties and health claims', in MCCLEARY B V and PROSKY L, *Advanced dietary fibre technology*, Blackwell Science, Oxford, UK, 315–27.

WOOD P J (2002), 'Relationships between solution properties of cereal β-glucans and physiological effects—a review', *Trends Food Sci Technol*, **13**, 313–20.

WOOD P J (2007), 'Cereal β-glucans in diet and health', *J Cereal Sci*, **4**, 230–8.

WOOD P J, BRAATEN J, SCOTT FW, RIEDEL K D, WOLYNETZ M S and COLLINS M W (1994), 'Effect of dose and modification of viscous properties of oat gum on plasma glucose and insulin following an oral glucose load', *Br J Nutr*, **72**, 731–43.

YADAV B S, SHARMA A and YADAV R B (2009), 'Studies on effect of multiple heating/cooling cycles on the resistant starch formation in cereals, legumes and tubers', *Int J Food Sci Nutr*, **60**, 258–72.

11

Performance of resistant starches in baking: a case study on fibre-rich and wholegrain muffins

A. Salvador and S. Fiszman, Instituto de Agroquímica y Tecnología de Alimentos (CSIC), Spain

DOI: 10.1533/9780857095787.3.236

Abstract: The chapter begins by discussing the basic concepts of resistant starches as a source of fibre and their application in bakery products. It then reviews the physical properties of muffins, including rheology, colour and texture characteristics, and the effects of addition of resistant starches on these properties. The chapter also includes a study of sensory shelf-life during storage, sensory descriptive analysis and consumer acceptability of muffins made with resistant starch.

Key words: resistant starch, fibre, muffins, rheology, texture, sensory.

11.1 Introduction

Many fibre-enriched foods have been developed with the aim of increasing the fibre consumed in the diet. However, one general problem of these products is their low sensory quality, which makes them less acceptable to consumers. Resistant starch (RS) is a recently recognized source of fibre. RS is defined as the sum of starch and the products of starch degradation not absorbed in the small intestine of healthy individuals (Asp and Björck, 1992). According to the latest definition of dietary fibre (De Vries, 2003), RS is considered dietary fibre, and it is included in the official method for measuring Total Dietary Fibre (TDF), AOAC 991.43 (Haralumpu, 2000). Some of the benefits of RS resemble those of traditional fibre and others are unique. RS possesses remarkable health benefits. One of its interesting characteristics is its pattern of fermentation in the colon, principally its short chain fatty acid profile. In particular, butyrate production during colonic fermentation of RS is higher than during the fermentation of other dietary fibres. Also, RS has been found to reduce the glycaemic response.

RS has been classified into four types (Champ, 2004). RS type 1 refers to physically inaccessible starch found in starchy foods that have not been fractionated and refined. RS type 2 comprises native RS granules, such as those that are present in green bananas or raw potatoes. RS type 3 refers to retrograded starch. Since the first commercial RS was introduced in Australia in 1993 (Sajilata *et al.*, 2006), sources of RS2 and RS3 have been commercially available for use in foods. Of particular interest is the high thermal stability of RS3, which allows it to remain stable during most normal cooking operations. Finally, RS type 4 corresponds to highly chemically modified starch. RS4 is not authorized in Europe, although it is in Japan. On the European market, commercial sources of RS2 and RS3 are available. Among the newest developments in RS is an RS2 that remains resistant after mild food processing. Compared with conventional fibres, it has many advantageous features. It is white and has a bland flavour and a fine particle size between 10 and 15 µm. It also has a reduced caloric content and may be used as a bulking agent to complement reduced sugar or reduced fat formulations. With a TDF content of approximately 40%, RS2 can be used alone or as a functional complement to other fibre sources and can be labelled simply as 'cornstarch'. Commercial RS has a much lower water-holding capacity than various traditional fibres, because it absorbs less water, and adjustments in product formulations and processing are substantially minimized.

Apart from the potential health benefits of RS, another advantage is its lower impact on the sensory properties of the food in comparison to traditional sources of fibre such as whole grains or bran. This makes RS a more suitable option for producing fibre-enriched food with high consumer acceptability. In order for a novel, nutritionally functional ingredient to be accepted by the food industry and consumers, beneficial physiological effects as well as high sensory acceptability need to be demonstrated (Australian National Food Authority, 1994).

11.1.1 Uses of RS in bakery products

Scientific research on how RS affects the physical and sensory properties of foods is scarce. However, some studies on bread, cookies and muffins have been conducted. The effects of pea starch with high level of RS on wheat dough functionality were evaluated by Sanz-Penella *et al.* (2010). Flour substitution by pea starch with a high level of RS, up to 20%, allowed the mechanical, extensional and viscometric parameters to be retained without significant hindering of dough machinability. However, Ozturk *et al.* (2009) found that loaf volumes of the breads decreased and firmness increased with RS supplementation above 10–20%. Aparicio-Sanguilán *et al.* (2007) used an experimental RS-rich product obtained from lintnerized banana in cookies and found no difference in preference between the RS cookies and the control sample without RS. In short-dough biscuits, addition of a RS-rich ingredient increased the breaking strength and crumbliness and reduced the resistance to penetration (Laguna *et al.*, 2011). They found that RS concentrations below 40% produced biscuits with the same sensory acceptability and consumption intention as the control sample. In muffins, several studies have been developed taking into account rheological, textural and sensorial aspects. This chapter reviews the technological aspects of adding RS2 to a sweet bakery product such as muffins or cakes, studying the effects of RS both in the batter and in the final properties of the baked products.

11.2 Muffin batter

11.2.1 Flow properties of the batter

The viscosity of the batter system is a controlling factor for the final product volume, due to its effects on bubble incorporation and movement (Bath *et al.*, 1992; Handleman *et al.*, 1961; Kim *et al.*, 2001). The rate at which bubbles rise due to buoyancy (related to the tendency to float) is inversely proportional to viscosity. Thus, rapidly rising bubbles in a low viscosity muffin batter may result in final volume loss. Higher muffin batter viscosities help to incorporate more air bubbles into the batter and keep them from escaping from the mass, giving the complete system more stability. Coalescence (the formation of a single bubble by the union of two or more colliding bubbles) is the most important process by which cells disappear in porous bakery products, and it too is prevented by increasing the viscosity of the medium.

The effect of replacing wheat flour with different amounts of RS on the performance of a muffin batter formulation during baking and the relationship between this effect and the linear viscoelastic properties of the raw batter before, during and after heating have been studied by Baixauli *et al.* (2008a). They found that an increase in RS content (from 5% to 20%) caused a progressive decrease in the apparent viscosity values (Fig. 11.1).

Their data showed a good fit ($r > 0.99$) to the power-law equation $\eta = k \cdot \dot{\gamma}^{n-1}$ (η = apparent viscosity, k = consistency index, $\dot{\gamma}$ = shear rate and n = flow index), within the experimental shear rate range studied (from 1 to 100 s^{-1}): increasing the RS content brought about a significant decrease in consistency (k) and in shear thinning behaviour (n value closer to 1), indicating that the structure was less complex and the shear thinning properties had become less pronounced (Table 11.1). This effect has been attributed to the dilution of the wheat flour protein in the system, an important component for structure development during mixing (Loewe, 1993), as the increased RS content of the muffin batter is associated with a lower wheat flour content. In fact, the decreased viscosity of the raw batter as RS levels increase is not a favourable factor for the stability of the batter and the quality of the final baked product. Many authors have related a decrease in batter viscosity to low final quality, mainly associated with an increase in the buoyancy of the air bubbles and a denser final texture (Lakshminarayan *et al.*, 2006). Lee *et al.* (2005) found that substituting Oatrim

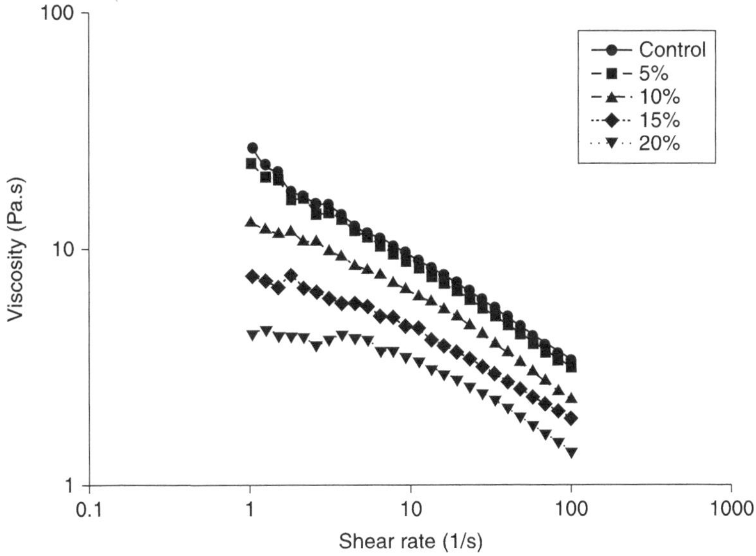

Fig. 11.1 Influence of RS level replacing flour on the flow properties of a muffin batter at 25°C. Control: no flour replacement.

Table 11.1 Consistency index (k) and flow behaviour index (n) at 25°C for muffin batters with increasing levels of resistant starch (RS)

RS (% w/w, d.b.)	k (Pas^n)	n
0 (control)	23.6[a] (2.9)	0.55[a] (0.01)
5	16.4[b] (1.8)	0.58[a,b] (0.03)
10	15.6[b] (0.8)	0.60[b] (0.02)
15	7.7[c] (0.9)	0.71[c] (0.02)
20	3.7[d] (0.3)	0.85[d] (0.03)

Notes: [a–d] Means in the same column without a common letter differ ($P < 0.05$) according to the least significant difference multiple range test.

Values in parentheses are standard deviations.
w/w, weight/weight; d.b., dry basis.

(20%, 40% and 60%) for shortening in a cake decreased the batter viscosity and the final volume, although the addition of up to 20% did not affect the general quality.

11.2.2 Viscoelastic properties of the batter

The determination of viscoelastic behaviour obtained through small amplitude oscillatory shear (SAOS) gives very valuable information about the structural properties of a system. A small sinusoidal strain (or stress) is applied and the resulting stress (or strain) is measured. Provided that these values are obtained within the linear viscoelastic domain, the results may be considered a sort of fingerprint of the material's structure.

In addition, the changes that the batter undergoes during heating are critical in determining the quality of the final baked product, and SAOS is highly suitable for studying structural changes during heating, since it allows the process to be monitored without altering the evolving sample structure.

Baixauli *et al.* (2008a) found that batters in which different proportions of wheat flour were replaced by RS behaved like a *soft gel*, that is to say, their elastic modulus G′ values were slightly higher than viscous modulus G″, and both moduli values were significantly frequency-dependent within the frequency range studied (Fig. 11.2). Increasing the RS content caused a (slight) decrease in both G′ and G″ values and no changes in the loss tangent values (loss tg = G″/G′) were found. These results indicate a (slight) decrease in the degree of structuring of the system due to the addition of RS, but without a significant effect on the type of structuring attributed to the proportional contribution of the elastic and viscous components. Different studies have shown a decrease in consistency and in viscoelastic properties when wheat flour is partially replaced with either wheat starch or modified corn starch in other types of batter system (for covering food to be fried); this effect has been attributed to the dilution of the wheat flour proteins (Sanz *et al.*, 2005). Similarly, a higher protein content in different types of wheat flour has been associated with higher G′ and G″ values (Navickis *et al.*, 1982), measured at room temperature.

The structural changes that take place during heating are further determining factors for bubble formation and stability and for the final baked texture (Shelke

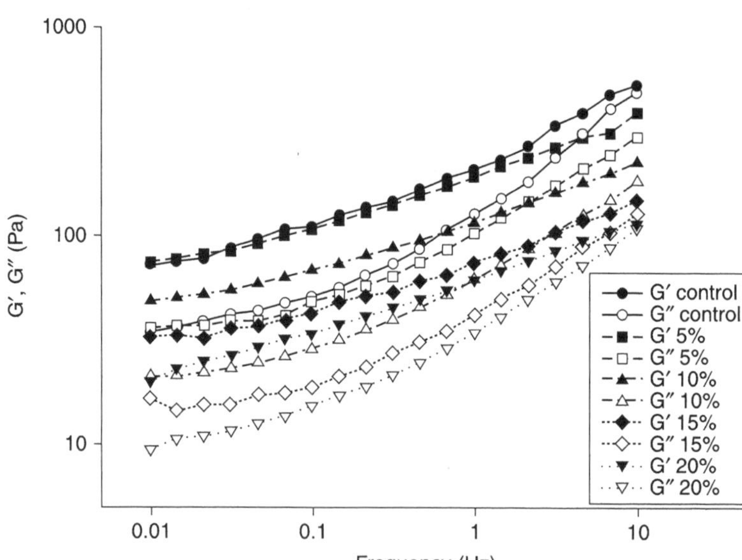

Fig. 11.2 Influence of RS level in muffin batters (%RS w/w, d.b.) on the frequency dependence of the elastic modulus G′ (solid symbols) and on the viscous modulus G″ (open symbols) at 25°C. Shear stress wave amplitude: 0.1 Pa.

et al., 1990). To simulate conditions during baking, Baixauli *et al.* (2008a) studied linear viscoelastic properties while applying a temperature sweep from 25 to 85°C. They found that increasing the amounts of RS in the muffin batter decreased the values of both viscoelastic moduli (Fig. 11.3). Initially, in the temperature

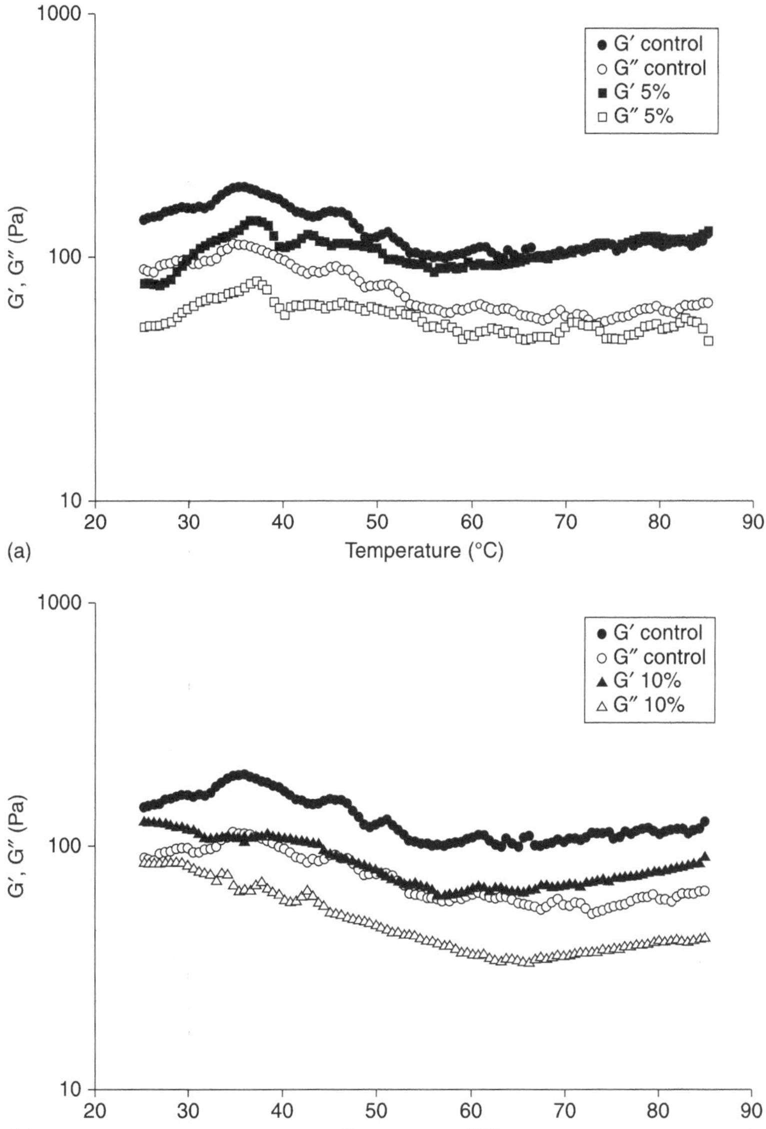

Fig. 11.3 Influence of RS level in the batter on the evolution of G′ (solid symbols) and G″ (open symbols) with temperature. Heating rate: 0.017 1C/s. Strain wave amplitude: 0.0007 (control, 5% and 10% RS) and 0.001 (15% and 20% RS). Frequency: 1 Hz: (a) control versus 5% RS; (b) control versus 10% RS. (*Continues overleaf.*)

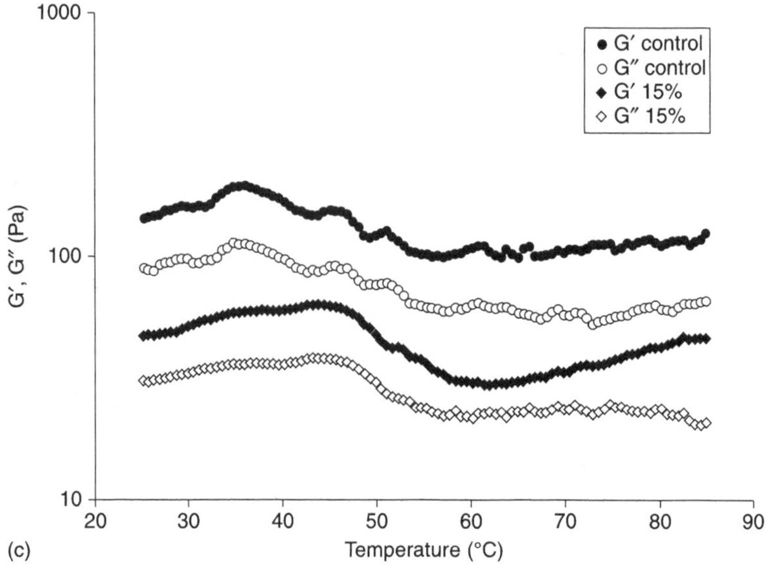

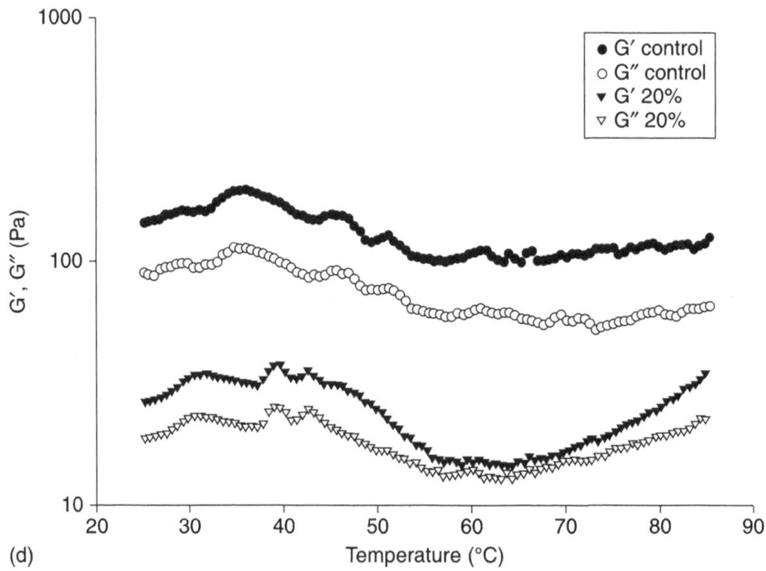

Fig. 11.3 (*Continued*) (c) Control versus 15% RS; and (d) control versus 20% RS.

range from 25 to 35–40°C, they observed that both viscoelastic moduli values showed a very slight tendency to increase, a trend that was also found by Ngo and Taranto (1986) and was attributed to protein–protein interactions. From 35–40°C to around 55°C, they found a decrease in both moduli values. These results agree with previous observations in cake batters by other authors (Lee *et al.*, 2005; Ngo and Taranto, 1986). In this temperature range, CO_2 is formed; it diffuses into occluded air bubbles and expands, producing a decrease in the density of the batter. Baixauli *et al.* (2008a) also found differences in the evolution of the loss tangent (tg δ) with temperature for the different RS contents of the batters (Fig. 11.4). While a slight decrease in tg δ values was registered in the control and the lower RS content samples in the temperature range studied, samples with 15% and 20% RS, especially from 50 to 70°C, showed an increase in the values of this parameter, which has to be interpreted as a decrease in the elastic contribution of the system.

In agreement with the results found in the temperature sweep, increasing the RS content lowered the values of both viscoelastic functions at 85°C (Fig. 11.5(a)). In addition, the tg δ values clearly grew steadily closer to 1 as the RS content of the muffin batter increased (Fig. 11.5(b)), reflecting a decrease in the elastic contribution to the viscoelastic behaviour of the system (more like a fluid) (Baixauli *et al.*, 2008a). Since the wheat flour content was reduced proportionately to the RS incorporated into the batter, the effects described may be attributed to a progressive decrease in the structuring effect of starch and wheat protein in the set structure. It should be pointed out that at the highest RS level (20%) only 6% of wheat flour was present in the system.

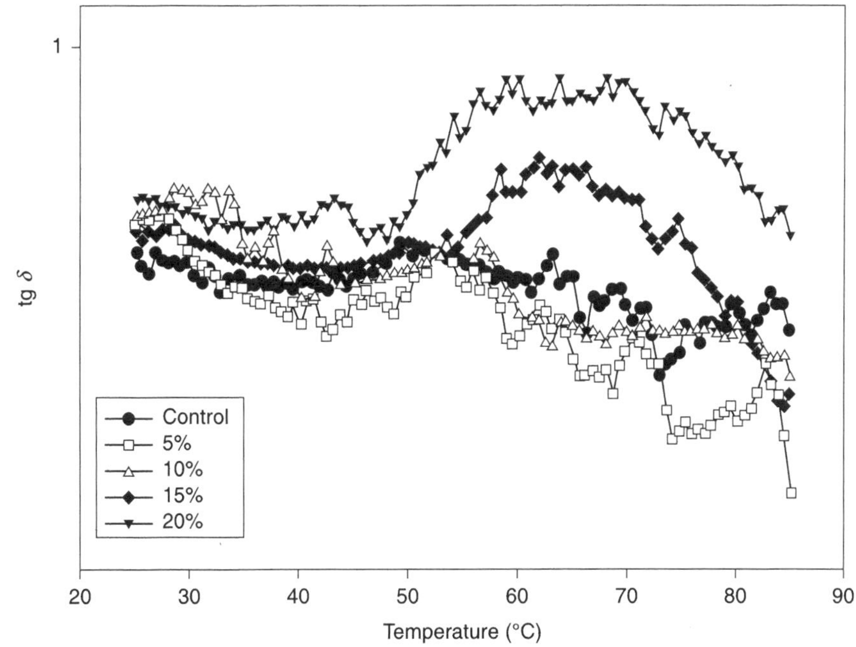

Fig. 11.4 Influence of RS level in the muffin batters on the evolution of loss tangent values (tg δ) with temperature. Heating rate: 0.017 1C/s. Strain wave amplitude: 0.0007 (control, 5% and 10% RS) and 0.001 (15% and 20% RS). Frequency: 1 Hz.

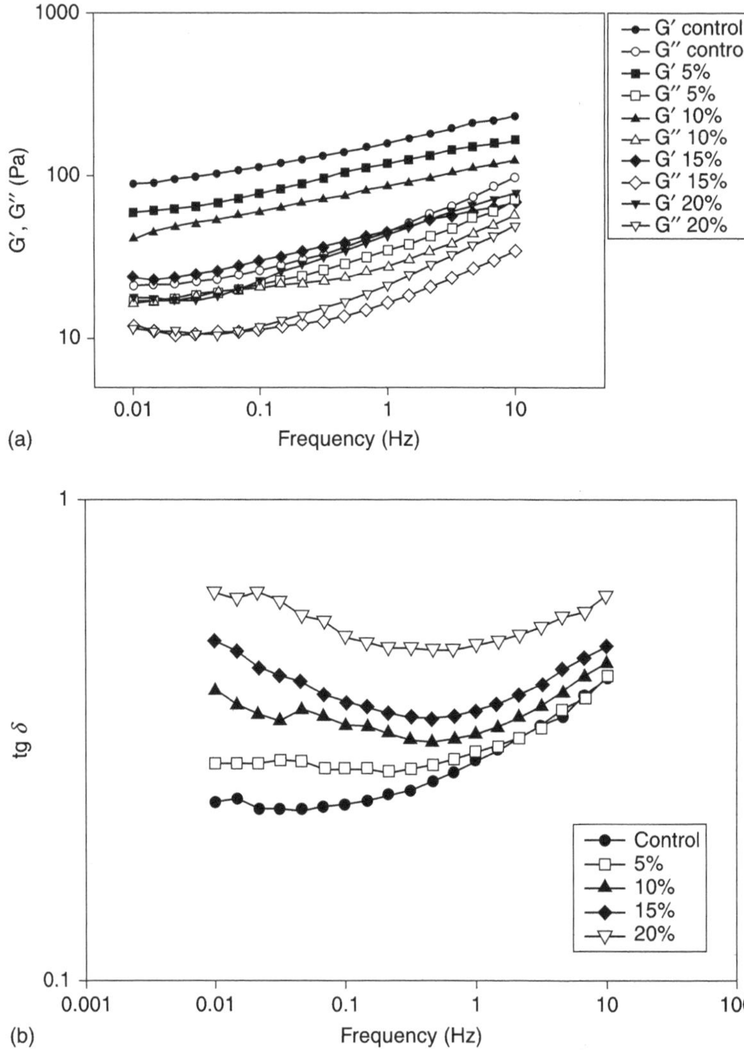

Fig. 11.5 (a) Influence of RS level in the batter on the frequency dependence of the elastic modulus G′ (solid symbols) and the viscous modulus G″ (open symbols) and (b) on the loss tangent values (tg δ) at 85 °C. Shear stress wave amplitude: 0.5 Pa (control), 0.4 Pa (5%, 10% and 15%), and 0.2 Pa (20%).

11.3 Muffin properties

11.3.1 Colour properties

During muffin-making, which involves oven baking, a large quantity of Maillard reaction products is formed. These compounds are responsible for colour, as well as contributing to the flavour and texture properties (Pino and González-SanJosé,

2002). During cooking the humidity decreases, generating a decreasing humidity gradient from the inside part of the muffin towards its surface (Thorvasldsson and Skjöldebrand, 1998). In the external layer, the water content is quickly reduced as the temperature rises, the sugars are thermally degraded and the first Maillard reactions take place. These steps are a prelude to the formation of the typical dark crust of these products. In the interior of the muffins the water loss is lower, relatively high water activity continues and the temperature does not exceed 105°C. Under these conditions Maillard reactions progress more slowly; therefore the crumb is only slightly coloured (González-Mateo *et al.*, 2009).

Colour is directly related to the quality of final products, including consumer acceptance and preference. Variations in muffin formulation can affect the muffin colour. For example, adding RS to muffins produces changes in their colour, as Baixauli *et al.* (2008b) found. The higher the concentration of RS, the lower the redness, yellowness and, consequently, the chroma of the muffins. The 'white' colour of the RS dilutes the pigmented elements of the formulation. For the same reason, the brightness and hue values increase with RS concentration. In order to ascertain whether colour differences can be appreciated by the human eye, it can sometimes be important to calculate the total colour differences (ΔE^*), using Eq. 11.1:

$$\Delta E^* = ((\Delta L^*)^2 + (\Delta a^*)^2 + (\Delta b^*)^2)^{1/2} \quad [11.1]$$

The following values can be used to determine whether the total colour difference is visually obvious (Bodart *et al.*, 2008):

$\Delta E^* < 1$, colour differences are not obvious to the human eye
$\Delta E^* > 3$, colour differences are obvious to the human eye.

In the case of muffins with RS, the ΔE^* value increases as the concentration of RS rises. At 5% and 10% RS, the colour differences are probably not appreciated by the human eye ($1 < \Delta E^* < 3$), whereas at 15% and 20% RS the colour differences are obvious to the human eye ($\Delta E^* > 3$), as the samples are less yellow and have less colour (Baixauli *et al.*, 2008b).

11.3.2 Muffin texture analysis

Freshly baked muffins

Texture is one of the main characteristics of bakery products that can be affected by the addition of fibre. It can be determined by instrumental or sensory methods. Instrumental methods offer some advantage over sensory analysis because they are rapid and objective. Baeva *et al.* (2000) made a study of texture (sensory and instrumental) to compare normal and energy-reduced sponge cakes; Sahi and Alava (2003) studied the crumb structure of sponge cakes to evaluate the effect of different emulsifiers; texture profile analysis (TPA) of cake crumb was performed by Singh Gujral *et al.* (2003) to study the effect of the addition of sodium lauryl sulphate; and Kamel and Rasper (1988) investigated the effect on cake crumb firmness of reduced-calorie cakes with sorbitol or polydextrose to replace

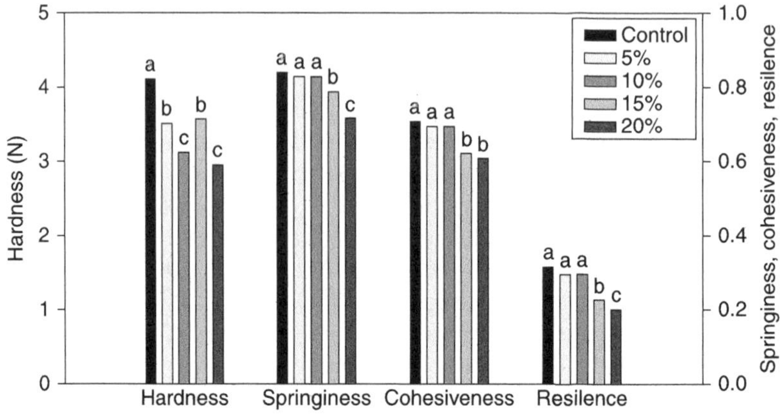

Fig. 11.6 Effect of different RS concentrations on TPA parameter values for muffins.

sugar. Baixauli *et al.* (2008b) compared the influence of replacing increasing proportions of wheat flour with four different levels of RS on the textural properties of freshly baked muffins and the changes that took place during two weeks' storage. They found that the 'hardness' values of the muffins with RS were significantly lower ($P < 0.05$) than those of the control muffins and that, although the decrease in hardness was not linear with wheat replacement, the lowest hardness value corresponded to the highest concentration of RS (20%). The springiness, cohesiveness and resilience of the muffins decreased as the RS rose, although this decrease was only clear and significant from 15% RS onwards (Fig. 11.6). A possible explanation of the lower resilience and springiness when RS is added is that the product matrix becomes denser: at higher RS levels the number and area of the gas cells and the height of the final baked muffins have been found to decrease (from 4.70 cm for the control to 3.84 cm for the muffin with 20% RS) (Baixauli *et al.*, 2006) and the samples lose the ability to recover after deformation. A volume reduction in bread with β-glucan addition has been attributed to gluten dilution resulting in an underdeveloped gluten network, which limits the extent of dough expansion and gas cell stability during proving and leads to reduced loaf volume (Symons and Brennan, 2004). Similar results were found by Tudorica *et al.* (2002) in pasta enriched with dietary fibre: the significantly reduced firmness and elasticity values obtained with fibre addition were related to the fibre's disruption of the protein–starch binding during pasta matrix formation.

Textural changes during muffin storage

Staling is one of the most important attributes in muffin quality. Muffin staling is a complex process that includes loss of flavour, changes in mouth texture, loss of tenderness, humidity redistribution and partial dryness. Baixauli *et al.* (2008b) studied textural changes (TPA) in muffins prepared with different RS levels over a 16-day storage period. They found that the 'hardness' value of the control muffin and muffins with 5, 10 and 15% RS tripled over 16 days of storage whereas muffins with 20% RS were softer than the other muffins, as their hardness value only doubled over the 16 days of storage (Fig. 11.7(a)). The 'springiness' parameter did not provide useful information (Fig. 11.7(b)), as the differences

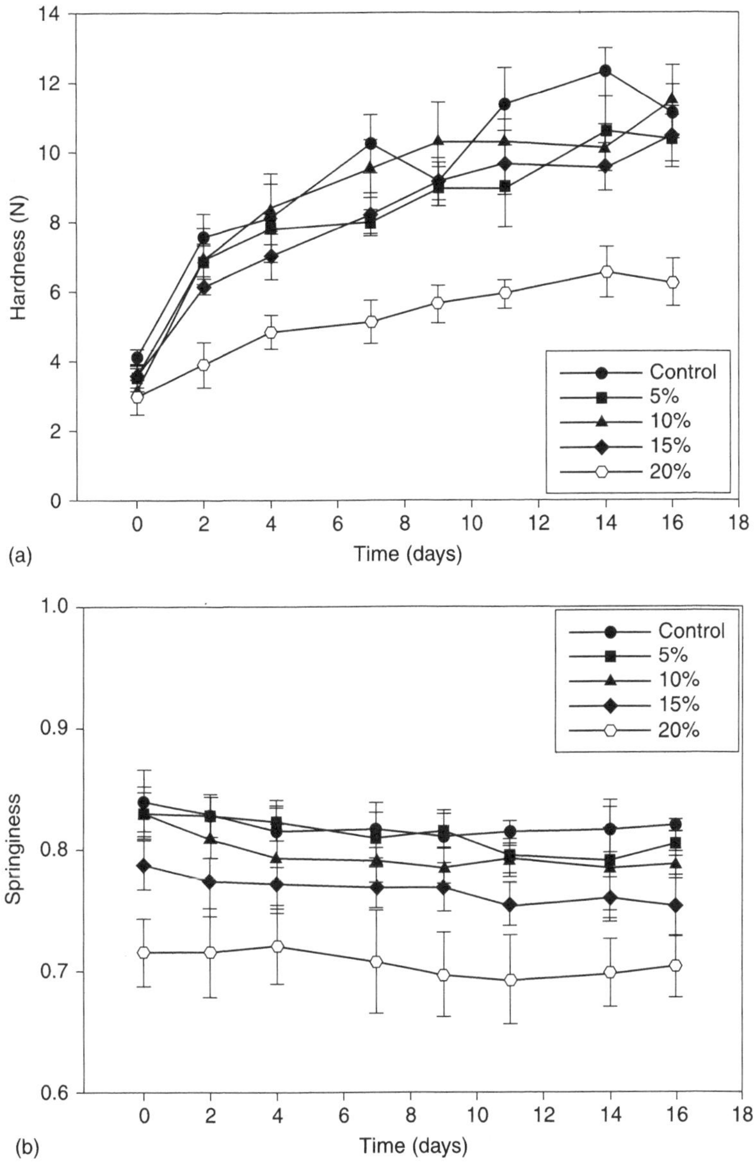

Fig. 11.7 TPA parameter values of muffins with different RS concentrations as a function of storage time: hardness (a), springiness (b). (*Continues overleaf.*)

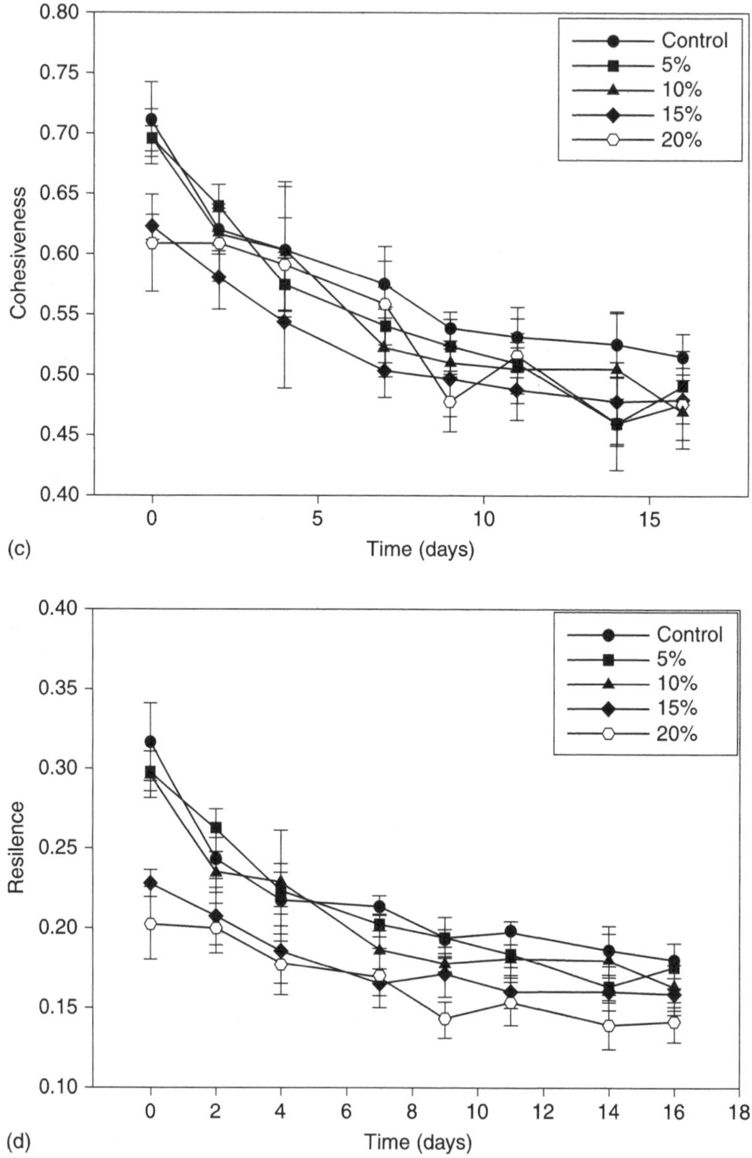

Fig. 11.7 (*Continued*) Cohesiveness (c) and resilience (d).

with storage time were not significant, but the values were lower in the presence of RS. 'Cohesiveness' and 'resilience' showed a significant fall over the storage period (Fig. 11.7(c), (d)), although these decreases were lower for the 15% and 20% RS samples. Consequently, higher concentrations of RS were effective in preventing a sharper drop in these parameters. These results are in agreement with

Yue and Waring (1998), who found that muffins formulated with 40% of RS remained softer than the control over a 2-week storage period.

11.4 Sensory shelf life of muffins

Storage stability or the shelf life of baked products could be defined as maintenance of the sensory and physical characteristics associated with freshness, such as crumb tenderness, compressibility and moistness, by preventing alterations associated with staling during storage (Guy, 1983; Paeschke, 1997). However, sensory methods are the only ones that make it possible to assess consumer acceptance. Consumers expect a product with a soft, spongy, tender crumb, but also a certain degree of resistance rather than crumbling easily; these characteristics worsen with storage time and, in general, consumer rejection of the product occurs before any microbiological spoilage makes it unsuitable for human consumption (Hough *et al.*, 2003). Different methods may be used to determine the sensory shelf life of a food product using consumer data. In the failure cut-off point method, shelf life is determined as the time when the first significant change in overall acceptability is detected. At this time, consumers detect a change in sensory characteristics compared with the fresh product. However, this does not mean that consumers would refuse to consume the product (Giménez *et al.*, 2007). In order to estimate the sensory shelf life based on consumer rejection of a food product, survival analysis can be applied. The use of survival analysis to study the shelf life of foods is quite a novel technique. Survival analysis, a branch of statistics, is extensively used in clinical studies, epidemiology, biology, sociology, and reliability studies (Kleinbaum, 1996; Klein and Moeschberger, 1997; Meeker and Escobar, 1998; Gómez *et al.*, 2001; Gómez, 2002). Hough *et al.* (2003) introduced this methodology into the study of food shelf life. Their key concept is to focus the shelf-life risk on the consumers' rejection of the product rather than on product deterioration. Survival analysis has been used to estimate the shelf life of some baked products, such as white pan bread (Gámbaro *et al.*, 2004), brown pan bread (Giménez *et al.*, 2007) and muffins (Baixauli *et al.*, 2008b).

Baixauli *et al.* (2008b) calculated the shelf life of muffins prepared with RS using survival analysis and the Weibull distribution. The percentage of rejection by consumers versus storage time is shown in Fig. 11.8. It will be seen that the shapes of the curves were different for the two different levels of RS (control and 20%). During the early days of storage, the rejection percentage was lower for the control muffins than for the 20% RS muffins, probably because the controls reminded the consumers more of a typical muffin flavour and texture. As time went on, however, the reverse was found: rejection was higher for the control muffins than for the 20% RS muffins. This could be because the texture of the 20% RS muffins changed less over time, as mentioned above. After 23 days of storage the predicted percentage of rejection by consumers for the muffins prepared with RS was lower than for the control sample.

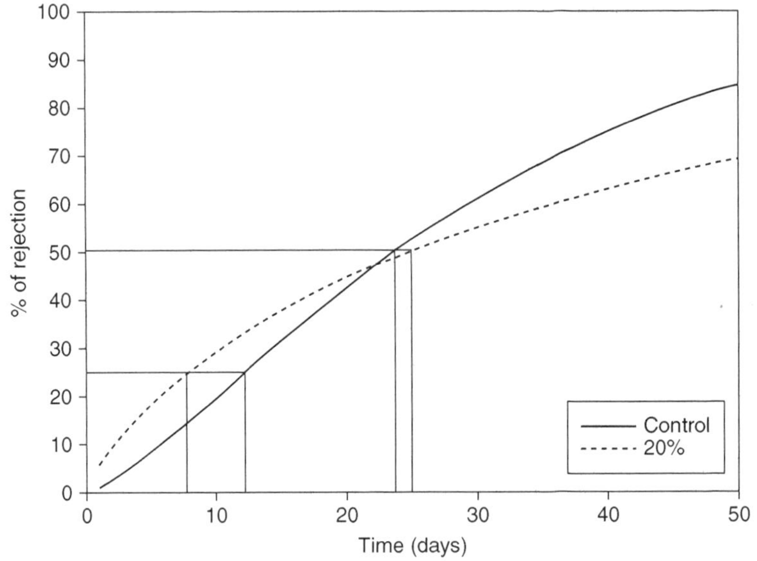

Fig. 11.8 Percentage of consumers rejecting control and 20% RS muffins versus storage time.

11.5 Sensory characteristics of muffins

11.5.1 Descriptive sensory analysis

Sensory evaluation of food products, especially by consumer panels, has re-emerged as an invaluable science in conjunction with nutritional research and functional food development (Scholtz and Bosman, 2005). However, sensory evaluation using a trained descriptive panel is also required for a fuller assessment of the effects of fibre use on the wide range of parameters involved (Meilgaard *et al.*, 1991).

The effect of adding different types of fibre on the sensory analysis of a baked product has been studied by several authors. Grigelmo-Miguel *et al.* (1999) evaluated the sensory characteristics of muffins in which high levels of peach dietary fibre replaced flour; these muffins had a good flavour and mouthfeel and were as spongy as traditional muffins, although slightly darker. Baixauli *et al.* (2008c) studied the attributes that describe muffins when RS is used as a fibre. They used a panel of eight assessors with wide experience in descriptive analysis to determine the sensory profile of muffins with RS. In their work, it is interesting to emphasize that from the preliminary sensory sessions, in addition to traditional attributes of bakery products such as 'sweetness', 'taste', 'odour', 'chewiness' or 'springiness', other new attributes appeared that were distinctive for muffins with RS as a fibre. These were 'number of gas cells', 'grittiness' and 'moisture'. These authors found significant differences for all the descriptors as the RS level in the samples increased. Six of the descriptors ('typical odour', 'number of gas cells', 'springiness', 'chewiness', 'cohesiveness' and 'typical taste') received

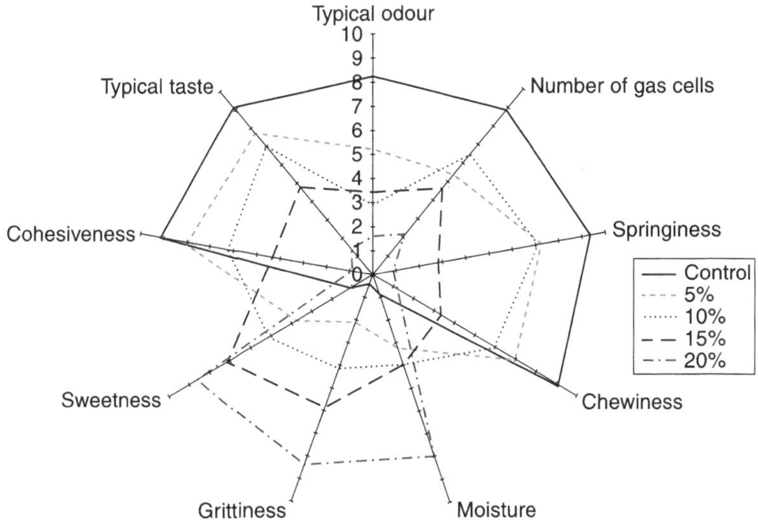

Fig. 11.9 Evolution of sensory attributes when RS was added to the muffins.

significantly lower scores compared with the control, while the 'grittiness', 'sweetness' and 'moisture' scores rose with the addition of RS (Fig. 11.9).

The higher 'grittiness' score for the addition of RS indicates that the perception of particles can be important as a textural characteristic. The ingredient used has a fine particle size, between 10 mm and 15 mm, yet despite this small size it was detected by the panellists. Fondroy *et al.* (1989) found that when an oat straw fibre fraction (fluffy cellulose) was added to a lean white cake the presence of the fibre altered the product by leaving a gritty mouthfeel after swallowing. Imai *et al.* (1995) reported that particle concentration, dispersion medium and particle size are all important factors that contribute to perceived grittiness; they also observed that the perceived grittiness decreased as the viscosity of the dispersion medium increased.

The panellists' scores for the 'moisture' descriptor rose with the addition of RS, whereas the instrumental measurement of moisture showed that the values fell. The perception of moisture could be related to the 'number of gas cells' descriptor. The panellists found fewer big gas cells as the RS in the formulations increased, but more small gas cells (Baixauli *et al.*, 2008c). In baked products, small cells in the crumb are directly related to the perception of an even surface and a fresh product (Cauvain *et al.*, 1999). This perception of a smooth surface could be the reason why the panellists perceived greater moisture as the RS concentration in the muffins increased.

11.5.2 Consumer acceptability

Consumer research in the early stages of new product development makes it possible to go farther and deeper into understanding consumer needs, often well beyond

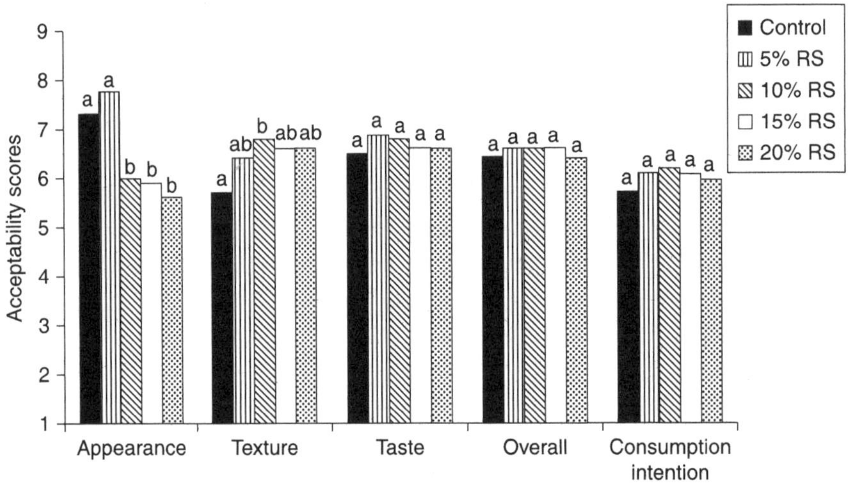

Fig. 11.10 Consumers' sensory scores of muffins containing resistant starch.

what could be understood without them (Van Kleef *et al.*, 2005). Clark and Johnson (2002) studied the sensory acceptability of muffins enriched with lupin kernel fibre, finding that the addition of this fibre did not change the consumer rating of the muffins' appearance significantly, although it lowered the consumer ratings for 'overall acceptability', 'flavour' and 'texture in mouth'. Ramcharitar *et al.* (2005) evaluated the consumer acceptability of muffins with flaxseed on sensory attributes such as 'appearance', 'colour', 'flavour', 'texture' and 'overall acceptability' by hedonic scoring; they obtained lower scores for all sensory attributes. Baixauli *et al.* (2008c) assessed the consumer acceptability of muffins enriched with RS on 'appearance', 'texture', 'taste', 'overall acceptance' and 'consumption intention'. They did not find significant differences in 'taste', 'overall acceptance' and 'consumption intention' (Fig. 11.10). However, although the 'appearance' attribute did not differ significantly between the control and 5% RS, probably due to the similarity of their external appearance, the scores were lower at higher RS concentrations; this could be related to the height of the final baked muffin, which falls as the RS in the formulation is increased (Baixauli *et al.*, 2008a). For 'texture', they reported that the RS muffins were rated higher than the control, demonstrating that the addition of RS improved the perception of this attribute. These results are in agreement with Yue and Waring (1998), who found that when RS type 2 and RS type 3 were added to cake-like muffins they acted as a texture modifier, imparting a favourable tenderness to the crumb.

11.6 Conclusion

Used as a muffin ingredient, RS modifies a number of properties of the batter and the final product. Generally speaking, the batters are technologically compatible with the manufacturing process, as their rheology is not radically altered, but the quantity and size of the air bubbles incorporated into them is affected, resulting in a denser batter. The final products are acceptable. Their colour is lighter and their height lower. A certain degree of graininess appears among the sensory characteristics, but the texture is perceived as being moister and more tender. Good communication of the characteristics and benefits of RS is important, as consumers can find their expectations confused by the differences compared with traditional fibres such as bran.

11.7 Acknowledgements

The authors are grateful to the Spanish Ministry of Science and Innovation for financial support (AGL 2009–12785-C02–01) and to Mary Georgina Hardinge for assistance with the English-language manuscript.

11.8 References

APARICIO-SANGUILÁN, A., SÁYAGO-AVENDI, S.G., VARGAS-TORRES, A., TOVAR, J., ASCENSIO-OTERO, T.E. and BELLO-PÉREZ, L.A., 2007. Slowly digestible cookies prepared from RS-rich lintnerized banana starch. *Journal of Food Composition and Analysis*, **20**, 175–81.

ASP, N.G. and BJÖRCK, I., 1992. Resistant starch. *Trends in Food Science and Technology*, **3**(5), 111–14.

AUSTRALIAN NATIONAL FOOD AUTHORITY, 1994. *Australian National Food Authority, functional foods policy discussion paper*. National Food Authority, Canberra, p. 42.

BAEVA, M.R., PANCHEV, I.N. and TERZIEVA, V.V., 2000. Comparative study of texture of normal and energy reduced sponge cakes. *Nahrung*, **44**(4), 242–6.

BAIXAULI, R., SANZ, T., SALVADOR, A. and FISZMAN, S.M., 2006. CONGRESS: bubbles in food 2: novelty, health and luxury.

BAIXAULI, R. SANZ, T. SALVADOR, A. and FISZMAN, S.M., 2008a. Muffins with resistant starch: Baking performance in relation to the rheological properties of the batter. *Journal of Cereal Science*, **47**, 502–9.

BAIXAULI, R., SALVADOR, A. and FISZMAN, S.M., 2008b. Textural and colour changes during storage and sensory shelf life of muffins containing resistant starch. *European Food Research and Technology*, **226**, 523–30.

BAIXAULI, R., SALVADOR, A., MARTÍNEZ-CERVERA, S. and FISZMAN, S.M., 2008c. Distinctive sensory features introduced by resistant starch in baked products. *LWT – Food Science and Technology*, **41**, 1927–33.

BATH, D.E., SHELKE, K. and HOSENEY, R.C., 1992. Fat replacers in high-ratio layer cakes. *Cereal Foods World*, **37**(7), 495–500.

BODART, M., DE PEÑARANDA, R., DENEYER, A. and FLAMANT, G., 2008. Photometry and colorimetry characterisation of materials in daylighting evaluation tools. *Building and Environment*, **43**, 2046–58.

CAUVAIN, S.P., WHITWORTH, M.B. and ALAVA, J.M., 1999. The evolution of bubble structure in bread doughs and its effect on bread structure. In: G.M. CAMPBELL, C. WEBB, S.S. PANDIELLA and K. NIRAJAN, eds. *Bubbles in food*. Minnesota, USA. AACC, pp. 85–8.

CHAMP, M., 2004. Resistant starch. In: ELIASSON A.C., ed. *Starch in food: structure, function and applications*. Woodhead, Cambridge.

CLARK, R. and JOHNSON, S., 2002. Sensory acceptability of foods with added lupin (*Lupinus angustifolius*) kernel fiber using pre-set criteria. *Journal of Food Science*, **67**, 356–62.

DE VRIES, J.W., 2003. On defining dietary fibre. *Proceedings of the Nutrition Society*, **62**, 37–43.

FONDROY, E.B., WHITE, P.J. and PRUSA, K.J., 1989. Physical and sensory evaluation of lean white cakes containing substituted fluffy cellulose. *Cereal Chemistry*, **66**(5), 402–4.

GÁMBARO, A., FISZMAN, S.M., GIMÉNEZ, A., VARELA, P. and SALVADOR, A., 2004. Consumer acceptability compared with sensory and instrumental measures of white pan bread: sensory shelf-life estimation by survival analysis. *Journal of Food Science*, **69**(9), S401–S405.

GIMÉNEZ, A., VARELA, P., SALVADOR, A., ARES, G., FISZMAN, S.M. and GARITTA, L., 2007. Shelf life estimation of brown pan bread: A consumer approach. *Food Quality and Preference*, **18**, 196–204.

GÓMEZ, G., 2002. Análisis de Supervivencia. *Apuntes del curso de la Licenciatura en Ciencias y Técnicas Estadísticas de la Facultat de Matemàtiques I Estadística.* Barcelona: Univ. Politècnica de Catalunya.

GÓMEZ, G., CALLE, M.L. and OLLER, R., 2001. A walk through interval-censored data. *Technical Report, 2001/16, Dept. Statistics and Operations Research.* Barcelona: Univ. Politècnica de Catalunya.

GONZÁLEZ-MATEO, S., GONZÁLEZ-SANJOSÉ, M.L. and MUÑIZ, P., 2009. Presence of Maillard products in Spanish muffins and evaluation of colour and antioxidant potential. *Food and Chemical Toxicology*, **47**, 2798–805.

GRIGELMO-MIGUEL, N., CARRERAS-BOLADERAS, E. and MARTÍN-BELLOSO, O., 1999. Development of high-fruit-dietary-fibre muffins. *European Food Research and Technology*, **210**, 123–8.

GUY, R.C.E., 1983. Factors affecting the staling of madeira slab cake. *Journal of the Science of Food and Agriculture*, **34**, 477–91.

HANDLEMAN, A.R., CONN, J.F. and LYONS, J.W., 1961. Bubble mechanics in thick foams and their effects on cake quality. *Cereal Chemistry*, **38**, 294–305.

HARALUMPU, S.G., 2000. Resistant starch—a review of the physical properties and biological impact of RS3. *Carbohydrate Polymers*, **41**, 285–92.

HOUGH, G., LANGOHR, K., GÓMEZ, G. and CURIA, A., 2003. Survival analysis applied to sensory shelf-life of foods. *Journal of Food Science*, **68**, 359–62.

IMAI, E., HATAE, K. and SHIMADA, A., 1995. Oral perception of grittiness: effect of particle size and concentration of the dispersed particles and the dispersion medium. *Journal of Textural Studies*, **26**, 561–76.

KAMEL, B.S. and RASPER, V.F., 1988. Effects of emulsifiers, sorbitol, polydextrose, and crystalline cellulose on the texture of reduced-calorie cakes. *Journal of Texture Studies*, **19**, 307–20.

KIM, H.Y., HYEON, W.Y., LIM, H.S. and LIM, S.T., 2001. Replacement of shortening in yellow layer cakes by corn dextrins. *Cereal Chemistry*, **78**(3), 267–71.

KLEIN, J.P. and MOESCHBERGER, M.L., 1997. *Survival analysis, techniques for censored and truncated data.* New York: Springer-Verlag.

KLEINBAUM, D.G., 1996. *Survival analysis, a self-learning text.* New York: Springer-Verlag.

LAGUNA, L., SALVADOR, A., SANZ, T. and FISZMAN, S.M. 2011. Performance of a resistant starch rich ingredient in the baking and eating quality of short-dough biscuits. *LWT – Food Science and Technology* **44**, 737–46.

LAKSHMINARAYAN, S.M., RATHINAM, V. and KRISHNARAU, L., 2006. Effect of maltodextrin and emulsifiers on the viscosity of cake batter and on the quality of cakes. *Journal of the Science of Food and Agriculture*, **86**, 706–12.

LEE, S., KIM, S. and INGLETT, G.E., 2005. Effect of shortening replacement with Oatrim on the physical and rheological properties of cakes. *Cereal Chemistry*, **82**(2), 120–4.

LOEWE, R., 1993. Role of ingredients in batter systems. *Cereal Foods World*, **38**(9), 673–7.

MEEKER, W.Q. and ESCOBAR, L.A., 1998. *Statistical methods for reliability data*. New York: John Wiley & Sons.

MEILGAARD, M., CIVILLE, G.V. and CARR, B.T., 1991. *Sensory evaluation techniques* (2nd ed.). Boca Raton, FL: CRC Press Inc.

NAVICKIS, L.L., ANDERSON, R.A., BAGLEY, E.B. and JASBERG, B.K., 1982. Viscoelastic properties of wheat flour doughs: variation of dynamic moduli with water and protein content. *Journal of Texture Studies*, **13**, 249–64.

NGO, W.H. and TARANTO, M.V., 1986. Effect of sucrose level on the rheological properties of cake batters. *Cereal Foods World*, **31**(4), 317–22.

OZTURK, S., KOKSEL, H. and NG, P.K.W. (2009). Farinograph properties and bread quality of flours supplemented with resistant starch. *International Journal of Food Sciences and Nutrition*, **60**(6), 449–57.

PAESCHKE, T., 1997. Shelf life extension of reduced-fat baked goods using fruit powders. *Cereal Foods World*, **42**(5), 391–5.

PINO, R. and GONZÁLEZ-SANJOSÉ, M.L., 2002. Effects of brown pigments on the texture properties of bakery products. *Meeting Cost–919*.

RAMCHARITAR, A., BADRIE, N., MATTFELDT-BEMAN, M., MATSUO, H. and RIDLEY, C., 2005. Consumer acceptability of muffins with flaxseed (*Linum usitatissimum*). *Journal of Food Science*, **70**, S504–S507.

SAHI, S.S. and ALAVA, J.M., 2003. Functionality of emulsifiers in sponge cake production. *Journal of the Science of Food and Agriculture*, **83**, 1419–29.

SAJILATA, M.G., SINGHAI, R.S. and KULKARNI, P.R., 2006. Resistant starch. A Review. *Comprehensive Reviews in Food Science and Food Safety*, **5**, 1–17.

SANZ, T., SALVADOR, A., VÉLEZ, G., MUÑOZ, J. and FISZMAN, S.M., 2005. Influence of ingredients on the thermo-rheological behaviour of batters containing methylcellulose. *Food Hydrocolloids*, **19**(5), 869–77.

SANZ-PENELLA, J.M., WRONKOWSKA, M., SORAL-S'MIETANA, M., COLLAR, C. and HAROS, M. (2010). Impact of the addition of resistant starch from modified pea starch on dough and bread performance. *European Food Research and Technology*, **231**, 499–508.

SCHOLTZ, S.C. and BOSMAN, M.J.C., 2005. Consumer acceptance of high-fibre muffins and rusks baked with red palm olein. *International Journal of Food Science and Technology*, **40**, 857–66.

SHELKE, K., FAUBION, J.M. and HOSENEY, R.C., 1990. The dynamics of cake baking as studied by a combination of viscosimetry and electrical resistance oven heating. *Cereal Chemistry*, **67**(6), 575–80.

SINGH GUJRAL, H., ROSELL, C.M., SHARMA, S. and SINGH, S., 2003. Effect of sodium lauryl sulphate on the texture of sponge cake. *Food Science and Technology International*, **9**(2), 89–93.

SYMONS, L.J. and BRENNAN, C.S., 2004. The influence of (1→3) (1→4)-β-D-glucan-rich fractions from barley on the physicochemical properties and in vitro reducing sugar release of white wheat breads. *Journal of Food Science*, **69**(6), 463–7.

THORVASLDSSON, K. and SKJÖLDEBRAND, C., 1998. Water diffusion in bread during baking. *Lebensm. Wiss. Technol.*, **31**(7–8), 658–63.

TUDORICA, C.M., KURI, V. and BRENNAN, C.S., 2002. Nutritional and physicochemical characteristics of dietary fiber enriched pasta. *Journal of Agriculture and Food Chemistry*, **50**, 347–56.

VAN KLEEF, E., VAN TRIJP, H.C.M. and LUNING, P., 2005. Consumer research in the early stages of new product development: a critical review of methods and techniques. *Food Quality and Preference*, **16**, 181–201.

YUE, P. and WARING, S., 1998. Functionality of resistant starch in food applications. *Food Australia*, **50**(12), 615–21.

12

Fibre in extruded products

N. Sozer and K. Poutanen, VTT Technical Research Centre of Finland, Finland

DOI: 10.1533/9780857095787.3.256

Abstract: This chapter discusses the effects of dietary fibre (DF) and outer grain parts on extrusion processing of expanded foods and summarizes the ongoing research in development of high DF foods with improved structural and sensory profile. The chapter first outlines the basics of extrusion processing and the influence of both fibre addition and fibre type on the product quality and then discusses how the extrusion processing can be used to tailor fibre properties.

Key words: dietary fibre, extrusion, extrudate quality.

12.1 Introduction

There is a remarkable demand worldwide to design foods with high nutritional profile. Research evidence on the health benefits of dietary fibre (DF) has brought with it the need to increase DF content in food products. The challenge is to combine high fibre and wholegrain content with low saturated fat, sugar and salt contents and nevertheless produce acceptable sensory appeal. Extruded food products are one of the cereal product categories in which an increased fibre level would offer a nutritional benefit. According to the Nutrition Labeling and Education Act of 1990 USA, extruded snacks can be labelled as 'good source' or 'high fibre source' if the DF amount per serving is at least 2.5 or 5 g, respectively (Eastman *et al.*, 2001). Implementing the data from Healthy Eating Index 2005 and MyPyramid, the US developed a classification system based on the nutrient composition of foods (http://www.health.gov/DietaryGuidelines/dga2005/document/). In the Nutrition and Health Claims directive of the European Union (EU), foods can be claimed to be a source of fibre at the level of 3 g DF/100 g and a good source at 6 g/100 g, provided they fulfil the other nutritional profile requirements (Annex I, EC No 1924/2006).

Extrusion technology is one of the processing techniques to design expanded food matrices. Food extrusion applications can be found as early as the 1930s for processing of cereals, snack foods and texturized foods (Ilo *et al.*, 2000). Extrusion technology enables formulation and design of a large variety of food products. It can be used either to form ready-to-eat foods (snacks, cereals, pasta, confectionery) or to modify food ingredients which can form solid, semi-solid and liquid products after preparation steps for consumption. Structure–texture properties of the expanded food products strictly depend on the operational parameters.

The structural elements of an extruded food product are formed *via* the physicochemical changes occurring in the raw materials. It is known that extrusion processing results in irreversible changes in starch granules and polymers, denaturation of proteins and formation of starch–lipid, protein–lipid and protein–protein complexes (Lai and Kokini, 1991; Cremer and Kaletunç, 2003, Hagenimana *et al.*, 2007). Cereal extrudates consist of a continuous starch matrix and a discontinuous protein phase (Hermansson, 1988). It has been suggested that structural segregation within the extruded material occurs due to formation of protein fibrils (Noguchi, 1989). It is a food engineering challenge to design palatable extruded foods containing a large amount of DF, since polymer matrices with high levels of DF have low expansion capability. The majority of high DF products exhibit poor textural (high hardness and low crispiness) and morphological (small pores, high density) properties. In this chapter the aim is to review the effects of DF and outer grain parts on extrusion processing of expanded foods, and summarize the ongoing research into development of high DF foods with enhanced palatability.

12.2 Extrusion cooking

12.2.1 Extruders in cereal processing

Extruders are screw reactors, and extrusion is a series of processes which includes mixing, forming, puffing and drying. Single and twin screw extruders are the two main types of extruders based on screw configuration. Twin screw extruders can be co-rotating or counter-rotating depending on direction of rotation. The screws help in conveying and mixing of raw materials, and finally transform the dry mix into plastic melt, which is forced through a die. In general, there are three different zones where structural transformations take place (Fig. 12.1). The first one is the feeding section, where the raw materials are fed to the extruder. At this stage initial mixing occurs, with or without water. In the second part, which is called the compression section, pressure is built up due to increase in temperature by either heating coils or friction. The final transformation takes place in the metering zone, where the dry mixture forms a homogeneous viscoelastic material. The transitions in this zone control the structure, texture, colour and flavour of the product. Expansion occurs right after this stage at the die exit due to temperature and pressure drop (Eastman *et al.*, 2001). Table 12.1 summarizes some features of both single and twin screw extruders.

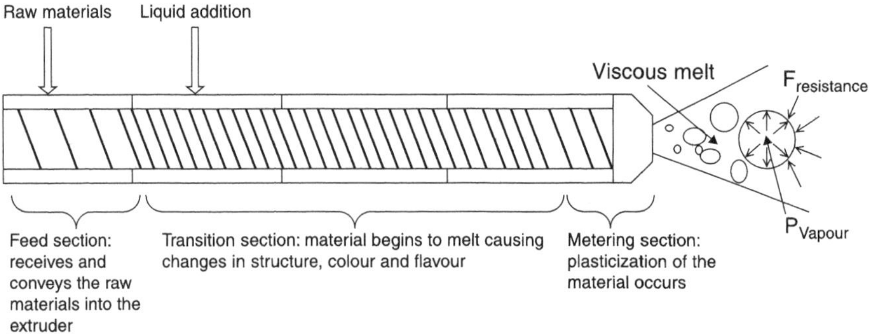

Fig. 12.1 Sections of an extruder and expansion mechanism.

Table 12.1 Comparison of single and twin screw extruders

Single screw extruder	Twin screw extruder
Simple/economic	Expensive
Easy to operate	Difficult to operate
Suitable for foods with < 4% fat, 10% sugar and 30% water	Better mixing capability, extended product range < 20 % fat, 40% sugar, 65% moisture

Source: Adapted from Chen and Rosenthal (2009).

12.2.2 Operational parameters important for product properties

Product quality of extruded food products depends on integrated factors such as screw configuration, die design and process variables, besides ingredient properties and preconditioning steps. Figure 12.2 summarizes the paths describing how each of these parameters influences the final product quality.

Feed moisture content, screw speed and temperature are the factors which control the density of the extrudate. Increased feed moisture rates reduce the elasticity of both the dough and the final material obtained, which is a highly plasticized melt with reduced specific mechanical energy and degree of gelatinization. This will cause low expansion rate, resulting in dense products. Increased barrel temperatures will form superheated water in the extruder, which promotes bubble formation and reduces the product density. Increased feed rates at low water content, or increasing water content at low feed rate, were reported to result in extrudates with a hard texture (Ding *et al.*, 2006). Extrudate expansion is strongly influenced by the melt rheology and biopolymer interactions, as reviewed recently by Xie *et al.* (2012). Melt viscosity in conjunction with moisture content controls the expansion profile during extrusion. High melt viscosity at high moisture content levels results in products with low expansion, whereas high melt viscosity at low moisture content levels results in improved expansion due to higher stored energy of biopolymers (Xie *et al.*, 2012). Chen and Rizvi (2006) reported that higher expansion rates can be achieved from high viscosity melts. High melt viscosity causes reduction in gas diffusion rates, which improves

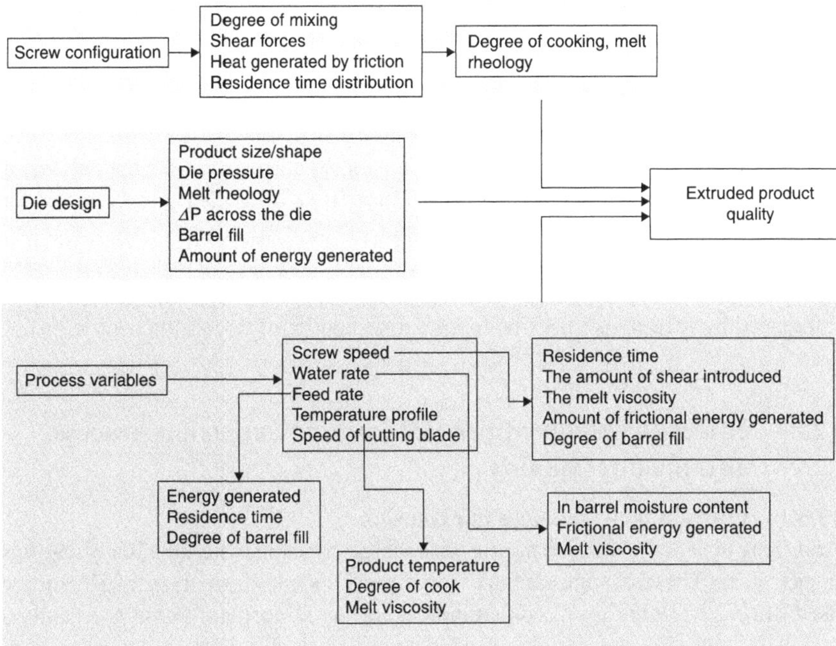

Fig. 12.2 Operational variables controlling extruded product quality (based on Guy, 2001).

bubble growth. Elastic properties of polymer melts can be evaluated by extensional viscosity measurements (Cogswell, 1994). In order to simulate the extrusion processing conditions, a pre-shearing rheometer can be used to collect rheological data of starch polymer melts. Also, in-line rheometers allow real time rheological characterization during processing. Under the same thermal conditions different shear rates can result in varying expansion rates (Vergnes *et al.*, 1987). High shearing regimens will form low viscosity melts due to shear thinning and extension thinning behaviour of starch.

The operational parameters of screw speed, torque input and barrel temperature are the factors which determine the final product quality and also DF functionality in the product. Extrusion processing at temperatures above 150°C and below 180°C with a moderate screw speed of 200 rpm was found not to influence total DF content (Gualberto *et al.*, 1997). Under high shearing of wheat bran and wholegrain wheat at high temperature and barrel pressure profiles, insoluble DF was found to be solubilized (Camire *et al.*, 1990; Björck *et al.*, 1984; Aoe *et al.*, 1989).

Increasing the screw speed increased longitudinal expansion and lowered radial expansion in DF-containing extrudates. An increase in screw speed will apparently cause a decrease in melt viscosity and an increase in elasticity, creating a more homogeneous moisture distribution. High screw speed rates lowered residence times, which resulted in decreased starch gelatinization in corn starch and grit extrusion (Chinnaswamy and Hanna, 1988; Fletcher *et al.*, 1985; Lue *et al.*, 1991). Combination of high DF levels (30%) and high screw speed rates resulted in formation of surface distortion, called 'sharkskin' in polymer extrusion (Lue *et al.*, 1991). This is a common cause of failure for extrusion of non-food polymer melts, which generally occurs at high stretching rates where the surface structure fails (Miller and Rothstein, 2004).

The glass transition (Tg) property is an important process-dependent factor which is associated with physicochemical properties of foods and influences, for example, product stability. After expansion in the extruder, the material under cooling crosses to the glassy region. Lazou and Krokida (2011) showed that in extruded corn–lentil snacks the glass transition temperature of the products was influenced by feed rate, extrusion temperature and lentil to corn flour ratio.

12.3 Effects of dietary fibre (DF) on the extrusion process and product quality

12.3.1 Fibre-induced changes in extrusion

Addition of DF to the reaction mixture has a large effect on material transformations in extrusion. These changes are also largely dependent on the type of DF source used. Jin *et al.* (1995) observed that increasing soy DF content (10–40%) resulted in close-textured, less expanded products with thick cell walls in soy fibre–corn meal extrudates. Lue *et al.* (1990) found a similar trend with oat bran and corn meal extrudates. Increasing bran content can cause structural defects of air cell rupture, which will affect the expansion rate (Mendonca *et al.*, 2000; Moore *et al.*, 1990). Typically about 10–30% of cereal brans have been used in extrusion studies. Increasing the amount of DF results in reduced expansion, tough and non-crisp textures. Increasing the sugar beet fibre content in corn meal (0–30%) resulted in decreased diameter but longer extrudates, meaning that radial expansion decreased whereas longitudinal expansion increased (Lue *et al.*, 1991). The size of air cells was directly related to the radial expansion rate. Pectin addition (10%) in corn extrudates also reduced the radial expansion, which was due to an increase in melt viscosity (Yanniotis *et al.*, 2007). The increase in melt viscosity is associated with the water absorption index at high barrel temperatures ($T > 150°C$).

The interaction between DF and water occurs through polar and hydrophobic interactions. The type and degree of interaction vary with the nature of the DF preparation. Cereal brans are challenging DF ingredients due to their insoluble nature. Wheat bran, commonly used as a DF source, consists of insoluble particles containing protein and starch in addition to DF. Due to the incompatibility of bran particles with other raw materials, they act as fillers, and so their presence influences the characteristic properties of the system, such as mechanical and physical properties, particle size distribution, and orientation of polymers within the food matrix (Robin *et al.*, 2011a). Particle size distribution of bran was shown to influence the expansion rate (Guy, 1985). Most of the insoluble fibres go through minor structural changes during extrusion, causing structural anisotropy, which increases extensional viscosity. It can be hypothesized that the extent of the structural anisotropy can be reduced by reducing the bran particle size. Coarse particle-sized fibre preparations can interrupt the matrix, disrupt the bubble wall film and result in failure of gas cells before expansion (Guy, 1985). However, Blake (2006) found that reduction of cellulose particle size to less than 60 μm did not improve the sectional expansion.

Chassagne-Berces *et al.* (2011) studied the effects of adding oat and wheat bran (0, 10, and 20%) to wholegrain and white wheat flours on extrusion. Regardless of DF source, the addition of bran caused a decrease in expansion rate and the cell size, and an increase in cell wall thickness. Water absorption capacity of the DF preparation influences the expansion rate. The available water within the food matrix also controls the extent of starch gelatinization.

For the majority of food processing techniques, water is known to be an excellent plasticizer. For starch-based extruded products it promotes both rupture and formation of new hydrogen bonds. Different types of DF ingredients have different tendencies towards water absorption. They compete for water with starch and protein in the food matrix and inhibit its availability for starch gelatinization. Reduced rate of starch gelatinization has a negative influence on expansion rate (Yanniotis *et al.*, 2007; Chevanan *et al.*, 2009; Stojceska *et al.*, 2010). Pai *et al.* (2009) compared unmodified corn bran, alkali-treated bran and alkali-soluble bran at the level of 26% DF as additives in extrusion of cornmeal. Alkali-soluble bran, with molecularly dispersed highly branched DF polymers of lower molecular weight, resulted in expansion almost as high as the control without DF, whereas the insoluble bran gave limited expansion due to presence of high content of cross-linked non-dispersed molecules. Pai *et al.* (2009) concluded that, to obtain good extrudate expansion, the shear viscosity of the melt should be low enough to promote bubble growth and expansion, but high enough to prevent bubble collapse. The type of DF has an important effect here.

Robin *et al.* (2011a–d) recently reported a detailed study about the inclusion of wheat bran in wheat flour extrusion to achieve DF levels of 12.6 and 24.4% in the product. Regardless of the bran concentration, Robin *et al.* (2011b) found that increasing both the barrel temperature and the screw speed increased the number of cells, while, on the other hand, increasing the water content decreased the number of cells. Under the same operating conditions it was found that bran concentration had an adverse effect on the volumetric expansion rate. At the same time, the influence of extrusion operating conditions was found to be less effective as the bran concentration increased. The combination of low barrel temperature, water content and screw speed gave favourable conditions for sectional expansion of wheat bran-enriched extrudates (Robin *et al.* 2011b). According to Robin *et al.* (2011b), the nucleation mechanisms for fibre-containing extrudates are slightly different from those of their counterparts. The authors claim that adding nucleation agents such as bran would decrease the free energy barrier and result in early nucleation in the die, favouring longitudinal expansion. The higher amount of bran was found to cause early bursting of air bubbles, which resulted in shrinkage. It was concluded that the overall changes were associated with not only the rheological differences between the continuous starch matrix and the filler bran particles, but also their low compatibility and interacting effects.

12.3.2 Effect of fibre type on extrudate quality

Dietary fibre sources are highly variable, and both chemical and physical properties and the presence of associated compounds can vary significantly. Cereal DF preparations typically contain cellulose, lignin and hemicelluloses as well as polyphenolics as DF components, and most often also contain starch and protein as impurities, whereas fruits and vegetables are sources of gums, pectin and mucilage. The purity, solubility and other polymer properties largely influence the performance of DF preparations in various food applications, as well as in extrusion (Elleuch *et al.*, 2011). Molecular weight, together with degree and pattern of branching, controls polymer functionality. High molecular weight fibre polymers with large hydrodynamic radii result in high viscosity dispersions. The molecular weight of soluble DF preparations (corn fibre gum, arabinogalactan and Carboxymethyl cellulose (CMC) was found to play a significant role in determining the degree of expansion (Kale *et al.*, 2010).

Various DF sources have been studied in extrusion, the main ones being wheat, oat and corn brans, and soya and beet fibres (Table 12.2). The different performance of two different types of DF ingredients was demonstrated by Yanniotis *et al.* (2007), who used commercial pectin obtained from a mixture of vegetable and fruit sources and wheat fibre (94.5% insoluble fibre and 2.5% soluble fibre) alone and in combination in the production of extruded cornstarch snacks. These very different types of fibres had different effects on mechanical and structural properties. For instance, the insoluble wheat fibre decreased the radial expansion, whereas pectin was found to have less effect. Pectin reduced the fracture of air cell walls by increasing the extensibility. The extrudates produced with higher amounts of wheat fibre and less pectin showed instability on the surface of extrudates, which is a major problem in polymer extrusion. The melt fracture caused periodic spiral formation (Fig. 12.3). In order to avoid the problem, the critical wall shear stress at the die exit has to be determined and should not be exceeded.

Wheat fibre and pectin had opposite effects on hardness and porosity of the extruded samples (Yanniotis *et al.*, 2007). Wheat fibres increased hardness and reduced porosity, whereas pectin decreased hardness and increased porosity. Thus it was claimed that the undesired effects of insoluble fibre on product texture can be overcome with the addition of soluble fibres. On the other hand, there were no data on the interaction between the two types of fibres. The superior performance of solubilized and partially hydrolysed corn fibre as compared with insoluble corn bran as an extrusion ingredient (Pai *et al.*, 2009) is discussed in Section 12.3.1.

Particle size of insoluble DF ingredients is probably one criterion influencing extrusion parameters. For instance, the particle size reduction of wheat bran to an

Table 12.2 Examples of fibre-rich ingredients used in extrusion

Fibre type	Starch ingredients	Authors
Whole grain	Wheat flour	Björck *et al.*, 1984
Wheat bran		Caprez *et al.*, 1986
Wheat bran	Corn starch	Aoe *et al.*, 1989
Wheat bran and oat fibre	Corn meal	Lue *et al.*, 1990
Sugar beet fibre	Corn meal	Lue *et al.*, 1991
Soy fibre	Corn meal	Jin *et al.*, 1994 and 1995
Wheat/Oat/Rice bran	–	Gualberto *et al.*, 1997
Apple pomace	–	Hwang, 1998
Oat	Corn flour	Liu *et al.*, 2000
Corn bran	Corn meal	Mendonca *et al.*, 2000
Cassava bran	Cassava starch	Hashimoto and Grossmann, 2003
Orange pulp	–	Larrea *et al.*, 2005
Rye bran	–	Gumul and Korus, 2006
Pectin and wheat bran	Corn starch	Yanniotis *et al.*, 2007
Wholewheat flour	–	Cheng and Friis, 2008
Wheat bran	Wheat flour	Gajula *et al.*, 2008
Distillers dried grains	Soy and corn flour	Chevanan *et al.*, 2009
Blueberry pomace	White sorghum	Khanal *et al.*, 2009
Corn fibre	Corn meal	Pai *et al.*, 2009
Corn bran	–	Kale *et al.*, 2010
Oat and wheat bran	Wholewheat flour	Chassagne-Berces *et al.*, 2011
Oat bran, inulin	Corn starch	Lobato *et al.*, 2011
Guar gum	Maize, potato, rice and wheat flour	Parada *et al.*, 2011
Quinoa	–	Repo-Carrasco-Valencia and Serna *et al.*, 2011
Wheat bran	Wheat flour	Robin *et al.*, 2011a,b,c,d
Beta glucan	Oat flour	Yao *et al.*, 2011
Oat bran	–	Zhang *et al.*, 2009, 2011

average of 345 nm caused a decrease in hydration properties (Zhu *et al.*, 2010), and the hydration properties of coconut fibre increased when the particle size decreased from 1127 to 550 μm, whereas they decreased when it was reduced from 550 to 390 μm (Raghavendra *et al.*, 2006). The hydration properties influence melt properties, and also the particle properties may have an influence on the bubble cell wall homogeneity.

12.3.3 Role of other ingredients in fibre-enriched extrusion

Understanding the interaction mechanisms within different ingredients is important in design of high quality nutritious healthy snacks. A basic expanded snack formulation generally includes starch, sugar, salt, protein, fat and water. Optimizing

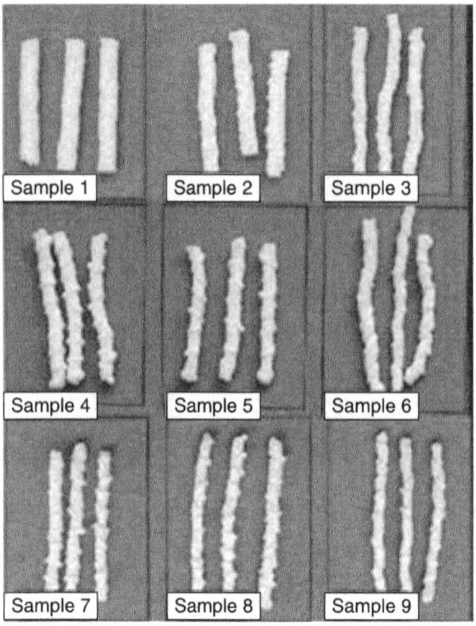

Sample	Starch %	Wheat bran %	Pectin %
1	100	0	0
2	95	0	5
3	90	0	10
4	95	5	0
5	90	5	5
6	85	5	10
7	90	10	0
8	85	10	5
9	80	10	10

Fig. 12.3 Samples of extrudates with different percentages of corn starch, wheat fibre and pectin (Yanniotis *et al.*, 2007).

the type and source of starch can help to improve textural properties and expansion ratios. There should be 60–70% of starch in the formulation for good expansion characteristics and good gas-holding properties of fibre-enriched extrudates. Sugar, fat and fibre interfere with the expansion of the starch matrix (Yao *et al.*, 2011). Expansion rates at high fibre levels can be improved by addition of extrusion aids such as monoglycerides, modified starches, modified gelatin, oligofructose and inulin. The two latter are soluble non-digestible oligo- and polysaccharides, which are nowadays included in the definition of DF. These ingredients will not only improve expansion rates but also provide additional functional properties.

Starch and proteins are the two dominating ingredients that contribute to the solid matrix in extruded food products. Proteins can affect the expansion rate based on differences in macromolecular structure and conformation, as well as differences in their water-binding affinities. High temperature and shear occurring during extrusion processing destabilize the tertiary and quaternary structures of proteins, leading to denaturation. During extrusion, protein molecules unfold and align themselves in the direction of flow and form new intermolecular bonds, disulphide bonds being the major form (Camire, 1991). Fourier transform infrared (FTIR) spectra of corn/oat flour extrudates revealed that extrusion caused changes in the protein bands and the distribution of protein occurred heterogeneously within a discontinuous phase. It was claimed that the protein phase was destroyed during extrusion, producing aggregates that formed fibrous networks (Cremer and Kaletunç, 2003).

Lobato *et al.* (2011) developed a functional puffed product with defatted soy flour, oat bran, corn starch and inulin. An increase in corn starch content from 200 to 300 g/kg total weight in the formulation decreased hardness to 200 N, a critical threshold hardness value for consumer acceptance. Increase in screw speed increases the mechanical damage to starch molecules. The damaged starch which is formed during extrusion is less cohesive than gelatinized starch, resulting in small pores with less expansion. Increasing levels of sugar and soy fibre formed extrudates with thick cell walls and smaller air cells with high breaking strength values (Jin *et al.*, 1995). Extrudates with low sugar levels were found to have thin cell walls and large air cell size.

Núñez *et al.* (2010) studied the effect of shear on elongational properties of extruded breakfast cereals made of oat and rice flour. The high lipid content of oat flour resulted in polymer stick-slip transition, which caused instabilities during processing. The majority of end products contain low levels of lipid (< 7%) because higher levels of lipid prevent expansion. On the other hand, addition of low levels of lipid (5%) favours expansion and improves texture (Cheftel, 1986). During extrusion lipids can be either entrapped or encapsulated as droplets. They also have a tendency to interact with starch and protein.

In order to produce snack foods with enhanced nutrient profile, the content of protein and/or DF should be increased. However, both these ingredients have a critical concentration, beyond which the important quality control parameters (expansion, brittleness etc.) are adversely affected. Addition of both DF and protein causes low expansion rate with increased bulk density, which will eventually lead to hard and crunchy rather than crispy product textures. A new approach is to use supercritical fluid extrusion (SCFX) instead of the conventional steam-based extruders. With the help of SCFX the detrimental effects of heat on the structural properties will be avoided by using low temperature profiles (< 100°C) (Cho and Rizvi, 2009; Cho and Rizvi, 2010). The SCFX of starch-based products consists of three processes in which melt formation takes place because of starch gelatinization and mixing; the supercritical CO_2 addition at this step creates melt–CO_2 solution. Diffusion of CO_2 through the cells causes expansion of product in the die exit. In general, the SCFX is followed by baking or frying for further expansion and improvement of flavour and appearance. Alavi *et al.* (1999) showed that the SCFX products have a non-porous surface and uniform cell size distribution (50–250 μm) with a high polydispersity index (0.95), which provides better flavour encapsulation.

12.4 Effects of extrusion on dietary fibre (DF) properties

12.4.1 Changes in DF polymers

The DF content usually does not greatly decrease in extrusion, whereas the ratio of insoluble to soluble DF often decreases due to depolymerization and solubilization of insoluble fibre components. If depolymerization of the soluble DF occurs to such an extent that the hydrolysis products are no longer analysed as DF, the DF content may decrease. Under harsh extrusion conditions, the DF content may also increase due to formation of resistant starch or some undigestible Maillard reaction products. The polysaccharide–lipid complexes formed during extrusion cannot be separated either chemically or enzymatically, and thus they were found to contribute to the insoluble fibre fraction, together with resistant starches (Gualberto *et al.*, 1997). Variable results have been obtained in studies on the effects of extrusion on DF polymers, depending on extrusion conditions and also to a large extent on the DF ingredients used, as reviewed, for example, by Singh *et al.* (2007) and Camire *et al.* (1990).

Zhang *et al.* (2009; 2011) showed that the extrusion of oat bran altered the molecular weight distribution of soluble DF fractions of oat bran, and the amount of soluble DF was increased from 8.9% to 14% by extrusion. Extrusion was also reported to promote the extraction of high molecular weight DF from oat bran and improve the properties of the soluble oat DF, but the effects of feed moisture and temperature during extrusion were significant. On the other hand, extruded breakfast cereals made of oat flours with elevated β-glucan contents had higher peak molecular weight than the corresponding raw materials (Yao *et al.*, 2011).

Solubilization of DF in wheat, oat and rice brans was also shown by Gualberto *et al.* (1997), who related it to screw speed and barrel pressure profiles. For instance, an increase in soluble fractions of DF was detected by increasing the screw speed. The shear stress exerted by the turning of the screws puts a strain on the DF molecules, causing chemical cleavage. Pressure builds up in the barrel at low screw speeds because of higher rate of barrel fill. In some cases pressure might have more effect than the screw speed on the solubilization rate of DF. Larrea *et al.* (2005) extruded an orange pulp preparation and detected a remarkable decrease in total and insoluble DF and increase in soluble DF content. Temperature in the barrel was the most important factor influencing the changes in the orange peel pectin, followed by the screw speed.

Extrusion-induced changes in wheat bran properties have been reported, for example, by Aoe *et al.* (1989) and Gajula *et al.* (2008). Both reported increased soluble DF content. The latter reported that the decrease of insoluble dietary fibre fraction was higher than the increase in the soluble fraction, and suggested that the fragmentation of cellulose or lignin by the shearing action of extrusion results in formation of lower molecular weight soluble DF residues, which can degrade further to low molecular weight fragments and also to sugar derivatives. Scanning electron microscopy (SEM) images revealed structural changes in the extruded bran as thinning out of the cell wall and either folding or curling of the pericarp layers (Aoe *et al.*, 1989), also modifying the physicochemical form of DF and its fermentability in rats.

12.4.2 Changes in associated compounds

The majority of the plant DF preparations are also rich in bioactive phytochemicals. The outer parts of the cereal kernel, which contain bran and germ, are rich in phenolic acids, lignans and phytosterols (Liukkonen *et al.*, 2003; Inglett and Chen, 2011; Jonnala *et al.*, 2010). The amount and bioaccessibility of bioactive compounds, in particular phenolics, in DF preparations can be altered during processing, as recently reviewed by Brennan *et al.* (2011). The amount of polyphenols has been shown to decrease with extrusion in cereal extrudates fortified with vegetable/fruit by-products (Yagci and Gogus, 2009; Khanal *et al.*, 2009; White *et al.*, 2010). However, the levels increased in extrusion of rye, quinoa and wheat flour/cauliflower-based snacks (Gumul and Korus, 2006; Repo-Carrosco-Valencia and Serna, 2011; Stojceska *et al.*, 2008). Better extractability of bioactive compounds has been associated with the release of phenolic acids by extrusion (Brennan *et al.*, 2011).

12.4.3 Changes in nutritional properties

DF addition *per se* improves the nutritional quality of the product. The physiological effects of DF and the product can further change due to extrusion-induced changes, as indicated above. The nutritional consequences of changes in DF due to extrusion have been discussed in the review by Singh *et al.* (2007), who indicated that there are conflicting results with respect to cholesterol-lowering properties in animal studies. Taking into consideration the large variation in raw materials and processing conditions, this actually seems quite natural.

In a recent study by Parada *et al.* (2011), various levels of guar gum as a soluble fibre source were used in extruded foods made from maize, potato, rice and wheat flour. Starch digestibility *in vitro* did not decrease with addition of guar gum; instead a small increase in rapidly available glucose was observed. This was suggested to be due to softer texture and more open microstructure of the products.

12.5 Conclusion and future trends

The demand for 'natural' and 'nutritionally enhanced' foods is increasing. The daily supply of fibre has been reduced by the consumption of ready-made or processed foods. The importance of DF intake for human health has been recognized for the past 40 years, and the DF terminology, definitions and analytics have evolved over time (Raninen *et al.* 2011).

The world snack food market was worth around $55 billion by the year 2000. The largest snack food market is in the US, followed by Japan and the UK (http://www.managementparadise.com/forums/marketing-research-mr/218772-marketing-research-whirlpool-corporation.html). Today's consumer has an increasing demand for healthy snacking with low salt and fat and high dietary fibre and protein values. The healthy food market, consisting of functional, good/better-for-you and organic foods, has also influenced the snack food market to design next generation healthy snack foods. In Europe, the savoury snacks market (potato chips, nuts, biscuits, extruded snacks) was worth €12.4 billion in 2009, with an annual growth rate of 0.54% for the 2009–12 period (http://foodmarkets.wordpress.com/2011/02/08/savoury-snacks-europe-potato-crisps-nuts-biscuits).

After all the attempts during the past decades, extrusion processing is still considered to be more of an art than a science. In order to have better control over the entire process, scientists have to explore the interrelationship among ingredients, processing conditions and structural factors such as molecular weight in interdisciplinary collaboration between rheology, polymer physics and chemistry. Quantitative modelling of extrusion processing will allow efficient product development stages with reduced time and cost. Cheng and Friis (2010) used a new phenomenological model that links expansion and operation parameters of a twin screw extruder of wholewheat flour and fish feed. The model was developed based on dimensional analysis theory and aimed to understand the physical meaning of interactions among raw material mixing, particle size condition, ingredients and operation parameters.

Cell wall strength and elasticity have a great impact on the mechanical properties of porous DF-rich extrudates. Thus, understanding the factors that affect composition and thermal properties will guide scientists to engineer structural features of the food matrix. Improvement of three-dimensional non-destructive analysis methods will provide data to evaluate the relationship between cell architecture, texture and operational parameters (Corradini and Peleg, 2007).

Following the early work in the 1990s, DF-enriched extrusion is currently a vibrant research topic. Snack foods are an obvious carrier of dietary fibre, and healthier options in this product category are warranted. It can be expected that the active research will gradually be translated to new types of cereal snacks, and also that extrusion will increasingly be used to functionalize DF preparations to enhance their applicability.

12.6 References

ALAVI, S.H., GOGOI, B.K., KHAN, M., BOWMAN, B.J., and RIZVI, S.S.H. (1999). Structural properties of protein-stabilized starch-based supercritical fluid extrudates. *Food Res. Int.*, **32**: 107–18.

ANNEX I (EC) No: 1924/2006 of 30 Dec 2006 lastly amended by Regulation (EC) No 1116/2010. REGULATION (EC) No 1924/2006 OF THE EUROPEAN PARLIAMENT AND OF THE COUNCIL of 20 December 2006 on nutrition and health claims made on foods.

AOE, S., NAKAOKA, M., IDO, K., TAMAI, Y., OHTA, F. and AYANO, Y. (1989) Availability of dietary fibre in extruded wheat bran and apparent digestibility in rats of coexisting nutrients. *Cereal Chem.*, **66**(4):252–6.

BJÖRCK, I., NYMAN, M. and ASP, N.G. (1984) Extrusion cooking and dietary fibre: Effects on dietary fibre content and on degradation in the rat intestinal tract. *Cereal Chem.*, **61**(2):174–9.

BLAKE, O.A. (2006) *Effect of molecular and supramolecular characteristics of select dietary fibres on extrusion expansion* (PhD Thesis). Purdue University, Indiana, US.

BRENNAN, C., BRENNAN, M., DERBYSHIRE, E. and TIWARI, B.K. (2011) Effects of extrusion on the polyphenols, vitamins and antioxidant activity of foods. *Trends Food Sci. Tech.*, **22**:570–5.

CAMIRE, M.E., CAMIRE, A., KRUMHAR, K. (1990) Chemical and nutritional changes in foods during extrusion. *Crit. Rev. Food Sci. Nutr.*, **29**:35–57.

CAMIRE, M.E. (1991) Protein functionality modification by extrusion cooking. *JAOCS*, **68**(3): 200–5.

CAPREZ, A., ARRIGONI, E., AMADO, R. and ZEUKOM, H. (1986) Influence of different types of thermal treatment on the chemical composition and physical properties of wheat bran. *J. Cereal Sci.*, **4**:233–9.

CHASSAGNE-BERCES, S., LEITNER, M., MELADO, A., BARREIRO, P., CORREA, E.C., *et al.* (2011) Effect of fibres and whole grain content on quality attributes of extruded cereals. *Proceedings of ICEF 2011, International Congress of Engineering and Food, ICEF 2011*, International Congress of Engineering and Food, 22–26 May 2011, Athens, Greece.

CHEFTEL, J.C. (1986) Nutritional effects of extrusion-cooking. *Food Chem.*, **20**(4):263–83.

CHEN, J. and ROSENTHAL, A. (2009) Food processing. In: G. CAMPBELL-PLATT (Ed.) *Food Science and Technology*. Wiley-Blackwell, West Sussex, UK, pp. 232–3.

CHEN, K.H. and RIZVI, S.S.H. (2006) Rheology and expansion of starch-water-CO_2 mixtures with controlled gelatinization by supercritical fluid extrusion. *Int. J. Food Prop.*, **9**:863–76.

CHENG, H. and FRIIS, A. (2008) Expansion of the whole wheat flour extrusion. *Proceedings of the 5th International Conference on Simulation and Modelling in the Food and Bio-Industry – FoodSim 2008*, Dublin, Ireland, 26–28 June 2008. http://orgprints.org/19729/2/19729.pdf (date accessed 18 October 2012).

CHENG, H. and FRIIS, A. (2010) Modelling extrudate expansion in a twin-screw food extrusion cooking process through dimensional analysis methodology. *Food Bioprod. Process.*, **88**:188–94.

CHEVANAN, N., MUTHUKUMARAPPAN, K. and ROSENTRATER, K.A. (2009) Extrusion studies of aquaculture feed using distillers dried grains with solubles and whey. *Food Bioprocess. Technol.*, **2**:177–85.

CHINNASWAMY, R. and HANNA, M.A. (1988) Optimum Extrusion-Cooking Conditions for Maximum Expansion of Corn Starch. *J. Food Sci.*, **53**(3):834–6.

CHO, K.Y. and RIZVI, S.S.H. (2009) 3D microstructure of supercritical fluid extrudates I: Melt rheology and microstructure formation. *Food Res. Int.*, **42**: 595–602.

CHO, K.Y. and RIZVI, S.S.H. (2010) New generation of healthy snack food by supercritical fluid extrusion. *J. Food Process Preserv.*, **34**: 192–218.

COGSWELL, F.N. (1994) *Polymer melt rheology: a guide for industrial practice*. Woodhead Publishing Ltd, Cambridge, UK.

CORRADINI, M.G. and PELEG, M. (2007) Solid food foams. In: J.M. AGUILERA and P.J. LILLFORD (Eds) *Topics in Food Materials Science*. Springer, New York, NY, pp. 169–202.

CREMER, D.R. and KALETUNÇ, G. (2003) Fourier transform infrared microspectroscopic study of the chemical microstructure of corn and oat flour-based extrudates. *Carbohydr. Polym.*, **52**:53–65.

DING, Q.B., AINSWORTH, P., PLUNKETT, A., TUCKER, G. and MARSON, H. (2006) The effect of extrusion conditions on the functional and physical properties of wheat-based expanded snacks. *J. Food Eng.*, **73**:142–8.

EASTMAN, J., ORTHOEFER, F. and SOLORIO, S. (2001) Using extrusion to create breakfast cereal products. *Cereal Foods World*, **46**(10):468–71.

ELLEUCH, M., BEDIGIAN, D., ROISEUX, O., BESBES, S., BLECKER, C. and ATTIA, H. (2011). Dietary fibre and fibre-rich by-products of food processing: characterisation, technological functionality and commercial applications: A review. *Food Chem.*, **124**:411–21.

FLETCHER, S.I., RICHMOND, P. and SMITH, A.C. (1985) An experimental study of twin-screw extrusion-cooking of maize grits. *J. Food Eng.*, **4**(4):291–312.

GAJULA, H., ALAVI, S., ADHIKARI, K. and HERALD, T. (2008) Precooked Bran-Enriched Wheat Flour Using Extrusion: Dietary Fibre Profile and Sensory Characteristics. *J. Food Sci.*, **73**(4):S173–179.

GUALBERTO, D.G., BERGMAN, C.J., KAZEMZADEH, M.C. and WEBER, C.W. (1997) Effect of extrusion processing on the soluble and insoluble fibre, and phytic acid contents of cereal brans. *Plant Foods Hum. Nutr.*, **51**:187–98.

GUMUL, D. and KORUS, J. (2006) Polyphenol content and antioxidant activity of rye bran extrudates produced at varying parameters of extrusion process. *Electronic J. Polish Agr. Univ.*, **9**(4):1–9.

GUY, R. (2001) Raw materials for extrusion cooking. In: R. GUY (Ed.) *Extrusion cooking technologies and applications*. Woodhead Publishing Ltd, Cambridge, UK, pp. 5–28.

GUY, R. C. E. (1985). The extrusion revolution. *Food Manufacture*, **60**:26–7, 29.

HAGENIMANA, A., DING, X., YING, D. and GU, W. (2007) Steady state flow behaviours of extruded blend of rice flour and soy protein concentrate. *Food Chem.*, **101**:241–7.

HASHIMOTO, J.M. and GROSSMANN, M.V.E. (2003) Effects of extrusion conditions on quality of cassava bran/cassava starch extrudates. *Int. J. Food Sci. Tech.*, **38**:511–17.

HERMANSSON, A.-M. (1988) Gel structure of food biopolymers. In: J.M.V. BLANSHARD and J.R. MITCHELL (Eds) *Food structure—Its creation and evaluation*. Butterworths, London, p. 25.

HWANG, J.K. (1998) Solubilization of apple pomace by extrusion. *J. Food Process. Pres.*, **22**:477–91.

ILO, S., SCHOENLECHNER, R. and BERGHOFE, E. (2000) Role of lipids in the extrusion cooking processes. *Grasas Y Aceites*, **51**(1–2):97–110.

INGLETT, G.E. and CHEN, D. (2011) Antioxidant Activity and Phenolic Content of Air-Classified Corn Bran. *Cereal Chem.*, **88**(1):36–40.

JIN, Z., HSIEH, F. and HUFF, H. E. (1994) Extrusion cooking of corn meal with soy fibre, salt, and sugar. *Cereal Chem.*, **71**(3):227–34.

JIN, Z., HSIEH, F. and HUFF, H.E. (1995) Effects of Soy Fibre, Salt, Sugar and Screw Speed on Physical Properties and Microstructure of Corn Meal Extrudate. *J. Cereal Sci.*, **22**:185–94.

JONNALA, R.S., IRMAK, S., MACRITCHIE, F. and BEAN, S.R. (2010) Phenolics in the bran of waxy wheat and triticale lines. *J. Cereal Sci.*, **52**:509–15.

KALE, M.S., PAI, D.A., HAMAKER, B.R. and CAMPANELLA, O.H. (2010) Structure–function relationships for corn bran arabinoxylans. *J. Cereal Sci.*, **52**:368–72.

KHANAL, R.C., HOWARD, L.R., BROWNMILLER, C.R. and PRIOR, R.L. (2009) Influence of extrusion processing on procyanidin composition and total anthocyanin contents of blueberry pomace. *J. Food Sci.*, **74**(2):H52–H58.

LAI, L.S. and KOKINI, J.L. (1991) Physicochemical Changes and Rheological Properties of Starch during Extrusion (A Review). *Biotech. Progress*, **7**(3):251–66.

LARREA, M.A., CHANG, Y.K. and MARTINEZ-BUSTOS, F. (2005) Some functional properties of extruded orange pulp and its effect on the quality of cookies. *LWT*, **38**:213–20.

LAZOU, A. and KROKIDA, M. (2011) Thermal characterisation of corn–lentil extruded snacks. *Food Chem.*, **127**:1625–33.

LIU, Y., HSIEH, H., HEYMANN, H. and HUFF, H. E. (2000). Effect of processing conditions on the physical and sensory properties of extruded oat-corn puff. *J. Food Sci.*, **65**(7):1253–9.

LIUKKONEN, K.H., KATINA, K., WILHELMSON, A., MYLLYMÄKI, O., LAMPI, A.M., *et al.* (2003). Process-induced changes on bioactive compounds in whole grain rye. *Proc. Nutr. Soc.*, **62**:117–22.

LOBATO, L.P., ANIBAL, D., LAZARETTI, M.M. and GROSSMANN, M.V.E. (2011) Extruded puffed functional ingredient with oat bran and soy flour. *LWT*, **44**:933–9.

LUE, S., HSIEH, F., PENG, I.C. and HUFF, H.E. (1990) Expansion of corn extrudates containing dietary fibre: a microstructure study. *Lebensmittel-Wissenschaft Und-Technologie*, **23**(2):165–73.

LUE, S., HSIEH, F. and HUFF, H.E. (1991). Extrusion cooking of corn meal and sugar beet fibre: Effects on expansion properties, starch gelatinization, and dietary fibre content. *Cereal Chem.*, **68**(3):227–34.

MENDONCA, S., GROSSMANN, M.V.E. and VERHE, R. (2000). Corn bran as a fibre source in expanded snacks. *Lebensmittel-Wissenschaft und-Technologie*, **33**:2–8.

MILLER, E. and ROTHSTEIN, J.P. (2004) Control of the sharkskin instability in the extrusion of polymer melts using induced temperature gradients. *Rheol. Acta*, **44**:160–73.

MOORE, D., SANEI, A., VAN HECKE, E., and BOUVIER, J.M. (1990) Effect of ingredients on physical/structural properties of extrudates. *J. Food Sci.*, **55**(5):1383–402.

NOGUCHI, A. (1989) Extrusion cooking of high moisture foods. In: KOKINI, J.L., HO, C. and KARWE, M.V. (Eds) *Food Extrusion Science and Technology*. Marcel Dekker, Inc., New York, pp. 343–70.

NÚÑEZ, M., DELLA VALLE, G. and SANDOVAL, A.J. (2010) Shear and elongational viscosities of a complex starchy formulation for extrusion cooking. *Food Res. Int.* **43**:2093–100.

PAI, D.A., BLAKE, O.A., HAMAKER, B.R. and CAMPANELLA, O.H. (2009) Importance of extensional rheological properties on fibre-enriched corn extrudates. *J. Cereal Sci.*, **50**:227–34.

PARADA, J., AGUILERA, J.M. and BRENNAN, C. (2011) Effect of guar gum content on some physical and nutritional properties of extruded products. *J. Food Eng.*, **103**:324–32.

RAGHAVENDRA, S.N., SWAMY, S.R., RASTOGI, N.K., RAGHAVARAO, K.S.M.S., KUMAR, S. and THARANATHAN, R.N. (2006) Grinding characteristics and hydration properties of coconut residue: A source of dietary fibre. *J. Food Eng.*, **72**:281–6.

RANINEN, K., LAPPI, J., MYKKÄNEN, H. and POUTANEN, K. (2011) Dietary fiber type reflects physiological functionality: comparison of grain fiber, inulin, and polydextrose. *Nutrition Reviews*, **69**(1): 9–21.

REPO-CARRASCO-VALENCIA, R.A.M. and SERNA, L.A. (2011) Quinoa (*Chenopodium quinoa*, Willd.) as a source of dietary fibre and other functional components. *Ciênc. Tecnol. Aliment.*, Campinas, **31**(1):225–30.

ROBIN, F., DUBOIS, C., CURTI, D., SCHUCHMANN, H.P. and PALZER, S. (2011a) Effect of wheat bran on the mechanical properties of extruded starchy foams. *Food Res. Int.*, **44**:2880–8.

ROBIN, F., DUBOIS, C., PINEAU, N., SCHUCHMANN, H.P. and PALZER, S. (2011b) Expansion mechanism of extruded foams supplemented with wheat bran. *J. Food Eng.*, **107**(1):80–9.

ROBIN, F., THÉODULOZA, C., GIANFRANCESCOA, A., PINEAUB, N., SCHUCHMANN, H.P. and PALZERD, S. (2011c) Starch transformation in bran-enriched extruded wheat flour. *Carbohydr. Polym.*, **85**:65–74.

ROBIN, F., BOVET, N., PINEAU, N., SCHUCHMANN, H.P. and PALZER, S. (2011d) Online Shear Viscosity Measurement of Starchy Melts Enriched in Wheat Bran. *J. Food Sci.*, **76**(5):E405–E412.

SINGH, N. and SMITH, A.C. (1997) A comparison of wheat starch, whole wheat meal and oat flour in the extrusion cooking process. *J. Food Eng.*, **34**:15–32.

SINGH, S., GAMLATH, S. and WAKELING, L. (2007) Nutritional aspects of food extrusion: a review. *Int. J. Food Sci. Tech.*, **42**(8):916–29.

STOJCESKA, V., AINSWORTH, P., PLUNKETT, P., IBANOGLU, E. and IBANOGLU, S. (2008) Cauliflower by-products as a new source of dietary fibre, antioxidants and proteins in cereal based ready-to-eat expanded snacks. *J. Food Eng.*, **87**:554–563

STOJCESKA, V., AINSWORTH, P., PLUNKETTA, A. and IBANOĞLU, S. (2010) The advantage of using extrusion processing for increasing dietary fibre level in gluten-free products. *Food Chem.*, **121**(1):156–64.

VERGNES, B., VILLEMAIRE, J.P., COLONNA, P. and TAYEB, J. (1987) Interrelationships between thermomechanical treatment and macromolecular degradation of maize starch in a novel rheometer with preshearing. *J. Cereal Sci.*, **5**:189–202.

WHITE, B.L., HOWARD, L.R. and PRIOR, R.L. (2010) Polyphenolic composition and antioxidant capacity of extruded cranberry pomace. *J. Agric. Food Chem.*, **58**(7):4037–42.

XIE, F., HALLEY, P.J. and AVÉROUS, L. (2012) Rheology to understand and optimize processibility, structures and properties of starch polymeric materials. *Progress Poly. Sci.*, **37**(4):595–623.

YAGCI, S. and GOGUS, F. (2009) Effect of incorporation of various food by-products on some nutritional properties of rice-based extruded foods. *Food Sci. Technol. Int.*, **15**(6):571–81.

YANNIOTIS, S., PETRAKI, A. and SOUMPASI, E. (2007) Effect of pectin and wheat fibres on quality attributes of extruded cornstarch. *J. Food Eng.*, **80**:594–9.

YAO, N., WHITE, P.J. and ALAVI, S. (2011) Impact of β-glucan and other oat flour components on physico-chemical and sensory properties of extruded oat cereals. *Int. J. Food Sci. Technol.*, **46**:651–60.

ZHANG, M., LIANG, Y., PEI, Y., GAO, W.W. and ZHANG, Z.S. (2009) Effect of process on physicochemical properties of oat bran soluble dietary fibre. *J. Food Sci.*, **74**:C628–C636.

ZHANG, M., BAI, X. and ZHANG, Z. (2011) Extrusion process improves the functionality of soluble dietary fibre in oat bran. *J. Cereal Sci.*, **107**(1):98–103.

ZHU, K., HUANG, S., PENG, W., QIAN, H. and ZHOU, H. (2010) Effect of ultrafine grinding on hydration and antioxidant properties of wheat bran dietary fibre. *Food Res. Int.*, **43**:943–8.

13

Fibre-enriched and wholewheat pasta

C. S. Brennan, Lincoln University, New Zealand

DOI: 10.1533/9780857095787.3.273

Abstract: Pasta is a commonly consumed food product, which makes it ideal for the inclusion of wholegrain and dietary fibre material. However, technological and processing issues surround the use of these ingredients in pasta. These tend to revolve around hydration dynamics of ingredients and the development of a homogeneous starch–protein matrix during dough formation. From a nutritional point of view it is clear that the inclusion of whole grains and dietary fibre has significant positive effects in controlling satiety and the postprandial glycaemic response. These issues are discussed in this chapter.

Key words: pasta, dietary fibre, whole grains, starch gelatinisation, glycaemic index.

13.1 Introduction

Pasta is a very generic term used to describe a commonly consumed food group which encompasses noodles, spaghetti and similar commodities. The word 'pasta' is derived from the Latin word meaning 'dough/pastry cake', which describes its constitution very well. Traditionally pasta has been made using two basic ingredients – wheat (*Triticum durum* – durum wheat), semolina, and water. Indeed, in the past Italian law has insisted that the manufacture of pasta has to be from *Triticum durum* and not *Triticum aestivum* (GazzettaUfficiale, 1967; Cubadda and Carcea, 2000). The purity of pasta processing has been maintained in some European countries, where any incorporation of *Triticum aestivum* into pasta was classed as adulteration and considered illegal. The history and origins of pasta are worthy of a book of their own. Unfortunately space does not exist in this volume to do the history of pasta justice. Its past appears to lie in the production of noodles in China, which have been shown to date back to at least 300 BC (Lu *et al.*, 2005; Gong *et al.*, 2011). However, it is clear that there has been a heavy Italian influence, not only on the popularity and widespread use of pasta but on the development of different forms of pasta shapes.

In its simplest form, the durum wholegrain/wholewheat flour and water are mixed into a crumb-like dough before being formed. The mixing and forming can be conducted either by manual manipulation or, more commercially, using extrusion technology. The resulting dough sheet or extruded product is then cut into appropriate shapes. Two main types of pasta are produced: fresh (wet) pasta, which is only minimally dried and has a high moisture content and hence has a relatively short shelf life, or dried pasta – pasta dried to between 4 and 8% moisture, which is therefore more shelf-stable. The ease of pasta manufacture and the simplicity of raw material formulation make pasta a relatively inexpensive food product to manufacture, which has led to its popularity as a convenient food.

This insistence on pasta being produced from durum wholegrain and refined wheat flour has led to a plethora of research into the various factors contributing to pasta quality maintenance. These studies examine areas ranging from the physical and chemical properties of durum grains to the effect of water and the milling of durum into wholemeal or refined flour. Pasta quality and cooking characteristics have been shown to be dependent upon the protein–starch matrix of the extruded pasta product. Characteristics such as firmness, cooking loss and stickiness of pasta can be associated with the protein content of the pasta (Oak *et al.*, 2006) as well as the starch composition (El-Khayat *et al.*, 2003; 2006). The even hydration of the starch and protein fractions in the semolina during the mixing stages of processing is responsible for ensuring the formation of a suitable pasta shape which is both resistant to stretching and manipulation and also elastic in nature. If the starch and protein are poorly hydrated, this disrupts the development of the cohesive matrix and leads to brittle or soft sticky pasta. Inclusion of wholegrain, wholemeal, or dietary fibre-rich components into pasta can also interfere with the development of the starch–protein matrix and lead to disruption of the structural integrity of the pasta as well as reduction in final quality and consumer acceptability (Tudorica *et al.*, 2002).

13.1.1 Understanding durum wheat flour characteristics

The physicochemical quality of the durum wheat kernel is a major determinant of the suitability of the crop for its end-use, and inevitably is responsible for the quality of pasta (Mariani *et al.*, 1995; El-Khayat *et al.*, 2003; 2006). Factors which have been shown to affect durum wheat quality include genotype (Troccoli *et al.*, 2000), environment (Kovacs *et al.*, 1997; Sharma *et al.*, 2002) and the interaction between genotype and environment. The hardness of the cereal grain is considered to be an important factor that determines end-use quality characteristics of durum wheat. This is particularly important when considering the milling process, in that grain hardness has a significant impact on the facture characteristics of kernels during milling (Symes, 1961). Subsequently, the milling properties of hard or soft grains have effects on factors such as the conditioning of wheat before milling, the particle size of flour, quantity of damaged starch, water absorption and milling extraction rate (Hoseney, 1987; Pomeranz and Williams, 1990; Delwiche, 1993), as well as the rheological properties of the flour produced (Pomeranz *et al.*, 1984).

Additionally, the milling quality of durum wheat is reflected in the total yield of flour from the milled grains. Milling can remove between 15 and 20% of grain weight (in the form of bran and germ). The hardness or softness of the grain affects the overall recovery of flour during milling and, inversely, the amount of bran, germ and dietary fibre lost during milling (El-Khayat *et al.*, 2003). Much of the research investigating the genetic basis of kernel hardness has been conducted on *Triticum aestivum*. Such work has illustrated the role of the starch granule proteins, sometimes named friabilins (Greenwell and Schofield, 1986; Brennan *et al.*, 1993) and other times puroindolines (Baldwin, 2001; Igrejas *et al.*, 2001), which inhibit starch–protein binding and hence govern grain softness. The scarcity of these puroindolines in durum wheats is often regarded as one of the factors which explain the high hardness of durum wheat kernels.

In durum wheat, the degree of vitreousness of the kernel is often used, in conjunction with kernel hardness, to predict the quality of the cereal crop. The degree of kernel translucency, and hence the apparent degree of vitreousness, is related to the degree of compactness of the kernel (Yamazaki and Donelson, 1983). The degree of vitreousness of kernels has been linked to the hardness of the kernel, and the amount of protein and starch within the kernel (Stenvert and Kingswood, 1977). Starchy kernels have been shown to have a discontinuous endosperm with many air spaces and appear white in colour (Dexter *et al.*, 1989). These air spaces, and the more porous nature of the kernel, appear to be related to softer texture of the starchy kernels. Many studies have shown that environmental factors, such as temperature and light intensity during grain development, determine whether the kernels will appear vitreous or starchy (Parish and Halse, 1968; Hoseney, 1987). Pomeranz and Williams (1990) observed that nitrogen fertilisation affects kernel protein content, and hence the hardness and appearance of kernels. So the degree of vitreousness is highly influenced by both genetic and environmental factors.

The degree of vitreousness of a grain has an important impact on the milling quality of durum wheat because of its effect on semolina yield, granulation and protein content (Matsuo and Dexter, 1980). By growing durum wheat in low protein environments one can manipulate the grain composition to decrease kernel protein content and increase starchiness (decrease of kernel vitreousness). This in turn has the effect of decreasing semolina yield (El-Khayat *et al.*, 2006). As mentioned before, as semolina yield decreases so too do the amount of bran and fibre content of the flour (milling yield being positively correlated with high starch contents). Thus protein content is one of the most important quality characteristics of durum wheat kernels in relation to determining milling yield, starch and fibre content, and overall pasta quality (Dexter and Matsuo, 1977; 1980; Autran and Galterrio, 1989). The initial research of Dexter and Matsuo (1977) was the starting point of our understanding of how protein from durum wheat can influence pasta quality. They investigated two Canadian durum wheat cultivars that differed in their protein contents, but were grown under the same environmental conditions, and found that the increase in protein content was associated with an increase in pigment content and improvement in cooking quality of the resulting pasta.

Although total protein content is a major factor in final pasta quality, research has also investigated the importance of the gluten components in determining the rheological and cooking quality of pasta (Damidaux *et al.*, 1980; Du Cros *et al.*, 1982; Carrillo *et al.*, 1990).

Ash content is also regarded as a quality characteristic for durum wheat kernels and has a direct influence on pasta colour. The faint colour of semolina is caused by high ash content, and may be due to high extraction rates (Cubadda, 1988). The resulting pasta tends to have a brown colour (Taha and Sagi, 1987; Borrelli *et al.*, 1999). Premium-grade semolina generally has ash content lower than 0.9% (Cubadda, 1988).

13.1.2 Nutritional quality of pasta

The nutritional quality of pasta is balanced as shown in Table 13.1. As can be seen from the table, the contribution of pasta to the diet is mainly in terms of carbohydrates (not surprisingly in terms of the composition of the raw materials used). Pasta also contains an appreciable level of protein, and in certain types (such as wholemeal spaghetti) can be a contributor of dietary fibre to our diet. From an energy intake point of view, pasta and spaghetti have a relatively low energy value when compared with other carbohydrate counterparts such as white or wholemeal bread (931 and 922 kJ, respectively). This in turn leads to pasta being considered a relatively low glycaemic index (GI) food compared with breads and biscuits (Table 13.2). Another contributing factor to the low GI of pasta compared with bread is the particle size of the flours after milling and the degree of starch damage during milling. High levels of starch damage increase the rate of starch digestibility, whereas large particle sizes of flour (above 300 μm) reduce the degree of hydration of the starch granules in the dough and hence lower the accessibility of starch degrading enzymes to the starch held within the starch–protein matrix of pasta.

Today's food industry is interested in low GI foods and foods containing high amounts of dietary fibre. The fact that pasta has a limited number of raw ingredients

Table 13.1 Chemical composition of cooked pasta (per 100 g)

Pasta type	Water (g)	Protein (g)	Fat (g)	Carbohydrate (g)	Starch (g)	Dietary fibre (g)	Energy value (kJ)
Macaroni	78.1	3.0	0.5	18.5	18.2	0.9	1483
Noodles (egg)	84.3	2.2	0.5	13.0	12.8	0.6	1656
Pasta (fresh)	61.5	6.6	1.5	31.8	30.7	1.9	677
Spaghetti (white)	73.8	3.6	0.7	22.2	21.7	1.2	442
Spaghetti (wholemeal)	69.1	4.7	0.9	23.2	21.9	3.5	485

Source: Food Standards Agency (2002).

Table 13.2 Comparative glycaemic index (GI) and glycaemic loading (GL) of pasta

Pasta type	GI (Glucose = 100)	GL (per serving)	Serving size (g)
Bread (white fibre enriched)	68	9	30
Bread (wholemeal)	69	8	30
Barley bread	40	8	30
Oat bran bread	44	8	30
Rye bread	67	10	30
All Bran cereal	30	4	30
Cheerios	74	15	30
Coco-pops	77	20	30
Cornflakes	72	18	30
Maize pasta (gluten free)	78	32	180
Fettucine (egg)	40	18	180
Noodles (instant)	47	19	180
Macaroni	47	23	180
Spaghetti (white)	32	15	180
Spaghetti (wholemeal)	32	14	180

Source: Adapted from Foster-Powell *et al.* (2002)

(wheat and water) makes pasta an attractive model food system to manipulate so as to improve its nutritional content. Indeed, the simplicity of pasta ingredients has helped researchers to study starch–protein–fibre interactions in a controlled manner. The potential nutritional and technological effects of the incorporation of different bioactive ingredients such as dietary fibre into the food system, or incorporation of high levels of whole grain, have therefore been well studied, and the virtues of incorporating wholegrain material into food systems are comparatively well understood in pasta products (as will be illustrated later in this chapter).

13.2 Process variables affecting pasta production

In considering processing parameters, the selection of good quality ingredients is important. Semolina from durum wheat is considered the ideal wheat product for pasta production due to its colour, flavour and cooking quality (Feillet and Dexter, 1996). As mentioned before, the quality of semolina is directly correlated with the protein content of the grain and the quality of that protein. Researchers have used many methods to determine the protein quality of durum wheat (alverograph, mixograph, farinograph, gluten index, Sodium dodecyl sulfate (SDS) -sedimentation and rapid visco analyser), all of which look at the hydration properties of the grain and gluten components. The degree of milling, and hence total and damaged starch content, can contribute to variations in processing conditions (mainly due to changes in the hydration dynamics of the dough) and hence pasta quality (El-Khayat *et al.*, 2006).

As with any food production system, the processing parameters of pasta manufacture have to be considered when trying to incorporate novel ingredients. Traditional methods of pasta manufacture are based on hand mixing of durum wheat with water ingredients to form a dough, which is then rolled into sheets that, in turn, are cut or shaped to the desired geometry. Most commercial production of pasta uses extrusion technology to mix and form the ingredients into a dough-like material, which is then passed through a rotating auger to a die face and expelled at the die face into strands of continuous dough which are cut and shaped as required. During the extrusion process the dough is subjected to both shear and temperature (although generally the temperature of a pasta extruder is cool (40–60°C) compared with the hot extrusion (160–200°C) used in breakfast cereal manufacture). The effects of shear and temperature do contribute to the amount of starch disassembly and gelatinisation during extrusion, although, as the conditions used during pasta manufacture are normally at low temperatures and minimal water concentration, very limited starch gelatinisation occurs during pasta processing. This fact goes some way in helping to explain why pasta is a relatively low GI food compared with bread or breakfast cereals (Table 13.2).

Nevertheless, parameters such as the hydration dynamics of ingredients, mixing time, extrusion temperature, die geometry and drying conditions are all important in governing final pasta quality (Debbouz and Doekott, 1996; Sudha *et al.*, 2011). Each of these factors would have an effect on how the raw materials combine and form the product structure, with a resulting effect on product texture and digestibility. Optimisation of mixing time and conditions is crucial in developing hydrated starch–protein continuums in the form of dough (El-Khayat *et al.*, 2006). There is the potential to add other ingredients, such as egg, flavours and colours, and non-durum wheat material (for example, in the manufacture of gluten-free pasta), to manipulate the colour, flavour and texture of pasta. Again, understanding the water-absorbing/binding ability of the raw ingredients is of paramount concern, not only to ensure that the hydrated starch–protein matrix is stable but also to ensure that any other ingredients do not interfere with the structure of this dough and the development of protein networks.

13.2.1 Process variables, and sensorial and textural properties

Most durum semolina flour is milled to produce flour particles of between 300 and 500 μm. In the process of milling wheat flour to obtain a flour of particle size 300–500 μm, wheat bran and germ are removed from the flour. These fractions of the grain are rich in fibre, vitamins and minerals, and hence their removal has negative effects on the nutritional balance of the flour. One of the most common ways to counteract this is to incorporate wheat bran and germ back into the flour to produce a wholewheat or possibly a wholegrain flour.

There has been much discussion in this book regarding fibre and wholegrain materials and their relationship to health and nutrition. Wholegrain wheat products undoubtedly contain more vitamins, minerals, dietary fibre and antioxidants than refined wheat flours (Baic, 2005). In turn, the antioxidant properties of spaghetti and pasta can be enhanced by the inclusion of wholegrain material (Hirawan *et al.*, 2010). However, these wholegrain materials, rich in wheat bran and germ fractions, are often not homogeneous in size and hydration characteristics. This in itself leads to challenges when incorporating them into food systems. For instance, these homogeneous fractions can form isolated pockets of materials which interfere with the protein–starch matrix developing in pasta dough, thus reducing overall pasta quality (Manthey and Schorno, 2002; Tudorica *et al.*, 2002).

Pasta and cereal foods made from wholewheat and wholegrain foods have often been noted as being less acceptable than refined flour counterparts due to consumer attitude to colour, taste and cooking qualities (Edwards *et al.*, 1995; D'Egidio *et al.*, 1990; Sahlstrom *et al.*, 1993; Brennan, 2005; Cleary and Brennan, 2006; Brennan *et al.*, 2008a). The consumer perception may be that enrichment of pasta with wholegrain materials and fibres promotes a gritty mouthfeel; alternatively, a slimy, paste-like quality is observed due to a combination of the hydration factors of the fibres and increased starch gelatinisation. To this effect, the incorporation of wholemeal and dietary fibres into pasta mix has been shown to affect the tenacity of the protein–starch matrix binding and thus influence the cooking quality characteristics of pasta. For instance, research by Gautheir *et al.* (2006) and Tudorica *et al.* (2002) has illustrated that the incorporation of bran into durum wheat semolina can produce pasta products which are brittle and sticky and exhibit high cooking losses. A high level of cooking loss of pasta is a significant problem, with starch and protein solubilising in the cooking water, weakening the structure of the pasta, and creating increased stickiness and disintegration on cooking.

Table 13.3 illustrates the effects of incorporating some dietary fibres into pasta products and the results in terms of cooking properties. As can be seen, differences exist within the fibre components themselves in how they alter the textural properties of pasta. Inclusion of pea fibre, inulin and guar can reduce pasta firmness compared with a control pasta product, as well as increasing stickiness and adhesiveness. Inclusion of locust bean gum and xanthan gum had the opposite effect. Not all dietary fibres behave in the same way. The quantity of fibre added is also important: levels of 2.5–5% can be used without necessarily causing significant loss of textural characteristics compared with a control pasta, whereas incorporation of greater than 5% starts to cause problems in terms of product textural characteristics. Any change to the textural characteristics of pasta also alters the sensorial perception of the product by the consumer.

Aravind *et al.* (2012) followed on from the initial research of Tudorica *et al.* (2002) and incorporated wheat bran (insoluble fibres) into durum wheat spaghetti, evaluating the quality of pasta in terms of colour and sensory qualities (as well as nutritional qualities by *in vitro* analysis). Their findings illustrated that inclusion of fibre at a level above 10% had a significant effect in disrupting the structural arrangements of the pasta, hence negatively affecting its sensorial properties (grittiness and cohesiveness).

Such negative effects in terms of sensorial properties of the pasta can be related to the incomplete hydration of particulate material in the pasta and hence

Table 13.3 The effects of dietary fibre addition to the textural attributes of cooked pasta

Sample	Firmness (N)	Stickiness (N)	Adhesiveness (N*s)	Elasticity (N)
Effect of the type of DF				
Control	*1.6*	*2.96*	*0.22*	*0.17*
Pea fibre	$1.23^{c,d}$	$2.9^{c,d}$	0.17^{d}	$0.16^{b,c}$
Inulin	$1.17^{c,d}$	3.3^{c}	$0.31^{c,d}$	0.14^{c}
Guar gum	1.32^{c}	4.2^{b}	$0.38^{b,c}$	$0.15^{b,c}$
Bamboo fibre	1.31^{c}	2.6^{d}	0.19^{d}	$0.16^{b,c}$
Xanthan gum	2.09^{b}	2.4^{d}	0.22^{d}	0.22^{a}
Locust bean gum	2.38^{a}	4.0^{b}	0.53^{b}	0.18^{b}
Significance	***	***	***	***
SEM	0.046	0.14	0.015	0.008
Effect of the level of DF addition				
2.5%	1.71^{A}	3.6^{A}	0.40^{B}	0.18^{A}
5.0%	1.62^{A}	4.1^{B}	0.45^{B}	$0.16^{A,B}$
7.5%	1.47^{B}	4.1^{B}	0.37^{B}	0.15^{B}
10.0%	1.25^{C}	5.5^{C}	0.59^{A}	0.14^{B}
Significance	***	***	***	**
SEM	0.035	0.11	0.012	0.006

Notes: within the same column, the values with the same letter are not significantly different. ***$p < 0.001$; **$p < 0.01$; *$p < 0.05$; DF–dietary fibre; ND – not determined.

Source: Adapted from Tudorica *et al.* (2002).

the perception of grittiness by the consumer (Tudorica *et al.*, 2002). It is possible, by careful mixing and addition of water (as well as pre-conditioning ingredients), to avoid or at least reduce the impact of poor ingredient hydration on the textural and sensory characteristics of pasta. However, it is not enough simply to assume that if you include wholegrain or fibre-rich ingredients you need to add more water to the developing dough, or increase the mixing time of the pasta. For instance, Chillo *et al.* (2011) illustrated that, even using the same cereal fractions (in this case beta-glucans), very different pasta qualities can be obtained under similar processing conditions. Two beta-glucans derived from barley (Glucagel and Barley Balance) were studied at varying levels of incorporation and tested against a control pasta product. The authors found that incorporation of these two ingredients at similar levels gave drastically different cooking losses and sensorial properties (hardness, stickiness and adhesiveness) as well as glycaemic response (more discussion on the role of pasta and fibre in modulating the glycaemic response of individuals will follow in this chapter). This further illustrates that it is not sensible to assume from a food ingredient viewpoint that the incorporation of apparently similar phytochemicals from similar grain sources will yield similar product quality characteristics. The minefield of ingredient selection and utilisation is scattered with potentially novel added-value ingredients which fail to be incorporated into successful commercial products.

13.3 Enrichment of pasta with whole grains or dietary fibre

Previously we discussed the purity of pasta production (durum wheat and water as the main ingredients). It is the simple nature of the ingredients that makes pasta an excellent vehicle to manipulate nutritionally. In 1949 the Food and Drug Administration of the United States (FDA) authorised the enrichment of pasta with vitamins and iron. Since then researchers have endeavoured to improve the nutritional content of pasta by incorporating protein (Shogren *et al.*, 2006; Chillo *et al.*, 2008) and other nutrients such as dietary fibres and vitamins (Kordonowy and Youngs, 1985; Bahnassey *et al.*, 1986; Knuckles *et al.*, 1997; Tudorica *et al.*, 2002). Much attention has been given to the use of wheat bran, wheat germ or wholegrain material in nutrient-rich pasta streams (Buck *et al.*, 1987; Cara *et al.*, 1992). For instance, Chillo *et al.* (2008) developed pasta with the addition of buckwheat flour and wheat bran and found that, although inclusion rates of 15–20% were possible, changes to pasta colour and sensorial qualities limited the use of the additional ingredients from a consumer preference viewpoint (Sudha *et al.*, 2011).

Interest in incorporating wholegrain material (and dietary fibre) is based on the premise that these ingredients are nutritionally sound. Epidemiological studies have shown significant correlations between the consumption of wholegrain material and reduced risk of cardiovascular disease (Fraser, 1999; Jacobs *et al.*, 1998; Liu *et al.*, 1999) and diabetes (Liu *et al.*, 2000; Meyer *et al.*, 2000). These tend to be associated with not only the dietary fibre components in wholegrain materials but also the phytochemical co-passengers from the bran layer of the grain (Okarter and Liu, 2010).

Pasta itself appears to possess unique nutritional features, compared with other carbohydrate-rich foods, in that the starch is slowly digested and absorbed in the small intestine. The slow digestibility of starch in pasta results in a delaying of sugar release from the carbohydrate food and hence potential blood glucose response. It is partly for this reason that pasta has become even more popular, being regarded as a product with a low GI potential and featuring heavily in low GI diets (Jenkins *et al.*, 1983). Research has shown that pasta steadily liberates sugars that the body needs over a 2–3 hour digestion period, and it is this slow release of sugars as starch is digested that leads to its low postprandial blood glucose and insulin responses in humans (Jenkins *et al.*, 1983; Granfeldt *et al.*, 1994).

The slower release of starch degradation products from pasta in comparison with other cereal products such as breads and biscuits has been attributed to the compact structure of pastas resulting from the extrusion process, and characterised by a very close protein network which entraps starch granules and delays α-amylase activity (Fardet *et al.*, 1999; Tudorica *et al.*, 2002). The large particle size of the flour used in pasta production also limits the amount of starch degradation by reducing the accessibility of enzymes to starch and hence regulating starch digestion kinetics.

Interactions of starch with other components such as certain dietary fibres have also been suggested to further reduce the rate of starch digestion and thus to lower the glycaemic response (Ellis *et al.*, 1988; Tudorica *et al.*, 2002). One such example is that of Bustos *et al.* (2011), who investigated the use of resistant starches and oat bran to enrich pasta with fibre and illustrated the possible use of these ingredients in reducing the potential glycaemic response to some ingredients. For instance, oat bran inclusion reduced the digestibility of starch in a dose–response manner, whereas resistant starch increased the starch digestibility of the pasta. However, inclusion of both resistant starch and oat bran reduced consumer acceptability in terms of firmness, chewiness and overall acceptability of pastas compared with the control pasta. Tudorica *et al.* (2002) and Brennan *et al.* (2008 a, b) also illustrated this phenomenon with a range of dietary fibres in pasta and breakfast cereal products. Table 13.4 demonstrates the findings of Tudorica *et al.* (2002). Using simple *in vitro* starch digestion systems, they followed the digestion of starch over 180 minutes and used the evolution of sugars from the digested starch to determine potential GI of the pasta. It is clear that inclusion of dietary fibres had a significant reducing effect on the amount of starch digestion taking place between 0 and 150 minutes. However, this significance was reduced at 180 minutes. Nevertheless, pasta with dietary fibre inclusions did lower the predicted GI of the pastas (but not necessarily in a

Table 13.4 The effects of dietary fibre addition on the digestion characteristics of cooked pasta

Sample	Starch digested after 150 min (%)	Starch digested after 180 min (%)	Predicted GI (% against white bread standard)
Effect of the type of DF			
Control	12.91	19.19	45.0
Pea fibre	10.12[b]	15.62[a,b]	39.2[b,c]
Inulin	12.81[a]	17.83[a]	41.1[a,b,c]
Guar gum	7.70[c,e]	11.83[c,d]	37.9[b,c]
Bamboo fibre	8.33[b,c,d]	12.42[c,d]	37.1[c]
Xanthan gum	6.87[d,e]	10.22[d]	41.4[a,b]
Locust bean gum	8.79[b,c,d]	12.78[c,d]	37.0[c]
SEM	0.446	0.592	0.93
Significance	***	***	***
Effect of the level of DF addition			
2.5%	10.73[A]	15.13[A]	42.1[A]
5.0%	9.43[A]	14.33[A]	39.2[B,C]
7.5%	9.71[A]	14.12[A]	40.1[A,B,C]
10.0%	6.65[B]	10.01[B]	37.2[C]
SEM	0.337	0.446	0.70
Significance	***	***	***

Notes: Within the same column, the values with the same letter are not significantly different. ***$p < 0.001$; **$p < 0.01$; *$p < 0.05$; DF – dietary fibre; GI – glycaemic index; NS – not significant. Predicted GI measured against a white bread standard.

Source: Adapted from Tudorica *et al.* (2002).

dose-responsive manner, as can be seen when evaluating differences between the different inclusion levels).

It is also important to note that not all fibres behave in the same manner when reducing GI of foods. This was observed by Kristensen *et al.* (2010), who conducted research on 20 young adults in which wholemeal and refined wheat flour isocaloric meals of bread and pasta were consumed. Interestingly, the researchers found no significant differences between the meals from wholemeal and refined flour in terms of glucose response (pasta meals gave a lower glycaemic response than others). The wholemeal bread meal yielded a reduction in hunger and increased satiety rating compared with the refined flour bread. The different responses found in terms of bread and pasta suggest that food product form (i.e. in this case bread or pasta) can have a dramatic effect in terms of satiety and glycaemic response, and that different whole grains or dietary fibre ingredients could exert different characteristics in different food forms.

When considering satiety regulation, it is useful to note that many studies have demonstrated the link between whole grain and dietary fibre consumption and the feeling of satiety (Grandfelt *et al.*, 1994; Liljeberg *et al.*, 1999; Solah *et al.*, 2007). Schroedar *et al.* (2009) investigated the potential benefits of whole grain consumption on satiety and energy intake by studying 47 subjects consuming a wholegrain enriched breakfast. Interestingly, they showed that intake of the wholegrain rich foods had no effect on overall energy intake, but that consumption of barley wholegrain foods as part of the breakfast reduced the feeling of hungriness before lunch. In observing this, they are also indicating that generalising all whole grains as having a similar effect is an oversimplification of the issue and that some grains, and some dietary fibres, behave differently from others. A similar observation was made by Berti *et al.* (2005) in studying wheat and oat wholegrain material. However, there remains a body of evidence which suggests that both insoluble (Porikos and Hagamen, 1986; Delargy *et al.*, 1997) and soluble dietary fibre components (Williams *et al.*, 2006; Chow *et al.*, 2007) have been shown to affect satiety.

13.4 Relationship between ingredient selection, processing and nutrition

So what is the relationship between whole grain/dietary fibre, processing and human nutrition? Most extrusion processes subject the raw material (in this case, starch and other carbohydrates) to relatively high pressures, temperature fluctuations and high shear (Jin *et al.*, 1994; Wang *et al.*, 1993). All of these have a significant effect on starch and carbohydrate degradation. It is well known that extrusion technologies can be used to pre-digest starch molecules so that reductions in the molecular weight of the amylose and amylopectin content of starch can be seen after extrusion. This degradation of the starch molecule and reduction in molecular weight to shorter and simpler sugar units could explain the significance of extrusion in the GI of extruded breakfast cereal products. Although the extrusion process used for the production of pasta is less harsh (in terms of having a lower processing temperature, and potentially less mechanical energy input) than that of breakfast cereal production, some modification of the starch molecule may occur during production. This modification would be related to the particle size of the semolina used in the raw materials, the amount of water present in the system and the control of barrel temperatures during processing, all of which would affect overall pasta quality (eating and nutritional quality). In particular, the role extrusion plays in 'filming' the outer surface of pasta products still needs to be explored adequately. This film formation on the outer surfaces of the pasta during extrusion would significantly affect the ease of water penetration during cooking.

The filming around the starch granule can not only limit the degree of starch gelatinisation, and hence glycaemic response, but also affect the physical characteristics of pasta. For instance, Tudorica *et al.* (2002) illustrated that the firmness of dietary fibre-enriched pastas was generally lower than that of the control, correlating this reduction in firmness with the increased moisture content and swelling index of these products in comparison to the control. However, some pastas containing locust bean gum or xanthan gum had moisture values similar to or higher than the control pasta, and at the same time their firmness showed increased values. The suggestion was that locust bean gum and xanthan gum contributed to the structure's strength. The authors further illustrated that these pasta products showed low values obtained for cooking losses, indicating a well-formed structure from which a small amount of solids is released during cooking. Similar results have been reported by Edwards *et al.* (1995), reporting an improvement in pasta firmness without the alteration of cooking qualities when xanthan gum was added at levels of 1% or 2%. Additionally, results reported by Fardet *et al.* (1999) for pasta made from freeze-dried flour fractions in which soluble fibres accounted for 7% indicated that the firmness of pasta increased (and cooking loss decreased) with inclusion. The proposed explanation was the formation of a network by the soluble fibre around the starch granules, leading to a stronger cohesiveness between starch and protein within the pasta structure.

It is clear that raw material qualities such as wheat flour, semolina particle size, level of water addition and protein content will all affect pasta quality. Much research has been conducted on the importance of starch type, starch damage, protein content, semolina quality and starch gelatinisation on cooking time and quality of pasta (Dexter and Matsuo, 1977; 1980; Cubadda, 1988; Chung *et al.*, 2003; El-Khayat *et al.*, 2003; 2006; Samaan *et al.*, 2006). Part of this is related to dough hydration (water absorption from both the starch and protein components of the dough) and how hydration dynamics is associated with the final structure of the pasta, the degree of starch swelling, gelatinisation and hence accessibility of degrading enzymes into the pasta structure. Addition of raw ingredients which have the ability to compete for moisture, and hence minimise starch hydration and gelatinisation during processing, would have an effect on the glycaemic impact of pasta. Wholegrain material and dietary fibre have hydration characteristics which have the potential to alter the water-holding capacity of a product and compete for water with protein and starch during dough development.

Much of our previous understanding of how fibre and wholegrain material contribute to manipulation of starch digestion and GI has concentrated on the interactions of fibre, protein and starch in altering the viscosity profile of dough, the product structure and hence the rheological behaviour of digesta. Indeed, dietary fibre has been used for many years to modulate the extent of starch swelling, gelatinisation and hence carbohydrate digestibility. For instance, soluble fibres from pulses, vegetables, whole fruits, oats and barley form gelatinous gels within the stomach which appear to delay gastric emptying and enzymatic digestion (Jenkins *et al.*, 1983), whereas insoluble fibres have little effect on gastric emptying and no effect on glucose absorption. This may in part explain why high fibre/wholegrain diets alone are not necessarily synonymous with low GI foods (Jenkins *et al.*, 1983).

More recently, research from the King's College group (Roder *et al.*, 2009; Butterworth *et al.*, 2011) has suggested that the main contribution to the potential glycaemic response of a product is related to substrate limiting events. For instance, Butterworth *et al.* (2011, 2012) suggest that all starch granules (and products) have the same glycaemic potential, with the rate of reaction being limited by the accessibility of amylolytic enzymes to starch components. Taking that further, Roder *et al.* (2009) have suggested that modulation of the glycaemic response of individuals to starchy foods is largely dependent on water mobility and the effects of water mobility on starch gelatinisation events. To this end, water appears to be the key component to investigate in future research. From a purely biochemical background, it is commonly believed that enzymes require water to function; thus, by limiting the water mobility in a food system during digestion, one can manipulate the enzyme kinetics of that food system and reduce the effectiveness of enzymes. Wholegrain material and dietary fibre change the water mobility properties of foods, and in this way will contribute to the control of starch digestion and hence glycaemic response.

13.5 Conclusion and future trends

Wholegrain material and dietary fibres are well documented in terms of exerting potential glycaemic response reductions when incorporated into food systems. Pasta represents a food system into which wholegrain material and dietary fibre can be incorporated relatively simply. Pasta is also a commonly consumed food product and has the potential to reach a large consumer base. There is no doubt that pasta represents a good vehicle to enhance the dietary intake of whole grains and dietary fibre. This in turn could lead to the development of fibre-rich pasta food products. However, the implications of fibre for the technological/processing parameters of pasta production should not be oversimplified, and much research is still required to determine the effectiveness of individual dietary fibres or wholegrain fractions on both product sensorial quality and nutritional value.

13.6 References

ARAVIND, N., SISSONS, M., EGAN, N, and FELLOWS, C. (2012) Effect of insoluble dietary fibre addition on technological, sensory and structural properties of durum wheat spaghetti. *Food Chemistry* **130**, 199–309.

AUTRAN, J.C. and GALTERIO, G. (1989). Association between electrophoretic composition of protein, quality characteristics, and agronomic attributes of durum wheat. II. Protein quality associations. *Journal of Cereal Science* **9**, 195–215.

BAHNASSEY, Y., KHAN, K. and HARROLD, R. (1986) Fortification of spaghetti with edible legumes. Physiochemical anti-nutritional, amino acid and mineral composition. *Cereal Chemistry* **63**, 210–15.

BAIC, S. (2005) Whole grains – the way to go. In *The food fact sheet by the British Dietetic Association*. UK: The British Dietetic Association, pp. 1–2.

BALDWIN, P.M. (2001). Starch granule-associated proteins and polypeptides: A review. *Starch* **53**, 475–503.

BERTI, C., RISO, P., BRUSAMOLINO, A. and PORRINI, M. (2005) Effect on appetite control of minor cereal and pseudocereal products. *British Journal of Nutrition* **94**, 850–8.

BORRELLI, G.M., TROCCOLI, A., DI FANZO, N. and FARES, C. (1999) Durum wheat lipoxygenase activity and other quality parameters that affect pasta colour. *Cereal Chemistry* **76**, 335–40.

BRENNAN, C.S. (2005) Dietary fibre, glycaemic response, and diabetes. *Molecular Nutrition and Food Research* **49**, 560–70.

BRENNAN, C.S., SULAIMAN, B.D., SCHOFIELD, J.D. and VAUGHAN, J.G. (1993) The immunolocation of friabilin and its association with wheat endosperm texture. *Aspects of Applied Biology*, **36**: *Cereal Quality III*, pp. 69–74.

BRENNAN, M.A., MONRO, J.A. and BRENNAN, C.S. (2008a) Effect of inclusion of soluble and insoluble fibres into extruded breakfast cereal products made with reverse screw configuration. *International Journal of Food Science and Technology* **43**, 2278–88.

BRENNAN, M.A., MERTS, I., MONRO, J., WOOLNOUGH, J. and BRENNAN, C.S. (2008b) Impact of guar gum and wheat bran on the physical and nutritional quality of extruded breakfast cereals. *Starch-Starke* **60**, 248–56.

BUCK, J.S., WALKER, C.E. and WATSON, K. (1987) Incorporation of corn gluten meal and soy into various cereal-based foods and resulting product functional sensory and protein quality. *Cereal Chemistry* **64**, 264–9.

BUSTOS, M.C., PREEZ, G.T. and LEON, A.E. (2011) Sensory and nutritional attributes of fibre-enriched pasta. *LWT- Food Science and Technology* **44**, 1429–34.

BUTTERWORTH, P.J., WARREN, F.J. and ELLIS, P.R. (2011) Human α-amylase and starch digestion: An interesting marriage. *Starch – Stärke* **63**, 395–405.

BUTTERWORTH, P.J., WARREN, F.J., GRASSBY, T., PATEL, H. and ELLIS, P.R. (2012) Analysis of starch amylolysis using plots for first-order kinetics. *Carbohydrate Polymers* **87**, 2189–97.

CARA, L., BOREL, P., ARMAND, M., LAFON, H., LESGARDS, G. and LARION, D. (1992) Milling and processing of wheat and other cereals affect their capacity to inhibit pancreatic lipase *in vitro*. *Journal of Food Science* **57**, 466–469.

CARRILLO, J.M., VASQUEZ, M. and ORELLANA, J. (1990) Relationship between gluten strength and glutenin proteins in durum wheat cultivars. *Plant Breeding* **104**, 325–33.

CHILLO, S., LAVERSE, J., FALCONE, P.M., PROTOPAPA, A. and DE NOBILE, M.A. (2008) Influence of the addition of buckwheat flour and durum wheat bran on spaghetti quality. *Journal of Cereal Science* **47**, 144–52.

CHILLO, S., RANAWANA, D.V. and HENRY, C.J.K. (2011) Effect of two barley beta-glucan concentrates on in vitro glycaemic impact and cooking quality of spaghetti. *LWT- Food Science and Technology* **44**, 940–8.

CHOW, J., CHOE, Y.S., NOSS, M.J., ROBINSON, K.J., DUGLE, J.E. and ACOSTA, S.H. (2007) Effect of viscous fibre-containing nutrition bar on satiety of patients with type 2 diabetes. *Diabetes Research and Clinical Practice* **76**, 335–40.

CHUNG, O.K., OHM, J.B., LOOKHART, G.L. and BRUNS, R.F. (2003) Quality characteristics of hard winter and spring wheats grown under an over-wintering condition. *Journal of Cereal Science* **37**, 91–9.

CLEARY, L.J. and BRENNAN, C.S. (2006) Effect of beta-glucan on pasta quality. *International Journal of Food Science and Technology* **41**, 910–18.

CUBADDA, R. (1988) Evaluation of durum wheat, semolina and pasta in Europe. In: FABRIANI, G. and LINTUS, C. *Durum wheat: Chemistry and technology*. AACC, St Paul, Minnesota, USA, pp. 217–28.

CUBADDA, R. AND CARCEA, M. (2000) Pasta and Macaroni. Methods of Manufacture. In: *Encyclopedia of Food Sciences and Nutrition*, Academic Press, London, UK, pp. 4374–8.

DAMIDAUX, R., AUTRAN, J.C. and FEILLET, P. (1980) Gliadin electrophoregrams and measurements of gluten viscoelasticity in durum wheats. *Cereal Foods World* **25**, 754–6.

DEBBOUZ, A. and DOETKOTT, C. (1996) Effect of process variables on spaghetti quality. *Cereal Chemistry* **73**, 672–6.

D'EDIGIO, M.G., MARIANI, B.M., NARDI, S., NOVARO, P. and CUBADDA, R. (1990) Chemical and technological variables and their relationships: A predictive equation for pasta cooking quality. *Cereal Chemistry* **67**, 275–81.

DELARGY, H.J., O'SULLIVAN, K.R., FLETCHER, R.J. and BLUNDELL, J.E. (1997) Effects of amount and type of dietary fibre (soluble and insoluble) on short-term control of appetite. *International Journal of Food Sciences and Nutrition* **48**, 67–77.

DELWICHE, S.R. (1993) Measurement of single-kernel wheat hardness using Near-Infrared Transmittance. *Transactions of the ASAE*, **36**, 1431–7.

DEXTER, J.E. and MATSUO, R.R. (1977) Influence of protein content on some durum wheat quality parameters. *Canadian Journal of Plant Science* **57**, 717–27.

DEXTER, J.E. and MATSUO, R.R. (1980) Relationship between durum wheat proteins properties and pasta dough rheology and spaghetti cooking quality. *Journal of Agriculture and Food Chemistry* **28**, 899–902.

DEXTER, J.E., MARCHYLO, B.A., MACGREGOR, A.W. and TKACHUK, R. (1989) The structure and protein composition of vitreous, piebald and starchy durum wheat kernels. *Journal of Cereal Science* **10**, 19–32.

DU CROS, D.L., WRIGLEY, C.W. and HARE, R.A. (1982) Prediction of durum wheat quality from gliadin-protein composition. *Australian Journal of Agriculture Research* **33**, 429–42.

EDWARDS, N.M., BILIADERIS, C.G. and DEXTER, J.E. (1995) Textural characteristics of wholewheat pasta and pasta containing non-starch polysaccharides. *Journal of Food Science* **60**, 1321–4.

ELLIS, P.R., KAMALANATHAN, T., DAWOUD, F.M., STRANGE, R.N. and COULTATE., T.P. (1988) Evaluation of guar biscuits for use in the management of diabetes – tests of physiological effects and palatability in non-diabetic volunteers. *European Journal of Clinical Nutrition* **42**, 425–35.

EL-KHAYAT, G.H, SAMAAN, J. and BRENNAN, C.S. (2003) Evaluation of Vitreous and Starchy Syrian Durum Wheat Grains: The Effect of Amylose Content on Starch Characteristics and Flour Pasting Properties. *Starch* **55**, 358–65.

EL-KHAYAT, H.G., SAMAAN, J., MANTHEY, F.A., FULLER, M.P. AND BRENNAN, C.S. (2006) Durum wheat quality I: correlations between physical and chemical characteristics of Syrian durum wheat cultivars. *International Journal of Food Science and Technology* **41**, 22–9.

FARDET, A., ABECASSIS, J., HOEBLER, C., BALDWIN, P.M., BULEON, A., *et al.* (1999) Influence of technological modifications of the protein network from pasta on in vitro starch degradation. *Journal of Cereal Science* **30**, 133–45.

FEILLET, P. AND DEXTER, J.E. (1996) Quality requirements of durum wheat for semolina milling and pasta production. In *Pasta and Noodle Technology*, AACC, St Paul, Minnesota, USA pp. 95–132.

FOOD STANDARDS AGENCY (2002) *McCance and Widdowson's The Composition of Foods*, Royal Society of Chemistry, Cambridge, UK.

FOSTER-POWELL, K., HOLT, H.A. and BRAND-MILLER, J.C. (2002) International table of glycaemic index and glycaemic load values: 2002. *American Journal of Clinical Nutrition* **76**, 5–56.

FRASER, G.E. (1999) Associations between diet and cancer, ischemic heart disease and all-cause mortality in non-Hispanic white California Seventh-day Adventists. *American Journal of Clinical Nutrition* **70**, 532S–538S.

GAUTHIER, J., GELINAS, P. AND BEAUCHEMIN, R. (2006) Effect of stone-milled semolina granulation on the quality of bran-rich pasta made from khorasan (Kamut) and durum wheat. *International Journal of Food Science and Technology* **41**, 596–9.

Gazzettaufficiale (1967) Law number 580 Disciplina per la lavorazione e commerciodei cereal, deglisfarinati, del pane e delle paste alimentary. *GazzettaUfficiale* 189.

GONG, Y., YANG, Y., FERGUSON, D.K., TAO, D., LI, W., *et al.* (2011) Investigation of ancient noodles, cakes and millet at the subeixi site Xinjiang, China. *Journal of Archaeological Science* **38**, 470–9.

GRANDFELT, Y., LIJEBERG, H., DREWS, A., NEWMADN, R. and BJORK, I. (1994) Glucose and insulin responses to barley products: influence of food structure and amylase-amylopectin ratio. *American Journal of Clinical Nutrition* **59**, 1075–82.

GREENWELL, P. and SCHOFIELD, J.D. (1986) A starch granule protein associated with endosperm softness in wheat. *Cereal Chemistry* **63**, 379–80.

HIRAWAN, R., SER, W.Y., ARNTFIRLD, S.D. and BETA, T. (2010) Antioxidant properties of commercial, regular- and whole-wheat spaghetti. *Food Chemistry* **119**, 258–64.

HOSENEY, R.C. (1987) Wheat hardness. *Cereal Foods World* **32**, 320–2.

IGREJAS, G., MARTINANT, J.P., BOUGUENNEC, A., VILLAIN, A.C., SAULNIER, L., *et al.* (2001) Genetical, biochemical and technological parameters associated with biscuit quality. I. Prediction using grain hardness and water extractable arabinoxylans. *Journal of Cereal Science* **36**, 115–24.

ISAKSSON, H., ANDERSSON, R., OLSSON, J., FREDRIKSSON, H., WEBB, D.L. and AMAN, P. (2012) Whole grain rye breakfast – sustained satiety during three weeks of regular consumption. *Physiology and Behaviour* **105**, 877–84.

JACOBS, D.R., MEYER, K.A., KUSHI, L.H. and FOLSOM, A.R. (1998) Whole grain intake may reduce the risk of ischemic heart disease death in postmenopausal women: The Iowa Women's Health Study. *American Journal of Clinical Nutrition* **68**, 248–57.

JENKINS, D.J.A., WOLEVER, T.M.S., JENKINS, A.L., LEE, R., WONG, G.S. and JOSSE, R. (1983) Glycemic response to wheat products – reduced response to pasta but no effect of fiber. *Diabetes Care* **6**, 155–9.

JIN, Z., HSIEH, F. and HUFF, H.E. (1994) Extrusion cooking of corn meal with soy fiber, salt and sugar. *Cereal Chemistry* **71**, 227–34.

KNUCKLES, B.E., HUDSON, C.A., CHIU, M.M. and SAYRE, R.N. (1997) Effect of beta-glucan barley fractions in high-fibre bread and pasta. *Cereal Food World* **42**, 94–9.

KORDONOWY, R.K. and YOUNGS, V.L. (1985) Utilization of durum bran and its effect on spaghetti. *Cereal Chemistry* **62**, 301–8.

KOVACS, M.I.P., POSTE, L.M., BUTLER, G., WOODS, S.M., LEISLE, D., *et al.* (1997). Durum wheat quality: Comparison of chemical and rheological screening tests with sensory analysis. *Journal of Cereal Science* **25**, 65–75.

KRISTENSEN, M., JENSEN, M.G., RIBOLDI, G., PERTRONIO, M., BUGEL, S., *et al.* (2010) Wholegrain vs refined wheat breads and pasta. Effect on postprandial glycemia, appetite, and subsequent *ad libitum* energy intake in young healthy adults. *Appetite* **54**, 163–9.

LIJEBERG, H.G., AKERBERG, A.K. and BJORK, I.M. (1999) Effect of the glycaemic index content of indigestible carbohydrates of cereal-based breakfast meals in glucose tolerance at lunch in healthy subjects. *American Journal of Clinical Nutrition* **69**, 647–55.

LIU, S., MANSON, J.E., STAMPFER, M.J., HU, F.B., GIOVANNUCCI, E., *et al.* (2000) A prospective study of whole grain intake and risk of type 2 diabetes mellitus in US women. *American Journal of Public Health* **90**, 1409–15.

LIU, S., STAMPFER, M.J., HU, F.B., GIOVANNUCCI, E., RIMM, E., *et al.* (1999) Whole-grain consumption and risk of coronary heart disease: Results from the Nurses Health Study. *American Journal of Clinical Nutrition* **70**, 412–19.

LU, H.Y., YANG, X.Y., YE, M.L., LIU, K.B., XIA, Z.K., *et al.* (2005) Millet noodles in late Neolithic China. *Nature* **437**, 967–8.

MANTHEY, F.A. AND SCHORNO, A.L. (2002) Physical and cooking quality of spaghetti made from whole wheat durum. *Cereal Chemistry* **79**, 504–10.

MARIANI, B.M., D'EGIDIO, M.G. AND NOVARO, P. (1995) Durum wheat quality evaluation: Influence of genotype and environment. *Cereal Chemistry* **72**, 194–7.

MATSUO, R.R. and DEXTER, J.E. (1980) Relationship between some durum wheat characteristics and semolina milling properties. *Canadian Journal of Plant Science* **60**, 49–53.

MEYER, K.A., KUSHI, L.H., JACOBS, D.R., SLAVIN, J., SELLERS, T.A. and FOLSOM, A.R. (2000) Carbohydrates, dietary fibre and incident type 2 diabetes in older women. *American Journal of Clinical Nutrition* **71**, 921–30.

OAK, M.D., SISSONS, M., EGAN, N., TAMHANKAR, S. A., RAO, V.S. and BHOSALE, S.B. (2006) Relationship between gluten strength and pasta firmness in Indian durum wheats. *International Journal of Food Science and Technology* **41**, 538–44.

OKARTER, N. AND LIU, R.H. (2010) *Health benefits of whole grain phytochemicals* **50**, 193–208.

PARISH, J.A. and HALSE, N.J. (1968) Effects of light, temperature and the rate of desiccation on translucency in wheat grain. *Australian Journal of Agriculture Research* **19**, 365–72.

POMERANZ, Y. and WILLIAMS, P.C. (1990) Wheat hardness: Its genetic, structure and biochemical background, measurement and significance. In: POMERANZ, Y. *Advances in cereal science and technology*. AACC, St Paul, Minnesota, USA, pp. 471–557.

POMERANZ, Y., BOLLING, H. and ZWINGELBERG, H. (1984) Wheat hardness and baking properties of wheat flour. *Journal of Cereal Science* **2**, 137–43.

PORIKOS, K. and HAGAMEN, S. (1986) Is fibre satiating? Effects of a high fiber preload on subsequent food intake of normal-weight and obese young men. *Appetite* **7**, 153–62.

RODER, N., ELLIS, P.R. and BUTTERWORTH, P.J. (2009) Factors affecting the action of α-amylase on wheat starch: Effects of water availability. An enzymic and structural study. *Food Chemistry* **113**, 471–8.

SAHLSTROM, S., MOSLETH, E., BAEVRE, A.B., GLORIA, H. and FAYARD, G. (1993) Influence of starch, gluten proteins and extraction rate on bread and pasta quality. *Carbohydrate Polymers* **21**, 169–75.

SAMAAN, J., EL-KHAYAT, G.H., MANTHEY, F.A., FULLER, M.P. and BRENNAN, C.S. (2006) Durum wheat quality II: The relationship of kernel physicochemical composition to semolina quality and end product utilisation. *International Journal of Food Science and Technology* **41**, 47–55.

SCHROEDAR, N., GALLAHER, D.D., ARNDT, E.A. and MARQUART, L. (2009) Influence of whole grain barley, whole grain wheat, and refined rice based foods on short term satiety and energy intake. *Appetite* **53**, 363–9.

SHARMA, R., SISSONS, M.J., RATHJEN, A.J. and JENNER, C.F. (2002) The null-4A allele at the waxy locus in durum wheat affects pasta cooking quality. *Journal of Cereal Science* **35**, 287–97.

SHOGREN, R.L., HARELAND, G.A. and WU, Y.V. (2006) Sensory evaluation and composition of spaghetti fortified with soy flour. *Journal of Food Science* **71**, 428–32.

SOLAH, V.A., FENTON, H., KERR, D., CROSBIE, G.B. and SIRYANI, S. (2007) Measurement of satiety of wheat based bulgur by intervention and sensory evaluation. *Cereal Foods World* **52**, 15.

STENVERT, N.L. and KINGSWOOD, K. (1977) The influence of the physical structure of the protein matrix on wheat hardness. *Journal of the Science of Food and Agriculture* **28**, 11–19.

SUDHA, M.L., RAMASARMA, P.R. AND VENKATESWARA, R.G. (2011) Wheat bran stabilization and its use in the preparation of high fibre pasta. *Food Science and Technology International* **17**, 47–53.

SYMES, K. (1961) Classification of Australian wheat varieties based on the granularity of their wholemeal. *Australian Journal of Experimental Agriculture and Animal Husbandry* **1**, 18–23.

TAHA, S.A. and SAGI, F. (1987) Relationship between chemical composition of durum wheat semolina and macaroni quality. II. Ash, carotenoid pigments, and oxidative enzymes. *Cereal Research Communication* **15**, 123–9.

TROCCOLI, A., BORRELI, G.M., DE VITA, P., FARES, C. and DI FONZO, N. (2000) Durum wheat quality: A multidisciplinary concept. *Journal of Cereal Science* **32**, 99–113.

TUDORICA, C.M., KURI, V. and BRENNAN, C.S. (2002) Nutritional and physicochemical characteristics of dietary fibre enriched pasta. *Journal of Agriculture and Food Chemistry* **50**, 347–56.

WANG, S., CASULLI, J. and BOUVIER, J.M. (1993) Effect of dough ingredients on apparent viscosity and properties of extrudates in a twin-screw extrusion cooking. *International Journal of Food Science and Technology* **28**, 465–79.

WILLIAMS, G., NOAKES, M., KEOGH, J., FOSTER, P. and CLIFTON, P. (2006) High protein high fibre snack bars reduce food intake and improve short term glucose and insulin profiles compared with high fat snack bars. *Asia Pacific Journal of Clinical Nutrition* **15**, 443–50.

YAMAZAKI, W.T. and DONELSON, J.R. (1983) Kernel hardness of some US wheats. *Cereal Chemistry* **60**, 344–50.

14

Fibre-enriched and wholewheat noodles

A. S. Ross, Oregon State University, USA

DOI: 10.1533/9780857095787.3.291

Abstract: Asian noodles are traditional foods that have emanated from eastern Asia. In their most popular forms, many of these noodles have distinct quality attributes that may be somewhat at odds with the quality attributes of wholegrain or fiber-enriched alternatives. Wheat flour noodles can be supplemented with a range of materials that can boost fiber or resistant starch contents, with beneficial health outcomes for consumers. A key factor in promoting the fiber-enriched alternatives is to stop holding them to the standards of appearance and texture established for refined flour versions. Similarly, non-wheat noodles may be supplemented to increase fiber levels. Maybe more advantageously, there are opportunities to reformulate and to modify processing to increase the amount of resistant starch already available in some types of rice or starch noodles.

Key words: noodles, wheat, starch, fiber, resistant starch.

14.1 Introduction

By now we should all know about the benefits of a diet containing adequate levels of fiber. The trouble is that many of us, faced with choosing between a traditional product made with refined flour or a fiber-enriched alternative, may choose the former. Why is this? In many cases, sensory factors such as appearance, color, texture, and taste win out over nutritional considerations. In the case of the noodles of eastern Asia, appearance is a particularly strong driver of consumer buying decisions, and the inclusion of colored fiber-rich materials (e.g. bran) can be a barrier to consumer acceptance. For wheat flour noodles, there is a widespread consumer preference for clean and bright color attributes. In the non-wheat noodle sector, transparency (e.g. starch noodles) and whiteness (rice noodles) are among the desired attributes (Lu and Collado, 2010).

Cooked noodle texture is also a factor in consumer acceptance of noodle products, and the textural characteristics of many of the different noodle types are well established in culinary tradition. This leads to consumer expectations that a specific type of noodle should conform to the expected quality criteria, even if reformulated as a fiber-enriched analog. The texture of noodle products is primarily determined by the characteristics of the starch, the major solid raw material. This pertains regardless of whether the noodles are made from wheat flour with up to 12% or more protein or whether the noodles are made from a refined starch with only trace amounts of proteins. Given the importance of starch in defining noodle texture (Lu and Collado, 2010; Ross and Crosbie, 2010), it is logical to surmise that dilution of the starch with fiber will influence processing characteristics and product texture. In one study on paste viscosity, fiber was added to wheat flour at replacement levels of up to 13% for individual fiber preparations and up to 34% for combinations (Collar *et al.*, 2006). In all cases, the hot paste viscosity of the composite flours was lower than the control, as could be anticipated simply from the dilution effect. However, the authors suggested that the reduction in peak viscosity also reflected a reduction of starch granule swelling. This conclusion was in accordance with earlier work using barley β-glucan at a 5% replacement level (Symons and Brennan, 2004) and has implications for all sources of fiber added to noodle formulations. (The term 'β-glucan' will be used throughout this article to denote the mixed linkage β,1→3,1→4 glucans common in barley and oats, unless specified otherwise.)

The fiber content of existing noodle types varies greatly. Wheat flour noodles made from refined flour only have the limited amount of fiber contained in the wheat endosperm. Starch noodles, such as rice and mung bean noodles, appear to be full of digestible carbohydrates with little fiber, but research into their resistant starch (RS) content suggests otherwise. Other non-wheat noodles are models for high fiber content. For example, the dry solids component of shirataki (konjac flour noodles) is almost 100% indigestible polysaccharides, primarily de-acetylated glucomannans. The gelled glucomannans are effectively an analogue of a cellulose gel and the β-anomeric configuration of their glycosidic linkages makes the glucomannans also indigestible in the human gut.

Despite their currently small market share, wholewheat, wholegrain and fiber-enriched noodles are considered to have market potential. For example, in 2010 the Nestlé Corporation in Malaysia released Maggi® Tastylite™ Atta Whole Wheat Noodles®. The placement of these noodles in the instant noodle market sector, a sector strongly driven by price factors, is interesting, suggesting that fiber-related health messages have gained traction in this price-sensitive, rather than nutrition-sensitive, product category. In North America, an informal survey of local food markets and Asian food specialty stores revealed a disturbingly meager collection of wholewheat, wholegrain, or fiber-enriched noodles. There were a few examples of wholewheat udon and somen, wholegrain rice noodles, and a variety of soba (buckwheat) noodle products. Searching the web finds a better selection of wholegrain rice noodles, wholewheat udon and somen, and wholewheat durum 'udon' noodles. Outside their traditional markets in Asia, shirataki are also readily available in the western world. Clearly there are rich opportunities to enrich noodles with the diverse array of food-fiber materials available. Formulating them to be palatable while at the same time having enough fiber to provide a beneficial effect may not be so easy. We should take heart, though. Humanity's earliest surviving example of noodle products is the 2600-year-old Subeixi noodles made from millet 'flour' (Gong *et al.*, 2011; Lu *et al.*, 2005). This flour was most likely unrefined, despite suggestions that flour refinement by sifting could have been practiced in that era, at least in ancient Egypt (Samuel, 2009), leading to a food of relatively high fiber content. Apocryphal writings also suggest that woven grass sieves may have predated the Subeixi noodles by at least 4000 years. Still, the Subeixi noodles are probably an ancient model for modern fiber-enriched noodle products.

14.2 Noodle quality attributes

14.2.1 Quality of wheat flour noodles

The processing of Asian wheat flour noodles and their quality attributes have been extensively reviewed elsewhere, and readers are encouraged to seek these and other resources for further detail (Hou, 2010; Ross and Bettge, 2009; Fu, 2008; Crosbie and Ross, 2004; Hatcher, 2001; Corke and Bhattacharya, 1999). In summary, Asian wheat flour noodles are made from flour milled from both soft and hard common wheat and are commonly formulated with either or both salt (NaCl) and alkaline substances (e.g. Na_2CO_3), and water. In commercial practice, Asian wheat flour noodles are generally processed using a 'sheet and cut' process and differ in practice from European-style 'pasta' as a result of raw material selection, formulation, and processing. Pasta products are defined for the purposes of this chapter as extruded products made from durum wheat semolina and water, and these are covered in Chapter 13. Within the Asian noodle sector, products are differentiated by formulation (e.g. salted vs. alkaline), cross-sectional dimensions, and whether the cooked noodles are relatively firm or soft. Asian wheat flour noodles are also subject to a variety of processes prior to packaging and distribution, creating an array of types: fried instant, steamed and dried instant, fresh, dried, par-boiled, and frozen, among others.

Wheat flour noodle products should have an attractive appearance. Colors vary from nearly white to deep yellow when made from refined flours (Crosbie and Ross, 2004) and the desired hue is a function of noodle type, formulation, and regional preference. Good appearance in noodles made from refined flour is also associated with freedom from discoloration and lack of bran specks (Symons and Brennan, 2004; Kruger *et al.*, 1994). Discoloration increases as flour extraction rates increase as a result of the disproportionate concentration of polyphenol oxidase (PPO) in the bran (Every *et al.*; 2006, Hatcher and Kruger, 1993). The issue of PPO-mediated darkening is indeed relevant to wholewheat noodles. Unpublished work from the author's laboratory has demonstrated, unsurprisingly, that noodles made from low PPO varieties retain their freshly made hue for longer than noodles made from high PPO varieties. Indeed, it may be even more important to source low PPO wheat for milling when the destination target is wholewheat noodles.

Cooked noodle texture is the other primary quality attribute and is also likely to be affected by wholewheat or fiber-enriched formulations. Softer types of noodles ('soft-bite', e.g. udon) are generally formulated with flour, salt and water, and are made from flours with moderate protein content (9.0–10%), medium–strong dough characteristics, and high swelling starch. The high swelling starch has a reduced amylose content. This may be a factor in starch digestibility and, at least *in vitro*, higher starch digestibility has been observed for reduced amylose wheat starches (Mangalika *et al.*, 2003). In the absence of a source of high swelling wheat flour, it is common to add other starches such as potato starch to achieve the desired softness and elasticity. The soft-bite noodles at their optimum are characterized by a 'long' texture, quantified as a large fracture strain (Ross, 2006). The presence of bran particles from wholewheat flours probably has the effect of reducing the fracture strain, potentially giving the noodles a rather brittle mouthfeel.

The hard-bite noodle category encompasses a greater range of formulations that also include alkaline compounds and in some instances, especially in 'instant' noodles, additionally include gums and polyphosphates (Crosbie and Ross, 2004; Hou and Kruk, 1998). Hard-bite noodles are generally made from wheat flours of moderately high to high protein content (10.5% to >13.0%) that have moderately strong to strong dough characteristics, and may have either high or low swelling starches (Ross and Bettge, 2009; Crosbie and Ross, 2004; Crosbie *et al.*, 1999).

14.2.2 Quality of noodles from other botanical sources

Noodles are also made from flours or refined starches of plant species other than wheat, such as mung bean, sweet potato, pea, potato, corn, and rice. These noodles share a common need to be processed using a combination of ungelatinized and gelatinized flour or starch (Lu and Collado, 2010; Tan *et al.*, 2009). The gelatinized portion is needed as a result of the non-cohesive nature of 'dough' made from non-wheat sources. In traditional methods, the dough is either dropped by gravity into boiling water to gelatinize the starch to form the noodle strands, or formed into sheets over a rotating heated drum. The drum partially cooks the starch, forming a sheet that is then chilled and cut into strips. Modern methods may utilize extrusion and steam cooking to form the sheet and cook the starch. Chilled noodles are cut into strips in both modern and traditional processes. The chilling step is interestingly parallel to traditional routines in which cooked noodles were held at sub-freezing temperatures during the customary time for noodle processing in the winter months (Lu and Collado, 2010). Of course we know in the modern era that the chilling retrogrades the starch. This not only makes the noodle sheets strong enough to perform adequately in the cutting process but is also a process by which the formation of RS may be enhanced. All starch noodles are then dried to a moisture range of 10 to 14.5% (Tan *et al.*, 2009). The processes have been reviewed in detail (Lu and Collado, 2010; Tan *et al.*, 2009).

Quality of rice and starch noodles is relative to the product type. Fresh rice noodles should have smooth surface characteristics, which includes a glossy appearance, with a white color, a characteristic aroma depending on whether or not they are fermented, and a smooth, chewy and elastic, and 'non-gritty' mouthfeel (Lu and Collado, 2010). Grittiness may be related to dry-milled rice with a larger particle size distribution compared with the wet-milled raw material. Dried rice noodles have similar requirements for cooked texture to their fresh counterparts. Starch noodles should have 'absence of discoloration, high glossiness, and high transparency' and when cooked should be 'firm, chewy and not sticky on standing after cooking'. Low cooking losses and short cooking times are also desired traits (Tan *et al.*, 2009).

14.2.3 Quality assessment of composite flour noodles

It is typical of most studies investigating the use of higher-fiber flours or other fiber-rich materials in noodles to use the quality parameters of noodles made with refined flour or starch as the gold standard. Sometimes this flour is very refined, with some 'premium' wheat flour noodles made with specialized flours that effectively only use the central endosperm of the wheat. It is of value to consider the alternative of holding wholewheat- or, say, barley-enriched noodles to a different standard of texture and taste. For example, eastern Asian milling technology before the onset of the modern roller-mill era was stone milling, little, if at all, different from the stone milling technology of the west. Given the difficulty of separating out finely ground bran in these all-in-one milling processes, even the best sifted flours probably had a light brown color cast and the 'gold standard' of a gleaming white noodle was probably not attainable. So what was the gold standard, say in the Han Period 2300 years ago? This is when the modern form of the noodle is reputed to have first appeared (Corke and Bhattacharya, 1999) and the gold standard might better be described by the characteristics of the Subeixi noodles (Gong *et al.*, 2011).

14.3 Wholewheat noodles

Exhaustive searching in both formal and informal databases and search engines yields almost no peer-reviewed technical information about wholewheat Asian noodles. Indeed, the index of the most recent monograph on Asian wheat flour noodles has no entry for 'whole-wheat' (Hou, 2010). There has been some work in which noodles were made with very high (95%) extraction flours (Ambalamaatil *et al.*, 2006), but otherwise there is, unbelievably, almost nothing. There is a rich history and literature regarding wholewheat pasta, and the introduction to this article described the 'atta' instant noodles marketed in Malaysia. One possible aspect of the poor market penetration of wholewheat noodles is summarized in personal correspondence with Dr Gary Hou (December 2010): 'Although we have been promoting whole-wheat noodles and high-fiber noodles in recent years to noodle manufacturers, we have not seen much success yet, especially for the whole-wheat noodles. The main obstacle to the success of whole-wheat noodles is the noodle texture and mouth feel. Asian consumers are not ready to accept this type of product with rough and gritty texture. Another issue is discoloration for untreated fresh [whole-wheat] noodles . . .'. There are substantial challenges in formulating wholewheat Asian-style noodles that would parallel issues related to long goods in durum pasta production. Readers are encouraged to read Chapter 13 of this book to get insight into the main issues.

The first challenge is the issue of color. With the high value placed on bright, clean colors in the refined flour products, it would seem that the brownness of the wholewheat noodles may be an impediment. A starting point would be to use flour milled from white-grained wheat. Ambalamaatil *et al.* (2006) showed that 95% extraction flours from white-grained wheat were equally bright as or brighter than 74% extraction flours milled from red-grained wheat. It takes no leap of imagination to recommend additionally the use of wholewheat flour milled from varieties with very low PPO activity in order to minimize darkening, given the high concentration of PPO in the bran. A more radical suggestion is to use whole-durum flour. Durum's significantly lower kernel PPO level (Demeke and Morris, 2002) minimizes darkening. There have already been some investigations of durum flour for Asian noodle production (Hatcher *et al.*, 2009; 2008a) and these studies are a good starting point to further investigate its use in wholewheat Asian noodle products.

From a textural perspective there would also appear to be parallels with durum-based pasta long goods. Wholewheat pasta long goods are reported to be stronger when dried at low temperatures (temperatures typical of dried Asian noodle production), but that is really the end of the good news. Wholewheat pasta had weak dough properties, higher cooking losses, and reduced cooked firmness (Manthey and Schorno, 2002). The authors attributed the differences to the disruption of the gluten network by bran and germ particles. It seems unlikely that a different outcome would accrue in Asian noodles. A micro-fine bran (e.g. milled to flour particle size or smaller) might be of value.

In that vein, although not wholewheat *per se*, a recent study that added wheat bran to dry white Chinese noodles (DWCN) encapsulates the general challenges encountered in formulating wholewheat noodles (Chen *et al.*, 2011). In this study, bran was added at 0 to 20% replacement of the refined flour, placing it in the range of bran concentrations from straight-grade to wholewheat. Additionally, the researchers ground the bran to three different fineness grades, defined by their average particle sizes: 1.73 mm, 0.53 mm, and 0.21 mm. In general, processing performance and noodle quality declined with both the amount of included bran and increased particle size. Dough properties showed an overall decline in parameters related to dough strength as both bran concentration and particle size increased. Flour pasting peak (hot paste) and final (cooled paste) viscosities declined with added bran, but the amount of bran was the primary effect. Dry noodle strength declined with increased bran concentration and bran particle size. This pattern was repeated for cooked noodle hardness, springiness, cohesiveness, and chewiness. In all cases, the worst performance came from the noodles with 20% bran addition at the 1.72 mm particle size. As noted above, bran may impart a gritty mouthfeel. Grittiness was reported after the inclusion of a fine soft-white wheat bran (passing a 1 mm screen) at up to 8% flour replacement (Sievert *et al.*, 1990). Chen *et al.* (2011) showed clearly that bran with finer particle size was of technological value in the noodles, but what about the effect of particle size in the colon? It has been shown that smaller bran particle size increases short-chain fatty acid (SCFA) production but that the molar concentration of the beneficial SCFA butyrate is enhanced at larger particle sizes (e.g. Stewart and Slavin, 2009). There is some evidence that coarser bran increases stool weight compared with finer bran at the same feeding rate (reviewed by Papanikolaou and Fulgoni, 2010). However, there is no dispute, at least in this author's mind, that, for generally healthy individuals, any bran is better than none at all!

14.4 Fiber-enriched wheat flour noodles

14.4.1 Addition of high-fiber flours

There is a long history of combining wheat flour with other flours in Asian noodle manufacture. The most visible manifestations of this are 'soba' (Japan) and 'naengmyon' (Korea) (Hatcher, 2001). These are made with blends of wheat and buckwheat (*Fagopyrum* sp.) flours. Buckwheat has unique flavor and aroma and is cherished for these attributes. Buckwheat groats add dietary fiber at varying concentrations to the formulation depending on the milling process used for the buckwheat and the level of admixture. Soba were the most common source of fiber-enriched noodle products in an informal survey of fiber-enriched noodles in North America. The soba products that were examined varied in claimed dietary fiber percentages from 8 to 17%, despite evidence that, at around 7% (Hatcher *et al.*, 2008; Wijngaard and Arendt, 2006), whole buckwheat flour has less fiber than that claimed on most packages. However, Hatcher *et al.* (2008) did report that a dark buckwheat flour that included fine bran could have up to 22% dietary fiber.

Barley flour has also been added to wheat flour noodles in attempts to formulate products with better nutritional profiles. However, not all barley flours are the same. Prior to milling into flour, hulled barley needs to have the unpalatable (but insoluble fiber-rich) hull removed, most commonly by abrasion. The remaining dehulled or pearled kernel has varying amounts of bran retained depending on the extent of the dehulling operation. Hull-less (free-threshing) barley varieties have no need of abrasive dehulling and therefore retain all of their bran when milled as whole grains. But even pearled barley can retain useful amounts of the important soluble fiber component β-glucan, which has been reported to be fairly evenly distributed in the endosperm (Miller and Fulcher, 1994). There are other reports showing β-glucan concentrated in the sub-aleurone layer in lower β-glucan, hull-less types (Zheng *et al.*, 2000). If this is also true for low β-glucan hulled types, β-glucan might be reduced in concentration by abrasive dehulling. The demonstrated ability to concentrate β-glucan in selected milling fractions (Izydorczyk and Dexter, 2008) suggests that care should be given to the type of barley flour being sourced when fiber enrichment of the products is a goal, to ensure that fiber targets are met.

Barley–wheat composite flours have been investigated in a number of studies. Baik and Czuchajowska (1997) used up to 20% barley flour milled from hull-less varieties. They observed substantial effects on technological measures of flour quality (e.g. paste viscosity) but saw little difference in the mechanical properties of the cooked noodles when made with non-waxy barley. Waxy barley did soften the noodles, but it was not made clear whether this was to a detrimentally soft level. In another study, an array of pearled and roller-milled hull-less barley flours were used to make 20/80 and 40/60 composite barley–wheat flours for alkaline noodle production (Hatcher *et al.*, 2005). The results of the 40% addition were more straightforward and are summarized here. At 40% barley flour, the authors reported that the dough required more water for optimum handling and that all doughs required less work to sheet regardless of whether the barley flour had normal, waxy, zero-amylose waxy, or high-amylose starch. Significantly, the authors reported no sheet breakage or other handling difficulties, despite the dilution of wheat gluten in the 40/60 barley–wheat composite flours. All cooking times were reduced at 40% barley addition, with the two waxy flours reducing optimum cooking time from 6.5 to 3 min. The shorter cooking times were considered responsible for reducing cooking losses. Variations of the cooked noodle physical properties were considered to be interactions between the starch type in the barley flour and cooking time. For example, compared with the wheat flour control, the waxy barley flours gave higher maximum cutting stress (cooked noodles were harder) but much faster relaxation times in a stress relaxation test (the cooked noodles had a more fluid-like character). These are to some extent contradictory mechanical signals. Similar results were also reported in a study after addition of a fiber-rich barley fraction (Izydorczyk *et al.*, 2005). Neither study reports how the texture, as perceived as by human subjects, was affected by this interesting mix of physical properties. Alkaline noodle color was affected 'detrimentally', that is, the noodles were darker, redder, and less yellow at 40% barley addition (Hatcher *et al.*, 2005). I think that, once again, some thought on what constitutes the gold standard is required. Hatcher and colleagues addressed the issue directly: 'While color and appearance generally play an important role in consumer acceptance and choice of food, certain food markets are more open and skewed toward less conventional products. For example, the traditional buckwheat noodles of Japan (soba) and Korea (naengmyon), deviate significantly from the common bright yellow or white color, but offer highly desirable texture, taste, and nutritional values and therefore are well established in their respective marketplaces.' These authors again addressed this matter in their conclusions, and readers are directed to those comments as well (Hatcher *et al.*, 2005). Hatcher's research group also carried out a parallel study on dried salted noodles (Lagassé *et al.*, 2006). In general, the results for cooking times, cooking losses, and cooked noodle physical properties paralleled those seen in their prior study on alkaline noodles (although the stress relaxation test was not repeated). The shorter cooking times reported again bring up an important issue with regard to the health benefits of the added barley: what happens to the soluble β-glucan during cooking? It appears that the reported shorter cooking times are an advantage and that there are only small losses, in the order of 2 to 4% of the total β-glucan present before cooking. Low β-glucan losses were also observed when cooking dried noodles, which necessarily take longer to cook (Izydorczyk *et al.*, 2005). Rye flour has been added at 30% replacement with similar results for color and cooked noodle texture to those reported for barley (Kruger *et al.*, 1998). Kruger and co-workers highlighted the effect of the choice of the base wheat flour, showing, not surprisingly, better outcomes with a high-protein flour with stronger dough properties.

Green banana flour has been used at 30% replacement with positive effects on fiber, RS, and phenolic contents of the resultant noodles (Choo and Aziz, 2010). The banana flour composite noodles were harder than a comparable soba noodle sample. The authors did not compare the composite flour noodles with the 100% wheat flour as a control. The banana composite noodles also showed beneficially reduced glycemic index and carbohydrate digestibility rates. Many other flours have been tried in noodles, with the expected changes in color, texture, and nutritional value related to the composition of the supplemented flours. These have included sweet potato (Collins and Pangloli, 1997), soybean (Chen *et al.*, 2010), and garbanzo bean (Lee *et al.*, 1998).

14.4.2 Addition of specific fiber materials

Refined fiber sources have also been added to wheat flour noodle formulations with the implied expectation that enough fiber can be added to gain a beneficial dietary effect without the consumer actually noticing that they are consuming a fiber-enriched product: the fiber-by-stealth approach. A great variety of materials have been added that fit this broad definition of dietary fiber: 'dietary fiber consists of all carbohydrate components that are non-digestible to mammalian enzymes' (McBurney, 2010). These have included soy polysaccharides (Sievert *et al.*, 1990), psyllium (mostly arabinoxylan) (Czuchajowska *et al.*, 1992), fiber-enriched barley fractions (β-glucan and arabinoxylan) (Izydorczyk *et al.*, 2005), oat β-glucan (Inglett *et al.*, 2005), guar gum (galactomannan) (Yu and Ngadi, 2006), alginate (a block copolymer of guluronate and mannuronate), and curdlan (β,1→3 glucan) (Lee *et al.*, 2008), among others. Given the diversity of materials that have been applied, only a small selection will be reviewed in detail.

A number of investigations have looked into formulating wheat flour noodles with β-glucan-rich materials. The study of Izydorczyk *et al.* (2005), which used fiber-enriched barley fractions, showed similar effects to that of adding unfractionated barley flour. Oat-based β-glucan materials have also been investigated (Inglett *et al.*, 2005). Noodles were supplemented with 'Nutrim', a freeze-dried extract of oat solubles, including soluble β-glucan (Carriere and Inglett, 2000). The noodles investigated were not standard wheat flour noodles, but included rice flour. In salted noodles, Nutrim at 10%

addition had no effect on cooking loss with 20% rice flour addition but increased cooking loss at higher rice flour levels. Nutrim decreased salted noodle hardness at all rice flour levels. In alkaline noodles the effects were less pronounced, with smaller increases in cooking loss and variable effects on cooked noodle hardness, decreasing hardness at 20% rice flour addition but increasing it at 50% rice flour. Another study using Nutrim had the specific goal of formulating to 0.75 g soluble fiber per serving (Mohamed *et al.*, 2005). This was achieved at 20% addition of Nutrim. Nutrim at 20% addition level increased optimum water addition for dough formation and decreased dough mixing stability. Raw (uncooked) noodle color was substantially darker, slightly redder, and noticeably yellower after Nutrim addition. Cooked noodle hardness and chewiness were drastically reduced, although cohesiveness and resilience increased, and springiness remained the same. Overall, even the authors had to conclude that, at the addition levels needed to meet the US soluble fiber health claim of 0.75 g per serving, the Nutrim supplemented noodles were 'somewhat acceptable'. This highlights the challenges of getting sufficient fiber into a product without decreasing its culinary desirability.

Alginates are an interesting polysaccharide category, with the potential to both provide health benefits (expanded below with respect to rice noodles) and improve, rather than diminish, the culinary quality of noodle products. Evidence of this was shown after alginate was added to wheat flour noodles (Lee *et al.*, 2008). Up to the maximum level used, 1.5% addition on a flour basis, alginate addition improved cutting force and tensile strength and reduced cooking loss in salted noodles. Dough properties were affected, with increased development times and decreased stability, and these changes might be of some concern in commercial production. Noodle color was darker and slightly yellower. To achieve the 1.5 g per meal dose shown to decrease cholesterol uptake in obese individuals (Paxman *et al.*, 2008), consumers would need to eat around 200 g of cooked noodles at the 1.5% addition level. This is about two standard servings converted from a dry-basis serving size of 40 g (Mohamed *et al.*, 2005) (dry salted noodles have cooked noodle yields at least double the weight of the dried noodles). Indeed, rather than health factors, if alginate were sufficiently inexpensive, its addition could be considered a useful functional intervention for improving the cooking performance and cooked noodle texture when less expensive lower-protein flours are used for hard-bite styles of wheat flour noodles. Alginate, with and without curdlan and starch, has also been used to create structure and improve the texture in noodles made with a so-called hypoallergenic wheat flour, a product with a highly hydrolyzed gluten fraction (Oishi *et al.*, 2009). Although the products had higher cooking losses and were softer than the control noodles, they may have a role for gluten-sensitive individuals.

One study that may be of interest added green seaweed (Family: Chlorophyta) powder to salted noodles with and without added egg. The Chlorophyta seaweeds contain a family of sulfated polysaccharides named ulvans at 8–29% (dry weight basis) (Lahaye and Robic, 2007). These polysaccharides have molecular weight

(MW) up to the order of 10^6 and have been shown to have a range of pharmacological effects beyond their contribution as a fiber source (Karnjanapratum and You, 2011). Chang and Wu (2008) added powdered green seaweed up to 8% (flour basis) (up to ~0.8 to 2.4% ulvan, based on Lahaye and Robic, 2007). Seaweed noodles showed higher cooked noodle yields, reduced cooking losses, and reduced cooked noodle tensile breaking strength, springiness, and extensibility. Sensory evaluations concurred on the noodles' mechanical properties. However, panelists rated the seaweed noodles better for color than the white flour control when the high-quality anchor was a green tea soba, not the white flour noodles.

Polysaccharides are commonly added to instant noodle formulations at low levels for their functional attributes (Hou and Kruk, 1998). It is easy to envisage increasing the levels of these fiber materials to a level that invokes a health benefit at a reasonable serving size without substantially altering the physical properties or appearance of the product. In fact, a broader benefit might accrue if the added polysaccharides were formulated in such a way that they also reduced fat uptake during the frying of instant noodles, as has been demonstrated for some gums. For example, guar gum addition at 0.37% reduced fat uptake during frying of instant fried noodles by just over 3% (from 24% down to just under 21%) while concurrently increasing cooked noodle firmness (Yu and Ngadi, 2006). Cellulose gums (Cash and Caputo, 2010) and curdlan (Khan *et al.*, 2007) have also been suggested for fat reduction in instant noodles. Curdlan has also been shown to improve elasticity in cooked instant noodles (Khan *et al.*, 2007). Clearly, from a fiber intake perspective there are opportunities to further decrease fat uptake while at the same time increasing fiber content of instant noodles to levels of practical value.

14.5 Wheat flour noodles and resistant starch

Research into the abundance in or addition of RS to Asian wheat flour noodles is sparse. Gelroth and Ranhotra (2000) indicated that two types of Asian-style wheat flour noodles had 0.4 to 0.5 g/100 g of RS on an as-served basis. For comparison, white pan bread had 0.9 g/100 g of RS. There appears to be an opportunity for adding RS to wheat flour noodle formulations, particularly where the texture characteristics are expected to be firm and where the low swelling power of high-amylose starches could be a unique way of adding hidden fiber to the product while enhancing textural qualities. Rendón-Villalobos *et al.* (2008) added plantain banana (*Musa paradisiaca* L.) up to 30% replacement in salted noodles and showed a modest increase from 1.9 to 2.2% (dry basis) RS at a 30% banana addition. This was paralleled by a decrease of around 5% in *in vitro* digestibility of the noodles. Decreased starch digestibility has also been reported in alkaline noodles with green Cavendish banana flour (Saifullah *et al.*, 2009). Similarly, when plantain starch was added to salted noodles (Osorio-Diaz *et al.*, 2008) there was a modest increase in RS from 2.7 to 4.6% and a parallel modest decrease in available starch.

14.6 Wholegrain and fiber-enriched noodles from other botanical sources

14.6.1 Fiber enrichment of rice noodles

As has been the experience when researching addition of fiber materials to other types of noodles, the addition of fiber materials to rice noodles has primarily been done to improve the processing, storage, or culinary quality of the product. Only recently has this transformed to the idea that there may also be health benefits. Informal sensory evaluations of a commercial wholegrain (brown) rice noodle were conducted in the author's laboratories. This evaluation directly compared the brown rice noodles with white rice noodles from the same manufacturer. Both noodle types had the same cross-sectional dimensions. Perceived textural deficits were reduced tensile strength and a more brittle, less chewy mouthfeel. Although the bran appeared to have been ground very finely, it may be valid to speculate that it interfered with the three-dimensional polymeric (starch) network, leading to the diminished textural quality.

Alginates have also been proposed as additives for rice noodles, and noodles supplemented with alginate may, in addition to increased fiber content, also have improved texture if treated in a calcium bath during processing (Onsøyen, 2001). Alginate has been shown to have beneficial effects when consumed in the diet. For example, a 1.5 g dose reduced uptake of glucose and cholesterol in obese subjects (Paxman *et al.*, 2008). There is evidence that the effects of alginate on satiety may rely on gelation of the alginate in the gut (Hoad *et al.*, 2004). Nonetheless, alginate added to rice noodles and gelled during processing (before consumption) was shown to reduce *in vitro* starch digestibility, and at the same time reduce cooking loss and soluble starch leakage (Koh *et al.*, 2009). These attributes were more evident with a stronger gelling high-guluronate alginate sample. There was some darkening of rice noodle color related to alginate addition, but in the intended target product—instant rice noodles in soup—this may not be a significant factor in consumer choice. Using rice flour gels as analogs for rice noodles, Huaisan *et al.* (2009) added guar gum, high-methoxy pectin, and alginate. This study observed some beneficial effects of high-methoxy pectin on the stability of the frozen gel, and maybe by inference frozen rice noodles. However, at the highest level of addition used in this study of 0.6% (flour basis) this would make only a minor contribution to total fiber intake. Yalcin and Basman (2008) added xanthan and locust bean gums to rice noodle formulations up to a maximum level of 3% (w/w). Xanthan was more effective for most noodle quality-related parameters, showing decreased cooking loss and increased maximum cutting force. Color was little affected. Xanthan was rated by sensory analysis to have improved noodle surface and chewing properties, as well as taste.

Rice noodles and resistant starch

One perspective on starch-rich products such as rice noodles is to examine the potential for the presence or induction of a RS fraction that could then exert the known beneficial effects of RS in the gut of the consumer. Rice starch with >25% amylose is reported to be preferred for products that require an intact cooked product (Juliano, 2005) and can be a preferred raw material for rice noodles (Lu and Collado, 2010). Coincidentally, this is a useful starting material for the production of RS3 (retrograded starch).

Rice noodles in a broad sense have been identified as intermediate to low glycemic index foods, with glycemic index values ranging from 37 (Ranawana *et al.*, 2009) to 83 (Juliano, 2005). This occurs even without specific interventions to decrease starch digestibility. RS content of rice noodles was reported to be almost 10% of total starch (~ 2% on an as-eaten basis) (Chen *et al.*, 2010) but there are clearly both processing and formulation strategies that could increase RS levels and hence lower starch digestibility in rice noodles. For example, Lu and Collado (2010) report the use of *Cannaedulis* starch as an additive in rice noodles. Canna starch's reported amylose content (29% (Lu and Collado, 2010); 34% (Watcharatewinkul *et al.*, 2009)) suggests the potential for enhanced levels of RS under appropriate processing conditions. Other high-amylose starches such as pea starch may also be applicable either as native starches or after treatments (e.g. lintnerization) aimed at increasing RS3 content (Lehmann *et al.*, 2003). Caution needs to be exercised, though. The strong retrogradation properties of some starches may make them unsuitable for frozen rice noodles, as potentially poor freeze–thaw stability could affect quality. Similarly, for fresh rice noodles, even after a chilling step to make them amenable to cutting, further retrogradation and the consequent syneresis could make the noodles undesirable.

14.6.2 Fiber enrichment of starch noodles

In this category of noodles it is clear again that most of the work on fiber enrichment has been related to processing, storage, and culinary quality rather than health benefits. The use of polysaccharides in starch-based systems analogous to noodles was recently reviewed (Tan *et al.*, 2009). In this instance, most of the reviewed studies looked at gels as model systems for noodles. The reviewed studies covered konjac glucomannan, guar galactomannan, and a recently 'discovered' polysaccharide from a source that has been used in Chinese medicine for centuries. The 'new' polysaccharide complex comes from the seeds of *Artemisia sphaerocephala* in the family Asteraceae. *Asphaerocephala* is thought to have pectic polymers with arabinogalactan side chains and the putative presence of a 4-O-methyl glucuronoxylan, which is considered to be bioactive (Batbayar *et al.*, 2008). However, Zhang *et al.* (2007) only reported the presence of arabinose, xylose, lyxose, mannose, glucose, and D-galactose, but no acidic monosaccharides or methylated glucuronic acid. The reported ability of *Asphaerocephala* to improve chewing quality and elasticity in noodles (Xing *et al.*, 2009) may suggest an anionic polymer with gelling capabilities similar to alginate or low-methoxypectins. *Asphaerocephala* gum is reputed to be effective against diabetes and has a clinical record in animal studies to support that conjecture (e.g. Xing *et al.*, 2009). *Asphaerocephala* gum also has the interesting property of being able to aggregate sandy soil (Batbayar *et al.*, 2008).

Starch noodles and resistant starch

The situation with the other starch-based noodles is similar to that of rice noodles. There is already a need to retrograde starch in processing in order to achieve the desired storage and culinary attributes expected of the products. Lu and Collado (2010) indicate that 'processes are employed to enhance retrogradation such as the application of low temperature conditioning after gelatinization'. They went on to indicate that this step sets the noodle structure. If the retrogradation, and in particular amylose retrogradation, were not promoted, the noodles might simply dissolve in the soup: not a desired outcome. The resistance of retrograded amylose crystallites to melting at temperatures below 100°C (Delcour and Hoseney, 2010) is the basis of this persistent structure.

Specific studies have been done on RS and related digestibility factors in starch noodles. A recent study is used here as an example of the potential of starch noodles to contribute to improved glycemic outcomes, presumably as a result of having starch that is slowly digestible or resistant to digestion by amylase. Lin *et al.* (2010) investigated mung bean noodles. They observed in human feeding trials of equivalent carbohydrate portions that the mung bean noodles decreased peak blood glucose concentration by half compared with white bread and by about one-third compared with a *Japonica* brown rice. Of the foods tested, the mung bean noodles were most effective at decreasing the insulin response, decreasing it by nearly half compared with white bread, but also delaying the peak in plasma insulin by approximately 15 minutes. Adlay (*Coxi lachrymal-jobi*), brown rice, taro, and yam all had only modest reductions (~10%) in insulin response compared with the white bread sample. Even better, despite being made entirely of starch, the mung bean noodles combined low glycemic index, and reduced insulin response, with the lowest glycemic load of the tested foods.

14.7 Conclusion

Greater awareness of the value of an adequate fiber intake will drive consumers to demand high fiber variants of traditional products. This demand will lead to innovation that will create palatable and nutritious noodle products that meet the culinary expectations of consumers. Opportunities are abundant for the use of composite flours in wheat flour noodle types. These could not only boost the fiber content but also, with the advent of high-amylose wheat varieties, boost the RS content of these popular noodles. Of course, there are also abundant opportunities to enrich all noodle types with a variety of more or less refined fiber sources, ranging from green seaweed powder to cellulose gums, and to take steps to further decrease or slow starch digestibility. It is clear, though, that the culinary community needs to be enlisted to highlight the 'delicious *and* nutritious' potential of the next generation of nutritionally more valuable noodles.

14.8 References

AMBALAMAATIL, S., LUKOW, O. M. and MALCOLMSON, L. J. 2006. Quality attributes of Canadian hard white spring wheat. *Journal of Food Quality*, **29**, 151–70.

BAIK, B. K. and CZUCHAJOWSKA, Z. 1997. Barley in udon noodles. *Food Science and Technology International*, **3**, 423–35.

BATBAYAR, N., BANZRAGCH, D., INNGJERDINGEN, K. T., NARAN, R., MICHAELSEN, T. E. and PAULSEN, B. S. 2008. Polysaccharides from Mongolian plants and their effect on the complement system: I. Polysaccharides from plants of the *Asteraceae* family. *Asian Journal of Traditional Medicines*, **3**, 33–41.

CARRIERE, C. J. and INGLETT, G. E. 2000. Effect of processing conditions on the viscoelastic behavior of NutrimX: an oat based glucan rich hydrocolloidal extractive. *Journal of Texture Studies*, **31**, 123–40.

CASH, M. J. and CAPUTO, S. J. 2010. Cellulose Derivatives. *Food Stabilisers, Thickeners and Gelling Agents*. A. IMESON (ed.), Wiley-Blackwell, Oxford, UK, 95–113.

CHANG, H. C. and WU, L. C. 2008. Texture and Quality Properties of Chinese Fresh Egg Noodles Formulated with Green Seaweed (*Monostroma nitidum*) Powder. *Journal of Food Science*, **73**, S398–S404.

CHEN, J. S., FEI, M. J., SHI, C. L., TIAN, J. C., SUN, C. L., *et al.* Effect of particle size and addition level of wheat bran on quality of dry white Chinese noodles. *Journal of Cereal Science*, in press.

CHEN, L., LIU, R., QIN, C., MENG, Y., ZHANG, J., *et al.* 2010. Sources and intake of resistant starch in the Chinese diet. *Asia Pacific Journal of Clinical Nutrition*, **19**, 274–82.

CHOO, C. L. and AZIZ, N. A. A. 2010. Effects of banana flour and beta-glucan on the nutritional and sensory evaluation of noodles. *Food Chemistry*, **119**, 34–40.

COLLAR, C., SANTOS, E. and ROSELL, C. M. 2006. Significance of dietary fiber on the viscometric pattern of pasted and gelled flour-fiber blends. *Cereal Chemistry*, **83**, 370–6.

COLLINS, J. L. and PANGLOLI, P. 1997. Chemical, physical and sensory attributes of noodles with added sweetpotato and soy flour. *Journal of Food Science*, **62**, 622–5.

CORKE, H. and BHATTACHARYA, M. 1999. Wheat Products: 1. Noodles. *Asian Foods: Science and Technology*. C. Y. W. ANG, K. LIU and Y.-W. HUANG (eds). Technomic Publishing Company, Lancaster, PA, USA, 43–65.

CROSBIE, G. B. and ROSS, A. S. 2004. Asian wheat flour noodles. *The Encyclopedia of Grain Science, Vol 2*. C. W. WRIGLEY, H. CORKE and C. E. WALKER (eds). Elsevier Academic Press, Oxford UK, 304–12.

CROSBIE, G. B., ROSS, A. S., MORO, T. and CHIU, P. C. 1999. Starch and protein quality requirements of Japanese alkaline noodles (Ramen). *Cereal Chemistry*, **76**, 328–34.

CZUCHAJOWSKA, Z., PASZCZYNSKA, B. and POMERANZ, Y. 1992. Functional-properties of psyllium in wheat-based products. *Cereal Chemistry*, **69**, 516–20.

DELCOUR, J. A. and HOSENEY, R. C. 2010. *Principles of cereal science and technology*, AACC International.

DEMEKE, T. and MORRIS, C. 2002. Molecular characterization of wheat polyphenol oxidase (PPO). *Theoretical and Applied Genetics*, **104**, 813–18.

EVERY, D., SIMMONS, L. D. and ROSS, M. P. 2006. Distribution of redox enzymes in millstreams and relationships to chemical and baking properties of flour. *Cereal Chemistry*, **83**, 62–8.

FU, B. X. 2008. Asian noodles: History, classification, raw materials, and processing. *Food Research International*, **41**, 888–902.

GELROTH, J. A. and RANHOTRA, G. S. 2000. Determination of resistant starch in selected grain-based foods. *Journal of AOAC International*, **83**, 988–91.

GONG, Y., YANG, Y., FERGUSON, D. K., TAO, D., LI, W., *et al.* 2011. Investigation of ancient noodles, cakes, and millet at the Subeixi Site, Xinjiang, China. *Journal of Archaeological Science*, **38**, 470–9.

HATCHER, D. W. 2001. Asian noodle processing. *Cereals Processing Technology*. G. OWENS (ed.). Woodhead Publishing: Cambridge, UK, 131–57.

HATCHER, D. W. and KRUGER, J. E. 1993. Distribution of polyphenol oxidase in flour millstreams of Canadian common wheat classes milled to three extraction rates. *Cereal Chemistry*, **70**, 51.

HATCHER, D. W., LAGASSE, S., DEXTER, J. E., ROSSNAGEL, B. and IZYDORCZYK, M. 2005. Quality characteristics of yellow alkaline noodles enriched with hull-less barley flour. *Cereal Chemistry*, **82**, 60–9.

HATCHER, D. W., DEXTER, J. E. and FU, B. X. 2008a. Investigation of amber durum wheat for production of yellow alkaline noodles. *Journal of Cereal Science*, **48**, 848–56.

HATCHER, D. W., YOU, S., DEXTER, J. E., CAMPBELL, C. and IZYDORCZYK, M. S. 2008b. Evaluation of the performance of flours from cross- and self-pollinating Canadian common buckwheat (*Fagopyrum esculentum* Moench) cultivars in soba noodles. *Food Chemistry*, **107**, 722–31.

HATCHER, D. W., DEXTER, J. E. and FU, B. X. 2009. Refrigerated Storage of Yellow Alkaline Durum Noodles: Impact on Color and Texture 1. *Cereal Chemistry*, **86**, 106–12.

HOAD, C. L., RAYMENT, P., SPILLER, R. C., MARCIANI, L., ALONSO, B. D. C., *et al.* 2004. In Vivo Imaging of Intragastric Gelation and Its Effect on Satiety in Humans. *The Journal of Nutrition*, **134**, 2293–300.

HOU, G. and KRUK, M. 1998. Asian noodle technology. *AIB Technical Bulletin*, **20**, 1–10.

HOU, G. G. 2010. *Asian Noodles: Science, Technology, and Processing*, Wiley.

HUAISAN, K., URIYAPONGSON, J., RAYAS-DUARTE, P., ALLI, I., SRIJESDARUK, V. and AHMED, J. 2009. Effect of food additives on rheological and textural properties of frozen high amylose rice starch gels. *International Journal of Food Properties*, **12**, 145–61.

INGLETT, G. E., PETERSON, S. C., CARRIERE, C. J. and MANEEPUN, S. 2005. Rheological, textural, and sensory properties of Asian noodles containing an oat cereal hydrocolloid. *Food Chemistry*, **90**, 1–8.

IZYDORCZYK, M. S. and DEXTER, J. E. 2008. Barley β-glucans and arabinoxylans: Molecular structure, physicochemical properties, and uses in food products—a Review. *Food Research International*, **41**, 850–68.

IZYDORCZYK, M. S., LAGASSE, S., HATCHER, D. W., DEXTER, J. E. and ROSSNAGEL, B. G. 2005. The enrichment of Asian noodles with fiber-rich fractions derived from roller milling of hull-less barley. *Journal of the Science of Food and Agriculture*, **85**, 2094–104.

JULIANO, B. O. 2005. Overview of rice and rice-based products. *Rice is life: scientific perspectives for the 21st century. Proceedings of the World Rice Research Conference held in Tsukuba, Japan, 4-7 November 2004*, K. TORIYAMA, K. L. HEONG and B. HARDY (eds). International Rice Research Institute (IRRI), 268–70.

KARNJANAPRATUM, S. and YOU, S. 2011. Molecular characteristics of sulfated polysaccharides from *Monostroma nitidum* and their in vitro anticancer and immunomodulatory activities. *International Journal of Biological Macromolecules*, **48**, 311–18.

KHAN, T., PARK, J. and KWON, J.-H. 2007. Functional biopolymers produced by biochemical technology considering applications in food engineering. *Korean Journal of Chemical Engineering*, **24**, 816–26.

KOH, L. W., KASAPIS, S., LIM, K. M. and FOO, C. W. 2009. Structural enhancement leading to retardation of in vitro digestion of rice dough in the presence of alginate. *Food Hydrocolloids*, **23**, 1458–64.

KRUGER, J. E., ANDERSON, M. H. and DEXTER, J. E. 1994. Effect of flour refinement on raw Cantonese noodle color and texture. *Cereal Chemistry*, **71**, 177–82.

KRUGER, J. E., HATCHER, D. W. and ANDERSON, M. J. 1998. The effect of incorporation of rye flour on the quality of oriental noodles. *Food Research International*, **31**, 27–35.

LAGASSÉ, S. L., HATCHER, D. W., DEXTER, J. E., ROSSNAGEL, B. G. and IZYDORCZYK, M. S. 2006. Quality Characteristics of Fresh and Dried White Salted Noodles Enriched with Flour from Hull-less Barley Genotypes of Diverse Amylose Content. *Cereal Chemistry*, **83**, 202–10.

LAHAYE, M. and ROBIC, A. 2007. Structure and Functional Properties of Ulvan, a Polysaccharide from Green Seaweeds. *Biomacromolecules*, **8**, 1765–74.

LEE, L., BAIK, B.-K. and CZUCHAJOWSKA, Z. 1998. Garbanzo Bean Flour Usage in Cantonese Noodles. *Journal of Food Science*, **63**, 552–58.

LEE, S., BAE, I. Y., JUNG, J.-H., JANG, K.-I., KIM, Y. W. and LEE, H. G. 2008. Physicochemical, textural and noodle-making properties of wheat dough containing alginate. *Journal of Texture Studies*, **39**, 393–404.

LEHMANN, U., RÖSSLER, C., SCHMIEDL, D. and JACOBASCH, G. 2003. Production and physicochemical characterization of resistant starch type III derived from pea starch. *Food/Nahrung*, **47**, 60–3.

LIN, M. H. A., WU, M. C., LU, S. and LIN, J. 2010. Glycemic index, glycemic load and insulinemic index of Chinese starchy foods. *World Journal of Gastroenterology*, **16**, 4973–9.

LU, H., YANG, X., YE, M., LIU, K. B., XIA, Z., *et al.* 2005. Culinary archaeology: Millet noodles in late Neolithic China. *Nature*, **437**, 967–8.

LU, Z.-H. and COLLADO, L. S. 2010. *Rice and Starch-Based Noodles, Asian Noodles: Science, Technology, and Processing.* G. HOU (ed.). John Wiley & Sons, 393–432.

MANGALIKA, W. H. A., MIURA, H., YAMAUCHI, H. and NODA, T. 2003. Properties of starches from near-isogenic wheat lines with different wx protein deficiencies. *Cereal Chemistry*, **80**, 662–6.

MANTHEY, F. A. and SCHORNO, A. L. 2002. Physical and cooking quality of spaghetti made from whole wheat durum. *Cereal Chemistry*, **79**, 504–10.

MCBURNEY, M. I. 2010. Dietary fibres insights and opportunities. *Dietary fibre: new frontiers for food and health.* J.W. VAN DER KAMP, J.M. JONES, B.V. MCCLEARY and D.L. TOPPING (eds). Wageningen Academic Publishers, 153–66.

MILLER, S. S. and FULCHER, R. G. 1994. Distribution of (1→3),(1→4)-β-D-glucan in kernels of oats and barley using microspectrofluorometry. *Cereal Chemistry*, **71**, 64–8.

MOHAMED, A. A., RAYAS DUARTE, P., XU, J., PALMQUIST, D. E. and INGLETT, G. E. 2005. Hard Red Winter Wheat/Nutrim OB Alkaline Fresh Noodles: Processing and Texture Analysis. *Journal of Food Science*, **70**, S1–S7.

OISHI, Y., UDAGAWA, H., SHINOZAKI, Y., MORIYAMA, M., TANIGUCHI, H., *et al.* 2009. Preparation of Hypoallergenic Wheat Flour Noodles and Evaluation of Their Physical Properties. *Food Science and Technology Research*, **15**, 39–44.

ONSØYEN, E. 2001. Alginate. *Handbook of Dietary Fiber.* S. CHO and M. L. DREHER (eds). CRC Press, 659–74.

OSORIO-DIAZ, P., AGUILAR-SANDOVAL, A., AGAMA-ACEVEDO, E., RENDON-VILLALOBOS, R., TOVAR, J. and BELLO-PEREZ, L. A. 2008. Composite durum wheat flour/plantain starch white salted noodles: Proximal composition, starch digestibility, and indigestible fraction content. *Cereal Chemistry*, **85**, 339–43.

PAPANIKOLAOU, Y. and FULGONI, V. L. 2010. The effect of wheat bran on various measures of bowel function and regularity. *Dietary fibre: new frontiers for food and health.* J. W. VAN DER KAMP, J. M. JONES, B. V. MCCLEARY and D. L. TOPPING (eds). Wageningen Academic Publishers, 261–82.

PAXMAN, J. R., RICHARDSON, J. C., DETTMAR, P. W. and CORFE, B. M. 2008. Alginate reduces the increased uptake of cholesterol and glucose in overweight male subjects: a pilot study. *Nutrition Research*, **28**, 501–5.

RANAWANA, D. V., HENRY, C. J. K., LIGHTOWLER, H. J. and WANG, D. 2009. Glycaemic index of some commercially available rice and rice products in Great Britain. *International Journal of Food Sciences and Nutrition*, **60**, 99–110.

RENDÓN-VILLALOBOS, R., OSORIO-DÍAZ, P., AGAMA-ACEVEDO, E., TOVAR, J. and BELLO-PÉREZ, L. A. 2008. Composite wheat-plantain starch salted noodles. Preparation, proximal composition and in vitro starch digestibility. *Interciencia*, **33**, 658–62.

ROSS, A. S. 2006. Instrumental measurement of physical properties of cooked Asian wheat flour noodles. *Cereal Chemistry*, **83**, 42–51.

ROSS A. S. and BETTGE, A. D. 2009. Passing the test on wheat end-use quality. *Wheat: science and trade.* B. CARVER (ed.). Wiley-Blackwell Publishing, 455–93.

ROSS, A. S. and CROSBIE, G. B. 2010. Wheat-flour factors influencing noodle texture. *Asian Noodles: Science, Technology, and Processing*. G. HOU (ed.). John Wiley & Sons, 313–29.

SAIFULLAH, R., ABBAS, F. M. A., YEOH, S. Y. and AZHAR, M. E. 2009. Utilization of green banana flour as a functional ingredient in yellow noodle. *International Food Research Journal*, **16**, 373–9.

SAMUEL, D. 2009. Experimental Grinding and Ancient Egyptian Flour Production. *Beyond the Horizon: Studies in Egyptian Art, Archaeology and History in Honour of Barry J. Kemp*. S. IKRAM and A. DODSON (eds). American University in Cairo Press, 456–77.

SIEVERT, D., POMERANZ, Y. and ABDELRAHMAN, A. 1990. Functional properties of soy polysaccharides and wheat bran in soft wheat products. *Cereal Chemistry*, **67**, 10–3.

STEWART, M. L. and SLAVIN, J. L. 2009. Particle size and fraction of wheat bran influence short-chain fatty acid production in vitro. *British Journal of Nutrition*, **102**, 1404–7.

SYMONS, L. J. and BRENNAN, C. S. 2004. The Effect of Barley Glucan Fiber Fractions on Starch Gelatinization and Pasting Characteristics. *Journal of Food Science*, **69**, 257–61.

TAN, H. Z., LI, Z. G. and TAN, B. 2009. Starch noodles: History, classification, materials, processing, structure, nutrition, quality evaluating and improving. *Food Research International*, **42**, 551–76.

WATCHARATEWINKUL, Y., PUTTANLEK, C., RUNGSARDTHONG, V. and UTTAPAP, D. 2009. Pasting properties of a heat-moisture treated canna starch in relation to its structural characteristics. *Carbohydrate Polymers*, **75**, 505–11.

WIJNGAARD, H. H. and ARENDT, E. K. 2006. Buckwheat. *Cereal Chemistry*, **83**, 391–401.

XING, X.-H., ZHANG, Z.-M., HU, X.-Z., WU, R.-Q. and XU, C. 2009. Antidiabetic effects of *Artemisia sphaerocephala* Krasch. gum, a novel food additive in China, on streptozotocin-induced type 2 diabetic rats. *Journal of Ethnopharmacology*, **125**, 410–16.

YALCIN, S. and BASMAN, A. 2008. Effects of gelatinisation level, gum and transglutaminase on the quality characteristics of rice noodle. *International Journal of Food Science and Technology*, **43**, 1637–44.

YU, L. J. and NGADI, M. O. 2006. Rheological properties of instant fried noodle dough as affected by some ingredients. *Journal of the Science of Food and Agriculture*, **86**, 544–8.

ZHANG, J., WU, J., LIANG, J., HU, Z., WANG, Y. and ZHANG, S. 2007. Chemical characterization of Artemisia seed polysaccharide. *Carbohydrate Polymers*, **67**, 213–18.

ZHENG, G. H., ROSSNAGEL, B. G., TYLER, R. T. and BHATTY, R. S. 2000. Distribution of β-glucan in the grain of hull-less barley. *Cereal Chemistry*, **77**, 140–4.

Part IV

Improving the quality of fibre-enriched foods: other products

15

Fibre-enriched dairy products

H. D. Goff, University of Guelph, Canada

DOI: 10.1533/9780857095787.4.311

Abstract: Dairy products can be a suitable carrier food for fibre enrichment. Such products include beverages, puddings, yogurts, frozen desserts and others. Consumers have shown a willingness to consume such products as an avenue for enhanced fibre intake and health benefits. For highest concentration potential in high water-containing products, viscosity of the fibre should be low, provided that the fibre also contributes positively to a wide range of health benefits. Thus far, inulin, gum Arabic, polydextrose and soluble soybean polysaccharides have all been successfully fortified into various dairy products, while other gums also may have potential. Protein–polysaccharide phase separation in such products has to be controlled.

Key words: milk, dairy products, dietary fibre, soluble fibre, fortification.

15.1 Introduction

Milk is not a natural source of soluble or insoluble fibre in the human diet. Human milk and human colostrum may contain up to 12–13 and 22–24 g/l of oligosaccharides, respectively, many of which are not digested in the small intestine, whereas bovine colostrum contains only ~1 g/l and only trace amounts are found in mature milk (Urashima *et al.*, 2009). The fate of these human colostrum and human milk oligosaccharides is undoubtedly fermentation in the colon, as prebiotics to help establish a microflora rich in bifidobacteria and other beneficial species. Although this is a very interesting natural source of prebiotics in the diet of the human infant, for the general milk-consuming public any fibres that dairy products contain would be added for their health benefit by dairy processors and sold as such.

There is increasing interest from food processors and consumers in voluntary enrichment or fortification of soluble fibre in food products that are part of the human diet, to compensate for the deficiency in the diet of the general public due to lack of sufficient natural sources of fibre: fruits, vegetables, legumes, whole grains, and so on. Soluble fibres contribute a large number of health benefits to human diets, and, although recommendations for inclusion of both soluble and insoluble fibres in the diet are usually given by health-promoting governmental agencies (e.g. 38 g/day for men and 25 g/day for women in the Dietary Reference Intakes as established by the Institute of Medicine in North America), there tends to be a large gap (the 'fibre gap') between recommended amounts and those actually consumed. For example, in Canada, surveys of nutrient intakes from foods indicate that mean dietary fibre intakes ranged from 14.3 to 16.6 g/d for women and from 16.5 to 19.4 g/d for men (Health Canada and Statistics Canada, Canadian Community Health and Nutrition Survey). While a preferable strategy would be to consume fibre from whole food sources, fibre enrichment of foods would be a preferred strategy to fibre supplements, due to the nutrient density associated with appropriate carrier food selection (Marlett *et al.*, 2002; Redgwell and Fischer, 2005; Anderson *et al.*, 2009).

The health benefits of soluble fibres in the diet are well known and discussed in detail elsewhere in this book. Briefly, some of the main functions include reduction in the risk of developing cardiovascular diseases because they lead to a reduction in blood cholesterol levels, decreased rate of carbohydrate absorption from the small intestine and hence regulation of postprandial blood glucose and insulin levels, fermentation in the large intestine producing beneficial short-chain fatty acids (acetate, propionate and butyrate) and the promotion of a healthy balance of colonic microflora (Marlett *et al.*, 2002; Tungland and Meyer, 2002; Brennan, 2005; Delzenne and Cani, 2005; King, 2005; Aleixandre and Miguel, 2008; Slavin, 2008; Anderson *et al.*, 2009; Chawla and Patil, 2010; Gunness and Gidley, 2010; Viuda-Martos *et al.*, 2010). Hence, avenues to enhance dietary intake are attractive to both the consumer and, consequently, to the food processor.

Some dairy products may be viable carrier foods for fibre enrichment. When fortifying foods with a nutrient or nutraceutical, the carrier food has to be a good 'fit', as perceived by the consumer (Shahidi, 2004). The incorporation of soluble fibres into the aqueous phase of foods will generally enhance their viscosity. Many dairy products are thickened as a result of fermentation (e.g. yogurt, sour cream, cream cheese, etc.); others are thickened to provide textural characteristics (e.g. milkshake beverages, puddings, ice cream and other frozen dairy desserts). The addition of soluble fibres to contribute to this already-present thickened texture thus could be a good fit in these cases. Since dairy products are consumed widely, this may provide consumers with a convenient and enjoyable means to enhance their fibre intake.

15.2 Dairy product categories and formulations

Milk beverages are generally low-fat milks (1–2%) to which have been added sweeteners, thickening agents and flavours. They are generally not pre-aerated (foamed) but can be designed in such a way that shaking before consumption will develop sufficient foaminess to enhance the textural perception. The milk solids-not-fat is generally in the 11–12% range, and they can be formulated either with fresh milk fortified with milk solids or with reconstituted milk powder. Sweeteners are generally added, depending in part on the flavour that is used, to develop a sweetness equivalent to 4–6% sucrose. These products are usually thickened by the addition of polysaccharide gums, for example cellulose gum or guar gum at concentrations of 0.35–0.6%, and if foaming is a characteristic of the product then emulsifiers such as mono- and di-glycerides may also be added. Examples of flavours in these products could include vanilla, chocolate, banana, strawberry, and so on.

Dairy desserts, or puddings, have also been a common thickened dairy product in the market for many years. They are widely consumed by children and the elderly, two important target populations for fibre enhancement in their diet. These puddings have formulations not unlike those for the beverages above, milk solids-not-fat contents of 12–15%, milk fat contents of 0–4% and sweetness equivalent to 8–12% sucrose, but they have a gelling agent rather than a thickening agent, often a modified starch and/or κ-carrageenan. This results in a visco-elastic, spoonable texture. They are usually flavoured with a variety of suitable flavours, including vanilla, banana, strawberry, chocolate, butterscotch, and so on.

Frozen dairy desserts, including ice cream and other similar products, have a wide range of formulations, including milk fat, milk solids-not-fat, sweeteners, stabilizers, emulsifiers, water and flavours. The primary role of the stabilizer is to add viscosity to the mix, which results in a more full-bodied texture but also inhibits lactose crystallization and helps to reduce rates of ice recrystallization. These products are all characterized by being frozen rapidly, mostly under shear or agitation (some stick novelties excepted), and then stored, distributed and consumed while in the frozen state. The high content of ice during consumption, coupled with the freeze-concentration of the proteins and the polysaccharide stabilizers in the unfrozen phase, give rise to a very thick texture during consumption.

Yogurts and yogurt beverages are very popular fermented dairy products. The milk base, typically 0–4% milk fat, 12% milk solids-not-fat, and perhaps added sweeteners, is heated to a high temperature to sterilize any native microflora and also to generate appropriate protein structure; then the milk base is cooled and inoculated with *Streptococcus thermophilus* and *Lactobacillus delbruckii* sbsp. *bulgaricus*, and perhaps other probiotic cultures such as *Lactobacillus acidophilus, Bifidobacterium* spp. or *Lactobacillus casei*, and incubated to a suitable pH to develop a milk gel through the destabilization of the casein micelles and their interaction with denatured whey proteins. Incubation may be done in the package, perhaps with a fruit base pre-added to the bottom of the cup, or it may be done in an incubation tank. If the latter, then the gel is stirred and perhaps fruit is added before packaging. Yogurt drinks have lower milk solids-not-fat contents than yogurts, so the same extent of casein gel network is not developed. In addition, these beverages are typically homogenized to disrupt any flocs of aggregated proteins after fermentation. To stabilize this protein from precipitating, high-methoxyl pectin may be used due to the reduced pH environment.

Sour cream is fermented from a milk base that includes 10–20% fat, or lower, and 8–10% milk solids-not-fat. Fermentation is carried out with *Lactococcus lactis* or other suitable culture to generate a protein gel network. Cream cheese is often associated with sour cream, but is actually produced in a way more similar to curd cheese manufacture and includes a draining step.

All these products are described briefly as they are all thickened, either with additives, generally polysaccharide gums, or naturally through fermentation. Hence, all of these products may be appropriate candidates for fibre enrichment, as the fibre would have minimal impact on the characteristic texture. Further details of composition and manufacturing of these products can be found in dairy technology texts, for example Walstra *et al.* (2005).

15.3 Challenges of fibre enrichment

15.3.1 Protein and polysaccharide incompatibility and phase separation

Most polysaccharides that are added to dairy products to modify texture are incompatible with milk proteins in solution; hence at typical concentrations used phase separation may occur, resulting in a change of functional behaviour of the proteins and polysaccharides, a visual separation of a clear serum ('wheying off') and a loss of desired quality in the product. In situations where the polysaccharide concentration is high, that is, in fibre enrichment, this concentration will undoubtedly be above the separation threshold on a phase diagram (Doublier *et al.*, 2000). Phase separation can be attributed to depletion flocculation (Tolstoguzov, 1997). In casein polysaccharide mixed systems, depletion flocculation results from the difference in chemical potential (osmotic pressure) between the solvent and the space between the casein micelles, from which the polysaccharide is excluded for steric reasons; consequently the casein micelles become enriched in concentration within discrete volumes. This induces the mixture to easily reach the thermodynamic incompatibility threshold, resulting in phase separation (Syrbe *et al.*, 1998). A lower intrinsic viscosity or hydrodynamic molecular volume of polysaccharide leads to smaller occupied volumes, which contribute to less exclusion of polysaccharide in mixtures. Thus, depending on molecular conformation, the aggregation of milk proteins, especially casein micelles, and hence the kinetics of phase separation can be at varying rates (Dickinson and McClements, 1996; de Kruif and Tuinier, 2001).

To retard this phenomenon or prevent it from occurring, κ-carrageenan can also be added to most polysaccharide blends for use with milk proteins. In phase-separating milk protein (casein micelle)–polysaccharide systems containing κ-carrageenan, the protein and polysaccharide remain incompatible and will phase-separate at a microscopic scale into a water-in-water emulsion-like structure; however, κ-carrageenan prevents this phase separation from manifesting itself into a macroscopic event in which two distinct phases become visible. Both κ-carrageenan direct adsorption to the surface of the casein micelle and κ-carrageenan helix aggregation are involved in establishing a loosely aggregated network structure that inhibits diffusion and aggregation of phase-separated droplets (Spagnuolo *et al.*, 2005).

15.3.2 Rheology and texture

Polysaccharides (e.g. guar, locust bean gum, sodium alginate, sodium carboxymethyl cellulose and xanthan) have been used extensively in dairy products for many years as thickeners and gelling agents. While these are all soluble fibres, the concentrations at which they are used (typically 0.1–0.5%) mean that their contribution to daily fibre intake is low. To elevate these concentrations for fibre enrichment requires these rheological properties to be controlled. The parameter that relates molecular structure to solution viscosity is intrinsic viscosity, which is a measure of the volume occupancy of an individual molecule in solution (typically in dl/g). Generally, higher molecular weight polymers with little or no branching and stiff, elongated rather than coiled structures produce high intrinsic viscosity, which parlays into high solution viscosity and high pseudoplasticity (shear-thinning, in which viscosity decreases with increasing rates of shear in solution) (Cui, 2005).

High solution viscosity is easily detected orally as a thick, gummy texture. The shear rate of swallowing is often quoted as 50 s^{-1} (van Vliet, 2002), although Goff *et al.* (2008) found best correlations between perceived viscosity of a wide range of fibre-containing dairy beverages from 12 trained panelists and apparent viscosity at 200 s^{-1}. Yanes *et al.* (2002) examined the effect of hydrocolloid addition (0.02 or 0.04% κ-carrageenan; 0.2 or 0.5% sodium alginate) on flow behaviour and sensory properties of milk beverages to reduce milk fat content. Although these levels are too low to be considered as fibre enrichment, it was interesting to note from their study that sensory viscosity correlated well with apparent viscosity at 10 s^{-1} for the low-viscous samples, whereas it correlated better with apparent viscosity at 300 s^{-1} for the high-viscous samples, indicating perhaps a different mouth behaviour for swallowing when the samples become too thick.

Polysaccharides that produce gels are capable of forming intermolecular bonding in long regular areas along the backbone, so-called 'junction zones', that are interrupted by irregularities, such that the aggregates form three-dimensional networks capable of trapping and holding the solution into viscoelastic solid structures (Cui, 2005). Hence, polysaccharides best suited for fibre enrichment at high concentration would be those that have low intrinsic viscosity and are unable to form junction zones. These will be discussed in more detail below.

15.3.3 Bioavailability of other nutrients

A potential concern with fibre-enriched dairy products is that the fibre could reduce protein digestibility and hence reduce amino acid bioavailability. Mouécoucou *et al.* (2003) studied the effects of different levels of gum Arabic, low methoxyl pectin or xylan (0, 1, 10, 20, 30, 50%) on *in vitro* digestibility (pepsin, followed by trypsin and chymotrypsin for 1 to 6 hours) of β-lactoglobulin. The three plant gums significantly inhibited β-lactoglobulin digestibility as determined by amino acid diffusion through a 1000 Da molecular weight cutoff dialysis membrane, with xylan showing the greatest digestibility decrease. However, no differences were seen in any of the three gums when measured with an 8000 Da dialysis membrane. This suggested that peptides between 1000 and 8000 Da may interact with polysaccharides more than peptides with a greater molecular weight, and that the nature of the polysaccharide plays a role in this interaction.

The effect of dietary fibre on mineral bioavailability has been studied extensively over many years. Fibre can have an adverse effect on the uptake of several minerals, including, for example, calcium, magnesium, iron and zinc, and this could be of significant concern in dairy products, which are an important contributor of minerals, particularly calcium, to the diet. Most of the effects of mineral binding are due to the presence of phytate, although oxalates and tannins can also contribute. When isolated polysaccharides have been compared with wholegrain bran in several studies, mineral bioavailability was unaffected by the isolated polysaccharides but significantly reduced, particularly iron and zinc, by the wholegrain fibres, and this has been correlated significantly with the phytate content (Harland, 1989). On the other hand, inulin and oligofructose have been shown to have a positive impact on calcium bioavailability by altering the pH of the colon to enhance its absorptive efficiency (Chawla and Patil, 2010), and, given the significance of calcium from dairy products in the diet, this would be a very positive contribution from inulin fortification.

15.4 Potential dietary fibre supplements for dairy products

In selecting fibre sources for enrichment in dairy products, the first consideration has to be the actual definition of fibre, and this has not been easy to define for regulatory bodies (Phillips and Cui, 2011). The Institute of Medicine in the United States defined fibre in the Dietary Reference Intakes in 2005 as: 'Dietary Fibre consists of nondigestible carbohydrates and lignin that are intrinsic and intact in plants. Functional Fibre consists of isolated, nondigestible carbohydrates that have beneficial physiological effects in humans. Total Fibre is the sum of Dietary Fibre and Functional Fibre.' In 2009, Codex agreed on the following definition: 'Dietary fibre means carbohydrate polymers with ten or more monomeric units which are not hydrolysed by the endogenous enzymes in the small intestine of humans and belong to the following categories: edible carbohydrate polymers naturally occurring in the food as consumed; carbohydrate polymers, which have been obtained from food raw material by physiological, enzymic or chemical means and which have been shown to have a physiological effect of benefit to health as demonstrated by generally accepted scientific evidence to competent authorities; synthetic carbohydrate polymers which have been shown to have a physiological effect of benefit to health as demonstrated by generally accepted scientific evidence to competent authorities.' They also include the following footnote: 'The decision on whether to include carbohydrates with monomeric units from 3 to 9 should be left to National Authorities.' As a further comment, Codex defines the energy value of dietary fibre as: '70 percent of the fibre in traditional foods is assumed to be fermentable. Therefore, it is appropriate that the average energy value should be 8 kJ/g (2 kcal/g)' (Phillips and Cui, 2011). The important message here for processors is to ensure that the fibre source used has already been demonstrated through scientific means to exhibit a physiological benefit in order to be claimed as a fibre source.

In addition to beneficial health properties (physiological functionality), the fibre source must be easy to incorporate in formulations, providing little if any change in physical or textural properties (technological functionality) (Redgwell and Fischer, 2005). Often these two functionalities are competing, for example the high-viscous vs. low-viscous soluble fibres, in which some evidence suggests that physiological viscosity (viscosity of digesta, including the soluble fibre, in the small intestine) is correlated with reduction in glucose absorption rates and increased bile salt binding (Dikeman and Fahey, 2006), but, on the other hand, low-viscous fibres would be easier to incorporate into foods at higher concentrations (hence higher content claims on nutrition labels). At present, there is not sufficient information to be able to predict physiological functionality from molecular properties (size, conformation, structure), which makes it difficult to determine optimum fibres to target (Raninen *et al.*, 2011; Gemen *et al.*, 2011).

15.4.1 Insoluble fibre

Dairy products are aqueous-based systems, so there is less interest in fortification with insoluble fibres, such as cellulose or bran, compared with soluble fibres. Insoluble fibres would have to be pulverized to a sufficiently small particle size that chalky or gritty mouthfeel was not evident (Fernandez-Garcia and McGregor, 1997). Another example would be the resistant starches. These are starches that resist degradation and absorption in the small intestine, either due to their native conformation (bound or non-gelatinized) or as a result of extensive cross-linking through either retrogradation or chemical modification. The latter is being manufactured as a food ingredient from high amylose corn starch and is available as an insoluble fibre source, with claims of prebiotic potential and reduction in risk of colon cancer (Ares *et al.*, 2009). It is naturally white, bland, less gritty and shows better flavour in applications compared with other sources of insoluble fibre. So, although there are some perceived health benefits of insoluble fibres, particularly in colon transit times, faecal bulk and laxation, there seems to be much more interest at present in the soluble fibres, which are more suited for dairy product application.

15.4.2 Soluble fibre

There are numerous potential soluble fibres that could be utilized for fibre enrichment. Some of the gums for which there are published reports of their utilization in dairy products include inulin, gum Arabic, pectins, soy soluble polysaccharide, flaxseed gum, β-glucans from barley or oats, and polydextrose. There could be several others as well. Much information exists on the source, structure and functional properties of these gums, for example Phillips and Williams (2009). Hence the properties of only a few will be mentioned briefly here, focusing particularly on the low-viscosity gums with demonstrated health benefits. However, to avoid the clinical testing required for novel fibres to be declared as a fibre source according to the regulations above, it may be more pragmatic for processors to use fibres for which there has already been regulatory approval.

Inulin has perhaps received the most addition as a fibre-source in dairy products, partly due to its well-known prebiotic effects of aiding the stability/growth of probiotic bifidobacteria in the colon, when consumed with the prebiotic (Granato *et al.*, 2010). Native inulin from chicory has a degree of polymerization (DP) of ~9–12 with a span of up to DP 60, but it can be hydrolysed to make short chains or fractionated into short-chain and long-chain fractions. The short-chain oligofructose (fructooligosaccharide) is more soluble and sweeter than native inulin, although both native and short-chain inulin are very soluble and high concentrations in solution are possible. Long-chain inulin is more viscous in solution. The long-chain fraction is reported to have fat-replacing potential due to its capacity to form microcrystals that interact to form aggregates. These occlude water and create a colloidal particle that contributes creamy mouthfeel and texture. Inulin has been added to ice cream, yogurts, fresh cheese, beverages and dairy desserts (Villegas and Costell, 2007).

Gum Arabic is a natural exudate from the tree *Acacia senegal*. It is a high molecular weight polysaccharide consisting of branched arabinogalactan heteropolymers with a covalently linked protein moiety (2%). It is highly coiled in solution, giving it a very low viscosity at very high concentration. It has been shown to be highly fermentable in the colon, with numerous potential health benefits (Phillips and Phillips, 2011).

Water-soluble soybean polysaccharide (SSPS) is extracted from bean curd residue (okara), which is the by-product of tofu, soymilk and soybean protein isolate. SSPS has been reported to provide health benefits to humans through lowering of blood cholesterol, improving laxation and reducing the risk of diabetes. SSPS is highly soluble in both cold and hot water, such that high concentrations in solution are easily obtainable. Structurally, SSPS has a galacturonic acid backbone, which is made up of rhamnogalacturonan and homogalacturonan. SSPS also contains homogeneous galactosyl and arabinosyl neutral sugar side chains, which are longer than the galacturonosyl main backbone. The high solubility and low viscosity of SSPS in water result from its irregularity of molecular structure, which prevents the formation of network interactions (Chen *et al.*, 2010).

Polydextrose is also being marketed for soluble fibre applications with demonstrated health benefits. It is a synthetic, low molecular weight (average DP ~12) but highly branched glucose polymer with many types of glycosidic linkages created by heating dextrose with an acid catalyst and purifying the resulting water-soluble polymer. Polydextrose is used as a bulking agent because it is tasteless and is resistant to digestion. It is also highly soluble, exhibiting low viscosity at high concentration (Raninen *et al.*, 2011).

β-Glucans from oat or barley are another potential fibre supplement for dairy products with several demonstrated individual health properties. β-Glucan is a linear, non-branched polysaccharide (1-3, 1-4 mixed link β-D-glucopyranosyl units) that exhibits either thickening or gelling properties in solution depending on the molecular weight and solution conditions (Tudorica *et al.*, 2004). Thus, while it is currently highly recognized in the market (as oat bran), its properties may restrict its use in dairy applications to low concentrations.

15.5 Potential product applications

Table 15.1 provides an overview of example applications of dietary fibres into dairy products and the potential effects of these on the product, as found in the literature. Product categories include beverages, gelled products, frozen products and cheeses. Each of these will be discussed in detail below.

15.5.1 Beverages

Low-fat milk products in which the fibre source provides enhanced creaminess to resemble full-fat milks or milkshake-type dairy beverages that are thickened by a high concentration of soluble fibre could be appealing as a product category to consumers and hence a target product for development by processors. There are several existing products in the market already and several reports in the literature on the use of specific gums in such products. Villegas and Costell (2007) incorporated three types of inulin (DP 2–10, DP 9–12, DP >23) at 2, 4, 6, 8 or 10% into reconstituted whole or 2% fat milk beverages with 12% milk solids-not-fat, also with 0.02% or without κ-carrageenan, and studied their rheological properties. The flow behaviour of the beverages without κ-carrageenan remained Newtonian except for the long-chain oligomers at 8 or 10%, which were pseudoplastic. All beverages containing κ-carrageenan were also pseudoplastic. The viscosity of whole milk could be approximated by skim milk with 4–10% short-chain inulin, 6–8% DP 9–12 inulin or 4–6% long-chain inulin. Oliveira *et al.* (2009) examined the effect of inulin (1, 2 or 4%) as a prebiotic on the production of probiotic fibre-enriched fermented milk. The acidification rate during probiotic culturing increased and the fermentation time was reduced as a result of inulin addition, indicating that inulin stimulated probiotic culture growth during fermentation. Inulin addition also increased the firmness of the product.

Goff *et al.* (2008) studied the sensory and rheological properties of dairy beverages fortified with two varieties of flaxseed gum as a soluble fibre source. Dairy beverages contained 14% reconstituted skim milk powder, 6% sucrose and 0.25%, 0.5%, 0.75% or 1.0% of flaxseed gum. Controls were prepared with no

Table 15.1 Applications of dietary fibres in dairy products as found in the literature

Dairy product	Fibre added	Impact of addition	Reference
Dairy beverage	Inulin	Fibre supplementation; fat replacement; Newtonian viscosity	Villegas and Costell, 2007
	Novel fibre	Fibre supplementation; acceptable sensory scores at optimal levels	Goff *et al.*, 2008
	Polydextrose	Fibre supplementation; reduced insulinaemic response	Lummela *et al.*, 2009
	Soy soluble polysaccharide	Fibre supplementation; acceptable viscosity and texture at optimal levels	Chen *et al.*, 2010
Fermented dairy beverage	Inulin	Prebiotic; enhanced acidification; enhanced firmness	Oliveira *et al.*, 2009
Dairy pudding	Inulin	Increased viscosity, elasticity, thickness and creaminess	Tárrega and Costell, 2006
	Novel fibres	Fibre supplementation; reduced glycaemic response; acceptable texture when optimized	Au, 2010
	Resistant starch	Fibre supplement; enhanced thickness and decreased creaminess if too high	Ares *et al.*, 2009
	Soy soluble polysaccharide	Fibre supplementation; acceptable viscosity and texture at optimal levels	Chen *et al.*, 2010
Yogurt	Inulin	Prebiotic; reduced syneresis; enhanced body and texture	Aryana *et al.*, 2007
		Fat replacement; fibre supplement; reduced syneresis; enhanced texture	Brennan and Tudorica, 2008
	β-Glucans	Prebiotic; enhanced viscosity; reduced flavour acceptability	Fernandez-Garcia *et al.*, 1998
		Normal pH development; depolymerization if lactose limiting	Gee *et al.*, 2007
		Fat replacement; fibre supplement; reduced syneresis; enhanced texture	Brennan and Tudorica, 2008

	Novel fibres	Fibre supplement; acceptable sensory scores	Dello Staffolo *et al.*, 2004
		Normal acidification; enhanced texture; decreased acceptability if too high	Hashim *et al.*, 2009
		Higher viscosity and yield stress; reduced syneresis; acceptable texture	Ramirez-Santiago *et al.*, 2010
	Insoluble fibres	Accelerated acidification; higher apparent viscosity; gritty texture	Fernandez-Garcia and McGregor, 1997
Frozen dairy dessert	Inulin	Probiotic; acceptable sensory properties	Di Criscio *et al.*, 2010
		Fat replacement; reduced melting rate; enhanced viscosity	Karaca *et al.*, 2009
	Novel fibres	Fibre supplement; reduced melting rate	Dervisoglu and Yazici, 2006
		Fibre supplement; cryoprotective action	Soukoulis *et al.*, 2009
	Soy soluble polysaccharide	Fibre supplementation; acceptable viscosity and texture at optimal levels	Chen *et al.*, 2010
Cheese	β-Glucans	Shorter coagulation time; higher yield; fat replacement	Tudorica *et al.*, 2004

gum, and with 0.25%, 0.5% or 0.75% of either guar or xanthan. Sensory evaluation was conducted by 12 trained panellists for 27 attributes using quantitative descriptive analysis. Significant differences were seen in 15 of the 27 attributes. Increasing gum concentrations, regardless of type, led to increases in astringency, viscosity, mouthcoating and presence of particulates, and decreases in sweetness, nutty aroma and flavour, and vanilla flavour. Both flaxseed gum varieties at 0.75% showed less sensory viscosity than guar or xanthan at 0.5%, which were not significantly different from each other. This suggested potential for flaxseed gum, as it could be used at elevated concentrations.

Lummela *et al.* (2009) studied the effects of a polydextrose-enriched (1.5%), fat-free, lactose-free milk drink on insulin and glucose levels. The insulin response was significantly lower for the fibre-enriched milk drink than it was for the skim milk control. The fibre-containing milk beverage was very low in carbohydrate content, so no difference in glucose response was seen. There was also no effect of the fibre on subjective satiety ratings compared with skim milk.

From an epidemiological perspective, people with diets that are either high in dairy calcium or higher in fibre/lower in glycaemic index tend to be less obese than those with low dairy calcium and low fibre/high glycaemic index diets. It is sometimes difficult to isolate effects from epidemiological data, since high fibre/low glycaemic index diets may be associated with enhanced fruit and vegetable or whole grain intake, in which other nutrients may play a role. In controlled studies, diets high in dairy calcium have also been shown to be beneficial for weight loss during periods of calorie restriction. Thompson *et al.* (2005) combined high dairy and high fibre/low glycaemic index diets, all of which provided a calorie deficit of 500 kcal/d, to study the effects of dairy and fibre on weight loss in obese subjects compared with a normal diet. There was substantial fat and weight loss with all diets, but the high dairy diet or high dairy/high fibre diets did not result in further weight loss compared with the control. They concluded that high dairy calcium diets and high fibre diets are beneficial in weight loss, but the lack of significant differences resulted from treatment diets that may have been too high in calorie restriction.

15.5.2 Gelled products

The category of gelled dairy products includes both dairy-based puddings that typically utilize a polysaccharide gelling agent and fermented products such as yogurts that are gelled by fermentation. Both of these products have been used as carriers for fibre enrichment in the market and reports of specific fibres utilized in these types of products are also present in the literature. Tárrega and Costell (2006) incorporated 6% inulin (DP > 23) into fat-free dairy puddings containing 2.5, 3.25 or 4% starch and compared these with a full-fat control. Inulin addition increased both storage modulus and complex viscosity values and decreased tan δ. Adding inulin to the fat-free desserts increased sweetness, vanilla flavour, thickness and creaminess at the lower concentrations of starch, but at 4% starch the effect of inulin was overwhelmed. They concluded that inulin addition to low-fat puddings would improve their texture, to the point of offering similar sensory characteristics to the full-fat pudding. Ares *et al.* (2009) utilized high-amylose resistant starch (RS) at 1, 2, 3, or 4% in milk puddings containing 9% reconstituted whole milk powder, 8% sugar, 4.2% waxy maize starch and 0.02% κ-carrageenan. A maximum of 1.4% RS was considered optimum for sensory properties and consumer acceptability. Higher levels of RS degraded sensory attributes (decrease in creaminess, melting and sweetness, appearance of chalky textures). They reported from their survey of participants that consumers more interested in consuming functional foods enriched with fibre were more tolerant of the sensory changes caused by the addition of RS to the milk puddings.

SSPS was incorporated by Chen *et al.* (2010) into thickened milkshake-style beverages and puddings, to the maximum amount without over-texturing the food. Rheological measurements and sensory tests were used to develop desirable SSPS-enriched products. From the rheological data, 4% SSPS-enriched dairy beverages and 4% SSPS-enriched puddings were in the range of commercial products. From sensory analyses, 4% SSPS-enriched dairy beverage with 0.015% κ-carrageenan, 4% SSPS-enriched pudding with 0.1% κ-carrageenan and 2% SSPS-enriched low-fat ice cream gained the highest scores in consumer hedonic rating. Panellists also indicated their willingness to consume those products if they were available commercially.

Au (2010) incorporated 1% SSPS and 1% flaxseed gum into dairy beverages and dairy-based puddings and studied the associations between soluble fibre concentration, product viscosity, and the postprandial glycaemic and insulinaemic responses in 12 healthy males. The glycaemic responses for all the dairy-based study treatments were lower than for the glucose reference. The fibre-enriched dairy-based study treatments were lower than those for the control products without fibre, and the flaxseed gum treatments, which had higher viscosity, were lower than the SSPS treatments. No differences were observed between the fluid and gelled dairy-based study treatments. From this study, it appeared that apparent viscosity of the product correlated more strongly with reduced glycaemic response than fibre concentration.

Yogurts are naturally thickened through the effect of the acidification on casein micelles, so they could be a very good carrier for dietary fibres that may contribute to this thickness, or the natural thickness could mask their presence. There are numerous reports in the literature of the effect in yogurt of inulin (Aryana *et al.*, 2007; Brennan and Tudorica, 2008; Dello Staffolo *et al.*, 2004), oat or barley bran or β-glucan (Fernandez-Garcia *et al.*, 1998; Gee *et al.*, 2007; Brennan and Tudorica, 2008) and other novel sources of fibres (Fernandez-Garcia and McGregor, 1997; Dello Staffolo *et al.*, 2004; Hashim *et al.*, 2009; Ramirez-Santiago *et al.*, 2010). All indicate a reasonable degree of success, with no negative effects on fermentation rate or syneresis. Texture will greatly affect sensory quality and consumer acceptability, so has to be controlled carefully. Yogurts bring the added complexity of an acidic environment, in which the fibres must be stable, not leading to enhanced syneresis.

15.5.3 Frozen dairy desserts

Frozen dairy desserts have also been targeted for fibre enrichment, both in the marketplace and as a subject of research. Chen *et al.* (2010) incorporated 1–4% SSPS into a low-fat ice cream formulation and reported that 2% SSPS gained the highest scores in consumer hedonic rating. Dervisoglu and Yazici (2006) examined the incorporation of citrus fibre at 0.4, 0.8 or 1.2% into ice cream of varying stabilizer levels. They concluded that citrus fibre alone did not offer stabilizing properties (improvement in viscosity, overrun and sensory properties) but together with stabilizer enhanced several physical and sensory properties, and so could be utilized as a source of dietary fibre enrichment. They reported the optimum concentration to be 0.8%.

Karaca *et al.* (2009) utilized native inulin at 4, 6 or 8% in a Maras-type ice cream (from Turkey) containing 8, 4, 2 or 1% milk fat, 9% milk solids-not-fat, 22% sugar, 0.5% salep, 0.2% gelatin and 0.3% guar. They reported that inulin increased the viscosity and the pseudoplasticity of the mix and reduced the melting rate in the ice cream. The inulin did not, however, impart creaminess to the reduced-fat and low-fat ice creams. Akalm *et al.* (2008) also incorporated inulin at 4% into regular (10%), reduced-fat (6%) and low-fat (3%) ice cream mixes. They found that inulin increased hardness in comparison with regular ice cream, but the products made with inulin melted significantly faster than the other samples.

Di Criscio *et al.* (2010) utilized native chicory inulin (DP 9) at 0, 2.5, 5 or 10% into a standard ice cream formulation that contained probiotic organisms *Lactobacillus casei* and *L. rhamnosus*. Cell counts of $> 10^7$ were preserved after frozen storage for up to 16 weeks at −20°C and were not affected by the presence of inulin. At 2.5% inulin, no adverse effects in sensory or physical properties were seen, although some degradation in properties (especially increased firmness) was apparent at higher concentrations. Thus, they recommended an incorporation level of 3% inulin to provide sufficient quantity in an 80 g serving of ice cream to provide > 40% of the 5 g/day requirement of prebiotic to support a probiotic intake of 10^7/day.

Soukoulis *et al.* (2009) examined the enrichment of ice cream at 6% milk fat with 2 or 4% of four fibre sources: oat fibre (93% insoluble), wheat fibre (93% insoluble), apple fibre (15% soluble) and long-chain inulin (90% soluble). The insoluble fibres increased the viscosity and pseudoplasticity of the mix while the soluble fibres reduced freezing point depression and increased the glass transition temperature of the mix, indicating potential cryoprotective action. Thus, they indicated that appropriate choice or blending of fibre sources could optimize both nutritional and technical functionality.

15.5.4 Cheeses

Although enrichment of cheese with soluble fibres is difficult due to the potential loss of fibre with the whey, some reports of fibre incorporation into cheese are available. Tudorica *et al.* (2004) incorporated barley β-glucan at 0.5, 1.0, 1.5

or 2.0% into whole milk, 1% fat milk or skim milk and proceeded to make rennet curd with coagulation at 32°C. They reported that coagulation time of the milk was reduced, curd yield increased and viscoelastic properties of the curd (G' and firmness) were reduced in the presence of increasing β-glucan. Higher moisture content in the curd was associated with the weaker structures observed. They concluded that β-glucan addition had positive effects in the lower-fat systems, thus providing an opportunity to utilize β-glucan as a fat replacer in milk destined for cheese manufacture. At the same time, if this is feasible, the β-glucan would also provide positive beneficial effects as a source of dietary fibre.

15.6 Future trends

There is no doubt that, from a nutrition and health perspective, people need to consume more fibre. Dietary fibre has, in general, been shown to provide numerous health benefits, and data from many countries suggest that people do not consume sufficient quantity of fruits, vegetables, whole grains and legumes to achieve recommended daily intakes for these benefits to occur. Thus, enrichment of foods with fibre provides enhanced choice for consumers and product development opportunities for manufacturers. It is clear both from the research literature and from already existing products in the market that dairy products can provide an excellent carrier food for fibre enrichment. Consumers have shown a willingness to consume such products as an avenue for enhanced fibre intake and health benefits. As public awareness of the food–health link, in general, and specifically fibre-for-health grows, so should opportunities for more product development and market introductions, and the dairy industry can become a stakeholder in this market.

The dairy product that is targeted for fibre enrichment has to be widely consumed across several demographic groups of consumers and at potentially significant daily levels. It also has to be seen by the consumer as a good fit for fibre enrichment, so beverages, puddings and yogurts may be the most obvious, and frozen desserts, cheeses and other dairy products perhaps less so. Many of the technical challenges for dairy product development can be overcome, but the most significant challenge to address is the fact that dairy products are aqueous-based systems with high water content, so the fibre utilized needs to function appropriately in that environment, not leading to over-texturization of the product when incorporated at significant concentration. This implies that low-viscous fibres would be the most appropriate. Thus far, various dairy products have been successfully fortified with inulin, gum Arabic, polydextrose and soluble soybean polysaccharides, while other gums also may have potential. However, the fibre that is utilized must also show specific physiological functionality, and ideally across a range of health benefits in both the small and the large intestines. Not all fibres contribute to all health benefits, so the fibre that is utilized in product fortification and the claims that are made for that product must be chosen carefully to achieve a balance of technological and physiological functionality.

15.7 References

AKALM A S, KARAGÖZLÜ C and ÜNAL G (2008), 'Rheological properties of reduced-fat and low-fat ice cream containing whey protein isolate and inulin', *Eur Food Res Technol*, **227**, 889–95.

ALEIXANDRE A and MIGUEL M (2008), 'Dietary fiber in the prevention and treatment of metabolic syndrome: A review', *Crit Rev Food Sci Nutr*, **48**, 905–12.

ANDERSON J W, BAIRD P, DAVIS R H JR, FERRERI S, KNUDTSON M, *et al.* (2009), 'Health benefits of dietary fiber', *Nutr Rev* **67**, 188–205.

ARES G, BAIXAULI R, SANZ T, VARELA P and SALVADOR A (2009), 'New functional fibre in milk puddings: Effect on sensory properties and consumers' acceptability', *LWT Food Sci Technol*, **42**, 710–16.

ARYANA K J, PLAUCHE S, RAO R M, MCGREW P and SHAH N P (2007), 'Fat-free plain yogurt manufactured with inulins of various chain lengths and *Lactobacillus acidophilus*', *J Food Sci*, **72**, M79–M84.

AU M (2010), *Effects of soluble fibre on the glycemic and insulinemic responses to dairy products and glucose solutions in healthy adult males*, MSc Thesis, University of Guelph, Canada.

BRENNAN C S (2005), 'Dietary fibre, glycaemic response, and diabetes', *Mol Nutr Food Res*, **49**, 560–70.

BRENNAN C S and TUDORICA C M (2008), 'Carbohydrate-based fat replacers in the modification of the rheological, textural and sensory quality of yoghurt: comparative study of the utilization of barley beta-glucan, guar gum and inulin', *Internat J Food Sci Technol*, **43**, 824–33.

CHAWLA R and PATIL G R (2010), 'Soluble dietary fiber', *Comp Rev Food Sci, Food Safety*, **9**, 178–96.

CHEN W, DUIZER L, CORREDIG M and GOFF H D (2010), 'Addition of soluble soybean polysaccharides to dairy products as a source of dietary fiber', *J Food Sci*, **75**, C478–C484.

CUI W S (2005), *Food Carbohydrates: Chemistry, Physical Properties and Applications*, Boca Raton, FL, Taylor and Francis.

DE KRUIF, C G and TUINIER R (2001), 'Polysaccharide protein interactions', *Food Hydrocoll*, **15**, 555–63.

DELLO STAFFOLO M, BERTOLA N, MARTINO M and BEVILACQUA Y A (2004), 'Influence of dietary fiber addition on sensory and rheological properties of yogurt', *Internat Dairy J*, **14**, 263–8.

DELZENNE N M and CANI P D (2005), 'A place for dietary fibre in the management of the metabolic syndrome', *Curr Opin Clin Nutr Met Care*, **8**, 636–40.

DERVISOGLU M and YAZICI F (2006), 'The effect of citrus fibre on the physical, chemical and sensory properties of ice cream', *Food Sci Technol Internat*, **12**, 159–64.

DICKINSON E and MCCLEMENTS D J (1996), 'Protein-polysaccharide interactions', in *Advances in Food Colloids*, New York, Blackie Academic and Professional, 81–101.

DI CRISCIO T, FRATIANNI A, MIGNOGNA R, CINQUANTA L, COPPOLA R, *et al.* (2010), 'Production of functional probiotic, prebiotic and symbiotic ice creams', *J Dairy Sci*, **93**, 4555–64.

DIKEMAN C L and FAHEY G C (2006), 'Viscosity as related to dietary fiber: A review', *Crit Rev Food Sci Nutr*, **46**, 649–63.

DOUBLIER J L, GARNIER C, RENARD D and SANCHEZ C (2000), 'Protein-polysaccharide interactions', *Curr Opin Coll Interface Sci*, **5**, 202–14.

FERNANDEZ-GARCIA E and MCGREGOR J U (1997), 'Fortification of sweetened plain yogurt with insoluble dietary fiber', *Z Lebensm Unters Forsch A*, **204**, 433–7.

FERNANDEZ-GARCIA E, MCGREGOR J U and TAYLOR S (1998), 'The addition of oat fiber and natural alternative sweeteners in the manufacture of plain yogurt', *J Dairy Sci*, **81**, 655–63.

GEE V L, VASANTHAN T and TEMELLI F (2007), 'Viscosity of model yogurt systems enriched with barley β-glucan as influenced by starter cultures', *Internat Dairy J*, **17**, 1083–8.

GEMEN R, DE VRIES J F and SLAVIN J (2011), 'Relationship between molecular structure of cereal dietary fiber and health effects: focus on glucose/insulin response and gut health', *Nutr Rev*, **69**, 22–33.

GOFF H D, MUELLER A E, CAPEL F, FINDLAY C J and CUI W S (2008), 'Sensory and rheological properties of a flaxseed gum-fortified dairy beverage', in WILLIAMS P A and PHILLIPS G O, *Gums and Stabilisers for the Food Industry 14*, London, Royal Society of Chemistry, 203–8.

GRANATO D, BRANCO G F, GOMES CRUZ A, FONSECA FARIA J and SHAH N P (2010), 'Probiotic dairy products as functional foods', *Comp Rev Food Sci Food Safety*, **9**, 455–70.

GUNNESS P and GIDLEY M J (2010), 'Mechanisms underlying the cholesterol-lowering properties of soluble dietary fibre polysaccharides', *Food Funct*, **1**, 149–55.

HARLAND, B F (1989) 'Dietary fibre and mineral bioavailability', *Nutr Res Rev*, **2**, 133–47.

HASHIM I B, KHALIL A H and AFIFI H S (2009), 'Quality characteristics and consumer acceptance of yogurt fortified with date fiber', *J Dairy Sci*, **92**, 5403–7.

HEALTH CANADA AND STATISTICS CANADA (2004), *Canadian Community Health and Nutrition Survey*, Ottawa, ON, Canada.

KARACA O B, GÜVEN M, YASAR K, KAYA S and KAHYAOGLU T (2009), 'The functional, rheological and sensory characteristics of ice creams with various fat replacers', *Internat J Dairy Technol*, **62**, 93–9.

KING D E (2005), 'Dietary fiber, inflammation, and cardiovascular disease', *Mol Nutr Food Res*, **49**, 594–600.

LUMMELA N, KEKKONEN R A, JAUHIAINEN T, PILVI T K, TUURE T, *et al.* (2009), 'Effects of a fibre-enriched milk drink on insulin and glucose levels in healthy subjects', *Nutr J*, **8**, 45, doi:10.1186/1475-2891-8-45.

MARLETT J A, MCBURNEY M I and SLAVIN J L (2002), 'Position of the American Dietetic Association: Health implications of dietary fiber', *J Amer Dietetic Assn*, **102**, 993–1000.

MOUÉCOUCOU J, SANCHEZ C, VILLAUME C, MARRION O, FRÉMONT S, *et al.* (2003), 'Effects of different levels of gum Arabic, low methylated pectin and xylan on *In vitro* digestibility of β-lactoglobulin', *J Dairy Sci*, **86**, 3857–65.

OLIVEIRA R P S, PEREGO P, CONVERTI A and OLIVEIRA M N (2009), 'The effect of inulin as a prebiotic on the production of probiotic fibre-enriched fermented milk', *Internat J Dairy Technol*, **62**, 195–203.

PHILLIPS G O and CUI S W (2011), 'Evolution and finalisation of the regulatory definition of dietary fibre', *Food Hydrocoll*, **25**, 139–43.

PHILLIPS A O and PHILLIPS G O (2011), 'Biofunctional behaviour and health benefits of a specific gum Arabic', *Food Hydrocoll*, **25**, 165–9.

PHILLIPS G O and WILLIAMS P A (2009), *Handbook of Hydrocolloids*, 2nd ed., Cambridge, Woodhead Publishing Ltd.

RAMIREZ-SANTIAGO C, RAMOS-SOLIS L, LOBATO-CALLEROS C, PENA-VALDIVIA C, VERNON-CARTER E J and ALVAREZ-RAMIREZ J (2010), 'Enrichment of stirred yogurt with soluble dietary fiber from *Pachyrhizus erosus* L. Urban: effect on syneresis, microstructure and rheological properties', *J Food Eng*, **101**, 229–35.

RANINEN K, LAPPI J, MYKKÄNEN H and POUTANEN K (2011), 'Dietary fiber type reflects physiological functionality: comparison of grain fiber, inulin, and polydextrose', *Nutr Rev*, **69**, 9–21.

REDGWELL R J and FISCHER M (2005), 'Dietary fiber as a versatile food component: An industrial perspective', *Mol Nutr Food Res*, **49**, 521–35.

SHAHIDI F (2004), 'Functional foods: their role in health promotion and disease prevention', *J Food Sci*, **69**, 146–9.

SLAVIN J L (2008), 'Position of the American Dietetic Association: Health implications of dietary fiber', *J Amer Dietetic Assn*, **108**, 1716–31.

SOUKOULIS C, LEBESI D and TZIA C (2009), 'Enrichment of ice cream with dietary fibre: Effects on rheological properties, ice crystallization and glass transition phenomena', *Food Chem*, **115**, 665–71.

SPAGNUOLO P, DALGLEISH D G, GOFF H D and MORRIS E R (2005), 'Kappa-carrageenan interactions in systems containing casein micelles and polysaccharide stabilizers', *Food Hydrocoll*, **19**, 371–7.

SYRBE A, BAUER W J and KLOSTERMEYER H (1998), 'Polymer science concepts in dairy systems. An overview of milk protein and food hydrocolloid interaction', *Internat Dairy J*, **3**, 179–93.

TÁRREGA A and COSTELL E (2006), 'Effect of inulin addition on rheological and sensory properties of fat-free starch-based dairy desserts', *Internat Dairy J*, **16**, 1104–12.

THOMPSON W G, HOLDMAN N R, JANZOW D J, SLEZAK J M, MORRIS K L and ZEMEL M B (2005), 'Effect of energy-reduced diets high in dairy products and fiber on weight loss in obese adults', *Obesity Res*, **13**, 1344–53.

TOLSTOGUZOV V B (1997), 'Protein–polysaccharide interactions' in DAMODARAN S and PARAF A, *Food Proteins and their Applications*. New York, Marcel Dekker, 171–98.

TUDORICA C M, JONES T E R, KURI V and BRENNAN C S (2004), 'The effects of refined barley β-glucan on the physico-structural properties of low-fat dairy products: curd yield, microstructure, texture and rheology', *J Sci Food Agric*, **84**, 1159–69.

TUNGLAND B C and MEYER D (2002), 'Nondigestible oligo- and polysaccharides (dietary fiber): Their physiology and role in human health and food', *Comp Rev Food Sci Food Safety*, **1**, 90–109.

URASHIMA T, KITAOKA M, ASAKUMA S and MESSER M (2009), 'Milk oligosaccharides', in MCSWEENEY P L H and FOX P F, *Advanced Dairy Chemistry Vol. 3 Lactose, water, salts and minor constituents*, 3rd ed., New York, Springer, 295–349.

VAN VLIET T (2002), 'On the relation between texture perception and fundamental mechanical parameters for liquids and time dependent solids', *Food Quality and Preference*, **13**, 227–36.

VILLEGAS B and COSTELL E (2007), 'Flow behaviour of inulin-milk beverages. Influence of inulin average chain length and of milk fat content', *Internat Dairy J*, **17**, 776–81.

VIUDA-MARTOS M, LOPEZ-MARCOS M C, FERNANDEZ-LOPEZ J, SENDRA E, LOPEZ-VARGAS J H and PEREZ-ALVAREZ J A (2010), 'Role of Fiber in Cardiovascular Diseases: A Review', *Comp Rev Food Sci Food Safety*, **9**, 240–58.

WALSTRA P, WOUTERS J T M and GEURTS T J (2005), *Dairy science and technology*, 2nd ed., Boca Raton, FL, Taylor and Francis.

YANES M, DURÁN L and COSTELL E (2002), 'Effect of hydrocolloid type and concentration on flow behaviour and sensory properties of milk beverages model systems', *Food Hydrocoll*, **16**, 605–11.

16

Fibre-enriched meat products

F. Jiménez-Colmenero and G. Delgado-Pando, Instituto de Ciencia y Tecnología de Alimentos y Nutrición (ICTAN-CSIC) (formerly Instituto del Frío), Spain

DOI: 10.1533/9780857095787.4.329

Abstract: This chapter discusses different aspects of the use of dietary fibre (DF) in the development of fibre-enriched meat products. It begins by discussing the importance of healthier meat and meat products from the standpoint of the industry and of consumers, and possible strategies for their development. It then describes the technological properties of DFs of interest for meat processing and identifies potential health benefits. Finally, it reviews the use of DF and fibre-rich ingredients in the formulation of different types (fresh, cooked and fermented) of meat products.

Key words: healthier meat product strategies, technological properties of fibre in meat processing, fibre-enriched fresh, cooked and fermented meat products.

16.1 Introduction

Dietary fibre (DF) is defined as the remnants of the edible part of the plant and analogous carbohydrates that are resistant to digestion and absorption in the human small intestine with complete or partial fermentation in the human large intestine (Prosky, 1999). DF as a class of compounds includes a mixture of plant carbohydrate polymers, both oligosaccharides and polysaccharides, for example cellulose, hemicelluloses, pectic substances, gums, resistant starch and inulin, which may be associated with lignin and other non-carbohydrate components (e.g. polyphenols, waxes, saponins, cutin, phytates and resistant protein) (Elleuch *et al.*, 2011). For several decades, interest in the role of DFs in health and nutrition has prompted a wide range of research and received considerable public attention. Various studies have shown that a fibre-rich diet has a number of beneficial effects: it reduces the risk of coronary heart disease, diabetes, obesity and some forms of cancer, and also helps regulate constipation (WHO, 2003; Verma and Banerjee, 2010). Additionally, DF possesses technological properties that are useful for food processing, and since it can be recovered (from industrial processing residue) its use in value-added products provides a means of upgrading co-products.

Because of the numerous health benefits that they offer, interest in fibre-rich products has grown in recent years. This is especially important since the recommended total DF intake is more than 25 g/day (WHO, 2003), whereas current intake levels are lower in more developed societies. There has been a considerable upsurge in the development of fibre-enriched foods in recent years in an effort to palliate this deficit, which is especially important in the case of meat products in view of their specific characteristics.

Meat and meat products are an important group of nutritionally dense foods consumed by broad sectors of the population around the world. Consumption levels, although varying from country to country, are generally high; for example, meat intake ranges from 47 to 106 g/day in women and from 79 to 170 g/day in men in European countries, while in the USA the figures are 168 and 260 g/day, respectively (Wyness *et al.*, 2011). The meat industry is extremely important for the economies of many countries. Meat also accounts for a considerable portion of consumer spending on food; in the case of the European Union, for example, it is more than 22%. Meat and meat products are important sources of a wide range of nutrients (proteins, lipids, vitamins, minerals, etc.), and make up considerable proportions of the dietary intakes of various nutrients that are essential for growth and development.

However, in recent years recommendations for a reduction in meat consumption have been made. The role of meat in health is being reconsidered by nutritionists as well as consumers. Among the factors that help to explain this erosion are the following: a) associations between some meat constituents (e.g. fat, saturated fatty acids, cholesterol, sodium, etc.) and the risk of major chronic diseases in our society (e.g. ischaemic heart disease, cancer, hypertension and obesity); b) frequent meat safety crises (e.g. bovine spongiform encephalitis or avian flu); c) growing concern about ethical aspects of meat production practices (animal welfare); and d) concern about the impacts of animal production on the environment (due to their large contribution to greenhouse gas emissions) (Jiménez-Colmenero *et al.*, 2012). However, it would appear that reducing meat consumption poses serious nutritional challenges for some key nutrients (Millward and Garnett, 2010).

Changes in consumer demand and growing market competition have prompted a need to improve the quality and image of meat, not only to prevent the loss of market share attendant on a negative perception of meats, but also to achieve a much-needed diversification in the activity of the sector, through the development of products with health-beneficial properties (Jiménez-Colmenero *et al.*, 2012). Fibre-enriched meat products (as potential meat-based functional foods) are seen as an opportunity to improve 'meat image' as well as to update the recommendations related to DF goals. Given that these are frequently consumed foods, such goals could be achieved without any great changes in consumer habits.

This chapter describes different aspects of the use of DF as an ingredient for the development of healthier (fibre-enriched) meat products and highlights the health benefits of the fibres. It also looks at the use of DF in the formulation of fresh, cooked and fermented meat products and technological aspects relating to the type and proportion of fibre used, the purpose of its addition and the consequences for product characteristics.

16.2 Strategies for the development of healthier meat products

In order to develop healthier foods, different strategies can be used that increase the presence of beneficial compounds and limit those with negative health implications in meat and meat products. These strategies may basically affect animal production (genetic and nutritional) and meat transformation systems (reformulation process); however, aspects relating to meat processing, storage and consumption conditions can also affect product composition and hence the contents in terms of healthy/unhealthy compounds. Through the changes effected in the ingredients (raw meat material and non-meat ingredients) used in the making of meat products, the reformulation process offers an excellent opportunity to remove, reduce, increase, add and/or replace different components, including those with health implications (Jiménez-Colmenero *et al.*, 2001; Arhiara, 2006). In this respect, many non-meat ingredients (from animal and vegetal sources of terrestrial or marine origin) have been used in the preparation of healthier meat products. DF or fibre-rich materials constitute a very important sector of these (Fig. 16.1). The use of DFs for their technological properties and health benefits opens up interesting possibilities in functional meat product development (Jiménez-Colmenero, 2007; Jimenez-Colmenero *et al.*, 2001; Verma and Banerjee, 2010).

Fat reduction has generally been seen as an important strategy to produce healthier products. This aspect is especially relevant to the meat industry, since some meat products contain high proportions of fat, and fat from meats has often been assumed to be a risk factor in consumer health (Ferguson, 2010; Williamson *et al.*, 2005; McAfee *et al.*, 2010). In industrialized countries, approximately 36–40% of the total calories in the food supply come from fat, nearly half of which is from meat intake (Byers *et al.*, 1993; Sheard *et al.*, 1998).This is more

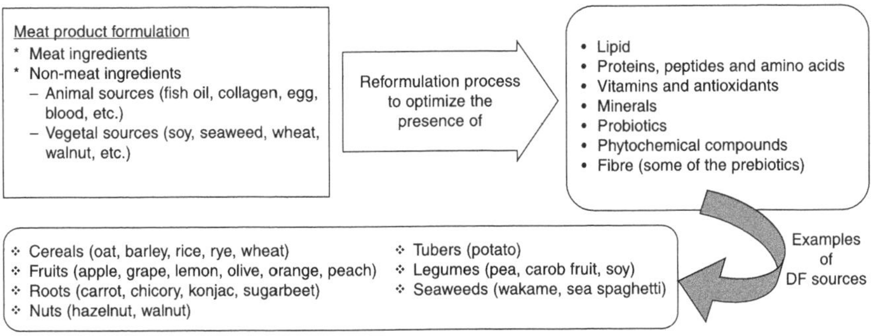

Fig. 16.1 Strategies for development of healthier meat products.

than recommended, and DF plays an important role in attempts to produce lower-fat foods.

16.3 Fibre as an ingredient in meat product formulation

DF and fibre-rich ingredients from cereals (oats, rice, wheat, etc.), fruits (apple, lemon, orange, etc.), legumes (soy, peas, etc.), roots (carrot, sugar beet, konjac, etc.), tubers (potato) and seaweeds (red and brown algae) have been used as additives/ingredients in the manufacture of meat products essentially for technological purposes. More recently, however, there has been renewed interest in their use in health-related applications, also encouraging the use of new DF sources. In the following are some brief considerations regarding technological and health properties.

16.3.1 Technological properties of fibre for meat processing

DFs have been incorporated into meat products as non-caloric bulking agents, as enhancers of water and oil retention, to help modify texture, to improve emulsion or oxidative stability or to help overcome the effects produced by composition changes, for example the fat reduction process, on the characteristics of meat products.

The hydration properties of DFs are related to the chemical structure of the component polysaccharides and to other factors such as porosity, particle size, ionic form, pH, temperature, ionic strength, type of ions in solution and stresses upon fibres (Elleuch *et al.*, 2011). Depending on type and conditions of use, fibres can bind considerable amounts of water; for example, konjac can bind more than 100 times its weight (Tye, 1991). As well as their hydration properties, fibres possess the capacity to hold oil. The ability of fibres to bind water and fat has been used in the manufacture of processed meat products. These properties contribute not only to final cook yield and purge or drip loss in chilling storage, freezing and thawing, but also to the final quality of the product (appearance, texture, colour, juiciness, flavour, etc.). DF constituents have been used by the meat industry for their gelling properties. Many soluble fibres form gels, for instance carrageenans, pectins, konjac, and so on. The capacity to form a gel and the characteristics of that gel will depend on a number of factors, including concentration, temperature, presence of certain ions and pH.

Because of their ability to form highly viscous solutions, fibres have been used as thickeners in meat systems; in this respect, the substances most widely used as thickeners are plant-derived gums. Fibres can help to modify textural properties in meat processing, including restructured meats. Thermo-irreversible gels, which form in the presence of calcium ions, are used to bind comminuted or diced meat pieces (cold-set binders) and make restructured meat products. Some fibre components possess antioxidant properties, which can be exploited as potential novel antioxidants and as such may be used as ingredients to improve the oxidative stability and prolong the shelf life of meat products. Because of their technological properties, fibres have also been added to meat products to reduce caloric content by fat substitution (Keeton, 1994; Jiménez-Colmenero *et al.*, 2001; Elleuch *et al.*, 2011). Fat reduction in meat products is usually based on two main criteria: the use of leaner meat raw materials and the reduction of fat density (dilution) by adding water (at higher levels than traditional products) and other ingredients with little or no caloric content. These ingredients, among them DF, are added to modulate the product's water-binding capacity, texture and sensory properties.

16.3.2 Healthy properties of fibre for meat-based functional foods

DFs may be considered functional ingredients since they also provide various potential beneficial physiological effects. DF has been associated with various health benefits, including maintenance of gut health (by facilitating excretion), prevention of carcinogenesis, reduced risk of coronary heart disease (hypocholesterolaemic effects), prevention of diabetes type 2 (ability of the fibre to reduce the glycaemic response) and reduction of obesity (by imparting a sensation of satiety). For more information on DF and health benefits in the context of muscle food applications, see Borderías *et al.* (2005) and Verma and Barnerjee (2010). Chapter 3 of this book deals with these aspects in detail.

16.4 Dietary fibre in meat products

While the possibilities of using DF or fibre-rich ingredients (e.g. type and amount) in meat processing depend on factors associated with the nature of the DF (technological and sensory properties), these are very much dependent on the meat product concerned. It is aspects relating to composition (fat, moisture and protein content), appearance or processing conditions (degree of structural disintegration or subjection to cooking, fermentation, smoking, etc.) that determine the technological and sensory viability of reformulated products. In view of this, the following subsections examine the use of DF separately for fresh, cooked and fermented meat products, with particular stress on technological and sensory effects on meat products.

16.4.1 Fibre-enriched fresh meat products

Several types of DF have been used in fresh meat products, in principle for fat reduction, but in some cases also for purposes of nutritional improvement (Table 16.1). Carrageenans (mostly ι and κ) have been widely used as fat replacers because of their ability to retain moisture. Ground beef, sausages, pork nuggets and mutton kofta are some examples of carrageenan-added low-fat fresh meat products (Egbert *et al.*, 1991; Bullock *et al.*, 1995; Solheim and Ellekjaer, 1993; Modi *et al.*, 2009a; 2009b; Berry, 1994). These studies confirmed the excellent water-binding characteristics of carrageenans (especially ι-carrageenan), and their

Table 16.1 Fresh meat products enriched with different DFs and fibre-rich materials

Product	Ingredients	Added as	Fibre content (g/100g)	Source
Ground beef	Carrageenan	Fat replacer	na[c]	Egbert *et al.*, 1991
Ground beef and pork sausages	Oat bran	Fat replacer	na[c]	Pszczola, 1991
Ground beef patties	Sugar beet, oat, pea fibre, Polydextrose®	Fat replacer	3.5–6.0[d]	Troutt *et al.*, 1992
Beef sloppy-joes	Wheat and barley bran	Fat replacer, functional ingredient	5.0–10.0[d]	Vosen *et al.*, 1993
Breakfast sausages	CMC[a], MCC[b]	Fat replacer	na[c]	Mittal and Barbut, 1993
Sausages	Carrageenan, guar and xanthan gum	Fat replacer	0.3–0.7[d]	Solheim and Ellekjaer, 1993
Pork nuggets	Carrageenan	Fat replacer	0.5[d]	Berry, 1994
Pork sausage	Konjac flour	Fat replacer	10–20[d]	Osburn and Keeton, 1994
Ground beef patties	ι,κ-carrageenans	Fat replacer	na[c]	Bullock *et al.*, 1995
Ground beef patties	Xanthan, locust bean gum	Fat replacer	na[c]	Bullock *et al.*, 1995
Ground beef patties	Pea flour	Fat replacer	na[c]	Bullock *et al.*, 1995
Beefburger	Apple fibre	Fat replacer	1.2[e]	Carballo *et al.*, 1996
Beefburger	Wheat bran, red and white beeswing hydrated	Fat replacer, functional ingredient	5.0–15.0[d]	Mansour and Khalil, 1997
Beefburger	Oat fibre	Fat replacer	0.4–2.0[d]	Desmond *et al.*, 1998a; 1998b
Beefburger	Carrageenan, locust bean gum	Fat replacer	na[c]	Desmond et al., 1998a
Beefburger	Maltodextrin, vegetable fibre	Fat replacer	na[c]	Desmond *et al.*, 1998a
Beefburger	MCC[b], maltodextrin, xanthan gum	Fat replacer	na[c]	Desmond *et al.*, 1998a
Beefburger	Pectin	Fat replacer	na[c]	Desmond *et al.*, 1998a
Beef patties	Inner pea fibre	Fat replacer	1.6[d]	Anderson and Berry, 2000
Ground beef	Inner pea fibre	Fat retainer	9.9–17.4	Anderson and Berry, 2001

Meatballs	Oat bran	Fat replacer, functional ingredient	5.0–20.0[d]	Yilmaz and Daglioglu, 2003
Pork patties	Barley flour	Fat replacer	4.0–10.0[d]	Kumar and Sharma, 2004
Meatballs	Rye bran	Fat replacer, functional ingredient	5.0–20.0[d]	Yilmaz, 2004
Meatballs	Wheat bran	Fat replacer, functional ingredient	5.0–20.0[d]	Yilmaz, 2005
Beefburger	Hazelnut pellicle	Fat replacer, functional ingredient	0.6–3.0[e]	Turhan *et al.*, 2005
Beef patties	Oat flour	Fat replacer	2.0–4.0[d]	Serdaroglu, 2006
Re-structured beef steak	Walnut	Functional ingredient	10.0–20.0[d]	Serrano *et al.*, 2006
Beef patties	Oats soluble fibre (β-glucan)	Fat replacer, functional ingredient	1.4[e]	Piñero *et al.*, 2008
Beef patties	Flaxseed flour	Functional ingredient	0.8–4.2[e]	Elif Bilek and Turhan, 2009
Chicken hamburgers	Grape DF	Functional ingredient, antioxidant	0.4–1.6	Sáyago-Ayerdi *et al.*, 2009
Mutton kofta	Carrageenan, oat flour	Fat replacer, functional ingredient	0.5[e] and 8.0[d]	Modi *et al.*, 2009a; 2009b
Meatballs	Inulin	Functional ingredient	5.0–20.0[d]	Yilmaz and Geçgel, 2009
Meatballs	DF from olive mill wastewater	Fat replacer, functional ingredient	0.4–0.6	Galanakis *et al.*, 2010
Meatballs	Potato flour	Fat replacer, functional ingredient	0.4	Galanakis *et al.*, 2010
Meatballs	Carrot	Fat replacer, functional ingredient	0.5	Galanakis *et al.*, 2010
Beef patties	Wakame	Functional ingredient	3.0[d]	López-López *et al.*, 2010
Beef patties	Inulin and insoluble fibre (Jelucell®)	Functional ingredient	4.0–5.3	Martínez *et al.*, 2011
Chicken patties	Oyster mushroom	Functional ingredient, meat replacer	3.4–4.9	Wan-Rosli *et al.*, 2011
Beefburger	Cashew apple	Functional ingredient, meat replacer	0–7.7	Xerez-Pinho *et al.*, 2011

Notes: [a]Carboxymethyl cellulose, [b]microcrystalline cellulose, [c]data not available, [d]% of added ingredient, [e]estimated from the composition data.

final low-fat products exhibited acceptable sensory and textural characteristics. Oat bran (with seasonings and flavourings) has been used to produce low-fat ground beef and pork sausage with the texture, flavour and juiciness of full-fat meat products (Pszczola, 1991). Texture characteristics of low-fat ground beef patties have been improved with a blend of fibres (sugar beet, oat and pea), starch and polydextrose, although juiciness was reduced most by added ingredients (Troutt *et al.*, 1992). The use of different blends of carrageenan, fibres and modified starches provided tenderness to low-fat ground beef patties (Bullock *et al.*, 1995). Desmond *et al.* (1998a) studied 17 different blends (containing widely available fibre sources) used in the manufacture of low-fat beefburgers, reporting that low-fat beef burgers containing oat fibre, modified starch and maltodextrin with vegetable fibre had improved palatability.

Vosen *et al.* (1993) reported on the use of fibre as a functional ingredient and a fat replacer in low-fat beef sloppy-joes. According to the authors, organoleptic characteristics were depleted by fat reduction and the incorporation of fibre (wheat and barley bran). Mansour and Khalil (1997) developed low-fat beefburgers with lower cholesterol and caloric content but similar sensory properties to control burgers. In that study, addition of white and red beeswings produced better texture and overall results than wheat bran. Addition of wheat bran has been found to produce a deterioration of sensory properties in low-fat meatballs (Yilmaz, 2005), but acceptable sensory properties have been achieved with the incorporation of rye bran and oat bran (Yilmaz, 2004; Yilmaz and Daglioglu, 2003).

Chemically modified celluloses have also been used in fresh meat products. Addition of carboxymethyl cellulose (CMC) and microcrystalline cellulose (MCC) as fat replacers in low-fat breakfast sausages reduced lightness and tenderness and improved moisture retention (especially MCC) (Mittal and Barbut, 1993). A combination of different fibres including MCC produced good sensory results in low-fat beefburgers, but good sensory quality was not achieved by addition of MCC alone (Desmond *et al.*, 1998a).

Inner pea fibre has been used in low-fat beef patties to improve tenderness and cooking yield, without negative effects on juiciness and flavour (Anderson and Berry, 2000). In a further study, Anderson and Berry (2001) reported that the addition of at least 10% inner pea fibre to high-fat ground beef increased fat retention and cooking yield when endpoint temperature reached 85–95°C. Water- and fat-binding properties of low- and high-fat beefburgers were enhanced by the addition of apple fibre (Carballo *et al.*, 1996). Turhan *et al.* (2005) obtained darker (reduced yellowness and redness) low-fat beefburgers by adding hazelnut pellicle as a DF. According to the authors, addition of 1–2% hazelnut pellicle can be recommended as a DF source in low-fat beefburger production. Oat soluble fibre (β-glucan) has been added to low-fat beef patties to achieve a sensorially satisfying product with increased cooking yield and fat and moisture retention (Piñero *et al.*, 2008). Several types of flour have been used as fibre sources to improve the cooking yield of fresh meat products. Barley flour used as a fat substitute in low-fat pork patties produced improved cooking yield but some loss of flavour and texture (Kumar and Sharma, 2004); however, overall acceptability and quality during storage were good when 4% was added. Moisture and fat retention in beef patties have been improved with the addition of oat flour (Serdaroglu, 2006). Flaxseed flour have been used as a functional ingredient in beef patties, enhancing their nutritional status with minimal composition and sensory changes (Elif Bilek and Turhan, 2009). Konjac has been used to develop acceptable low-fat prerigor fresh pork sausages with equal or improved cooking yield (Osburn and Keeton, 1994).

The development of new sources of DF has opened up new prospects in the field of fibre-enriched fresh meat products. Inulin (a long-chain fructooligosaccharide – FOS) has been used as a functional ingredient in meatballs and beef patties; the meatballs were lighter and yellower and sensory properties were not affected by 5% inulin (Yilmaz and Geçgel, 2009). n-3 Polyunsaturated fatty acids and fibre-enriched (inulin and insoluble fibre) beef patties were successfully developed by Martínez *et al.* (2011). Sayago-Ayerdi *et al.* (2009) added a grape antioxidant DF, obtained from red grape pomace, to chicken burgers, thus incorporating not only the health-beneficial properties of the fibre but its antioxidant potential and so increasing the stability and shelf life of the food. Galanakis *et al.* (2010) used a DF source recovered from olive mill wastewater as a potential fat replacer in meatballs; when combined with carrot (to supply insoluble fibres), this improved water retention and oil uptake. Powdered cashew apple waste was used in the production of low-fat hamburgers as a partial substitute for the beef and a source of fibre (Xerez Pinho *et al.*, 2011). Also, grey oyster mushrooms have been used as meat substitutes and fibre sources in chicken patties (Wan Rosli *et al.*, 2011). Fibre-rich ingredients such as walnut or seaweeds have also been used to produce fibre-enriched fresh meat products. The addition of both ingredients not only enhanced the technological properties of the meat system but also augmented the presence of DF; for example, the addition of 20% walnut furnished around 1% of DF in restructured beef steak (Jiménez-Colmenero *et al.*, 2010b), while the DF content in low-fat beef patties containing 3% Wakame was around 1.6% (López-López *et al.*, 2009).

16.4.2 Fibre-enriched cooked meat products

Different types of DF materials have been used in the formulation of cooked meat products to improve their nutritional and health quality (Table 16.2); as in the case of fresh meat products, these ingredients were used in principle mainly as fat replacers, but more recently attention has focused on their role as sources of bioactive compounds. Foegeding and Ramsey (1986) evaluated the addition of various gums to low-fat frankfurters and found that all low-fat treatments were similar and comparable to a full-fat control when evaluated by a sensory panel. Low-fat, high added water bologna sausages have been formulated with oat fibre and pea fibre; although they exhibited different physicochemical and sensory characteristics, the DF had beneficial effects on properties of the reformulated products (Claus and Hunt, 1991). Fat content of chicken frankfurters has been

Table 16.2 Cooked meat products enriched with different DFs and fibre-rich materials

Products	Ingredient	Added as	Fibre content (g/100g)	Source
Bologna sausages	Oat and pea fibre	Fat replacer	3.5[b]	Claus and Hunt, 1991
Pork nuggets	ι-carrageenan	Fat replacer	0.5[b]	Berry, 1994
Frankfurters	Oat bran	Fat replacer, functional ingredient	2.0–6.0[b]	Chang and Carpenter, 1997
Frankfurters	Oat fibre	Fat replacer	2.0[b]	Hughes *et al.*, 1997; Cofrades *et al.*, 2000
Frankfurters	λ, κ-carrageenan	Fat replacer	1.0[b]	Hughes *et al.*, 1997; Cofrades *et al.*, 2000
Bologna sausages	Konjac flour	Fat replacer	0.5–1.0	Chin *et al.*, 1998a, b; 1999; 2000
Frankfurters	Peach DF	Fat replacer	0.9–7.0[b]	Grigelmo-Miguel *et al.*, 1999
Low-fat pork bologna	Waxy hull-less barley	Fat replacer	4.0[b]	Shand, 2000
Low-fat pork bologna	κ-carrageenan	Fat replacer	0.3[b]	Shand, 2000
Re-structured beef roast	Rice fibre	Functional ingredient	3.0[b]	Kim *et al.*, 2000
Fat-free frankfurters	Oat fibre	Fat replacer, functional ingredient	1.0–3.0[b]	Steenblock *et al.*, 2001
Light bologna	Oat fibre	Fat replacer, functional ingredient	1.0–3.0[b]	Steenblock *et al.*, 2001
Bologna sausages	Citrus fibre	Functional ingredient	0.0–0.2	Fernández-Ginés *et al.*, 2003
Bologna sausages	Lemon albedo	Functional ingredient	0.2–2.0	Fernández-Ginés *et al.*, 2004
Frankfurters	Sugar beet fibre	Functional ingredient	1.0[b]	Vural *et al.*, 2004
Cooked sausage	FOS[a]	Functional ingredient	2.0–12.0	Cáceres *et al.*, 2004
Low-fat frankfurters	Locust bean, xanthan gum	Fat replacer	0.5–0.6[b]	Lurueña-Martínez *et al.*, 2004
Turkish-type salami	Sugar beet fibre	Functional ingredient	2.0[b]	Javidipour *et al.*, 2005
Cooked meat sausages	Inulin	Functional ingredient	2.5–7.5[b]	Selgas *et al.*, 2005; García *et al.*, 2006
Cooked meat sausages	Apple, orange, peach fibres	Functional ingredient	1.5–3.0[b]	García *et al.*, 2007

Low-fat bologna	Pea fibre-rich fraction	Functional ingredient	4.0[b]	Pietrasik and Janz, 2010
Frankfurters	Seaweed (sea spaghetti)	Functional ingredient	2.5[b]	López-López *et al.*, 2009
Meat emulsion	Rice bran fibre	Fat replacer, functional ingredient	1.1[c]	Choi *et al.*, 2009
Pork meat system	Carob fruit	Antioxidant, functional ingredient	1.3[c]	Bastida *et al.*, 2009
Frankfurters	Walnut	Functional ingredient	1.0[b]	Jiménez-Colmenero *et al.*, 2010a
Frankfurters	Konjac gel	Fat replacer	10.5–19.3[b]	Jiménez-Colmenero *et al.*, 2010b
Bologna sausages	Orange DF	Antioxidant, antimicrobial, functional ingredient	1.0[b]	Viuda-Martos *et al.*, 2010
Chicken nuggets	Apple pulp	Functional ingredient	1.8–2.5[c]	Verma *et al.*, 2010
	Chickpea hull flour	Functional ingredient	5–10[b]	Verma *et al.*, 2012
Pâté	Konjac gel	Fat replacer, functional ingredient	7.0–15.0[b]	Delgado-Pando *et al.*, 2011
Frankfurters	Rice bran	Functional ingredient	2.5[b]	Álvarez *et al.*, 2011
	Walnut	Functional ingredient	2.5[b]	Álvarez *et al.*, 2011

Notes: [a]Fructooligosaccharides; [b]% of added ingredient; [c]estimated from the composition data; DF, dietary fibre.

reduced using oat bran (and added water); the authors found that the products formulated with higher proportions of oat bran (6%) were rated less juicy and more grainy by tasting panellists (Chang and Carpenter, 1997). Addition of carrageenan and oat fibre can partially offset some of the changes that occur in low-fat frankfurters when added water replaces fat and the protein level remains constant (Cofrades *et al.*, 2000; Hughes *et al.*, 1997).

The ability of oat fibre to increase moisture retention and modify textural characteristics has been used to produce light bologna and fat-free frankfurters (Steenblock *et al.*, 2001). Similarly, the incorporation of rice bran fibre (along with vegetable oils) helps to reduce animal fat in frankfurters (Álvarez *et al.*, 2011) and low-fat meat emulsion systems (Choi *et al.*, 2009). Konjac flour has been used as a fat replacer in low-fat bologna, producing similar textural characteristics to control full-fat bologna (Chin *et al.*, 1998a, b; 1999; 2000). Konjac gel has been added to potentially functional cooked meat products such as frankfurters (with olive oil and seaweed) and pâtés (with a healthier oil combination) as a fat replacer (Jiménez-Colmenero *et al.*, 2010a; Delgado-Pando *et al.*, 2011).

Wheat flour and apple fibre have been used to induce changes in the process of gelation in two low-fat meat emulsion systems (Fernández *et al.*, 1996). Verma *et al.* (2010; 2012) reported the use of apple pulp and chickpea hull flour in the formulation of low-salt, low-fat and high-fibre chicken nuggets (meat emulsion). Addition of peach DF and water to low-fat high DF meat frankfurters has been reported to help retain the sensory properties of traditional products. However, drastic reductions of fat content (to below 10%) reduced the sensory quality of the products (Grigelmo-Miguel *et al.*, 1999). Citrus fibres (lemon albedo and orange fibre powder) have been added at different concentrations to cooked sausages; bologna sausage with added citrus fibres exhibited improved fibre content, reduced residual nitrite and delayed lipid oxidation, with generally satisfactory quality scores (Fernández-Ginés *et al.*, 2003; Fernández-López *et al.*, 2004; Viuda-Martos *et al.*, 2010). Oxidative stability and nutritional properties of precooked restructured beef roast can be improved by the addition of rice fibre (Kim *et al.*, 2000); these authors reported that this beef product can be considered a functional food in that it incorporates several components containing health-promoting ingredients.

García *et al.* (2007) reported the combined effect of fat reduction and fruit fibre addition (peach, apple, orange) on the sensory characteristics of bologna-type sausage. According to these authors, it is possible to manufacture cooked sausages (30% less energy value) containing fruit DF without sacrificing their sensory quality, and some of them may be considered functional foods, since they are hypocaloric and enriched in DF. The influence of pea fibre-rich fraction on technological and sensory characteristics of low-fat bologna sausage has been reported by Pietrasik and Janz (2010).

The effect of addition of waxy hull-less barley (containing β-glucan and DF) on textural, water-holding and sensory properties of low-fat pork bologna was studied by Shand (2000), who reported that barley meal made a positive contribution to the control of product purge loss. Sugar beet fibre has been used to increase the DF level in frankfurters and Turkish-type salami containing interesterified vegetable oils (Javidipour *et al.*, 2005; Vural *et al.*, 2004). FOS have been used to make fibre-enriched reduced-fat cooked sausages with good sensory and textural properties and overall acceptability, suggesting that this fibre is a good fat replacer (Cáceres *et al.*, 2004). Inulin has been added to normal and reduced-fat cooked meat sausages (bologna-type products). This kind of product can be fibre-enriched with inulin (5–7.5%) while retaining good sensory quality (García *et al.*, 2006; Selgas *et al.*, 2005).

Fibre-rich ingredients such as walnut or seaweed have also been used to produce fibre-enriched cooked meat products. As well as enhancing the technological properties of the meat system, the addition of both ingredients to frankfurters augments the presence of DF; for example, the addition of 20% walnut furnishes around 1% of DF (Jiménez-Colmenero *et al.*, 2010b), while the consumption of 100 g of frankfurters containing 5% sea spaghetti would supply around 10% of the recommended daily DF intake (López-López *et al.*, 2009).

16.4.3 Fibre-enriched fermented meat products

It is only in the past 10 years, and to a very limited extent, that there have been reports of studies on the use of fibres in fermented meat products (Table 16.3). During ripening, a large amount of water is lost, increasing the relative proportions of the other components, including fibre. This feature, which is absent in cooked and fresh meat products, can limit the amount of fibre that the product will admit. In order to improve the nutritional and health quality of this type of product, fibre (from wheat, peach, apple, orange, lemon and carrot, as well as inulin, short-chain FOS and carrageenan) has been added mainly as a fat replacer and/or as a functional ingredient. Fat reduction strategies are of particular interest, since the fat content of fermented meat products is usually high (over 30%) and modification of that content affects product characteristics. In 'sobrassada', a dry-fermented sausage traditionally made in Mallorca (Spain), fat is the principal component, accounting for as much as 75% after ripening. When carrot fibre was added to sobrassada, the resulting products had good physicochemical and sensory

Table 16.3 Fermented meat products enriched with different DFs and fibre-rich materials

Product	Ingredients	Added as	Fibre content (g/100g)	Source
Dry-fermented sausages	Inulin	Fat replacer, functional ingredient	9.3–16.9	Mendoza *et al.*, 2001
Dry-fermented sausages	Wheat, oat, peach fibre	Fat replacer, functional ingredient	2.0–4.0	García *et al.*, 2002
Dry-fermented sausages	Apple, orange fibre	Fat replacer, functional ingredient	2.0	García *et al.*, 2002
Dry-cured sausages	Raw lemon albedo	Functional ingredient	0.3–0.4	Aleson-Carbonell *et al.*, 2003
Dry-cured sausages	Cooked lemon albedo	Functional ingredient	0.3–0.4	Aleson-Carbonell *et al.*, 2003
Fermented sausages	ι-carrageenan	Fat replacer	1.0–3.0[b]	Koutsopoulos *et al.*, 2008
Fermented sausages	κ-carrageenan	Fat replacer	1.0–3.0[b]	Koutsopoulos *et al.*, 2008
Dry-fermented sausage (sobrassada)	Carrot fibre	Functional ingredient	3.0–12.0[b]	Eim *et al.*, 2008
Dry-fermented sausages	sc-FOS[a]	Fat replacer, functional ingredient	2.9–8.7	Salazar *et al.*, 2009

Notes: [a]Short-chain fructooligosaccharides; [b]% of added ingredient; DF, dietary fibre.

properties when fibre addition did not exceed 3% (Eim *et al.*, 2008). Aleson-Carbonell *et al.* (2003) added raw and cooked lemon albedo to dry cured sausages to produce sausages with 0.26–0.43 g fibre/100 g product and good overall acceptability. Active biocompounds of lemon albedo may also generate additional health benefits given a range of added lemon albedo between 2.5 and 10%. Of these benefits, perhaps the most striking is a reduction in the residual nitrite level.

Over 4% inulin and short-chain FOS have been added with good acceptability to reduced-fat fermented meat products (Mendoza *et al.*, 2001; Salazar *et al.*, 2009). Both types of fibre are considered excellent fat replacers. Cereal (oat and wheat) and fruit fibres (apple, peach and orange) have also been used to develop a low-fat, fibre-enriched fermented product (García *et al.*, 2002). The amount and type of added fibre influenced the textural and sensory parameters; scores were worst with 4% fibre content (in the final product) and were acceptable with 2%. Fruit fibres, particularly orange fibre, gave the best results, closer to conventional products. However, when carrageenans (ι, κ) were assayed as fat replacers to improve the quality of low-fat fermented sausages (by increasing water binding and lipid oxidation stability), the sensory scores were lower, with ι-carrageenan producing a better effect than κ-carrageenan (Koutsopoulos *et al.*, 2008).

16.5 Future trends

The addition of DF to meat products is of great interest from a technological point of view. In meat processing, DFs were initially used as non-caloric bulking agents, to enhance water and oil retention and to improve emulsion and oxidative stability. However, the scope for their use has very much expanded in recent years due to the health benefits they can confer. The possibilities for their use may be enhanced by the development of new DFs, better understanding of these and improvements in meat manufacturing systems. Research is needed to improve the application of traditional fibres, considering the changes in composition that are being introduced in meat derivative reformulation processes associated with the development of healthy meat products.

The development of new DFs (from traditional and non-traditional sources) with technological and sensory properties redesigned for new meat products with new formulations may open up unexplored avenues in food processing. Research aimed at a fuller understanding of the presence and functions of associated bioactive compounds, their technological possibilities and their potential health implications, within the context of a meat matrix, could provide new opportunities for the formulation of healthier meat products. This could be of particular interest if the possibilities of using DF to develop healthier meat products were investigated in association with other ingredients; this would involve searching for more complex formulations with optimized combinations of different functional ingredients (e.g. low-fat, low-sodium, unsaturated-enriched, fibre-enriched and probiotic-enriched). Finally, for purposes of health claims it is essential to carry out research that demonstrates the functional effect associated with the presence of fibre in meat products conceived as potential functional foods. Foods promoted with such claims may be perceived by consumers as having an overall nutritional, physiological or other health advantage over similar or other products. Functional foods have progressed very fast in the past few years and are contributing to the development of new foods, including meats.

16.6 Acknowledgements

Projects AGL2008-04892-CO3-01 and the Consolider Ingenio 2010: CARNISENUSA CSD2007-00016, Ministerio de Ciencia y Tecnología (Spain).

16.7 References

ANDERSON E T and BERRY B W (2000), 'Sensory, shear, and cooking properties of low-fat beef patties made with inner pea fiber', *J Food Sci*, **65**(5), 805–10.

ANDERSON E T and BERRY B W (2001), 'Effects of inner pea fiber on fat retention and cooking yield in high fat ground beef', *J Food Sci*, **34**(8), 689–94.

ALESON-CARBONELL L, FERNÁNDEZ-LÓPEZ J, SAYAS-BARBERA E, SENDRA E and PÉREZ-ÁLVAREZ J A (2003), 'Utilization of lemon albedo in dry-cured sausages', *J Food Sci*, **68**(5), 1826–30.

ÁLVAREZ D, DELLES R M, XIONG Y L, CASTILLO M, PAYNE F A and LAENCINA J (2011), 'Influence of canola-olive oils, rice bran and walnut on functionality and emulsion stability of frankfurters', *LWT-Food Sci Technol*, **44**(6), 1435–42.

ARHIARA K (2006), 'Strategies for designing novel functional meat products', *Meat Sci*, **74**, 219–29.

BASTIDA S, SÁNCHEZ-MUNIZ F J, OLIVERO R, PEREZ-OLLEROS L, RUIZ-ROSO B and JIMÉNEZ-COLMENERO F (2009), 'Antioxidant activity of Carob fruit extracts in cooked pork meat systems during chilled and frozen storage', *Food Chem*, **116**(3), 748–54.

BERRY B W (1994), 'Properties of low-fat, nonbreaded pork nuggets with added gums and modified starches', *J Food Sci*, **59**(4), 742–6.

BORDERÍAS A J, SÁNCHEZ-ALONSO I and PÉREZ-MATEOS A (2005), 'New applications of fibres in foods: Addition to fishery products', *Trends Food Sci Tech*, **16**(10), 458–65.

BULLOCK K B, HUFFMAN D L, EGBERT W R, BRADFORD D D, MIKEL W B and JONES W R (1995), 'Nonmeat ingredients for low-fat ground beef patties', *J Muscle Foods*, **6**(1), 37–46.

BYERS F M, TURNER N D and CROSS H M (1993), 'Meat products in low-fat diet' in ALTSCHUL, A. M., ed. *Low-calorie foods handbook*, New York: Marcel Dekker, Inc., 343–75.

CÁCERES E, GARCÍA M L, TORO J and SELGAS M D (2004), 'The effect of fructooligosaccharides on the sensory characteristics of cooked sausages', *Meat Sci*, **68**(1), 87–96.

CARBALLO J, FERNÁNDEZ P and JIMÉNEZ-COLMENERO F (1996), 'Incorporation of apple fibre to low- and high-fat beef burgers' in HILDRUM, K. I., ed. *Meat for the consumer. 42nd International Congress of Meat Science and Technology*, Lillehammer (Norway), MATFORSK, Norwegian Food Research Institute, 363–4.

CHANG H C and CARPENTER J A (1997), 'Optimizing quality of frankfurters containing oat bran and added water', *J Food Sci*, **62**(1), 194–197, 202.

CHIN K B, KEETON J T, LONGNECKER M T and LAMKEY J W (1998a), 'Functional, textural and microstructural properties of low-fat bologna (model system) with a konjac blend', *J Food Sci*, **63**(5), 801–7.

CHIN K B, KEETON J T, LONGNECKER M T and LAMKEY J W (1998b), 'Low-fat bologna in a model system with varying types and levels of konjac blends', *J Food Sci*, **63**(5), 808–13.

CHIN K B, KEETON J T, LONGNECKER M T and LAMKEY J W (1999), 'Utilization of soy protein isolate and konjac blends in a low-fat bologna (model system)', *Meat Sci*, **53**(1), 45–57.
CHIN K B, KEETON J T, MILLER R K, LONGNECKER M T and LAMKEY J W (2000), 'Evaluation of konjac blends and soy protein isolate as fat replacements in low-fat bologna', *J Food Sci*, **65**(5), 756–63.
CHOI Y S, CHOI J H, HAN D J, KIM H Y, LEE M A, *et al.* (2009), 'Characteristics of low-fat meat emulsion systems with pork fat replaced by vegetable oils and rice bran fiber', *Meat Sci*, **82**(2), 266–71.
CLAUS J R and HUNT M C (1991), 'Low-fat, high added-water bologna formulated with texture-modifying ingredients', *J Food Sci*, **56**(3), 643–647, 652.
COFRADES S, HUGHES E and TROY D J (2000), 'Effects of oat fibre and carrageenan on the texture of frankfurters formulated with low and high fat', *Eur Food Res Technol*, **211**(1), 19–26.
DELGADO-PANDO G, COFRADES S, RODRÍGUEZ-SALAS L and JIMÉNEZ-COLMENERO F (2011), 'A healthier oil combination and konjac gel as functional ingredients in low-fat pork liver pâté', *Meat Sci*, **88**(2), 241–8.
DESMOND E M, TROY D J and BUCKLEY D J (1998a), 'Comparative studies of nonmeat adjuncts used in the manufacture of low-fat beef burgers', *J Muscle Foods*, **9**(3), 221–41.
DESMOND E M, TROY D J and BUCKLEY D J (1998b), 'The effects of tapioca starch, oat fibre and whey protein on the physical and sensory properties of low-fat beef burgers', *Food Sci Technol-Leb*, **31**(7–8), 653–7.
EGBERT W R, HUFFMAN D L, CHEN C M and DYLEWSKI D P (1991), 'Development of low-fat ground beef', *Food Technology*, **45**(6), 64–73.
EIM V S, SIMAL S, ROSSELLO C and FEMENIA A (2008), 'Effects of addition of carrot dietary fibre on the ripening process of a dry fermented sausage (sobrassada)', *Meat Sci*, **80**(2), 173–82.
ELIF BILEK A and TURHAN S (2009), 'Enhancement of the nutritional status of beef patties by adding flaxseed flour', *Meat Sci*, **82**(4), 472–7.
ELLEUCH M, BEDIGIAN D, ROISEUX O, BESBES S, BLECKER C and ATTIA H (2011), 'Dietary fibre and fibre-rich by-products of food processing: Characterisation, technological functionality and commercial applications: A review', *Food Chem*, **124**(2), 411–21.
FERGUSON L R (2010), 'Meat and cancer', *Meat Sci*, **84**(2), 308–13.
FERNÁNDEZ P, BARRETO G, CARBALLO J and COLMENERO F J (1996), 'Rheological changes during thermal processing of low-fat meat emulsions formulated with different texture modifying ingredients', *Z Lebensm Unter Fors*, **203**(3), 252–4.
FERNÁNDEZ-GINÉS J M, FERNÁNDEZ-LÓPEZ J, SAYAS-BARBERA E, SENDRA E and PÉREZ-ÁLVAREZ J A (2003), 'Effect of storage conditions on quality characteristics of bologna sausages made with citrus fiber', *J Food Sci*, **68**(2), 710–15.
FERNÁNDEZ-GINÉS J M, FERNÁNDEZ-LÓPEZ J, SAYAS-BARBERÁ E, SENDRA E and PÉREZ-ÁLVAREZ J A (2004), 'Lemon albedo as a new source of dietary fiber: Application to bologna sausages', *Meat Sci*, **67**(1), 7–13.
FERNÁNDEZ-LÓPEZ J, FERNÁNDEZ-GINÉS J M, ALESON-CARBONELL L, SENDRA E, SAYAS-BARBERA E and PÉREZ-ÁLVAREZ J A (2004), 'Application of functional citrus by-products to meat products', *Trends Food Sci Technol*, **15**(3–4), 176–85.
FOEGEDING E A and RAMSEY S R (1986), 'Effect of gums on low-fat meat batters', *J Food Sci*, **51**(1), 33–36.
GALANAKIS C M, TORNBERG E and GEKAS V (2010), 'Dietary fiber suspensions from olive mill wastewater as potential fat replacements in meatballs', *LWT-Food Sci Technol*, **43**(7), 1018–25.
GARCÍA M L, CÁCERES E and SELGAS M D (2006), 'Effect of inulin on the textural and sensory properties of mortadella, a Spanish cooked meat product', *Int J Food Sci Tech*, **41**(10), 1207–1215.
GARCÍA M L, DOMÍNGUEZ R, GÁLVEZ M D, CASAS C and SELGAS M D (2002), 'Utilization of cereal and fruit fibres in low fat dry fermented sausages', *Meat Sci*, **60**(3), 227–36.

GARCÍA M L, CÁCERES E and SELGAS M D (2007), 'Utilisation of fruit fibres in conventional and reduced-fat cooked-meat sausages', *J Sci Food Agr*, **87**(4), 624–31.

GRIGELMO-MIGUEL N, ABADÍAS-SEROS M I and MARTÍN-BELLOSO O (1999), 'Characterisation of low-fat high-dietary fibre frankfurters', *Meat Sci*, **52**(3), 247–56.

HUGHES E, COFRADES S and TROY D J (1997), 'Effects of fat level, oat fibre and carrageenan on frankfurters formulated with 5, 12 and 30% fat', *Meat Sci*, **45**(3), 273–81.

JAVIDIPOUR I, VURAL H, OZBAS O O and TEKIN A (2005), 'Effects of interesterified vegetable oils and sugar beet fibre on the quality of Turkish-type salami', *Int J Food Sci Tech*, **40**(2), 177–85.

JIMÉNEZ-COLMENERO F (2007), 'Healthier lipid formulation approaches in meat-based functional foods. Technological options for replacement of meat fats by non-meat fats', *Trends Food Sci Tech*, **18**, 567–78.

JIMENEZ-COLMENERO F, CARBALLO J and COFRADES S (2001), 'Healthier meat and meat products: their role as functional foods', *Meat Sci*, **59**(1), 5–13.

JIMÉNEZ-COLMENERO F, COFRADES S, LÓPEZ-LÓPEZ I, RUIZ-CAPILLAS C, PINTADO T and SOLAS M T (2010a), 'Technological and sensory characteristics of reduced/low-fat, low-salt frankfurters as affected by the addition of konjac and seaweed', *Meat Sci*, **84**(3), 356–63.

JIMÉNEZ-COLMENERO F, SÁNCHEZ-MUNIZ F J, OLMEDILLA-ALONSO B, *et al.* (2010b), 'Design and development of meat-based functional foods with walnut: Technological, nutritional and health impact', *Food Chem*, **123**(4), 959–67.

JIMÉNEZ-COLMENERO F, HERRERO A, COFRADES S and RUIZ-CAPILLAS C (2012), 'Meat and functional foods' in HUI, Y. H., ed. *Handbook of meat and meat processing*, 2nd Edition, Colchester, UK: Taylor and Francis. 225–248.

KEETON J T (1994), 'Low-fat meat products – technological problems with processing', *Meat Sci*, **36**(1–2), 261–76.

KIM J S, GODBER J S and PRINAYWIWATKUL W (2000), 'Restructured beef roasts containing rice bran oil and fiber influences cholesterol oxidation and nutritional profile', *J Muscle Foods*, **11**(2), 111–27.

KOUTSOPOULOS D A, KOUTSIMANIS G E and BLOUKAS J G (2008), 'Effect of carrageenan level and packaging during ripening on processing and quality characteristics of low-fat fermented sausages produced with olive oil', *Meat Sci*, **79**(1), 188–97.

KUMAR M and SHARMA B D (2004), 'Quality and storage stability of low-fat pork patties containing barley flour as-fat substitute', *J Food Sci Tech Mys*, **41**(5), 496–502.

LÓPEZ-LÓPEZ I, COFRADES S, RUIZ-CAPILLAS C and JIMÉNEZ-COLMENERO F (2009), 'Design and nutritional properties of potential functional frankfurters based on lipid formulation, added seaweed and low salt content', *Meat Sci*, **83**(2), 255–62.

LÓPEZ-LÓPEZ I, COFRADES S, YAKAN A, SOLAS M T and JIMÉNEZ-COLMENERO F (2010), 'Frozen storage characteristics of low-salt and low-fat beef patties as affected by Wakame addition and replacing pork backfat with olive oil-in-water emulsion', *Food Res Int*, **43**(5), 1244–54.

LURUEÑA-MARTÍNEZ M A, VIVAR-QUINTANA A M and REVILLA I (2004), 'Effect of locust bean/xanthan gum addition and replacement of pork fat with olive oil on the quality characteristics of low-fat frankfurters', *Meat Sci*, **68**(3), 383–9.

MANSOUR E H and KHALIL A H (1997), 'Characteristics of low-fat beefburger as influenced by various types of wheat fibers', *Food Res Int*, **30**(3–4), 199–205.

MARTÍNEZ B, MIRANDA J M, FRANCO C M, CEPEDA A and VÁZQUEZ M (2011), 'Evaluation of transglutaminase and caseinate for a novel formulation of beef patties enriched in healthier lipid and dietary fiber', *LWT-Food Sci Technol*, **44**(4), 949–56.

MCAFEE A J, MCSORLEY E M, CUSKELLY G J, MOSS B W, WALLACE J M W, *et al.* (2010), 'Red meat consumption: An overview of the risks and benefits', *Meat Sci*, **84**(1), 1–13.

MENDOZA E, GARCÍA M L, CASAS C and SELGAS M D (2001), 'Inulin as fat substitute in low fat, dry fermented sausages', *Meat Sci*, **57**(4), 387–93.

MILLWARD D J and GARNETT T (2010), 'Food and the planet: nutritional dilemmas of greenhouse gas emission reductions through reduced intakes of meat and dairy foods', *P Nutr Sc*, **69**(1), 103–18.

MITTAL G S and BARBUT S (1993), 'Effects of various cellulose gums on the quality parameters of low-fat breakfast sausages', *Meat Sci*, **35**(1), 93–103.

MODI V K, YASHODA K P and MAHENDRAKAR N S (2009a), 'Low-fat mutton kofta prepared by using carrageenan as fat replacer: Quality changes in cooked product during storage', *J Food Sci Tech Mys*, **46**(4), 316–19.

MODI V K, YASHODA K P and NAVEEN S K (2009b), 'Effect of Carrageenan and Oat Flour on Quality Characteristics of Meat Kofta', *Int J Food Prop*, **12**(1), 228–42.

OSBURN W N and KEETON J T (1994), 'Konjac flour gel as fat substitute in low-fat prerigor fresh pork sausage', *J Food Sci*, **59**(3), 484–9.

PIETRASIK Z and JANZ J A M (2010), 'Utilization of pea flour, starch-rich and fiber-rich fractions in low fat bologna', *Food Res Int*, **43**(2), 602–8.

PIÑERO M P, PARRA K, HUERTA-LEIDENZ N, ARENAS DE MORENO L, FERRER M, *et al.* (2008), 'Effect of oat's soluble fibre (β-glucan) as a fat replacer on physical, chemical, microbiological and sensory properties of low-fat beef patties', *Meat Sci*, **80**(3), 675–80.

PROSKY L (1999), 'What is fibre? Current controversies', *Trends Food Sci Tech*, **10**(8), 271–5.

PSZCZOLA D E (1991), 'Oat-bran based ingredient blend replaces fat in ground beef and pork sausage', *Food Tech*, **6**(1), 37–46.

SALAZAR P, GARCÍA M L and SELGAS M D (2009), 'Short-chain fructooligosaccharides as potential functional ingredient in dry fermented sausages with different fat levels', *Int J Food Sci Tech*, **44**(6), 1100–7.

SAYAGO-AYERDI S G, BRENES A and GONI I (2009), 'Effect of grape antioxidant dietary fiber on the lipid oxidation of raw and cooked chicken hamburgers', *LWT-Food Sci Technol*, **42**(5), 971–6.

SELGAS M D, CÁCERES E and GARCÍA M L (2005), 'Long-chain soluble dietary fibre as functional ingredient in cooked meat sausages', *Food Sci Tech Int*, **11**(1), 41–7.

SERDAROGLU M (2006), 'The characteristics of beef patties containing different levels of fat and oat flour', *Int J Food Sci Tech*, **41**(2), 147–53.

SERRANO A, COFRADES S and JIMENEZ-COLMENERO F (2006), 'Characteristics of restructured beef steak with different proportions of walnut during frozen storage', *Meat Sci*, **72**(1), 108–15.

SHAND P J (2000), 'Textural, water holding, and sensory properties of low-fat pork bologna with normal or waxy starch hull-less barley', *J Food Sci*, **65**(1), 101–7.

SHEARD P R, WOOD J D, NUTE G R and BALL R C (1998), 'Effects of grilling to 80°C on the chemical composition of pork loin chops and some observations on the UK national food survey estimate of fat consumption', *Meat Sci*, **49**(2), 193–204.

SOLHEIM R and ELLEKJAER M (1993), 'Sensory quality of low-fat sausages affected by fat substitutes', *Food Qual Prefer*, **4**, 127–31.

STEENBLOCK R L, SEBRANEK J G, OLSON D G and LOVE J A (2001), 'The effects of oat fiber on the properties of light bologna and fat-free frankfurters', *J Food Sci*, **66**(9), 1409–15.

TROUTT E S, HUNT M C, JOHNSON D E, CLAUS J R, KASTNER C I and KROPF D H (1992), 'Characteristics of low-fat ground beef containing texture-modifying ingredients', *J Food Sci*, **57**(1), 19–24.

TURHAN S, SAGIR I and USTUN N S (2005), 'Utilization of hazelnut pellicle in low-fat beef burgers', *Meat Sci*, **71**(2), 312–16.

TYE R J (1991), 'Konjac flour – properties and applications', *Food Tech*, **45**(3), 82–6.

VERMA A K and BANERJEE R (2010), 'Dietary fibre as functional ingredient in meat products: a novel approach for healthy living – a review', *J Food Sci Tech Mys*, **47**(3), 247–57.

VERMA A K, SHARMA B D and BANERJEE R (2010), 'Effect of sodium chloride replacement and apple pulp inclusion on the physico-chemical, textural and sensory properties of low fat chicken nuggets', *LWT-Food Sci Tech*, **43**(4), 715–19.

VERMA A K, BANERJEE R and SHARMA B D (2012), 'Quality of low fat chicken nuggets: effect of sodium chloride replacement and added chickpea (*Cicer arietinum* L.) hull flour', *Asian-Aust J Anim Sci*, **25**(2), 291–8.

VIUDA-MARTOS M, RUIZ-NAVAJAS Y, FERNÁNDEZ-LÓPEZ J and PÉREZ-ÁLVAREZ J A (2010), 'Effect of orange dietary fibre, oregano essential oil and packaging conditions on shelf-life of bologna sausages', *Food Control*, **21**(4), 436–43.

VOSEN T R, ROGERS R W, HALLORAN J D, MARTIN J M and ARMSTRONG T (1993), 'Effects of bran on sensory, storage, and compositional properties of low fat beef sloppy-joes', *J Muscle Foods*, **4**(1), 71–9.

VURAL H, JAVIDIPOUR I and OZBAS O O (2004), 'Effects of interesterified vegetable oils and sugarbeet fiber on the quality of frankfurters', *Meat Sci*, **67**(1), 65–72.

WAN ROSLI W I, SOLIHAH M A, AISHAH M, NIK-FAKURUDIN N A and MOHSIN S S J (2011), 'Colour, textural properties, cooking characteristics and fibre content of chicken patty added with oyster mushroom (*Pleurotus sajor-caju*)', *Int Food Res J*, **18**(2), 612–18.

WHO (2003) 'Diet, Nutrition and the Prevention of chronic diseases', *Technical Report Series*, No. 916.

WILLIAMSON C S, FOSTER R K, STANNER S A and BUTTRISS J L (2005), 'Red meat in the diet', *Nutr B*, **30**(4), 323–55.

WYNESS L, WEICHSELBAUM E, O'CONNOR A, WILLIAMS E B, BENELAM B, *et al.* (2011), 'Red meat in the diet: an update', *Nutr B*, **36**(1), 34–77.

XEREZ-PINHO L, RODRIGUES-AMORIM A M, BESERRA-CARIOCA J O, CORREIA DA COSTA J M and MOTA-RAMOS A (2011), 'The use of cashew apple residue as source of fiber in low fat hamburgers', *Cienc Tecnol Aliment*, **31**(4), 941–5.

YILMAZ I (2004), 'Effects of rye bran addition on fatty acid composition and quality characteristics of low-fat meatballs', *Meat Sci*, **67**(2), 245–9.

YILMAZ I (2005), 'Physicochemical and sensory characteristics of low fat meatballs with added wheat bran', *J Food Eng*, **69**(3), 369–73.

YILMAZ I and DAGLIOGLU O (2003), 'The effect of replacing fat with oat bran on fatty acid composition and physicochemical properties of meatballs', *Meat Sci*, **65**(2), 819–23.

YILMAZ I and GEÇGEL U (2009), 'Effect of inulin addition on physico-chemical and sensory characteristics of meatballs', *J Food Sci Tech Mys*, **46**(5), 473–6.

17

Fibre-enriched seafood

A. J. Borderías and M. Pérez-Mateos, Instituto de Ciencia y Tecnología de Alimentos y Nutrición (ICTAN-CSIC) (formerly Instituto del Frío), Spain, and I. Sánchez-Alonso, Instituto de Estructura de la Materia (IEM-CSIC), Spain

DOI: 10.1533/9780857095787.4.348

Abstract: The chapter reviews addition of soluble, semi-soluble and insoluble dietary fibre (DF) of various origins to restructured seafood products. It pays particular attention to the effect of non-soluble or partially soluble ones, since soluble DF has been more extensively studied and more frequently used for many years in the processing industry. The main purpose of this addition is technological, but its presence may have a positive effect on health. A compromise needs to be found in order to meet functional and technological requirements while offering consumers healthy, tasty and attractive seafood products.

Key words: seafood, dietary fibre, seaweeds, polysaccharides, oligosaccharides.

17.1 Introduction

Restructured seafood products are foods made from minced and/or chopped muscle which are used, with or without additives/ingredients, to make other products with new appearance and texture (Borderías *et al.*, 2005; Ramírez *et al.*, 2011). Different types of matrices can be used depending on the integrity of the muscle: from pieces of fillets to minced fish or *surimi*, which is a paste of stabilized myofibrillar proteins with long frozen storage stability and unique gel-forming abilities. These restructured products are good carriers for functional ingredients. Thus, fish muscle as a food vehicle for bioactive ingredients has considerable potential for tailoring foods with the required functional and sensory characteristics.

Many of the dietary fibres (DFs) currently used for technological purposes in seafood products are highly soluble and come from algae, such as carrageenans, or from seeds, such as locust bean, guar, xanthan and inulin, and others from bulbs, like glucomannan. On the other hand, there is very limited experience in the use of insoluble DF, such as cereal DF or partially insoluble DF, for example from peas, in seafood products. The advantages of DF are that they are practically calorie-free and for technological purposes they provide good water-binding capacity and can be used to modify texture. There are many references in the literature to addition of insoluble or partially insoluble DFs to meat and other food products, but there are hardly any references to addition of this type of DF to seafood products (Borderías *et al.*, 2005; Ramírez *et al.*, 2011). Another type of DF of particular interest for addition to fish products is antioxidant DF (ADF), obtained mainly from some fruits which contain both well-balanced soluble/insoluble DF (more than 50%) and natural constituents with specific antioxidant capacity (Saura-Calixto, 1998).

In most of the studies found in the references, DF was added to seafood products for technological purposes and therefore the amount added was small. From a functional point of view, according to the EU regulation (EC, 2006), a product can be labelled as a 'source of dietary fibre' if it contains a minimum of 3% fibre or a minimum of 1.5 g fibre per 100 kcal, and as having 'high content of fibre' if it contains 6% fibre or a minimum of 3 g of fibre per 100 kcal. Given that the calorie content of fish muscle is low (around 70–120 kcal/100 g in white species and 130–200 kcal/100g in fatty species), most of the studies cited in this chapter would meet the first requirement, with about 1–2.5% of fibre.

The technological and functional characteristics of these fortified products are very important, but they must also be compatible with sensory properties. For instance, they have to be attractive products to market, and therefore the product development process should incorporate consumer studies from the outset (Careche *et al.*, 2008). This chapter is organized on the basis of DF origin while addressing the technological importance of different types of DFs added to restructured seafood products.

17.2 Fortification with dietary fibres of aquatic origin

17.2.1 Seaweeds

Seaweeds contain significant amounts of insoluble and soluble polysaccharides, and hence offer potential for fortification of food products with DF for technological and physiological purposes. Seaweed is particularly suitable for enriching muscle-based restructured products. Some papers have been published on its use as an ingredient in meat products (Chun *et al.*, 1999; López-López *et al.*, 2010; Cofrades *et al.*, 2011), but there is scant information about addition to fish muscle.

Most seaweeds are useful dietary supplements because they are important sources of polysaccharides, minerals and vitamins. Many types of seaweed contain high concentrations of DF and omega-3 fatty acids, which are beneficial to health (Norziah and Chio, 2001). Seaweeds are also a source of other bioactive compounds, such as phytochemicals, sterols, tocopherols and phycocyanins, that are recognized to possess health benefits for humans, such as antitumoural, anticholesterolaemic, antiviral and antioxidant activities of seaweed constituents (Jiménez-Escrig and Sánchez-Muñiz, 2000; Venugopal, 2009).

One seaweed that has been extensively studied is *Fucus vesiculosus* L. (*Phaeophyta*). This is an edible brown-coloured perennial dioecious seaweed which contains protein, minerals, iodine, vitamins and mono- and polyunsaturated fats (Rupérez, 2002; Morel *et al.*, 2005). However, the components most directly responsible for the reported health effects of *Fucus* are non-digestible polysaccharides (DF) and polyphenols. This DF is composed of fucans, alginates, laminaranes, cellulose and fucoidan, the predominant polysaccharide. In fact, fucoidan (a sulphated polysaccharide) has been found to possess high antioxidant capacity (Jiménez-Escrig *et al.*, 2001; Rupérez *et al.*, 2002; Morel *et al.*, 2005) due to the presence of phenolic compounds and the synergic effect of phlorotannins, vitamin E and certain carotenoids (Rupérez *et al.*, 2002). Díaz-Rubio *et al.* (2011) studied the technological effect of ADFs from *Fucus vesiculosus* added to minced horse mackerel (*Trachurus trachurus*) during frozen storage. Minced fish samples supplemented with 1 and 2% ADF were compared with ADF-free control samples. The mince with ADF had lower lipid oxidation than those without addition of ADF, and the total drip (after thawing + cooking) was reduced after 3 months of frozen storage. When it was supplemented with 1% ADF, its flavour did not differ from the control. When it was supplemented with 2% ADF, the flavour did differ from the control, but it was still acceptable. Since 100 g horse mackerel muscle had 139 kcal, the fish sample could only be considered a source of fibre when it contained at least 2 g of ADF per 100 g fish muscle.

17.2.2 Seaweed hydrocolloids

Seaweeds are a good source for extraction of hydrocolloids. Seaweed hydrocolloids are the most widely used in the food industry after starch. They are currently used for technological purposes as thickening, emulsifying and gelling agents. They may also be considered as a source of soluble DF if used in adequate quantities.

Alginates are soluble DF from seaweed, usually used as food additives, especially in the production of gel-like foods. One of the particular characteristics of alginate is that it is capable of thermostable cold gelation (below 10°C) when a source of Ca^{2+} is added. Alginates are usually used mainly as gelling agents by incorporating minced fish in an alginate gel. In this way, the flaky internal appearance of fish fillets can be simulated by alginate layering (Glicksman, 1987). Recently, it has been used to develop a restructured fish product having the flaky appearance of raw fresh fish, from fish fillet trimmings and minced hake (*Merluccius capensis*) muscle (Moreno *et al.*, 2008; 2010). Also, alginates can be used as a thickening agent without addition of Ca^{2+}. In this case, Pérez-Mateos and Montero (2000) reported that the gel properties tended to be weakened by increasing concentrations in a range of 0.5–4% alginate in blue whiting (*Micromesistius poutassou*) mince (Table 17.1). Differential scanning calorimetry (DSC) analysis detected strong synergistic interactions when blended with carrageenan, but that did not affect the rheological properties of blue whiting

Table 17.1 Hardness (N) (mean ± standard deviation) of blue whiting minced gel containing hydrocolloid at different levels (0.5–4%), 1% NaCl and 80% moisture

	0.5%	1%	2%	3%	4%	Group mean
Guar gum	109.5 ± 6.0^{a}	110.7 ± 4.8^{a}	103.4 ± 1.9^{a}	86.1 ± 1.8^{b}	66.5 ± 3.1^{c}	95.2 ± 17.7
Xanthan	105.3 ± 4.7^{a}	$24.7 \pm 2.2^{b,d}$	33.5 ± 3.7^{bc}	39.4 ± 1.9^{c}	23.0 ± 2.5^{d}	45.2 ± 31.9
κ-Carrageenan	173.0 ± 3.6^{a}	215.3 ± 5.5^{b}	247.0 ± 9.0^{c}	251.7 ± 14.0^{c}	311.0 ± 6.3^{d}	239.6 ± 47.6
CMC	132.0 ± 1.7^{a}	86.6 ± 1.5^{b}	54.0 ± 1.0^{c}	30.3 ± 1.5^{d}	34.5 ± 1.5^{d}	67.5 ± 39.2
Alginate	144.0 ± 11.5^{a}	132.0 ± 4.6^{a}	124.3 ± 5.5^{a}	96.0 ± 6.0^{b}	75.7 ± 2.5^{c}	114.4 ± 26.5

Source: Adapted from Pérez-Mateos and Montero (2000).

Notes: Different letters (a, b, c) in each row indicate significant difference ($p \leq 0.05$). CMC, carboxymethylcellulose.

mince gels (Pérez-Mateos *et al.*, 2001). Besides, the gel-forming ability of blue whiting mince gels containing 0.5% alginate can be modified by applying high pressure during the gelation process (Pérez-Mateos *et al.*, 2002). Alginate has also been found to have a cryoprotective effect (about 0.5%) in cod *surimi* and red hake (*Urophycis chuss*) mince, preventing muscle fibre interaction and hence the dispersibility of the mince, but this effect was weaker than that produced by carbohydrates or polyalcohols (Sych *et al.*, 1990; Lian *et al.*, 2000).

Others sources of soluble DF from seaweed are sulphated polysaccharides (κ- and ι-carrageenans). In a concentration range of 0.2–5%, these can modify the properties of restructured fish products, such as texture, water-holding properties and colour, as a result of their gel-forming capacity and their ability to interact with the myofibrillar protein due to their anionic nature. According to Ortiz and Aguilera (2004), the enhancement in the textural properties of horse mackerel *surimi* gels containing κ-carrageenan are very similar to those observed in other hydrocolloids such as starch and form 'packed' microgels within the protein gel network through different mechanisms. In studies carried out in blue whiting mince, κ-carrageenan addition produced the hardest gels (Table 17.1), in direct proportion to the amount added (Pérez-Mateos and Montero, 2000). A mixture of κ- and ι-carrageenan was used to increase hardness in formulations containing proteins recovered from cape hake by-products ('sawdust') to prepare a frankfurter-type fish sausage (Pires *et al.*, 2009). Other products in which carrageenan has been used to enhance gel-forming capacity are: 'sawdust' from hake muscle (*Merluccius australis*) (Borderías *et al.*, 1996); minced chum salmon flesh (Gao *et al.*, 1999); sardine (*Sardina pilchardus*) mince (Gómez-Guillén and Montero, 1996; Gómez-Guillén *et al.*, 1997); and fish burgers from spotted croaker (*Protonibea diacantha*) (Kasapis *et al.*, 2004). Also, κ-carrageenan has been used to stabilize a *surimi* emulsion blended with tofu powder to produce a smoother and more compact gel network (Panyathitipong and Puechkamut, 2010). In the case of blue whiting mince, the gelling coadjutant effect of carrageenans can be explained by the fact that they are distributed throughout the mince matrix, and the size of the cavities formed and the volume occupied are such as to form a continuous structure inside the gel cavity (Montero *et al.*, 2000). In giant squid (*Dosidicus gigas*) mince, ι-carrageenan forms an independent network which supports the main structure after heat-treatment (Gómez-Guillén *et al.*, 1996). After high pressure gelation of blue whiting mince, 0.5% ι-carrageenan appears in globular form, indicating that it has not gelled; on the other hand, 0.5% κ-carrageenan forms small, fine reticular structures and noticeably increases water-holding capacity (WHC), as shown in Fig. 17.1 (Pérez-Mateos *et al.*, 2002).

κ-Carrageenans are also used in blends with other hydrocolloids (locust bean gum, guar gum, xanthan gum, carboxymethylcellulose (CMC), alginate) and even blends of different types of carrageenan (*kappa* plus *iota*) in order to modify the properties of heat-induced gels made from blue whiting mince (Pérez-Mateos *et al.*, 2001). Carrageenans (*lambda* and *iota*) have also been studied for their cryoprotective effect in cod *surimi* at 0.5%; however, as in the case of alginate, they were less effective than carbohydrates or polyalcohols (Sych *et al.*, 1990).

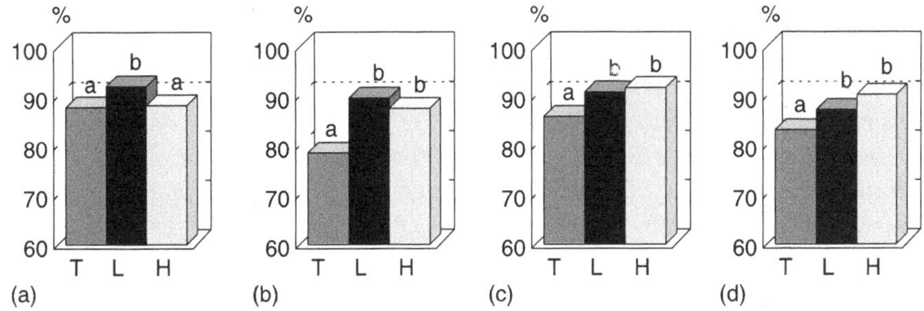

Fig. 17.1 Water-holding capacity (WHC) of blue whiting minced gels containing 0.5% of different hydrocolloids (a: alginate; b: κ-carrageenan; c: CMC; d: xanthan) under different gelling treatments (T: 37°C, 30 min/90°C 50 min at atmospheric pressure; L: 200 MPa, < 10°C, 10 min; H: 375 MPa, 3°C, 20 min). Different letters in each row (a, b) indicate significant difference ($p \leq 0.05$). Adapted from Pérez-Mateos *et al.* (2002) and Montero *et al.* (2001).

Agar, which is composed of 70% agarose and 30% agaropectin, is a soluble DF derived from a polysaccharide that accumulates in the cell walls of red algae and is a rich source of DF. Chen and Xue (2009) reported that the addition of agar can improve the gel-forming properties of horse mackerel *surimi* since it forms a dense and uniform three-dimensional network. Agar has also been used for its cryoprotectant effect in marlin fish *surimi* at 1–2% (Ueng and Chu, 1996).

17.2.3 Seafood waste polysaccharides

The term 'dietary fibre' includes not only non-digestible parts of vegetables but also DF polysaccharides of animal origin such as chitosan, which are derived from the chitin contained mainly in the exoskeletons of crustaceans, squid pens and in certain other organisms including many fungi, algae, and yeast. Chitosan, an aminopolysaccharide containing β-(1–4)-linkages as in cellulose, is known to possess numerous technological and physiological properties useful in foods (Koide, 1998; Shahidi *et al.*, 1999). As regards physiological activities, its highly polymerized oligomers show strong functionality (Jeon *et al.*, 2000). Studies on the use of chitosan in foods mainly address its antimicrobial and antioxidant capacity in solution, in powdered form and also in films and coatings (No *et al.*, 2007; Friedman and Juneja, 2010). Chitosan has been used in fish muscle or fish gels for its antioxidant capacity and its antimicrobial capacity, in a range that depends on the type of chitosan: from 50–200 ppm to about 0.5–1.5%. As mentioned above, to be considered a source of fibre a seafood would have to contain at least 1–1.8% per 100 g of muscle in lean species or about 2–3% per 100 g of muscle in fatty species. It has been used to reduce lipid oxidation in minced horse mackerel (*Trachurus* spp.) muscle under high pressure (Gómez-Guillén *et al.*, 2005) and in *kamaboko* gels made from grass carp (*Ctenopharyngodon idellus*) (Wu and Mao, 2009). Kamil *et al.* (2002) and Shahidi *et al.* (2002) reported that lower-viscosity chitosan (14 cP) was more effective than higher-viscosity chitosan in preventing lipid oxidation in cooked comminuted flesh of herring (*Clupea harengus*) and cod (*Gadus morhua*) after cooking. Chitosan has been reported to effectively inhibit microorganism growth in threadfin bream (*Nemipterus* spp.) (Kok and Park, 2007), in *kamaboko* gels made from grass carp (Wu and Mao, 2009), and in cod patties when applied as a coating but not when added in powdered form (López-Caballero *et al.*, 2005). As a texture modifier it has been used in concentrations of 1–1.5% in combination with calcium chloride, greatly improving the gelling properties of barred garfish (*Hemiramphus far*) (Benjakul *et al.*, 2001; 2003) and the low-quality walleye pollock (*Theragra chalcogramma*) *surimi* gels (Kataoka *et al.*, 1998). Chitosan (1% w/w) has been reported to have a cryoprotective effect on croaker fish (*Johnius gangeticus*) *surimi* similar to commercial cryoprotectants, both of which minimized the negative effects of frozen storage on physicochemical attributes of myofibrillar proteins (Dey and Dora, 2010). In lizardfish (*Synodontidae* spp.) *surimi*, chitin hydrolysates retard the effects of freeze-induced denaturation by stabilizing the hydrated water molecules that surround the protein (Somjit *et al.*, 2005).

17.3 Fortification with dietary fibres of terrestrial origin

17.3.1 Seeds

Guar gum, locust bean gum and tamarind gum are examples of water-soluble DFs extracted from seeds. They are used to enhance functional properties such as WHC and rheological properties at low concentrations (about 0.5–1%). Addition of 1% guar gum to minced fish muscle, which is the requirement to be considered as a source of fibre in lean fish, has been found to significantly increase the WHC of blue whiting mince gels (by about 15%). Higher concentrations (up to 4%) did not improve the effect and reduced folding test and hardness scores (Table 17.1) (Pérez-Mateos and Montero, 2000).

Locust bean gum (1%) has been found to increase the breaking deformation of blue whiting mince gels (Pérez-Mateos and Montero, 2000). However, other studies have reported that locust bean gum (1%) negatively affected the shear stress of myofibrillar protein gels from silver carp (*Hypophthalmichthys molitrixat*) (Ramírez *et al.*, 2002). Both gums (1% locust bean and 0.5% guar gum) behave differently in blue whiting mince gels under different gelling conditions (Fig. 17.2), probably because of the different structure that forms in the fish gel matrix: filamentous in pressurized gelation and more aggregated in heat gelation (Montero *et al.*, 2001). Chen and Xue (2009) reported that addition of tamarind gum improved the gelation properties of horse mackerel *surimi*, which formed a dense and uniform three-dimensional network.

17.3.2 Cereal dietary fibres

Wheat dietary fibre in surimi and surimi gels

Wheat DF (WDF) is one of the most widely used ingredients as dietary fibre sources. It is composed mainly of cellulose and hemicellulose, which makes it

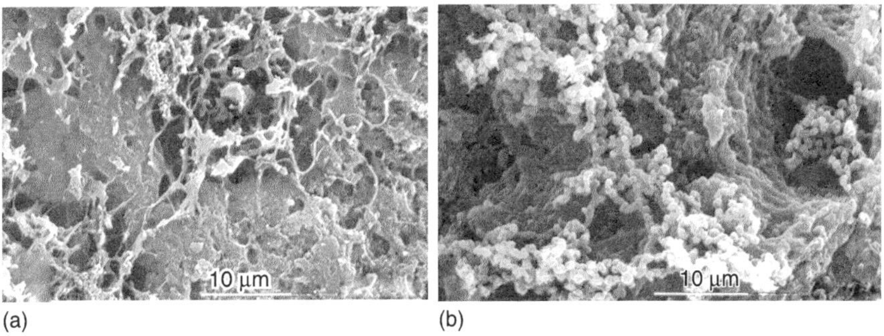

Fig. 17.2 Scanning electron microscopy images (× 1500 magnification) of blue whiting minced gels containing 0.5% guar gum. a: 200 MPa, 7°C, 10 min; b: 375 MPa, 37°C, 20 min. Adapted from Montero *et al.* (2001).

highly insoluble. It is white in colour and neutral in taste and smell, which is very important for use as an ingredient in fish products based on *surimi* and minced fish muscle.

Various authors (Sánchez-Alonso *et al.*, 2006; 2007a) carried out studies on the inclusion of WDF (Vitacel®) in gelled fish products. They were performed on two types of *surimi*, Alaska pollock and giant squid, at two concentrations (3% and 6%) and with two different WDF particle sizes (80 and 250 µm). The results in both types of *surimi* are similar, and from the point of view of gelation can be regarded as good quality, although water retention properties, and hence mechanical properties and texture, are significantly affected because the protein network becomes less homogeneous (Fig. 17.3) (Sánchez-Alonso *et al.*, 2006; 2007a). This porous structure has been described by other authors in *surimi* products to which hydroxylpropylmethylcellulose was added (Chen *et al.*, 2005). One of the reasons for lower gel strength (Sánchez-Alonso *et al.*, 2007a) may also

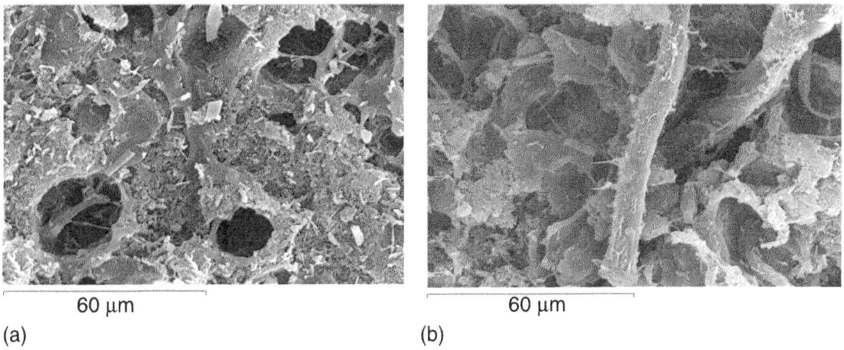

Fig. 17.3 Scanning electron micrographs (×1000 magnification) showing the arrangement of WDF in giant squid surimi gels. (a) Control sample without WDF; (b) sample with 6% WDF.

be that the inclusion of WDF involves a substitution of protein by DF and there is a well-known relationship between the actomyosin concentration and the ability to form a gel (Park, 2005). Sánchez-González *et al.* (2009) studied the interactions of DF with the water and protein in Alaska pollock gels with added WDF using Raman analysis. The authors of this study suggest that water transfer from protein to WDF can occur, either taking water that is delivered from the gel protein upon heat-mediated formation of β-sheets and hydrophobic bonds and/or acting as an active dehydrating agent. Furthermore, the addition of WDF to products made from Alaska pollock surimi increases gel brightness and luminosity.

The particle size of the added WDF is also relevant, since hydration properties and fat retention capacity decrease with decreasing particle size (Ang and Crosby, 2005). Decreasing DF particle size generally leads to changes at two levels: an increase in the surface area of particles and/or a decrease in the volume of internal holes (Nelson, 2001). The shorter particle WDF (80 μm) is denser than the longer particle WDF (250 μm), giving it a more compact structure in which less water can be retained (Miller, 1986). In gels made from giant squid *surimi*, both short and long particle DFs have the same water-binding effect, but after freezing short WDF binds more water than long WDF. This may be due to the disruption caused by the WDF particles in the protein network that forms the gel; this will be aggravated if the amount of WDF is increased, while a small particle size may cause less disruption. As regards texture, WDF makes gels softer and more deformable; this attenuates the gummy texture, which is not acceptable in western countries (Sánchez-Alonso *et al.*, 2007a).

Wheat dietary fibre in minced fish products

Sánchez-Alonso *et al.* (2007b) studied the incorporation of levels of 3–6% of WDF with a constant water percentage in minced muscle of two fish species: hake and horse mackerel. The results show that, when water is added to the formula to maintain the final moisture of the products, the presence of WDF reduces the water retention properties, but this loss is smaller when the particle size is small. However, when no water is added, more water is retained in minced fish muscle with WDF than without it. The presence of WDF significantly increases the WHC after thawing and cooking in minced fish muscle even when water is added to maintain the final moisture. Thus, if minced fish muscle is to be battered and fried, the addition of WDF will be useful, since it will prevent breakage of the coating and deformation of the fried portions (Nelson, 2001; Sánchez-Alonso *et al.*, 2007b). The incorporation of 3–6% WDF into minced fish muscle significantly affects product texture, as measured either instrumentally or by sensory analysis, making it less firm and cohesive (Sánchez-Alonso *et al.*, 2007b). There are no significant differences in shear strength of samples with and without WDF at the concentrations cited, irrespective of the particle size of the WDF, when water is added to maintain the final moisture. If water is not added to keep the moisture constant, shear strength increases. Hardness and cohesiveness of minced fish muscle are inversely proportional to the amount of WDF added (Sánchez-Alonso *et al.*, 2007b). The incorporation of WDF increased the whiteness of minced horse

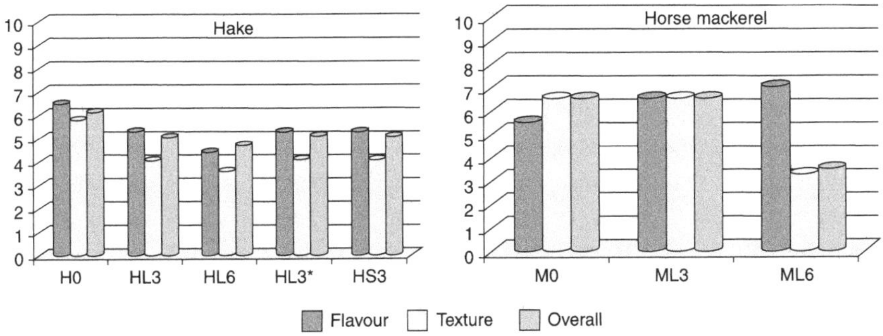

Fig. 17.4 Sensory evaluation: results of quantitative descriptive analysis carried out in cooked samples (H: hake; M: horse mackerel). 0: control without WDF; L3 and L6: 3% and 6% long particle WDF added, respectively (moisture adjusted to 81.5%); L3*: 3% long particle WDF added (final moisture not adjusted); S3: 3% short particle WDF added (moisture adjusted to 81.5%).

mackerel and hake muscle samples, in proportion to the amount of WDF added. This is important for consumers, as they value whiteness in fisheries products highly (Ang, 1993). Samples with WDF differed from the control in sensory aspects (Fig. 17.4), mainly related to texture. In the horse mackerel samples, the inclusion of WDF reduced the strong taste of the muscle, which is a feature characteristic. In both types of samples, those with 3% added WDF scored a little lower than the control, but samples with 6% were not acceptable (Sánchez-Alonso *et al.*, 2007b).

Other cellulose DFs used as ingredients in surimi *products*

The literature describes a trend of gradually declining hardness and gel strength in fish protein gels with increasing concentrations of added cellulosic DF (other than WDF); this is associated with discontinuity in the structure of the protein matrix that forms the gel, irregular distribution of water in the gel matrix due to competition affecting hydration of the DF, and lower protein content (Yoon and Lee, 1990; Tudorica *et al.*, 2002). When cellulose is added to moulded or fibreized seafood products, the tendency to acquire a dry, rubbery texture during frozen storage is reduced (Yoon and Lee, 1990).

Yoon and Lee (1990) examined the cryoprotective, texture-modifying and freeze-thaw stabilizing effects of 1–2% powdered cellulose (Solka Floc®) in red hake *surimi* products. These authors reported that cellulose effectively reduced the usage level of cryoprotectants, and hence sweetness. Cellulose also reduces the amount of modified starch needed in *surimi* products, thus achieving a non-starchy texture. It also prevents gelled products from becoming rubbery and dry during frozen storage by reducing freeze syneresis and improving water binding.

Other cellulose DFs used as ingredients in minced fish products

In order to develop a healthy low-fat fish sausage from minced hake (*Merluccius capensis*), Cardoso *et al.* (2008) added 4% pea DF (Swelite®) as an ingredient in fish sausages; this contains two-thirds cellulose. These authors concluded that it is possible to make a texturally acceptable sausage by combining lower fat content with increased Swelite® content.

CMC is a water-soluble polymer with different properties depending on the extent of modification of the cellulose ether structure. Addition of 1–4% CMC to minced blue whiting muscle produced a significant decrease in gel-forming ability and hardness, as shown in Table 17.1 (Pérez-Mateos and Montero, 2000). Chen and Xue (2009) reported that the addition of CMC modified the gelation properties of horse mackerel *surimi*, though to a lesser extent than other hydrocolloids (curdlan, tamarind gum, glucomannan and carrageenan). CMC needs large amounts of water to swell; not much water is released by the muscular protein, and therefore the CMC behaves as an inert filler in the fish–protein matrix of blue whiting minced gels, which are relatively water-constrained (Pérez-Mateos *et al.*, 2001). As noted earlier, the gelling treatment may produce an alteration in the hydrocolloid structure which could influence its behaviour as a texturizing additive and also as DF. As Fig. 17.1 shows, CMC significantly increases the WHC of gels after pressure gelling treatment (Montero *et al.*, 2001).

17.3.3 Fruits

Grape dietary fibre

The chief characteristics of the grape DF concentrates (GDF) obtained from wine industry by-products are high total DF content (> 70%), a relatively high ratio of soluble to total DF content, and the presence of associated polyphenolic compounds (> 5%) (Sánchez-Alonso *et al.*, 2007c; 2008). The effect of addition of these GDFs to minced fish muscle and their effect on suitability for frozen storage have been studied for technological purposes. Both white and red GDFs were used as ingredients in minced fish muscle in proportions of 2 and 4% (Sánchez-Alonso *et al.*, 2007c, d; 2008; Sánchez-Alonso and Borderías, 2008). However, GDF was not used in *surimi*, since the authors found a dramatic reduction of its gel-forming ability.

Water holding during frozen storage was higher in mince with added GDF than in control without GDF. GDF also reduced the thaw drip loss and increased the cooking yield, so here again GDF addition appears to be a good means of preventing the breadcrumb coating from breaking because of excessive drip release when frozen breaded portions are deep-fried. Also, mechanical properties were modified, reducing cohesiveness and hardness (Sánchez-Alonso *et al.*, 2007d; Sánchez-Alonso and Borderías, 2008). The main advantage of these GDFs was that they acted as strong antioxidants when added at 2% to frozen stored horse mackerel mince (Sánchez-Alonso *et al.*, 2007c; 2008). Their antioxidant properties come chiefly from extractable polyphenols (Sánchez-Alonso *et al.*, 2007e). The main drawback is that addition of more than 2% GDF produces some undesirable flavours and a colouring that is difficult to camouflage even in a strongly coloured muscle like horse mackerel.

Some consumer studies have been conducted on fish mince with added GDF. One recommendation arising from these was to use other sources of ADF, since it was shown that consumers did not like to mix terrestrial with seafood/fish DF but preferred DF of marine origin, for example seaweed DF (Careche *et al.*, 2008). Also, DF colour can be a problem for white seafood muscle; however, what is a disadvantage in a traditional product like the ones cited may be an advantage in the case of new, fancier products such as snacks or salad-bar products (Fig. 17.5) (Careche *et al.*, 2011).

Pectin

Pectins are another kind of soluble DFs found in fruits and vegetables, mainly citrus peels or apples. Pectin has been added as a cryoprotectant to cod and marlin fish *surimi*, though the *surimi* presented less freezing stability and gel-forming ability than when the traditional cryoprotectant sorbitol was used (Sych *et al.*, 1990; Ueng and Chu, 1996). There are only a few studies in which pectins have been used at 1–5% (w/w) in seafood products to increase the mechanical properties of the *surimi* gel (Barrera *et al.*, 2002; Uresti *et al.*, 2003a, b). In general, neither high- nor low-methoxyl pectins improve the mechanical properties of *surimi*; however, amidated pectins have been reported to improve its gelling properties. In fact, 25% amidated low methoxyl pectin can be added to restructured fish products at 1–5% to offer adequate textural properties with almost no perceptible changes in colour attributes (Ramírez *et al.*, 2007; Rodríguez *et al.*, 2008). However, some studies have reported that pectin had a negative effect on the gelation properties of horse mackerel *surimi*, causing the formation of an impacted network with huge holes (Chen and Xue, 2009). Besides textural modification, some researchers have used citrus pectin in fish burgers in order to improve organoleptic properties (Kasapis *et al.*, 2004).

17.3.4 Polysaccharide produced by microbial fermentation

Xanthan gum is a soluble DF produced from pure culture fermentation of the microorganism *Xanthomonas campestris*. Xanthan behaves differently from other anionic hydrocolloids, probably due to its large molecular size, producing softer fish mince gels, as shown in Table 17.1 (Pérez-Mateos and Montero, 2000). These authors also report that the addition of 1–4% xanthan gum to minced fish muscle produced a considerable decrease in hardness (Table 17.1), elasticity and adhesiveness of blue whiting gel (Pérez-Mateos and Montero, 2000). It is important to note that 0.5% xanthan gum significantly increased the WHC of the gels after high pressure gelling treatment (Fig. 17.1) (Montero *et al.*, 2001). Ramírez *et al.* (2002) reported a disruptive effect on the gel-forming ability of *surimi* with xanthan at 0.75–1%, though this negative effect was partially inhibited with addition of 0.4% calcium chloride. As noted earlier in the case of pectin, Chen and Xue (2009) also reported a negative effect of xanthan gum addition on the gelation properties of *surimi*, producing an impacted network with huge holes. In terms of fish gel microstructure, xanthan gum interacted with the fish–protein

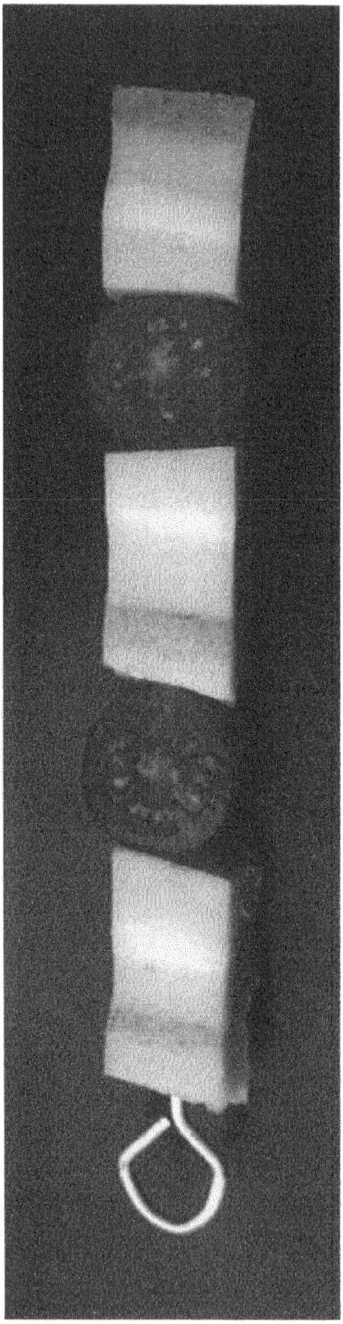

Fig. 17.5 Fancy brochette with added wheat DF and *Fucus* DF.

matrix (Pérez-Mateos *et al.*, 2001), forming a mesh of filaments inside the cavities of the heat-induced gel (Montero *et al.*, 2000). Addition of a blend of xanthan and locust bean gums (ratio 0.25/0.75) has been reported to enhance the mechanical properties of myofibrillar proteins from silver carp (*Hypophthalmichthys molitrixat*) (Ramírez *et al.*, 2002). As mentioned above, most of these levels of fibre addition are too low to be classified as fortification.

Curdlan, generic name β-(1–3)-D-glucan, is another microbial polysaccharide and an insoluble DF. Chen and Xue (2009) studied the addition of different hydrocolloids, of which curdlan produced the most beneficial effect on the gelation properties of horse mackerel *surimi*. When silver carp mince was mixed with curdlan at a concentration of 1–3%, the gel strength and hardness of the resulting gels increased (Yinghong *et al.*, 2003).

17.3.5 Others

Non-digestible oligosaccharides are potentially prebiotic soluble DF products. Protein cryoprotectants (such as trehalose, sorbitol and maltodextrin) are commonly used at concentrations of 4–8% in fish muscle to minimize thaw loss and texture changes of fish muscle (Nopianti *et al.*, 2011).

Inulin (Fibruline®), from chicory root, worsened textural quality and WHC when added at 4% (w/w) to restructured fish products made with South African hake mince (Cardoso *et al.*, 2007a, b; 2008). Following on from these studies, it was found that the textural quality of gels from Atlantic mackerel (*Scomber scombrus*) and chub mackerel (*Scomber japonicus*) *surimi* and from sea bass (*Dicentrarchus labrax*) trimmings, containing inulin, could be enhanced by addition of 1–2% carrageenan or 0.5% microbial transglutaminase (MTGase) (Cardoso *et al.*, 2009; 2010b; 2011a, b). The same authors successfully developed a healthy low-fat fish sausage containing inulin and South African hake mince as a pork meat replacer (Cardoso *et al.*, 2008), fortified with omega-3 fatty acids (Cardoso *et al.*, 2010a).

Park (1996) used glucomannan from konjac flour as an ingredient in both Alaska pollock and Pacific whiting *surimi*. Five per cent konjac flour reinforced the shear stress of gels 8–10-fold and exhibited an ability to maintain consistent shear strain values against repeated freeze/thaw abuse. This flour increased the lightness of gels at concentrations up to 2%, with a gradually increasing yellow hue from there up to 5%. Cardoso *et al.* (2011b) reported an increase of the hardness and elastic modulus of seabream (*Sparus aurata*) mince with 1% added konjac flour, but gels were less deformable and so of poorer quality. These authors also reported a mutual reinforcement of gel hardness when MTGase and konjac flour were added together. In the two papers cited, konjac flour was added as a filler and not as a gelling agent; the aim was to raise the pH in order to obtain thermostable gels after deacetylation. Iglesias-Otero *et al.* (2010) added konjac glucomannan to poor quality squid *surimi* in a final proportion of 0.1% in order to bring the pH up to around 10 and so improve the gelation quality of the *surimi* through the formation of a parallel thermostable network. Solo-de-Zaldivar *et al.*

(2012) studied glucomannan gelation with a view to making restructured seafood products based on a non-functional mince and an aqueous solution of glucomannan (at a final concentration of 1.5%) in order to achieve structures with non-functional mince, such as muscle which has been previously heated.

Glucomannan has also been studied as a cryoprotectant in *surimi* of grass carp (*Ctenophryngodon idella*) (Xiong *et al.*, 2009). These authors reported that the cryoprotective effect of 1% glucomannan was as good as that of a conventional cryoprotectant. They also reported that at this level the breaking force and deformation of gels increased, and that the water properties of *surimi* improved while whiteness decreased.

17.4 Conclusion

It is accepted that consumption of DF exerts a positive effect on human physiology through the gastrointestinal tract, in addition to certain metabolic activities. DF supplementation could thus considerably enhance the nutritional value of a very healthy food like fish. DF is not only a healthy complement in seafood products but is also useful for developing new seafood products, especially restructured products. To that end, a compromise needs to be found in order to meet functional and technological requirements while offering consumers healthy, tasty and attractive seafood products.

Soluble DFs have been used for many years and are essential ingredients in many seafood formulations. Other less widely used DFs, for instance from some cereals, fruits or seaweeds, have a good soluble/insoluble DF balance, which is better from a physiological point of view, and they also have useful technological properties for restructured seafood products. Also, antioxidant DFs offer a new way to prevent oxidation of highly unsaturated seafood lipids.

17.5 Future trends

The nutritional properties of DF can further complement the healthy characteristics of seafood with added beneficial effects such as reducing cholesterolaemia, modifying glycaemic response, reducing nutrient availability, prebiotic capacity, and so on. In many applications, the amounts of DF used may be too low to exert physiological effects; however, in the diet the sum of this and other DF from other sources can definitely be beneficial. Further intervention studies are needed to confirm the beneficial effects of DFs in general and balanced soluble/insoluble DFs in particular. As new ADFs are identified, they may be found suitable for addition to restructured fish products.

To date, DF has been added directly to restructured seafood products made from minced muscle. However, no other ways of adding DF ingredients, such as by injection in liquid dispersion into the whole fish muscle, have been reported.

Given the increasing awareness of health issues among consumers, the substitution of chemical for natural antioxidants like ADF is a sound argument in favour of future development. Another compelling argument is the replacement of polyphosphates and other additives for DFs to bind water and thus achieve a better texture.

The development of novel modified DFs with optimized properties for certain applications in particular products offers the prospect of better ingredients to bind water and probably improved gelation of muscle proteins in order to develop different kinds of textures.

The use of seaweed and seaweed DF as an ingredient in restructured seafood products offers the opportunity to create new fancy and healthy products which may be well received by consumers with the help of communication campaigns. Also, the sea-associated flavour imparted by seaweed, and the fact of its marine origin, are likely to enhance consumer acceptance.

Given the foreseeable need for the seafood industry to upgrade industrial by-products and by-catches through increasing development of restructured products, it will be necessary to use different ingredients such as traditional DFs – alginates, carrageenans and so on – and to design new ones to meet all kinds of technological requirements.

In general, DF fortification of seafood is still a largely empirical process. Clearly, then, further research into the effect of DF and associated substances and the development of new modified DFs targeting different technological effects will produce changes in seafood technology, especially in the field of processed seafood products.

17.6 Sources of further information and advice

Research and interest groups

- Institute of Food Science, Technology and Nutrition (ICTAN-CSIC), a part of the Spanish National Science Research Council (CSIC). The Research Departments of Products considers different aspects related to the design, recovery and innovation of restructured seafood products.
- West European Fish Technologists' Association (WEFTA) is a major European platform for institutes engaged in fish and food science and technology.
- Atlantic Fisheries Technology Conference (AFTC) promotes the application of science and engineering to the production, processing, packaging, distribution, preparation and utilization of fishery products.
- Seafood Science and Technology Society of the Americas (SST) is a professional and educational association of aquatic food product technologists focusing on tropical and subtropical species.
- The Pacific Fisheries Technologists (PFT) is a professional society for fisheries technologists that promotes better working relationships among companies, universities and government laboratories specifically involved in Pacific Fisheries, and also worldwide relationships.

Database and books

- The Global New Products Database (GNPD) facilitates searches for and analysis of ingredient trends in new consumer packaged goods, whether the search is for a specific emerging ingredient or for an overarching trend in ingredients.
- Seafood Network Information Center (SeafoodNIC) hosts a bibliographic database of citations in fish technology with a bias towards composition, quality, safety, quality assurance, inspection and regulation of fishery products.
- Book review: *Marine polysaccharides: food applications* (Venugopal, 2011) is a useful reference covering the nature, source, production and applications of these polysaccharides in food product development and other areas.

17.7 Acknowledgements

This work was carried out within the Projects AGL2011-24693ALI and AGL2008-00231ALI (Spanish Ministry of Science and Innovation). I. Sanchez-Alonso was supported by a Juan de la Cierva postdoctorate contract from the Spanish Ministry of Economy and Competitiveness.

17.8 References

ANG J F (1993), 'Reduction of fat in fried batter coatings with powdered cellulose', *JAOCS*, **70**(6), 619–22.

ANG J F and CROSBY G A (2005), 'Formulating reduced-calorie foods with powdered cellulose', *Food Technol*, **59**(3), 35–8.

BARRERA A M, RAMÍREZ J A, GONZÁLEZ-CABRIALES J J and VÁZQUEZ M (2002), 'Effect of pectins on the gelling properties of *surimi* from silver carp', *Food Hydrocolloids*, **16**(5), 441–7.

BENJAKUL S, VISESSANGUAN W, PHATCHRAT S and TANAKA M (2003), 'Chitosan affects transglutaminase-induced *surimi* gelation', *J Food Biochem*, **27**(1), 53–66.

BENJAKUL S, VISESSANGUAN W, TANAKA M, ISHIZAKI S, SUTHIDHAM R and SUNGPECH O (2001), 'Effect of chitin and chitosan on gelling properties of *surimi* from barred garfish (*Hemiramphus far*)', *J Sci Food Agric*, **81**(1), 102–8.

BORDERÍAS J, MONTERO P and MARTÍ DE CASTRO M A (1996), 'Gelling of hake (*Merluccius australis*) sawdust', *Food Sci Technol Int*, **2**(5), 293–9.

BORDERÍAS A J, SÁNCHEZ-ALONSO I and PÉREZ-MATEOS M (2005), 'New applications of fibres in foods: Addition to fishery products', *Trends Food Sci Tech*, **16**, 458–65.

CARDOSO C, MENDES R and NUNES M L (2007a), 'Dietary fibers' effect on the textural properties of fish heat-induced gels', *J Aquat Food Prod Technol*, **16**(3), 19–30.

CARDOSO C, MENDES R and NUNES M L (2007b), 'Effect of transglutaminase and carrageenan on restructured fish products containing dietary fibres', *Int J Food Sci Technol*, **42**(11), 1257–64.

CARDOSO C, MENDES R and NUNES M L (2008), 'Development of a healthy low-fat fish sausage containing dietary fibre', *Int J Food Sci Technol*, **43**(2), 276–83.

CARDOSO C, MENDES R, VAZ-PIRES P and NUNES M L (2009), 'Effect of dietary fibre and MTGase on the quality of mackerel *surimi* gels', *J Sci Food Agric*, **89**(10), 1648–58.

CARDOSO C, MENDES R, PEDRO S, VAZ-PIRES P and NUNES M L (2010a), 'Quality changes during storage of minced fish products containing dietary fiber and fortified with ω3 fatty acids', *Food Sci Technol Int*, **16**(1), 31–42.

CARDOSO C, MENDES R, SARAIVA J, VAZ-PIRES P and NUNES M L (2010b), 'Quality characteristics of high pressure-induced hake (*Merluccius capensis*) protein gels with and without MTGase', *J Aquat Food Prod Technol*, **19**(3), 193–213.

CARDOSO C, MENDES R, VAZ-PIRES P and NUNES M L (2011a), 'Production of high quality gels from sea bass: Effect of MTGase and dietary fibre', *LWT – Food Sci Technol*, **44**(5), 1282–90.

CARDOSO C, MENDES R, VAZ-PIRES P and NUNES M L (2011b), 'Effect of MTGase, dietary fiber and UV irradiation upon heat-induced gilthead seabream (*Sparus aurata*) gels', *Food Sci Technol Int*, **17**(2), 155–65.

CARECHE M, LUTEN J B, KOLE A, SCHELVIS R, SAURA-CALIXTO F, *et al.* (2008), 'Developing functional seafood products', in: BORRENSEN T, *Improving seafood products for the consumer*, Cambridge, CRC Press-Woodhead Publishing Limited, 331–62.

CARECHE M, BORDERÍAS A J, SÁNCHEZ-ALONSO I and LUND E K (2011), 'Functional seafood products', in SAARELA M, *Functional foods*, Oxford, Woodhead Publishing, 557–81.

CHEN H and XUE C (2009), 'Effect of hydrocolloids on the gel properties of horse-mackerel *surimi*', *Nongye Jixie Xuebao/Transactions Chin Soc Agric Machin*, **40**(2), 119–25 (in Chinese).

CHEN H H, FERNG L H, CHEN S D, SUN W C and LEE Y C (2005), 'Combination model for the spatial partition of *surimi* protein and hydroxylpropylmethylcellulose', *Food Hydrocolloids*, **19**, 761–8.

CHUN S S, PARK J R, PARK J C, SUH J S and AHN C B (1999), 'Quality characteristics of hamburger patties added with seaweed powder', *J Korean Soc Food Sci Nutr*, **28**(1), 140–4.

COFRADES S, LÓPEZ-LÓPEZ I, RUÍZ-CAPILLAS C, TREKI M and JIMÉNEZ-COLMENERO F (2011), 'Quality characteristics during chilling storage of low-salt restructured poultry with added microbial transglutaminase and seaweed', *Meat Sci*, **87**, 373–80.

DEY S S and DORA K C (2010), 'Suitability of chitosan as cryoprotectant on croaker fish (*Johnius gangeticus*) *surimi* during frozen storage', *J Food Sci Technol*, **48**(6), 699–705.

DÍAZ-RUBIO M E, SERRANO J, BORDERÍAS A J and SAURA-CALIXTO F (2011), 'Technological effect and nutritional value of dietary antioxidant *fucus* fibre added to minced fish muscle', *J Aquat Food Prod Technol*, **20**(3), 295–307.

EC (2006), Regulation (EC) No 1924/2006 of the European Parliament and of the Council of 20 December 2006 on nutrition and health claims made on foods. *Official Journal of the European Union*, **L404**, 9–25.

FRIEDMAN M and JUNEJA V K (2010), 'Review of antimicrobial and antioxidative activities of chitosans in food', *J Food Prot*, **73**(9), 1737–61.

GAO J C, PIGOTT G M and REINE B (1999), 'Gel forming additive effects on properties of thermally induced minced fish gel', *J Food Sci*, **64**(3), 414–17.

GLICKSMAN M (1987), 'Utilization of seaweed hydrocolloids in the food industry', *Hydrobiologia*, **151–2**(1), 31–47.

GÓMEZ-GUILLÉN M C and MONTERO P (1996), 'Addition of hydrocolloids and non-muscle proteins to sardine (*Sardina pilchardus*) mince gels: Effect of salt concentration', *Food Chem*, **56**(4), 421–7.

GÓMEZ-GUILLÉN C, SOLAS T, BORDERÍAS J and MONTERO P (1996), 'Effect of heating temperature and sodium chloride concentration on ultrastructure and texture of gels made from giant squid (*Dosidicus gigas*) with addition of starch, *i*-carrageenan and egg white', *Eur Food Res Technol*, **202**(3), 221–7.

GÓMEZ-GUILLÉN C, BORDERÍAS A J and MONTERO P (1997), 'Thermal gelation properties of two different composition sardine (*Sardina pilchardus*) muscles with addition of non-muscle proteins and hydrocolloids', *Food Chem*, **58**(1–2), 81–7.

GÓMEZ-GUILLÉN C, MONTERO P, SOLAS M T and PÉREZ-MATEOS M (2005), 'Effect of chitosan and microbial transglutaminase on the gel forming ability of horse mackerel (*Trachurus spp.*) muscle under high pressure', *Food Res Int*, **38**(1), 103–10.

HERRANZ B, SOLO-DE-ZALDIVAR B and BORDERÍAS A J (2012), 'Obtaining a restructured seafood product from non-functional fish muscle by glucomannan addition: first steps', *J Aquatic Food Product Technol*, in press (DOI:10.1080/10498850.2011.632114).

IGLESIAS-OTERO M A, BORDERÍAS J and TOVAR C A (2010), 'Use of konjac glucomannan as additive to reinforce the gels from low quality squid *surimi*', *J Food Eng*, **101**, 281–8.

JEON Y J, SHAHIDI F and KIM S K (2000), 'Preparation of chitin and chitosan oligomers and their applications in physiological functional foods', *Food Rev Int*, **16**(2), 159–76.

JIMÉNEZ-ESCRIG A and SÁNCHEZ-MUÑIZ F J (2000), 'Dietary fibre from edible seaweeds–chemical structure, physicochemical properties and effects on cholesterol metabolism', *Nutr Res*, **20**(4), 585–98.

JIMÉNEZ-ESCRIG A, JIMÉNEZ-JIMÉNEZ I, PULIDO R and SAURA-CALIXTO F (2001), 'Antioxidant activity of fresh and processed edible seaweed', *J Agric Food Chem*, **81**, 530–4.

JITTINANDANA S, KENNEY P B and SLIDER S D (2005), 'Cryoprotectants affect physical properties of restructured trout during frozen storage', *J Food Sci*, **70**(1), C35–C42.

KAMIL J Y V A, JEON Y J and SHAHIDI F (2002), 'Antioxidative activity of chitosans of different viscosity in cooked comminuted flesh of herring (*Clupea harengus*)', *Food Chem*, **79**(1), 69–77.

KASAPIS S, AL-OUFI H S, AL-MAAMARI S, AL-BULUSHI I M and GODDARD S (2004), 'Scientific and technological aspects of fish product development Part I: Handshaking instrumental texture with consumer preference in burgers', *Int J Food Prop*, **7**(3), 449–62.

KATAOKA J, ISHIZAKI S and TANAKA M (1998), 'Effects of chitosan on gelling properties of low quality *surimi*', *J Muscle Foods*, **9**(3), 209–20.

KOIDE S S (1998), 'Chitin-chitosan: Properties, benefits and risks', *Nutr Res*, **18**(6), 1091–101.

KOK T N and PARK J W (2007), 'Extending the shelf life of set fish ball', *J Food Quality*, **30**(1), 1–27.

LIAN P Z, LEE C M and HUFNAGEL L (2000), 'Physicochemical properties of frozen red hake (*Urophycis chuss*) mince as affected by cryoprotective ingredients', *J Food Sci*, **65**(7), 1117–23.

LÓPEZ-CABALLERO M E, GÓMEZ-GUILLÉN M C, PÉREZ-MATEOS M and MONTERO P (2005), 'A functional chitosan-enriched fish sausage treated by high pressure', *J Food Sci*, **70**(3), M166–M171.

LÓPEZ-LÓPEZ I, COFRADES S and JIMÉNEZ-COLMENERO F (2010), 'Frozen storage characteristics of low-salt and low-fat beef patties as affected by *Wakame* addition and replacing pork backfat with olive oil-in-water emulsion', *Food Res Int*, **43**, 1244–54.

MILLER W B (1986), 'Seeing the "light": Cellulose in reduced-calorie baked goods', *Bakers Digest*, **60**(1), 18–20.

MONTERO P, HURTADO J L and PÉREZ-MATEOS M (2000), 'Microstructural behaviour and gelling characteristics of myosystem protein gels interacting with hydrocolloids', *Food Hydrocolloids*, **14**(5), 455–61.

MONTERO P, SOLAS T and PÉREZ-MATEOS M (2001), 'Pressure-induced gel properties of fish mince with ionic and non-ionic gums added', *Food Hydrocolloids*, **15**(2), 185–94.

MOREL J M, PERREY F, LEJEUNE R and GOETZ P (2005), '*Fucus vesiculosus* L.', *Phytothérapie*, **3**(5), 218–21.

MORENO H M, CARBALLO J and BORDERÍAS A J (2008), 'Influence of alginate and microbial transglutaminase as binding ingredients on restructured fish muscle processed at low temperature', *J Sci Food Agric*, **88**(9), 1529–36.

MORENO H M, CARBALLO J and BORDERÍAS A J (2010), 'Use of microbial transglutaminase and sodium alginate in the preparation of restructured fish models using cold gelation: Effect of frozen storage', *Innov Food Sci Emerg*, **11**(2), 394–400.

NELSON A L (2001), *High-fiber ingredients. Practical guidelines for food industry*, Minnesota, USA, Eagan Press Handbook Series, AAC Chemists.

NO H K, MEYERS S P, PRINYAWIWATKUL W and XU Z (2007), 'Applications of chitosan for improvement of quality and shelf life of foods: A review', *J Food Sci*, **72**(5), R87–R100.

NOPIANTI R, HUDA N and ISMAIL N (2011), 'A review on the loss of the functional properties of proteins during frozen storage and the improvement of gel-forming properties of *Surimi*', *Am J Food Technol*, **6**(1), 19–30.

NORZIAH M H and CHIO Y C (2001), 'Nutritional composition of edible seaweed *Gracilaria changgi*', *Food Chem*, **68**(1), 69–76.

ORTIZ J and AGUILERA J M (2004), 'Effect of kappa-carrageenan on the gelation of horse mackerel (*T. murphyi*) raw paste *surimi*-type', *Food Sci Technol Int*, **10**(4), 223–32.

PANYATHITIPONG W and PUECHKAMUT Y (2010), 'Effect of tofu powder and carrageenan on functionality and physical characteristics of *surimi* emulsion gel', *Kasetsart J – Nat Sci*, **44**(4), 671–9.

PARK J W (1996), 'Temperature-tolerant fish protein gels using konjac flour', *J Muscle Food*, **7**, 165–74.

PARK J W (2005), 'Ingredient technology and formulation development', in PARK J W and DEKKER M, *Surimi and surimi seafood*, 2nd edition, New York, CRC Press, Taylor and Francis Group, 649–707.

PÉREZ-MATEOS M and MONTERO P (2000), 'Contribution of hydrocolloids to gelling properties of blue whiting muscle', *Eur Food Res Technol*, **210**(6), 383–90.

PÉREZ-MATEOS M and MONTERO P (2002), 'Effects of hydrocolloids and high-pressure-heating processing on minced fish gels', *Eur Food Res Technol*, **214**(2), 119–24.

PÉREZ-MATEOS M, HURTADO J L, MONTERO P and FERNÁNDEZ-MARTÍN F (2001), 'Interactions of κ-carrageenan plus other hydrocolloids in fish myosystem gels', *J Food Sci*, **66**(6), 838–43.

PÉREZ-MATEOS M, SOLAS T and MONTERO P (2002), 'Carrageenans and alginate effects on properties of combined pressure and temperature in fish mince gels', *Food Hydrocolloids*, **16**(3), 225–33.

PIRES C, BATISTA I, FRADINHO P and COSTA S (2009), 'Utilization of alkaline-recovered proteins from cape hake by-products in the preparation of frankfurter-type fish sausages', *J Aquat Food Prod Technol*, **18**(1–2), 170–90.

RAMÍREZ J A, BARRERA M, MORALES O G and VÁZQUEZ M (2002), 'Effect of xanthan and locust bean gums on the gelling properties of myofibrillar protein', *Food Hydrocolloids*, **16**(1), 11–16.

RAMÍREZ J A, RODRÍGUEZ N R, URESTI R M, VELÁZQUEZ G and VÁZQUEZ M (2007), 'Fiber-rich functional fish food from striped mullet (*Mugil cephalus*) using amidated low methoxyl pectin', *Food Hydrocolloids*, **21**(4), 527–36.

RAMÍREZ J A, URESTI R M, VELÁZQUEZ G and VÁZQUEZ M (2011), 'Food hydrocolloids as additives to improve the mechanical and functional properties of fish products: A review', *Food Hydrocolloids*, **25**(8), 1842–52.

RODRÍGUEZ N R, URESTI R M, VELÁZQUEZ G, VÁZQUEZ M and RAMÍREZ J A (2008), 'Effects of amidated low methoxyl pectin on healthy restructured fish food from Mexican flounder (*Cyclopsetta chittendeni*)', *J Food Process Eng*, **31**(2), 229–46.

RUPÉREZ P (2002), 'Mineral content of edible marine seaweeds', *Food Chem*, **79**(1), 23–6.

RUPÉREZ P, AHRAZEM O and LEAL J A (2002), 'Potential antioxidant capacity of sulphated polysaccharides from the edible marine brown seaweed *Fucus vesiculous*', *J Agric Food Chem*, **50**, 840–5.

SÁNCHEZ-ALONSO I and BORDERÍAS A J (2008), 'Technological effect of red grape antioxidant dietary fibre added to minced fish muscle', *Int J Food Sci Tech*, **43**, 1009–18.

SÁNCHEZ-ALONSO I, HAJI-MALEKI R and BORDERÍAS A J (2006), 'Effect of wheat fibre in frozen stored fish muscular gels', *Eur Food Res Technol*, **223**, 571–6.

SÁNCHEZ-ALONSO I, SOLAS M T and BORDERÍAS A J (2007a), 'Technological implications of addition of wheat dietary fibre to giant squid (*Dosidicus gigas*) *surimi* gels', *J Food Eng*, **81**, 404–11.

SÁNCHEZ-ALONSO I, HAJI-MALEKI R and BORDERÍAS A J (2007b), 'Wheat fiber as a functional ingredient in restructured fish products', *Food Chem*, **100**, 1037–43.

SÁNCHEZ-ALONSO I, JIMÉNEZ-ESCRIG A, SAURA-CALIXTO F and BORDERÍAS A J (2007c), 'Effect of grape antioxidant dietary fibre on the prevention of lipid oxidation in minced fish: Evaluation by different methodologies', *Food Chem*, **101**, 372–8.

SÁNCHEZ-ALONSO I, SOLAS M T and BORDERÍAS A J (2007d), 'Physical study of minced fish muscle with a white-grape by-product added as ingredient', *J Food Sci*, **72**(2), E94–E101.

SÁNCHEZ-ALONSO I, BORDERÍAS A J, LARSSON K and UNDELAND I (2007e), 'Inhibition of hemoglobin-mediated oxidation of regular and lipid-fortified cod mince by a white grape dietary fiber', *J Agric Food Chem*, **55**, 5299–305.

SÁNCHEZ-ALONSO I, JIMÉNEZ-ESCRIG A, SAURA-CALIXTO F and BORDERÍAS A J (2008), 'Antioxidant protection of white grape pomace on restructured fish products during frozen storage', *LWT – Food Sci Technol*, **41**, 42–50.

SÁNCHEZ-GONZÁLEZ I, RODRÍGUEZ-CASADO A, CARECHE M and CARMONA P (2009), 'Raman analysis of *surimi* by addition of wheat dietary fibre', *Food Chem*, **112**, 162–8.

SAURA-CALIXTO F (1998), 'Antioxidant dietary fiber product: A new concept and a potential food ingredient', *J Agric Food Chem*, **46**, 4303–6.

SHAHIDI F, ARACHCHI J K V and JEON Y J (1999), 'Food applications of chitin and chitosans', *Trends Food Sci Technol*, **10**(2), 37–51.

SHAHIDI F, KAMIL J, JEON Y J and KIM S K (2002), 'Antioxidant role of chitosan in a cooked cod (*Gadus morhua*) model system', *J Food Lipids*, **9**(1), 57–64.

SOMJIT K, RUTTANAPORNWAREESAKUL Y, HARA K and NOZAKI Y (2005), 'The cryoprotectant effect of shrimp chitin and shrimp chitin hydrolysate on denaturation and unfrozen water of lizardfish *surimi* during frozen storage', *Food Res Int*, **38**(4), 345–55.

SYCH J, LACROIX C, ADAMBOUNOU L T and CASTAIGNE F (1990), 'Cryoprotective effects of some materials on cod-*surimi* proteins during frozen storage', *J Food Sci*, **55**(5), 1222–7.

TUDORICA C M, KURI V and BRENNAN C S (2002), 'Nutritional and physicochemical characteristics of dietary fibre', *J Agric Food Chem*, **50**, 347–56.

UENG Y E and CHU Y J (1996), 'Effect of dietary fibers on cold resistance of *surimi*', *Food Sci Taiwan*, **23**, 266–75 (in Chinese).

URESTI R M, LÓPEZ-ARIAS N, GONZÁLEZ-CABRIALES J J, RAMÍREZ J A and VÁZQUEZ M (2003a), 'Use of amidated low methoxyl pectin to produce fish restructured products', *Food Hydrocolloids*, **17**(2), 171–6.

URESTI R M, LÓPEZ-ARIAS N, RAMÍREZ J A and VÁZQUEZ M (2003b), 'Effect of amidated low methoxyl pectin on the mechanical properties and colour attributes of fish mince', *Food Technol Biotech*, **41**(2), 131–6.

VENUGOPAL V (2009), 'Seaweed: nutritional value, bioactive properties and uses', in VENUGOPAL V, *Marine Products for Health care*, Florida, USA, CRC Press/Taylor & Francis, 261–89.

VENUGOPAL V (2011), *Marine polysaccharides: food applications*, Boca Raton, FL, USA, CRC Press.

WU T and MAO L (2009), 'Application of chitosan to maintain the quality of *kamaboko* gels made from grass carp (*Ctenopharyngodon idellus*) during storage', *J Food Process Pres*, **33**(2), 218–30.

XIONG G, CHENG W, YE L, DU X, ZHOU M, *et al.* (2009), 'Effect of konjac glucomannan on physicochemical properties of myofibrillar protein and *surimi* gels from grass carp (*Ctenopharyngodon idella*)', *Food Chem*, **116**, 413–18.

YINGHONG Q, YOKOYAMA M, HAYAKAWA F and SAITO M (2003), 'Effect of food additives on texture and smell of silver carp (*Hypophthalmichthys molitrix*) mince', *Food Sci Technol Res*, **9**(2), 176–9.

YOON K S and LEE C M (1990), 'Effect of powdered cellulose on the texture and freeze-thaw stability of *surimi*-based shellfish analog products', *J Food Sci*, **55**(1), 87–90.

18

Fibre-enriched beverages

L. Viscione, Dupont Nutrition and Health (formerly Danisco UK Ltd), UK

DOI: 10.1533/9780857095787.4.369

Abstract: The addition of fibre into products fulfils a role in improving the health positioning and nutritional content with a view to making a product claim. The purpose of this chapter is to introduce the important factors when fortifying non-dairy beverages with fibre, to introduce some fibre ingredients that are suitable for adding into non-dairy beverage systems and to provide some practical tips to ensure optimal stability and final product quality.

Key words: dietary fibre addition in beverages, quality, stability.

18.1 Introduction

There are many challenges to overcome when fortifying a beverage with dietary fibre. The objective of adding fibre into drinks is usually to improve the health positioning of a product and to make a product claim. Furthermore, when improving the health positioning, a reduction in the total level of sugars may also be an important objective. The challenge of adding fibre into non-dairy-based beverage systems is born out of the nature of the drink formula. Overall, non-dairy beverages typically exhibit a very low viscosity, and have a low pH. Within the beverage matrix, fibre addition can have a direct effect on the mouthfeel, texture and flavour release of the product. The type of fibre used to fortify non-dairy beverages must therefore be evaluated carefully to ensure that the desired texture and flavour profile are achieved or maintained. The fibre source must also have adequate scientific substantiation to support its use and/or fulfil the definition of fibre that exists in the target geographical market. The scope of this chapter includes all non-dairy beverages, including carbonates, juices and nectars, flavoured waters and powdered drinks.

18.1.1 Rationale for adding dietary fibre into beverages

Dietary fibre is present naturally in many different foods, such as wholegrain cereals, fruits and vegetables, and as such consumers are familiar with these foods. Traditionally, processed foods containing high amounts of fibre have been confined to products made from cereals such as breakfast cereals, rice and pasta. In addition to being high in fibre, grains exhibit physical properties that are suitable for use in breakfast cereals, breads, cakes, pasta and other similar products, but are less suitable for fibre fortification in aqueous products such as non-dairy beverages. However, it is possible to create cereal drinks, but these should be considered as a separate type of drink rather than being seen as fibre fortification in existing drinks (Angelov *et al.* 2006, Blandino *et al.* 2003, Gupta *et al.* 2010).

Today, with the extraction and manufacture of fibre from alternative sources, the prospect of fortifying drinks has become a reality. In general, the physical properties of many modern fibre ingredients are more suitable for use in aqueous systems such as beverages than traditional cereal- or fruit-based fibres due to their higher solubility and clarity in solution. This change in ingredient technology means that beverages can now be a valid source of dietary fibre. In a world where the consumption of manufactured beverages is high, adding dietary fibre into beverages could be a realistic option for consumers to make up for the shortfall in dietary fibre consumption and impact positively on their health (FSA 2008/9, Kendall *et al.* 2010). Furthermore, the reduction in sugars within a beverage could offset the cost of fibre addition and also further improve the health benefits of a drink.

There are many other important questions that should be asked when developing a product: what does this ingredient do, do consumers understand its benefits, does it fit with the application (from a consumer perspective), and does the ingredient have the right technical properties to make it work – or how can I make it work?

18.2 Adding fibres into drinks

Adding fibre into drinks is becoming more commonplace due to the appearance of new soluble fibre ingredients and the consumer benefit that adding fibre can bring. These new fibres allow a nutritionally significant amount of fibre to be added to a drink without causing high viscosity, slimy or gritty textures, or significant colour. Furthermore, due to the generally high solubility and dispersibility, there is no need for high shear equipment within the factory environment; simple mixing equipment is usually sufficient. Adding fibre into drinks can improve the nutritional profile and reduce the sugar content of the product per serving. Furthermore, concentrated and processed juice products can have very low fibre levels as a result of the processing, which largely removes the fibre from the starting material; therefore fruit juices made from concentrate are particularly good candidates for fibre fortification.

18.2.1 Aspects of formulating dietary fibres into drinks

This section will discuss the details that need to be considered when adding fibres into drinks. The intended characteristics of the final product will help to determine which dietary fibre is most suitable. The final composition and, therefore, parameters for the drink have a direct impact on the texture and the stability. Process parameters such as homogenisation, heat treatment (time and temperature) and filling temperature also play a key role. The physical properties of the fibres need to fit with the proposed drink. The particle size, bulk density, particle shape, solubility, dispersibility and hygroscopicity are all important parameters to control in powdered drinks, whereas solubility, dispersibility, acid stability and clarity/transparency are more important for ready-to-drink (RTD) formats. Furthermore, other properties such as digestive tolerance and nutritional composition are important factors that can determine consumer appeal and therefore the choice of fibre to fortify with. These aspects will be discussed below.

Physical properties

As introduced above, the physical properties of interest to the product developer will depend upon the format of the finished drink, with different considerations for RTD and powdered formats. These parameters can have a significant effect on the manufacturing process, the textural properties, final mouthfeel, flavour and appearance of the beverage. For beverages, it is preferable to add easily dispersible, soluble ingredients that require little or no additional processing. When adding less soluble ingredients, the particles need to be stabilised properly to avoid the perception of floury or grainy textures. Ingredients that cause colouration or cloudiness are more suitable for opaque beverages such as dairy beverages, cloudy fruit-based drinks, smoothies, or those containing a cloud. Ingredients that impart high viscosity at low usage levels are somewhat limited in their use as a sole dietary fibre ingredient. Ingredients that have high viscosity in solution tend to be gums and are typically used to stabilise and/or modify the mouthfeel of beverages. For example, guar gum, pectin, xanthan and cellulose gum can be used in this way. The high viscosity of gums prevents their use as a sole dietary fibre ingredient as they cannot be added in sufficient quantity to enable a claim. For example, typical use levels of gums are between 0.05 and 0.3%; in a 250 ml drink, this equates to approximately between 0.125 g and 0.75 g in the drink. To enable a claim, at least 2.5 g per serving is required in the USA or 3 g/100 g in the European Union (EU; EC 2006). For powder systems, it is preferable to add ingredients together that are well matched for particle size/shape and bulk density in order to prevent de-blending once mixed. Furthermore, ingredients that are non-hygroscopic improve the blending properties and shelf life and do not limit the choice of packaging options available. Lastly, it is important that the fibre ingredient can rapidly solubilise under the poor mixing conditions that are found within the consumption (home) environment.

Stability

The stability requirements for the beverage manufacturer are specific to each manufacturer and will depend on the quality of the ingredients used, the process and the shelf life of the intended product. For RTD beverages, instability in acidic conditions can result in hydrolysis of the fibre ingredient. The result is dependent on the source of dietary fibre; however, a dramatic loss in fibre content can result in the drink not fulfilling its nutritional panel or product claim throughout its intended shelf life. Any instability in a final product is undesirable and may cause other physical changes to the drink, such as increased sweetness level over time to a level not intended by the product developer, loss of mouthfeel, loss of stabilisation, loss of texture, increase in colouration or precipitation of the fibre, to mention a few. This, as you might expect, means a reduction in the amount of dietary fibre polymer present in the beverage, which has regulatory implications if a claim is being made. This loss can be reduced by modifying the manufacturing process, formulation, storage conditions and/or the intended shelf life. For powdered beverages, the issue of stability raises different questions. It is less related to acid stability over time but more related to hygroscopicity and the water activity (Aw) of individual ingredients. One result of increasing moisture levels is caking, reducing product flow/spoonability and so resulting in poor product performance.

Digestive tolerance

Digestive tolerance is a complex and important issue to consider when formulating a beverage in particular, due to the potential volume and speed of consumption that is possible. This is of course dependent on the actual product matrix, its viscosity, drinking occasion, price and marketing angle, but, nevertheless, a beverage has the potential to be consumed in fairly large quantities, very quickly, putting the consumers at risk of overconsumption. Although it is true that individuals consume fibre to improve digestive health, undesirable consequences of this will not be accepted. Factors that affect the digestion of a product include the physical properties of dietary fibre, such as particle size, viscosity, solubility, and so on (Guillon and Champ 2000). However, there are also other factors to take into to account: the dose in the product, the drink matrix, time taken for consumption, consumption frequency, whether or not the drink is consumed with other food, and individual sensitivities (Marteau and Flourie 2001). Furthermore, undesirable consequences of consuming too much dietary fibre include laxation and gastrointestinal (GI) effects, including abdominal discomfort, flatus, and diarrhoea, especially at higher or excessive intakes (Grabitske and Slavin 2008). However, the point of 'unacceptability' is very individual and therefore difficult to define. This subjectivity makes an acceptable dose difficult to evaluate (Roberfroid and Slavin 2000). It is important to note that there is usually a period of adjustment when ingesting new foods and ingredients and so tolerance usually improves over time, especially when dealing with low digestible carbohydrates. Such responses, though transient, affect the perception of the well-being of consumers and their acceptance of food products containing low digestable carbohydrates (LDCs) (Grabitske and Slavin 2008). In the following section, individual fibre ingredients will be discussed in relation to this topic.

18.3 Types of fibres suitable for fortifying non-dairy drinks: gums and beta-glucans

The physical properties of a fibre ingredient determine its suitability for easy addition into beverages. Some fibre ingredients can add texture and colour as well as fibre, while others are virtually undetectable at reasonably high doses. For high quality drinks and ease of addition, low viscosity functional fibre ingredients such as inulin, fructo-oligosaccharides, polydextrose, partially hydrolysed guar gum (PHGG) and resistant maltodextrins are most suitable.

The following fibre ingredients will be discussed further in this chapter:

- Acacia gum (Gum arabic)
- Cereal β-glucans
- Partially hydrolysed guar gum (PHGG)
- Inulin and fructo-oligosaccharides
- Polydextrose
- Resistant maltodextrins.

18.3.1 Acacia gum (Gum arabic)

Acacia gum or gum arabic is the natural resin released by various species of acacia tree. Acacia gum is a very complex, highly branched polysaccharide containing a mix of salts, protein and sugars (mainly galactose) (Anderson *et al.* 1990). It is this complexity that enables its use as a dietary fibre in beverages and is responsible for its stability in acid conditions. Acacia gum also has emulsification properties which enable its use as an emulsifier in the production of flavour oils for application in soft drinks. The fibre content of acacia gum is between 80% and 90% w/w (dependent on local legislation).

Solubility

Acacia gum is soluble in cold water (up to 43–48% v/v) but it is not soluble in ethanol. Acacia gum dissolves easily in cold water at low doses but requires higher shear at higher doses to enable complete dissolution. Solutions made with acacia gum do not require any pre-mixing with sucrose or other powder ingredients to facilitate hydration; however, when making a high dose solution (40%) or when using a granulated product, hydration for some hours may be necessary. Solutions made with standard acacia gum are not completely transparent, although recent advances have meant that clear versions of acacia gum are now available.

Viscosity

Acacia gum has a very low viscosity at high concentrations. At 40% w/w, with an average viscosity of 1000 mPa.s, solutions containing acacia gum show Newtonian behaviour (Williams and Phillips 2000). At low concentrations, acacia gum provides mouthfeel but has a very low viscosity that is difficult to measure (30% of acacia gum has lower viscosity than 1% of CMC at low shear rates) (Phillips and Williams 2000). Furthermore, a reduction in viscosity is seen at low pH due to the dissociation of carboxyl groups (Williams and Phillips 2009).

Stability
Acacia gum is stable at the low pHs that are required for non-dairy beverages, with no flocculation or colour formation over time (Williams and Phillips 2009).

Sensory properties
The flavour of acacia gum is minimal and considered to be bland at typical fibre claim usage levels (range of 1.5–6 g dependent on geographical location and legislation). Gum acacia has mouthfeel effects without masking the flavour release of drinks. Drinks containing acacia gum at fibre usage levels also have a good flavour release. As the sensory effects are minimal, acacia gum is suitable for fibre fortification in a variety of beverage products.

Tolerance
The acceptable toleration level for acacia gum is 50 g/day. The effects of increasing doses were monitored for frequency and severity of GI symptoms (Cherbut *et al.* 2003). Signs of flatulence began at doses higher than 50 g/day (Cherbut *et al.* 2003). The highly branched structure of acacia gum results in slow fermentation rates and good toleration. Acacia gum is fermented in the large intestine by the colonic microflora (Phillips 1998), providing energy for the colonocytes. Although acacia gum is highly fermentable by colonic bacteria, fermentation occurs slowly and progressively along the length of the colon. This is significant because the speed of fermentation is considered to be a factor in the ability to tolerate ingredients. Slow progressive fermentation rates are associated with low incidence of GI symptoms, as gas production occurs more slowly (Cherbut *et al.* 2003). Fast fermentation rates are associated with rapid gas production and, therefore, have greater potential to produce GI symptoms.

18.3.2 Cereal β-glucans

β-Glucans, although present in many cereals, such as wheat, rye, barley and oats, are usually only commercially available from oat or barley. This is due to the fact that oats and barley contain significant amounts of β-glucan. There are extracts of both oats and barley which can be used in beverage formulations today. The physical properties of β-glucans, such as solubility and rheological behaviour in solution, are controlled by the molecular structure, which in turn is responsible for the technological features and possibilities of the β-glucan ingredient.

β-Glucan is a linear polysaccharide composed of β 1-3 and β 1-4 linked glucosidyl subunits. β 1-3 links occur singly, linking together β 1-4 linked oligosaccharidyl subunits. Structurally related mixed linkage β-D-glucans differ in the ratio of tri- and tetrasaccharidyl residues: for β-glucan of oats this is 2.1–2.4, for barley 2.8–3.3 and for wheat 3.0–3.8 (Wood *et al.* 1991). Ingredients available commercially vary greatly from each other in terms of β-glucan content, viscosity, flavour and residual materials.

Solubility
The solubility of β-glucan depends on the molecular weight fraction and concentration. High molecular weight β-glucans tend to be more difficult to dissolve in water even for concentrations below 0.5% (Morgan 2000). Furthermore, the reduced solubility of high molecular weight β-glucans has been attributed to higher ratios of cellotriosyl/cellotetraosyl units (Skendi *et al.* 2003). Low molecular weight β-glucan is more soluble and is cloudy in solution. Dispersion of low molecular weight β-glucan is best carried out under high shear and at high (85°C) temperatures to enable full hydration.

Viscosity
The aqueous solution properties of β-glucan are dependent on molecular weight, structure and concentration (Wood 2002), and appear to be complex. β-Glucans with higher molecular weight form more viscous solutions than those with a lower molecular weight at a given concentration (Doublier and Wood 1995). β-Glucan derived from either oat or barley has a high viscosity in solution due in part to the other viscous materials present within the ingredient. The reported intrinsic or limiting viscosity values for cereal β-glucans vary between 0.28 and 9.6 dl/g, depending largely on the molecular weights of the isolated polysaccharides (Lazaridou, and Biliaderis 2007).

Due to this property, the particular drink chosen to fortify has to be selected carefully to avoid negative consumer opinion. High doses of β-glucan in drinks appear to have a deleterious effect upon mouthfeel and flavour profile (Lyly *et al.* 2007).

Stability
It is reported that there is some hydrolysis of β-glucan in model beverage systems, causing a decrease in viscosity over time (Kivela *et al.* 2009). During typical pasteurisation conditions (90°C, 5 minutes) of fruit and tomato juice fortified with β-glucan, it was noticed that a reduction in viscosity occurred. This was thought to be due to acid hydrolysis (Vaikousi and Biliaderis 2005). The effects of acid hydrolysis were dependent on pH, temperature and time, and were more pronounced for high molecular weight isolate than for low molecular weight isolate, indicating that differences in the flow behaviour of liquid products containing β-glucans of different molecular size may occur under different processing and formulation protocols. Furthermore, food processing and storage can alter the solubility and, thereby, the availability of β-glucans (Beer *et al.* 1991, Brummer *et al.* 2006). Furthermore, there are reports of the molecular weight decreasing in typical beverage manufacturing processes (Aman *et al.* 2004).

High-pressure homogenisation has also been reported to strongly affect the solution properties of β-glucan extracts (Kivela *et al.* 2010). With the reduction in viscosity, the flow properties also were affected and changed from shear thinning to Newtonian. This indicated that the concentration was reached as a result of the decreased size of β-glucan molecules. In addition, the viscosity of the homogenised solutions did not increase over the shelf life and remained more stable compared with the untreated solutions. The improved stability during storage is likely to be due to the enhanced dispersibility of smaller and uniform molecules or molecule aggregates, which may slow down the reaggregation and flocculation process (Kivela *et al.* 2010).

Organoleptic properties

Due to its highly viscous nature, β-glucan from barley or oats contributes to a full-bodied mouthfeel when added at doses of 0.5–0.7% (Temelli *et al.* 2004). At a higher dose of 1%, beverages were perceived to be thicker, more grainy and slimy when compared with those without addition of β-glucan, and these attributes strongly affected the likability (Lyly *et al.* 2007). Although β-glucan has very little inherent sweetness, it has a tendency to impart cereal notes within a beverage. This is dose and supplier dependent, with higher doses giving more cereal notes, and different brands giving different flavour profiles. Lyly *et al.* (2007) reported that beverages fortified with 1% β-glucan were found to contain more rancid notes, less flavour and acid notes compared with the control (no β-glucan) sample. On the other hand, Temelli *et al.* (2004) found that orange-flavoured beverages fortified with 0.3–0.7% barley β-glucan were not perceived to be significantly different in some attributes, including fruity orange aroma and peely flavour, when compared with pectin-thickened drinks. However, other attributes, such as the perception of acid, were decreased by the addition of 0.7% β-glucan, suggesting a dose-dependent sensory effect.

18.3.3 Guar gum derivatives

Guar gum is a galactomannan extracted from the endosperm of the guar plant (*Cyamopsis tetragonoloba*). Guar gum consists of a linear chain of mannose units linked by 1-4 β-D glycosidic bonds which have (statistically) a 1.6-bound galactose unit forming a side branch on every two mannose units. Due to this chemical structure, guar gum is cold water soluble. It is used as a pure thickener, with the main functionality of providing (or contributing to) viscosity and mouthfeel. Due to the high molecular weight of guar gum, the dose applied in drinks is very low, typically 0.05% to 0.1%, which achieves a viscous, smooth, mouth-coating effect. This efficient thickening property is desirable for thickening purposes; however, the ability to provide such efficient viscosity limits its use as a dietary fibre ingredient.

PHGG is an enzymatically hydrolysed guar gum product. Controlled enzyme hydrolysis of guar gum is an effective way to produce smaller chain lengths to reduce the viscosity, improve clarity and enable use of guar at higher dose levels. Therefore it optimises the use of guar gum for use as a dietary fibre in beverages. Despite the reduction in molecular weight during enzyme hydrolysis, the PHGG molecule is found to have the same chemical structure as native guar gum (Yoon *et al.* 2008). Dose levels up to 10% w/w are possible, and this enables a fibre when using PHGG. Even though the gum has been hydrolysed, it still is permitted as fibre for use within foods and drinks. PHGG has a fibre content of approx. 80–85% w/w; however, this is very dependent on the supplier.

Solubility

The physical properties of PHGG vary depending on grade and supplier. The degree and sites of hydrolysis determine the physical properties; however, PHGG, like guar gum, is cold water soluble. The main advantage of PHGG over native guar gum is the significantly decreased viscosity and improved solubility, which enable incorporation into beverages at higher levels (Yoon *et al.* 2008). Agglomerated versions of PHGG are available and allow instant use, such as in powdered drinks.

Viscosity

The viscosity of 5% PHGG is reported to be approximately 10.5 m.Pas.

Stability

The acid stability of PHGG is reported to be good and similar to standard guar products. Acid stability between pH 3 and 7 is reported to be good (Yoon *et al.* 2008). Use in powdered products is also possible as PHGG is not especially hygroscopic in nature.

Sensory properties

Native guar has beany notes that are detectable at relatively low doses in unflavoured drinks. However, PHGG is considered to be neutral tasting at low levels (5–10% w/w) (Greenberg *et al.* 1998). The degree of neutrality is rather dependent on the manufacturing process, and so differs between suppliers. Furthermore, PHGG is transparent in solution at 5% w/w. Therefore, it can be determined that PHGG is suitable for fortifying a wide range of beverages, including fruit juices, near waters and concentrates.

Tolerance

PHGG is considered to be well tolerated at relatively low doses. Consumption levels of approximately 20 g/day were well tolerated without adverse side effects when administered in humans over a period of 18 days or 4 weeks, respectively (Meier *et al.* 1993, Takahashi *et al.* 1993). PHGG is not digested in the small intestine by mammalian enzymes, but is readily and completely fermented in the colon by intestinal microflora (Balascio *et al.* 1981) which results in the increase of bacterial counts of beneficial *Bifidobacteria* spp. and *Lactobacillus* spp. (Okubo *et al.* 1994).

18.4 Types of fibres suitable for fortifying non-dairy drinks: fructans and glucose products

18.4.1 Fructo-oligosaccharides and inulin

Inulin and fructo-oligosaccharides (FOS) will be discussed together as they are related products based on fructose, collectively known as 'fructans'. Inulin is a linear molecule consisting of approx. 3–60 fructose units linked by β (2-1) bonds (Meyer 2009). FOS has 3–7 units of fructose and is either produced from controlled hydrolysis of inulin or synthesised from sucrose by the transfructosylating action of fungal fructofuranosidase (Tungland 2003). Inulin is found naturally in many fruits and vegetables such as bananas, artichokes and chicory. There are numerous commercial variants of inulin and FOS from a range of suppliers, differing with respect to chemical composition, sugar content, form and average degree of polymerisation (DP).

Solubility

There are many different inulin and FOS products available with different DP profiles that are suitable for different applications. Products with higher DP values tend to have lower solubility in water than those with lower DP. Higher DP inulin is more suited to beverages requiring weak gel structures, such as milk-based drinks and yogurt drinks. If they are used in water-based drinks there is a tendency for precipitation to form over time, especially when stored at low temperatures (5°C). Shorter chain inulin (approx. 10 DP) is suitable for aqueous beverages such as near water drinks. Some grades impart a mild yellow colour which at low fibre doses is almost imperceptible; however, transparent grades are also available. All FOS products are suitable for beverages due to the lower DP content, which results in a higher solubility. The dispersibility of powdered inulin and FOS is good and can be likened to the addition of crystalline sugar with respect to the ease of dissolution and the time taken for complete dissolution in aqueous solutions. Liquid products pose no dissolution problems. FOS is very soluble up to 80% w/w and is also available in liquid format (Meyer 2009). It, too, can have a very slight yellow colour in solution but is also available in transparent versions, so it can be used in a wide range of beverages.

Viscosity

The addition of inulin or fructo-oligosaccharides into a non-dairy beverage system does not provide a large increase in viscosity. According to Meyer (2009), a 20% solution of inulin has a viscosity of approximately 4.5 mPa.s at 20°C.

Stability

Inulin and FOS are relatively heat and process stable under normal beverage processing conditions. However, loss during processing can occur if high temperatures, combined with low pH and/or long processing times, are employed (Klewicki 2007). At low pH values associated with soft drinks (3.0–4.0), inulin and FOS products have a tendency to be susceptible to acid hydrolysis and may break down to fructose during shelf life (Klewicki 2007). At higher pH levels there is little breakdown to fructose. Meyer (2009) states that above pH 4.0 there is little breakdown of inulin. The degree of hydrolysis will depend on pasteurisation time and temperature. However, despite this it is still possible to formulate using inulin and FOS in soft drinks. Care must be taken to select the appropriate heating regime, product type, pH and shelf life to maximise the efficiency of inulin and FOS within the drink. There are no issues with adding inulin and FOS into drinks with pH above 4.0, and as such these are a popular choice for dairy-based drinks. Inulin and FOS can be added to acidic drinks such as premium refrigerated juices, despite the high acidity, as they have a relatively short shelf life. Furthermore, flavoured waters are also a good vehicle for these products. Inulin and FOS exhibit moderate to low hygroscopicity, and are therefore suitable for powdered drinks using both bulk containers and individual sachets.

Sensory properties

Inulin is slightly sweet and has a bland taste without any noticeable aftertaste. It can be added into beverages at relatively high levels, with limited changes in product attributes. Slight mouthfeel or body can be felt at 3–6% and it can be used to replace the mouthfeel and/or body lost with the reduction of sugars (Weidman and Jager 1997). However, it would be necessary to combine inulin with a bulk or high-potency sweetener to add sufficient sweetness to a beverage system. The sweetness value assigned to FOS depends on the commercial product in use. Sweetness can vary between 0.3 and 0.65 (dependent on grade), as a function of the sugars present (Weidman *et al.* 1997). When used in combination with high-potency sweeteners, it can modify the flavour profile to become more 'sucrose-like' and enhances fruit flavours similarly to fructose. Furthermore, FOS has been shown to mask the aftertaste of aspartame and acesulfame K, as well as providing a well-rounded flavour profile (Weidman and Jager 1997). Both inulin and FOS are suitable for use in a wide range of drinks, and are a popular choice for fibre fortification.

Tolerance

The process of digestion of inulin and FOS has been very well studied. They are well tolerated at doses around 20 g/day with only minor digestive complaints. This is supported by other studies conducted by Van Dokkum *et al.* (1999) and Ellegaard *et al.* (1997), which found that doses of 15–17g /day were well tolerated, whereas Bonnema *et al.* (2010) found that up to 10 g/day of native inulin and 5 g/day of FOS are well tolerated in healthy individuals, with higher doses substantially increasing GI symptoms. It has been established that doses higher than 20 g/day may result in GI symptoms such as flatulence, cramps and even diarrhoea, although these symptoms are transient and tend to reduce with a period of adjustment (Grabitske and Slavin 2009). Both inulin and FOS are completely fermented within the colon and in particular within the proximal colon shortly after entering. Furthermore, inulin and FOS have both been shown to stimulate *Bifidobacteria* spp., and so conform to the definition of a prebiotic (Bouhnik *et al.* 2007). Stimulation of bifidobacteria has been shown at doses of between 2.5 and 15 g/day (Wang and Gibson 1993, Van Dokkum *et al.* 1999, Bouhnik *et al.* 2007).

18.4.2 Polydextrose

Polydextrose is a low molecular weight polymer of glucose. Polydextrose is manufactured by bulk melt polycondensation of glucose and sorbitol in conjunction with small amounts of acid. It is a randomly bonded polysaccharide (of glucose) with all possible glycosidic linkages present. However, α and β 1,6 bonds predominate, resulting in a highly stable ingredient. It has an average DP of 12 and an average molecular weight of 2000 (with a range between 162 and approx. 20 000). Polydextrose was originally developed as a low calorie bulking agent, with the purpose of aiding the replacement of sugar in a variety of foods, but due to its indigestibility in the small intestine and incomplete fermentation in the large intestine it has also been recognised as a source of dietary fibre where the definition or legislation is based on physical effects or chemical composition (for example, in the EU). Polydextrose is, therefore, gaining popularity as a dietary fibre ingredient in a wide range of applications in many countries worldwide. Studies have shown that polydextrose has many of the features of dietary fibre, such as regularisation of bowel function, normalisation of blood lipid concentrations, and blood glucose attenuation (Jie *et al.* 2000, Vasankari and Ahotupa 2005, Foster-Powell *et al.* 2002, respectively). Studies have demonstrated increased faecal bulking and softening, decreased colonic pH and positive results on the colonic microflora (Jie *et al.*, 2000). Polydextrose has a calorie content of 1 kcal/g (4 kJ/g).

Solubility

Polydextrose is an amorphous ingredient and is highly soluble. Clear solutions of more than 80% w/w can be produced at 25°C in water (Allingham 1982). Polydextrose has good dispersibility and dissolution properties. Pre-blending with other ingredients (such as sugars) can improve dispersibility in poor mixing conditions, as in powdered drinks. As with many ingredients, good mechanical mixing is required to prepare concentrated solutions. Granulated polydextrose offers high dispersibility with minimum dusting.

Viscosity

Polydextrose solutions behave as a Newtonian fluid. A 70% solution of polydextrose at 25°C measures approximately 1800 cps (Auerbach *et al.* 2006). At this level (70% w/w), polydextrose solution has a higher viscosity than sucrose solution or high fructose corn syrup (HFCS) at similar concentrations. Despite the high viscosity elicited at 70% w/w, at typical beverage usage levels (1–5% RTD) polydextrose does not provide significant viscosity. However, it does contribute to the mouthfeel of the drink. This enables polydextrose to be used effectively to help retain mouthfeel in reduced-sugar, low-sugar and sugar-free beverages.

Stability

Polydextrose is very stable in solution as it is a complex branched molecule and contains a wide range of glycosidic bonds which are resistant to acid hydrolysis. Polydextrose contains predominantly 1-6 glycosidic bonds, which are two to four times more resistant to acid hydrolysis than 1-2, 1-3 or 1-4 bonds. Furthermore, the highly branched, complex, three-dimensional shape contributes to its acid stability and resistance to fermentation. Studies of model beverage systems containing polydextrose have shown resistance to hydrolysis over a broad range of pH and temperatures (Beer *et al.* 1991). Polydextrose has been shown to be stable throughout typical beverage process and storage conditions at pH 3 and 7 (Beer *et al.* 1991). Polydextrose is hygroscopic in nature and so care must be taken when using in powdered drinks. Use of flow agents and moisture absorbers limits caking; however, good packaging is necessary to prolong shelf life. Individual sachets are a good option when using polydextrose in powdered products. Furthermore, spray drying technology can enhance the shelf life of powdered products using polydextrose.

Sensory properties

Polydextrose has very little sweetness, with a relative sweetness of 0.15 compared with sucrose at 1. Polydextrose is very neutral in flavour and can be described as having little flavour of its own; however, in its most basic forms it can be described as mildly acidic. As described above, polydextrose can be used to provide the bulk and mouthfeel often lost with the removal of sugars as well as for fibre fortification. Furthermore, polydextrose can improve the flavour of beverages containing high-potency sweeteners by reducing bitter, acidic and metallic flavour notes and providing a more rounded sugar flavour. However, it may be necessary to combine polydextrose with a bulk or high-potency sweetener to achieve the desired sweetness in a beverage system. There are different grades to choose from which are suitable for different beverage applications.

As discussed above, polydextrose is an extremely flexible ingredient that can be used in a variety of beverages, including carbonated and non-carbonated, concentrated and RTD, and hot or cold beverages. Examples include juices, fruit and/or vegetable juice drinks, smoothies, meal replacements, milk, dairy and soy-based drinks, sport and energy drinks, tea and coffee, and near waters.

Tolerance

Extensive clinical studies have been carried out on polydextrose to evaluate GI toleration. These studies concluded that polydextrose is extremely well tolerated due to its high molecular weight, low osmotic potential and slow progressive fermentation rate. Flood *et al.* (2004) demonstrated that the mean laxative threshold for polydextrose is 90 g/day, or 50 g in a single dose. The fermentation profile of polydextrose has shown that fermentation takes place along the entire length of the colon, resulting in beneficial effects for the entire colon. Slow progressive fermentation rates are associated with reduced risk of GI effects such as bloating, wind and abdominal pain. Furthermore, studies have shown that polydextrose also exhibits prebiotic properties. Enhanced bifidobacteria and lactobacillus counts were demonstrated with the consumption of polydextrose at doses as low as 4 or 5 g/day (Jie *et al.* 2000, Tiihonen *et al.* 2008).

18.4.3 Resistant maltodextrins

Resistant starches (RS) are the starch fractions not digested in the small intestine in healthy individuals, due to inaccessibility of starch to digestive enzymes. They can be classified into four types – RS I, RS II, RS III and RS IV – and are classified in this way on the basis of their resistance to digestion. It has to be noted that, while most grades of RS are not readily soluble in water, solutions of RS IVs can easily be prepared. This section will therefore limit itself to discussing RS IV; that is, chemically modified cross-linked starch, otherwise known as 'resistant maltodextrins'. RS IVs have resistant linkages (α1-4, and α1-6) and are similar in functional properties to polydextrose and oligosaccharides (Kim *et al.* 2008).

Solubility

Resistant maltodextrins are readily soluble in water and are suitable for many types of beverages, including RTD, dry mixes and spray-dried powders.

Viscosity

The viscosity of resistant maltodextrins is low and similar to other functional fibre sources. Addition for mouthfeel and/or body is possible, and, similarly to other fibres discussed in previous sections, they can replace the mouthfeel and body of sugars.

Stability

Resistant maltodextrins as a group are resistant to high processing temperatures. High temperature processes such as sterilisation, retort and pasteurisation can be performed with minimal degradation. Resistant maltodextrins are stable to acidic conditions and do not show signs of hydrolysis (retrogradation) or haze over long storage times.

Organoleptic properties

Resistant maltodextrins have very low sweetness levels and can be considered essentially non-sweet. However, it has been reported that they have some flavour and mouthfeel modification properties.

Tolerance

Resistant maltodextrins are generally well tolerated. Studies have shown resistant maltodextrins to be well tolerated between 25 g and 45 g/day due to their high molecular weight and slow and progressive digestion (Van den Heuvel *et al.* 2004). The amount of RS that is absorbed in the small intestine and subsequently fermented depends on the chemical structure, as does the fermentation profile.

Some ingredients have fermentation up to 75% (Van den Heuvel *et al.* 2004) and others have approx. 50% fermentation (Ohkuma and Wakabayashi 2001). Studies also indicate that resistant maltodextrins have prebiotic effects with increased lactobacilli and bifidobacteria that are dose-dependent (Lefranc-Millot *et al.* 2006, Ohkuma and Wakabayashi 2001).

18.5 Typical beverage formulations containing fibre

As discussed in the sections above, adding fibre into non-dairy beverages can be very straightforward when using suitable fibres with high solubility and dispersibility. Formulations made with the suggested fibre sources are easy to incorporate within already existing processes. Some of these fibres are supplied in solutions/syrups that can be pumped and therefore easily incorporated. Some, however, require dissolution to enable usage. Table 18.1 contains a typical formulation for a juice drink containing 10% juice content. The exact level of fibre addition will depend on the type of fibre being added and the fibre content of the ingredient used, as well as the target. Table 18.2 contains a suggestion for a flavoured water formulation. The level of fibre added is lower than for juices, due to the bottle size being larger than for juices, typically 330 ml to 500 ml. The content of fibre in the example formulation is 6 g per 330 ml bottle and 9.2 g for a 500 ml bottle (for ingredients containing 80% of fibre). For ingredients containing more than 80% fibre, a reduction in dose will be needed to achieve the same target levels. Table 18.3 gives an example of a powdered drink formulation. The addition

Table 18.1 Example of a juice drink (15% juice) containing fibre

Ingredients	Percentage
Sucrose	8.0
Juice concentrate, tropical (55 brix)	2.1
Citric acid powder (anhydrous)	0.15
Fibre source (85% fibre)	3.75
Grindsted® JU 501 (Danisco)	0.1
Potassium sorbate	0.03
Colour	q.s.
Flavour	q.s.
Water	85.87

Process
Dissolve preservatives in the water.
Blend the sugar and stabiliser and add to hot water (approx. 85°C) under high shear mixing.
Once hydrated, dissolve the fibre source.
Add fruit concentrate using high shear mixer.
Add citric acid, colour and flavour.
Heat treatment: pasteurise at 90°C / 30 s.
Fill into bottles as required.

Table 18.2 Example of water with fibre

Ingredients	Percentage
Litesse® Ultra (Danisco)	2.3
Water	97.7

Process
Add Litesse® Ultra™ under good mixing conditions.
Pasteurise 105°C, 10 seconds.
Aseptic fill.

Table 18.3 Powdered mix containing fibre

Ingredients	Percentage
Sucrose (instant)	63.77
Fibre source	35.17
Citric acid	1.00
Tri-sodium citrate	0.06
Colour	q.s.
Flavour (strawberry)	q.s.

Process
Dry blend all ingredients.
Package into 20 g portions.
To reconstitute add 20 g mix into 200 ml water.

level of fibre per kg within the mix is considerably higher, as the desired parameter is dose per serving size or 100 ml in a RTD format.

18.6 Troubleshooting

Adding fibre into non-dairy beverages can be very straightforward when using suitable fibres with high solubility and dispersibility, and there should be only limited ingredient interactions as these fibres are all relatively stable and non-reactive. However, typical issues for all drinks are often a problem for fibre-enriched drinks as well. Common issues can include foaming on mixing, fobbing when carbonating, sedimentation/flocculation and colouration over time. Reducing the occurrence of these issues is largely solved by selecting the appropriate fibre source for the chosen drink, potentially through a process of trial and error.

18.7 Future trends

Recent trends have seen a move towards more natural formulations and products with as clean a label as possible over the food industry as a whole, and also within the non-dairy beverage category. Coupled with rising health problems associated with overconsumption and inadequate consumption of particular nutrients, it could be expected that there will be an increase in healthier, better-for-you drinks utilising natural sources of dietary fibres. These sources of dietary fibre should be able to perform well from a technical perspective as well as from a health benefits perspective. Furthermore, there are possibilities that these functional ingredients could even be developed *in situ* inside the drink, without the need for ingredient addition.

18.8 References

ALLINGHAM R (1982), Polydextrose – a new food ingredient: Technical Aspects, in *Chemistry of Foods and Beverages: Recent Developments,* edited by CHARALAMBOUS G and INGLETT G, Academic Press.

AMAN P, RIMSTEN L and ANDERSSON P (2004), Molecular weight distribution of β-glucan in oat-based foods, *Cereal Chemistry*, **81**, 356–60.

ANDERSON D M W, BROWN DOUGLAS D M, MORRISON N A and WEIPING W (1990), Specifications for gum arabic (*Acacia senegal*): analytical data for samples collected between 1904 and 1989, *Food Additives and Contaminants*, **7**, 303–21.

ANGELOV A, GOTCHEVA V, KUNCHEVA R and HRISTOZOVA T (2006), Development of an oat based probiotic drink, *International Journal of Food Microbiology*, **112**, 75–80.

AUERBACH M, CRAIG S and MITCHELL H (2006), Bulking agents: Multifunctional ingredients, in MITCHELL H, *Sweeteners and Sugar Alternatives in Food Technology*, Oxford, Blackwell Publishing, 367–97.

BALASCIO JR, PALLMER JK and SALYERS AA (1981), Degradation of guar gum enzymes produced by a bacterium from the human colon, *Journal of Biochemistry*, **5**, 271–82.

BEER M, ARRIGONI E, UHLMANN D, WECSHLER D and AMADO R (1991), Stability of polydextrose solutions to heat treatment and storage under acid conditions, **24**, 245–51.

BLANDINO A, AL-ASEERI M E, PANDIELLA S S, CANTERO D and WEBB C (2003), Cereal-based fermented foods and beverages, *Food Research International*, **36**, 527–43.

BONNEMA A L, KOLBERG LW, THOMAS W and SLAVIN JL (2010), Gastrointestinal Tolerance of Chicory Inulin Products, *Journal of American Dietetic Association*, **110**, 865–8.

BOUHNIK Y, FLOURIE B, D'AGAY-ABENSOUR L, POCHART P, GRAMET G, *et al.* (1997). Administration of transgalacto-oligosaccharides increases fecal Bifidobacteria and modifies fermentation metabolism in healthy humans. *Journal of Nutrition*, **127**, 444–8.

BOUHNIK Y, RASKINE L, CHAMPION K, ANDRIEUX C, PENVEN S, *et al.* (2007), Prolonged administration of low-dose inulin stimulates the growth of bifidobacteria in humans. *Nutrition Research*, **27**, 187–93.

BRIET F, ACHOUR L, FLOURIE B, BEAUGERIE L, PELLIER P and FRANCHISSEUR C (1995), Symptomatic response to varying levels of fructo-oligosaccharides consumed occasionally or regularly. *European Journal of Clinical Nutrition*, **49**, 501–7.

BRUMMER Y, WOOD P, TOSH S, LAN-PIDHAINY X and WOLEVER T (2006), Modification of molecular weight and solubility of beta glucan in oat bran muffins, and effect on the glycemic response. In *Book of Abstracts of AACC Meeting: World Grains Summit: Foods and Beverages*, San Francisco, USA, September, Abstract O-38, p. 84.

CHERBUT C, MICHEL C, RAISON V, KRAVTCHENKO T and MEANCE S (2003), Acacia gum is a bifidogenic dietary fiber with high digestive tolerance in healthy humans. *Microbial Ecology in Health and Disease*, **15**, 43–50.

DOUBLIER JL and WOOD PJ (1995), Rheological Properties of Aqueous Solutions of (1-3), (1-4)-β-D Glucan from Oats (*Avena sativa* L.), *Cereal Chemistry*, **72**(4), 335–40.

ELLEGARD L, ANDERSON H and BOSAEUS I (1997), Inulin and oligofructose do not influence the absorption of cholesterol, or the excretion of cholesterol, Ca, Mg, Zn, Fe or bile acids but increases energy excretion in ileostomy subjects. *European Journal of Clinical Nutrition*, **51** (1), 1–5.

EC (2006), REGULATION (EC) No 1924/2006 OF THE EUROPEAN PARLIAMENT AND OF THE COUNCIL of 20 December 2006 on nutrition and health claims made on foods.

FIGOR SK and BIANCHINE JR (1983), Calorie utilisation and disposition of [14C] polydextrose in man. *Journal of Agriculture and Food Chemistry*, **31**(2), 389–93.

FLOOD MT, AUERBACH MH and CRAIG SAS (2004), A review of the clinical toleration studies of polydextrose in food. *Food and Chemical Toxicology*, **42**, 1531–42.

FOOD STANDARDS AGENCY, National Diet and Nutrition Survey (2008/09), edited by BATES B, LENNOX A and SWAN G. *http://www.food.gov.uk/multimedia/pdfs/publication/ndnsreport0809.pdf*

FOSTER-POWELL K, HOLT SHA and BRAND-MILLER JC (2002), International table of glycemic index and glycemic load values. *American Journal of Clinical Nutrition*, **76** (1), 5–56.

FREMONT G (2007), Acacia gum, the natural multifunctional fibre. In SALOVAARA H, GATES F and TENKANEN M, *Dietary Fibre – components and functions*, The Netherlands, Wageningen Academic Publishers.

GRABITSKE HA and SLAVIN JL (2008), Low-digestible carbohydrates in practice. *Journal of the American Dietetic Association*, **108**, 1677–81.

GRABITSKE HA and SLAVIN JL (2009), Gastrointestinal effects of low-digestible carbohydrates. *Critical Reviews in Food Science Nutrition*, **49**, 327–60.

GREENBERG NA and SELLMAN D (1998), Partially hydrolyzed guar gum as a source of fiber. *Cereal Foods World*, **43**, 703.

GUILLON F and CHAMP M (2000), Structural and physical properties of dietary fibres, and consequences of processing on human physiology. *Food Research International*, **33**, 233–45.

GUPTA S, COX S and ABU-GHANNAM N (2010), Process optimization for the development of a functional beverage based on lactic acid fermentation of oats. *Biochemical Engineering Journal*, **52**, 199–204.

JIE Z, LUO B, XIANG M, LIU H, SHAI Z, *et al.* (2000), Studies on the effects of polydextrose on physiological function in Chinese people. *American Journal of Clinical Nutrition*, **72**, 1503–9.

JONES JM (2007), Dietary fibre or wholegrains or both? In SALOVAARA H, GATES F and TENKANEN M, *Dietary Fibre components and functions*, The Netherlands, Wageningen Academic Publishers, 13–30.

JUNEJA LR, SAKANAKA S and CHU DC (2001), Physiological and technological functions of partially hydrolysed guar gum (modified galactomannan), in MCCLEARY B V and PROSKY L, *Advanced Dietary Fibre Technology*, Oxford, Blackwell Science, 345–60.

KENDALL CWC, ESFAHANI A and JENKINS DJA (2010), The link between dietary fibre and human health. *Food Hydrocolloids*, **24**, 42–8.

KIM MJ, CHOI SJ, SHIN SI, SOHN MR, LEE CJ, *et al.* (2008), Resistant glutarate starch from adlay: Preparation and properties. *Carbohydrate Polymers*, **74**, 787–96.

KIVELÄ R, HYSTROM L, SALOVAARA H and SONTAG STROHM T (2009), Role of oxidative cleavage and acid hydrolysis of oat beta glucan in modelled beverage conditions. *Journal of Cereal Science*, **50**(2), 190–7.

KIVELÄ R, PITKÄNEN L, LAINE P, ASEYEV V and SONTAG-STROHM T (2010), Influence of homogenisation on the solution properties of oat β-glucan, *Food Hydrocolloids*, **24**, 611–18.

KLEWICKI R (2007), The stability of gal-polyols and oligosaccharides during pasteurisation at a low pH, *LWT*, **40**, 1259–65.

KRITCHEVSKY D (2001), in MCCLEARY B V and PROSKY L, *Advanced Dietary Fibre Technology*, Oxford, Blackwell Science, 149–61.

LAZARIDOU A and BILIADERIS CG (2007), Molecular aspects of cereal β-glucan functionality: Physical properties, technological applications and physiological effects. *Journal of Cereal Science*, **46**, 101–18.

LEFRANC-MILLOT C, WILS D and ROUTRIER D (2006), Effects of a soluble fibre with excellent tolerance, Nutriose 06, on the gut ecosystem: a review. *Proceedings of the Dietary Fibre Conference, 'Multifunctional Complex of Components'*, Helsinki, Finland, P34.

LYLY M, ROININEN K, HONKAPÄÄ K, POUTANEN K and LÄHTEENMÄKI L (2007), Factors influencing consumers' willingness to use beverages and ready to eat frozen soups containing oat B-glucan in Finland, France and Sweden. *Food Quality and Preference*, **18**, 242–55.

MARTEAU P and FLOURIE B (2001), Tolerance to low digestible carbohydrates: symptomatology and methods. *British Journal of Nutrition*, **85** Supplement 1, S17–21.

MITCHELL H, AUERBACH MH and MOPPETT FK (2001), Polydextrose, in NABORS E D and O'BRIEN L, *Alternative Sweeteners*, New York, Marcel Dekker Inc.

MEIER R, BEGLINGER C, SCHNEIDER H, ROWEDDER A and GYR K (1993), Effect of liquid diet with and without soluble fiber supplementation on intestinal transit and cholecystokinin release in volunteers. *Journal of Parenteral and Enteral Nutrition*, **17**, 231–5.

MEYER D (2009), Inulin, in PHILLIPS GO and WILLIAMS PA, *Handbook of Hydrocolloids*, 2nd edition, Cambridge, Woodhead, 829–48.

MORGAN K (2000), Cereal β-glucans, in PHILLIPS GO and WILLIAMS PA, *Handbook of Hydrocolloids*, Cambridge, Woodhead, 287–307.

OHKUMA K and WAKABAYASHI S (2001), Fibersol-2: a soluble, non-digestible, starch derived dietary fibre, in MCCLEARY BV and PROSKY L, *Advanced Dietary Fibre Technology*, Oxford, Blackwell Science, 509–22.

OKUBO T, ISHIHARA N, TAKAHASHI H, FUIJISAWA T, KIM M, *et al.* (1994), Effects of partially hydrolysed guar gum intake on human intestinal microflora and its metabolism. *Bioscience, Biotechnology and Biochemistry*, **58**, 1364–9.

PHILLIPS GO (1998), Acacia gum (gum Arabic): a nutritional fibre; metabolism and calorific value. *Food Additives and Contaminants*, **15**, 251–64.

PHILLIPS GO and WILLIAMS PA (2000), Gum Arabic, in PHILLIPS GO and WILLIAMS PA, *Handbook of Hydrocolloids*, Woodhead Publishing Ltd, Cambridge, 164, 167.

PHILLIPS GO, OGASAWARA T and USHIDA K (2008), The regulatory and scientific approach to defining gum arabic as a dietary fibre. *Food Hydrocolloids*, **22**, 24–35.

ROBERFROID M and SLAVIN J (2000), Non-digestible oligosaccharides. *Critical Reviews in Food Science and Nutrition*, **40**, 461–80.

SENSUS OPERATIONS CV, The Netherlands (2000), Frutafit® Inulin, in WILLIAMS PA and PHILLIPS GO, *Handbook of Hydrocolloids*, Cambridge, CRC Press/Woodhead, 397–403.

SKENDI A, BILIADERIS CG, LAZARIDOU A and IZYDORCZYK MS (2003), Structure and rheological properties of water soluble β-glucans from oat cultivars of *Avena sativa* and *Avena bysantina*. *Journal of Cereal Science*, **38**, 15–31.

TAKAHASHI H, YANG SI, HAYASHI C, KIM M and YAMAMOTO T (1993), Effect of partially hydrolysed guar gum on faecal output in human volunteers, *Nutrition Research*, **13**, 649–57.

TEMELLI F, BANSEMA C and STOBBE K (2004), Development of an orange-flavored barley β-glucan beverage. *Cereal Chemistry*, **81**, 499–503.

TIIHONEN K, SUOMALAINEN T, TYNKKYNEN S and RAUTONEN N (2008), Effect of prebiotic supplementation on a probiotic bacteria mixture: a comparison between a rat model and clinical trials, *British Journal of Nutrition*, **99** (4), 826–31.

TOMLIN J, READ NW, EDWARDS CA and DUERDEN BI (1986), The degradation of guar gum by faecal incubation system, *British Journal of Nutrition*, **55**, 481–6.

TOMLIN J, TAYLOR JS and READ NW (1989), The effects of mixed faecal bacteria on a selection of viscous polysaccharides *in vitro*. *Nutrition Research International*, **39**, 121–35.

TUNGLAND BC (2003), Fructooligosaccharides and other Fructans: Structures and Occurrence, Production, Regulatory Aspects, Food Applications and Nutritional Health

Significance, in *Oligosaccharides in Food and Agriculture*, edited by EGGLESTON G. ACS Symposium Series; American Chemical Society: Washington, DC, 2003.

VAIKOUSI H and BILIADERIS CG (2005), Processing and formulation effects on rheological behavior of barley β-glucan aqueous dispersions. *Food Chemistry*, **91**, 505–16.

VAN DEN HEUVEL E, WILSD, PASMAN WJ, BAKKER M, SANIEZ MH and KARDINAAL AFM (2004), Short term digestive tolerance of different doses of NUTRIOSE FB, a food dextrin, in adult men. *European Journal of Clinical Nutrition*, **S8**, 1046–55.

VAN DOKKUM W, VAN DEN HEUVEL EGHM, HAVENAAR R, SRIKUMAR TS, VAN AKEN P and WEZENDONK B (1995), The effect of non digestible oligosaccharides (NDO) on human physiology. *Report TNO*; (Zeist): TNO.

VAN DOKKUM W, WEZENDONK B, SRIKUMAR TS and VAN DEN HEUVEL EGHM (1999), Effect of non-digestible oligosaccharides on large bowel functions, blood lipid concentrations, and glucose absorption in young healthy male subjects. *European Journal of Clinical Nutrition*, **53**, 1–7.

VASANKARI TJ and AHOTUPA M (2005), Supplementation of polydextrose reduced a hamburger meal induced postprandial hypertriglyceridemia, American Heart Association (AHA) Congress, Dallas, 16th November, 2005. *AHA Congress Proceedings*, **112** (17), II–833.

WANG X and GIBSON GR (1993), Effects of the *in vitro* fermentation of oligofructose and inulin by bacteria growing in the human large intestine. *Journal of Applied Bacteriology*, **75** (4), 373–80.

WEIDMANN M and JAGER M (1997), Synergistic sweeteners. *Food Ingredients International*, November–December, 51–6.

WILLIAMS PA and PHILLIPS GO (2000), Gum Arabic, in WILLIAMS PA and PHILLIPS GO, *Handbook of Hydrocolloids*, Cambridge, CRC Press/Woodhead, 155–68.

WILLIAMS PA and PHILLIPS GO (2009), Gum Arabic, in WILLIAMS PA and PHILLIPS GO, *Handbook of Hydrocolloids* 2nd Edition, Cambridge, CRC Press/Woodhead, 252–73.

WOOD P (2002), Relationships between solution properties of cereal β-glucans and physiological effects – a review. *Trends in Food Science and Technology*, **13**, 313–20.

WOOD PJ, WEISZ J and MAHN W (1991), Molecular characterisation of cereal β-glucans. II. Size-exclusion chromatography for comparison of molecular weight. *Cereal Chemistry*, **68**, 530–6.

YOON SJ, CHU D and JUNEJA L (2008), Chemical and Physical Properties, Safety and Application of Partially Hydrolysed Guar Gum as Dietary Fibre. *Journal of Clinical Biochemistry and Nutrition*, **42**, 1–7.

19

Fibre-enriched snack foods

V. Stojceska, The Manchester Metropolitan University, UK

DOI: 10.1533/9780857095787.4.389

Abstract: This chapter investigates the health benefits of whole grains in the production of ready-to-eat expanded snacks. Extrusion technology is a popular and widely used continuous food processing technique that presents a great opportunity to produce ready-to-eat snacks with improved nutritional qualities. The incorporation of whole grains into expanded products has a beneficial effect in terms of dietary fibre, proteins, phytochemicals and vitamins, but it can also affect the physicochemical characteristics of the final product. Depending on the type of grain used, the product formulation and the extrusion conditions, considerable degradation could occur in terms of sensory appeal. Extrusion technology provides several ways in which these challenges can be overcome, by controlling extrusion conditions such as temperature, solid feed rate and screw speed combinations, and these will be discussed in this chapter.

Key words: whole grains, dietary fibre, ready-to-eat snacks, extrusion technology.

19.1 Introduction

19.1.1 Health benefits of consuming ready-to-eat snacks

Production of food snacks is increasing, and a variety of products are available to consumers. Cooke (2002) reports that, because consumers are showing an increasing preference towards snacking, over the past few years the market for savoury snacks has grown at a rate of 2–3% each year, and has increased in value as well as size. In 2001, £2.4 billion worth of savoury snacks were sold in the UK, amounting to 5.8 kg per person, or 344 000 tonnes in total (Huxley, 2003). According to Cooke (2002), cited by Huxley (2003), 344 000 tonnes of savoury snacks worth £2.4 billion were sold in the UK in 2001, which is equivalent to 5.8 kg snacks per person.

As people's lives become busier there is an increasing demand for tasty nutritious meals and snacks that can be eaten 'on the go'. Furthermore, snacks can be taken as a substitute for breakfast or between two main meals; therefore, good nutritional characteristics are essential. There is evidence to suggest that eating smaller, more frequent meals can lead to better weight, blood sugar and cholesterol control (Fabry and Tepperman, 1970) and improve the memory of school-aged children (Kurpad *et al.*, 2007).

The role of whole grain in increasing dietary fibre of ready-to-eat snacks is very well known. There are several types of technology that can be used, varying from the very basic, such as deep-frying (potato chips) or baking (different types of cakes, snacks and pizza), to drying (dried fruits) or extrusion technology (breakfast cereals and ready-to eat snacks).

In people aged 4–18 years living in Great Britain, breakfast cereals are the main source of whole grain intake, followed by bread, biscuits, pasta, rice, pizza, buns, cakes and pastries (Thane *et al.*, 2005). The dietary guideline for increasing the consumption of wholemeal cereal products presents a great opportunity to avoid too much fat and sugar, as appropriate to the main-meal-based consumption prototype, since snacks differ from meals in consisting of more carbohydrates and less fat and protein (Bellisle *et al.*, 2003). Wholemeal cereal products generally contain more carbohydrates and less fat and protein compared with main meals; therefore, consumption of those products is a great opportunity to improve healthy lifestyle.

Ready-to-eat snacks produced using extrusion technology are in great demand. Extruded snacks have been criticized for their 'empty calories' (Cheftel, 1986) and high level of fat (Neuhouser *et al.*, 2000), which contribute to poor diet quality. The addition of new sources of dietary fibres could significantly improve the nutritional content of these products.

In recent years, the extruded snack food market has grown rapidly, and in the UK alone is estimated to be worth between £2.1 and £2.5 billion per annum (Mintel, 2004; Datamonitor, 2004). In terms of volume, this equates to 486 000 tonnes of snack products purchased each year. Value sales of cereal, energy and snack bars reported double-digit growth in European countries between 2005 and 2009 (Mintel, 2010).

Table 19.1 summarizes the nutritional data of some breakfast cereals and ready-to-eat snacks commercially available in the UK. Dietary fibre varied from 1.5 to 15%. According to the Food Standards Agency's guidance on fibre claims, it is recommended that a 'source' of fibre should contain at least 3 g, or 3% of the 'reasonable expected daily intake of the food'. For a high-fibre claim, the food must contain at least 6%, or 6 g, in the reasonable expected daily intake of the food (British Nutrition Foundation, 2004).

This chapter is focused on the use of extrusion in developing high-fibre enriched ready-to-eat snacks or breakfast cereals through the incorporation of whole grains.

19.2 Extrusion processing of ready-to-eat snacks

Extrusion cooking is a high temperature, short time and continuous food processing technique, which is increasingly being used for generating snack products and breakfast cereals. It is very efficient, and enables manufacturers to process starchy grain flours, including rice, wheat, barley and oats, with various

Table 19.1 Nutritional composition of some processed breakfast cereals and snacks currently available on the market

	Manufacturers									
	Sainsbury's	Jacob's bakery	Penn State	Sainsbury's	Sainsbury's	Nestlé	Honey Monster Foods	Kellogg	Kellogg	Kellogg
	Name of the products									
	Salted pretzels	Twiglets	Salted pretzels	Potato swirls	Rice pops	Shreddies	Sugar puffs	Cornflakes	Special K	Bran Flakes
Protein (%)	10.3	12.7	10.5	2.8	7.5	8.2	5.3	7	14	10
Carbohydrate (%)	76.7	57.0	74.2	64.1	85.5	78.1	85.8	84	76	67
of which sugars (%)	1.8	0.7	23	10	0.6	30.2	35	8	17	22
Starch (%)	74.9			63.1						
Fat (%)	4.2	11.6	41	22.5	1.3	1.5	1.6	0.9	1.5	2
Fibre (%)	3.6	11.8	4.4	1.7	1.5	8.1	4.0	3	0.5	15
Salt (%)	1.50		3.0	3.13	0.74		Trace	1.3	1.15	1
Sodium (%)		0.7	1.2			0.2		0.5	0.45	0.4

combinations of ingredients. Residence time, temperature, pressure and shear rate are key parameters in extrusion cooking.

A number of physical and chemical changes occur during extrusion processing, including starch dextrinization, gelatinization, protein denaturation, complex formation and degradation of pigments, and these alterations affect the physical and functional properties of the end product (Ilo and Berghofer, 1999). For example, process conditions such as moisture content, feed rate and screw speed could greatly improve the quality of extruded snacks made from corn grits (Mazumder *et al.*, 2007).

Different raw ingredients, such as wheat, rice and corn, produce extruded snacks with different physiochemical characteristics due to variation in their composition, including proteins and starch levels. The extrusion behaviour of wheat starch, wholewheat meal and oat flour using a twin-screw extruder was observed by Singh and Smith (1997). The results revealed that wheat starch and wholewheat meal behaved differently from oats in terms of pressure, expansion, water solubility index (WSI), water absorption index (WAI), moisture content and material temperature. Selecting and combining appropriate ingredients are important factors in formulating acceptable extruded snack products.

Chávez-Jàuregi *et al.* (2000) studied the optimum process conditions for extruded amaranth grain. The most expanded products with acceptable textural properties were obtained at 150°C and 15% moisture, which also resulted in greater shearing force, greater extrudate surface, and reduced shearing stress at maximum shearing force. The consumption of extruded amaranth has been found to reduce total cholesterol levels in rabbits by 50% (Plate and Arêas, 2002).

However, the quality of the final product could vary considerably, depending on a number of factors. In particular, the formulation and process conditions, including extruder type, screw configuration, feed moisture, temperature profile in the barrel, screw speed, feed rate and die profile, can significantly affect product quality (Desrumaux *et al.*, 1999).

19.3 Nutritional benefits of extruded whole grains

The most important factors in developing high nutritional quality extruded snacks with good sensorial attributes are the proper selection of ingredients and optimization of extrusion parameters. Cereal grains offer a cheap source of binding agents and a great source of energy. Commonly consumed whole grains can be found in wheat, corn, oats, rice, rye and barley, and contain bran, germ and endosperm. Less fashionable whole grains include gluten-free cereals made from amaranth, buckwheat, millet, quinoa, sorghum and teff. They are low in saturated fat and cholesterol, rich in dietary fibre and proteins, and are a great source of energy (Table 19.2).

19.3.1 Formation of dietary fibre

The effect of extrusion cooking on the nutritional properties of snack foods has been studied by a number of authors (Englyst *et al.*, 1989; Lasekan *et al.*, 1996; Faraj

Table 19.2 Nutrient (g/100 g) and caloric (kcal/100 g) content of some grains

Content	Quinoa	Whole Wheat	Rye (whole grain)	Barley (whole grain)	Brown Rice	Corn (whole grain)
Caloric value	350.00	309.00	269.00	299.00	353.00	338.00
Protein	13.81	11.50	8.70	10.60	7.4	9.2
Fat	5.01	2.00	1.70	2.10	2.2	3.8
Carbohydrates	59.74	59.40	53.50	57.70	74.6	65.2
Water	12.65	13.20	13.70	11.70	13.1	12.5
Fibre	5.20	10.60	13.15	9.80	4.0	9.2

Source: adapted from Jacobsen and Sherwood (2002).

et al, 2004; Hagenimana *et al.*, 2006). Extrusion cooking increases total dietary fibre levels (TDF), soluble (SDF) and insoluble (IDF) (Table 19.3), probably as a result of the formation of resistant starch (Table 19.3), which is considered to be a form of functional fibre. Functional fibre has both physiological and health benefits in

Table 19.3 Resistant starch (RS3) content of native and selected extruded barley flours. [a]Barley flour produced by pin-milling of pearled (30–32%) grains. [b]Temperature (°C) moisture (%) used to produce extruded barley flour

Flour sample		RS3 (%, w/w)
CDC-Candle		
Native[a]		0
Extruded	90/20[b]	0
	100/20	0
	120/20	0
	140/20	0
	90/50	0
	100/50	0
	120/50	0
	140/50	0.58±0.20
Least Significant difference (LSD) (P<0.05)		–
Phoenix		
Native		0.83±0.15
Extruded	90/20	1.02±0.20
	100/20	1.08±0.15
	120/20	1.43±0.10
	140/20	1.10±0.21
	90/50	1.62±0.38
	100/50	1.75±0.25
	120/50	2.87±0.41
	140/50	1.94±0.33
LSD (P<0.05)		0.28

Source: adapted from Vasanthan *et al.* (2002).

humans (Björck *et al.*, 1984), and it is related to the product's functional qualities, such as expansion, volume, water solubility and colour (Vasanthan *et al.*, 2002; Stojceska *et al.*, 2010).

When starch is cooked, amylase resistant fractions are formed (Cheftel, 1986). These non-digestible polysaccharides contribute to increased insoluble dietary fibre levels. The formation of resistant starch is affected by the amylase to amylopectin ratios and processing conditions (Stojceska *et al.*, 2010). Changes in the profile of dietary fibre can also be attributed to the change of soluble dietary fibre (SDF) into insoluble. This can be accounted for because mechanical stress during the extrusion process breaks down the glucosidic bonds in polysaccharides, which leads to the release of oligosaccharides, and therefore to an increase in insoluble fibre (Esposito *et al.*, 2005; Stojceska *et al.*, 2010).

Björck *et al.* (1984) studied the effect of extrusion cooking on dietary fibre in wheat products, and found a slight increase in TDF with a significant redistribution from IDF into SDF, as a result of different extrusion conditions. The extruded wheat flour was used to feed rats and it was found that 'fecal excretion of dietary fibre constituents was lower than after raw flour, indicating higher fermentability due to extrusion' (Table 19.4). Caprez *et al.* (1986) found that extrusion cooking affected water-binding capacity and caused rheological changes in wheat bran, while dietary fibre and starch content remained unchanged, probably due to the mild conditions used (Table 19.4).

Table 19.4 Some figures from the literature showing the differences of various dietary fibre levels before and after extrusion processing

Sources	Grains	Samples	IDF (%)	SDF (%)	TDF (%)
Esposito *et al.* (2005)	Durum wheat bran by-product	Non-extruded	33.9–35	1.6–3.0	/
		Extruded	37.4–65.6	1.3–2.8	/
Vasanthan *et al.* (2002)	barley grains waxy (CDC)	Non-extruded	1.89	5.63	7.52
		Extruded	1.17–1.82	5.69–7.24	7.51–9.14
	Phoenix regular barley grains	Non-extruded	2.43	2.35	4.78
		Extruded	4.19–6.43	3.03–3.80	7.39–10.23
Østergård *et al.* (1989)	Barley flour	Non-extruded	17.3	2.6	19.8
		Extruded	17.4–19.5	3.3–3.8	20.8–22.5
Caprez *et al.* (1986)	Wheat bran	Non-extruded	56.3	5.6	61.9
		Extruded	52.9	6.1	59
Björck *et al.* (1984)	Wheat flour	Non-extruded	2.3	1.7	4.0
		Extruded	0.9–1.7	2.1–3.8	3.8–4.9

Østergård *et al.* (1989) reported a significant increase in the TDF content of barley during extrusion processing. This increase was a result of high starch gelatinization, which can be explained by the presence of enzymatically indigestible starch (Table 19.4). Vasanthan *et al.* (2002) examined the behaviour of two types of barley grain: waxy barley grains (CDC-Candle) and Phoenix regular barley grains. TDF, IDF, SDF, β-glucan and resistant starch contents were investigated during extrusion using various process conditions, including different temperature and moisture levels. The temperatures used ranged from 90°C to 140°C and the moisture content from 20% to 50%. It was found that SDF and TDF content increased during extrusion cooking, but IDF content depended on the type of barley grain (Table 19.4).

Stojceska *et al.* (2010) used Teff flour and a twin-screw extruder to increase dietary fibre in gluten-free ready-to-eat extruded snacks using the following process conditions: feed rate 15–25 kg/h, water feed of 12%, screw speed between 200 and 350 rpm and barrel temperatures of 80 and 150°C. Extrusion processing increased the level of dietary fibre from 3.37% up to 8.06–9.8%, depending on the extrusion parameters. This increase was more pronounced, probably due to the higher level of starch in the carbohydrate fraction, which contributed to the formation of resistant starch and consequently led to an increase in TDF.

19.3.2 Physicochemical changes in starches

Snack products are often based on starch, which plays a predominant role during extrusion processing. The presence of starch provides a number of functional benefits, including greater expansion and crispness. The transformation of different starchy flours during extrusion processing has already been very well documented. Changes to the structural properties of corn starch as a function of different process conditions, such as temperature, feed moisture content, residence time screw speed and feed moisture content, were studied by Thymi *et al.* (2005): 'The increase of residence time in a counter rotating twin-screw extruder caused a degradation of amylopectin molecular structure of the starch based materials and reduced the radial expansion, resulting in higher density values.'

A number of authors have studied extruded corn starches with varying levels of amylose and amylopectin (Xie *et al.*, 1995; Escarpa *et al.*, 1996; Della Valle *et al.*, 1997; Chanvrier *et al.*, 2007), and found that conversion of starch during extrusion depends on the amylopectin to amylase ratio, water content, process conditions and the presence of other ingredients. A literature review by Sajilata and Singhal (2005) showed that different starches could improve the quality of extruded snacks during production. Amylose cornstarch was used to obtain crisp and browned snack products, slightly degraded waxy pregels for crispy mouthfeel, and modified starches and high amylopectin flour to improve texture, crispness and expansion of the products. Carboxymethyl starch from waxy amaranth and pregel starches have been used to control extruded shapes.

Different amylose to amylopectin ratios in processed corn starches were investigated using a twin-screw extruder as a function of moisture content and temperature (Xie *et al.*, 1995). Amylose-rich corn starches exhibited higher viscosity and less Newtonian behaviour, which is probably a result of 'higher gelatinisation temperature, greater molecular entanglements between linear polymer chains, and less gel-balls and super-globes that are much easier to move than long linear chains'. Furthermore, the solubility and formation of resistant starch from starch depends on amylose/amylopectin ratios and the technological conditions during processing, including cooling (Escarpa *et al.*, 1996). High amylopectin starch exhibits a greater degree of gelatinization than high amylose starch (Kokini *et al.*, 1992), though parameters such as temperature and moisture content also have significant effects on gelatinization. The melting temperature of the amylopectin component of starch decreases with increasing water content, until critical moisture content is reached (Parker and Ring, 2001). In order to increase gelatinization in quinoa and oats, Chillo *et al.* (2010) used repeated extrusion. Davis and Arnold (1995) investigated *in vivo* digestibility of four different cereals, including whole wheat, corn flour, rice flour and milo, before and after extrusion, and found increased gelatinization in each case.

Della Valle *et al.* (1997) used starches with various amylase contents to examine the expansion indices, including volumetric expansion index, sectional expansion index and longitudinal expansion index of extruded products. At a constant moisture content and temperature, starches containing 0–70% amylase showed the same volumetric expansion, while at a higher moisture content and similar temperature starches were categorized according to their level of amylase.

Chanvrier *et al.* (2007) later studied the rheological properties of extrusion processed wheat flour with different starch/gluten ratios, investigating their contribution to the microstructure of the product. Five commercial wheat flours were hydrated at 28% moisture content and an extrusion temperature of 140°C. Figure 19.1 presents similar trends of flow behaviour for the flours, where shear viscosity decreased with increasing shear rate, and generally depended on the type of flour. No significant difference was found in terms of protein polymerization and starch transformation between different flours and shear rate. It was concluded that 'the effect of starch type on the shear viscosity of the samples studied was greater than that of gluten type', which was explained by the microstructure of the product.

19.3.3 Antioxidant activity

Whole grains are excellent sources of total antioxidants. This has been confirmed in a study by Adom and Liu (2002), in which corn grain was shown to have the highest total antioxidant activity, followed by wheat, oats and rice (Fig. 19.2).

A number of authors have investigated antioxidant changes in whole grains during extrusion processing. It was found that extrusion processing has a large impact on the level of antioxidants, with increased antioxidant activity occurring

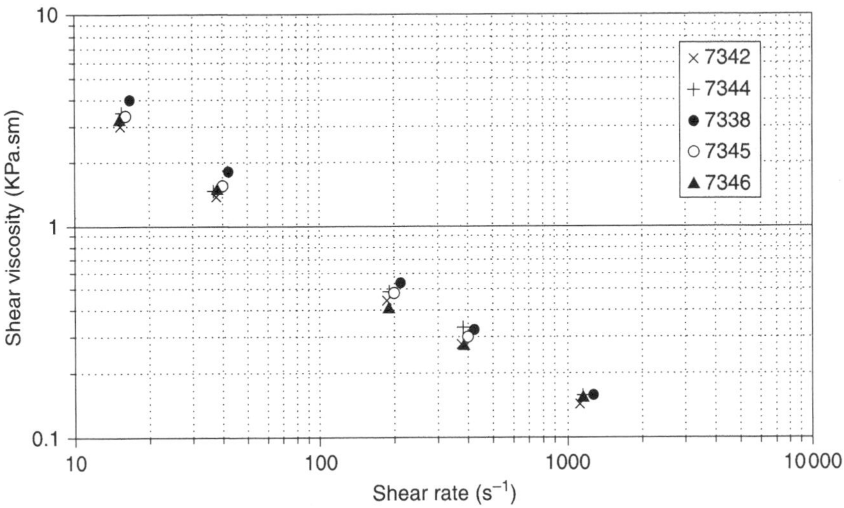

Fig. 19.1 Flow behaviour of the different wheat flours in the molten state (140°C, 28% moisture content), plotted as shear viscosity vs. shear rate (average viscosity values calculated from five replicates, standard deviation lower than 10%) (adapted from Chanvrier *et al.*, 2007).

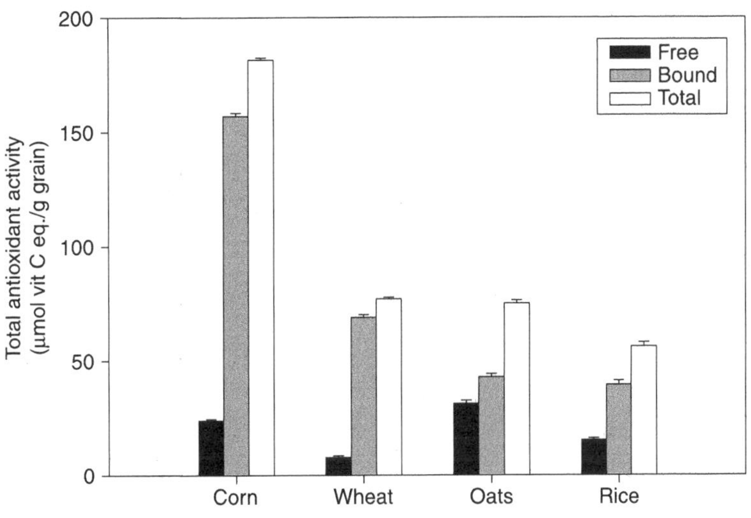

Fig. 19.2 Total antioxidant activity of grains (adapted from Adom and Liu, 2002).

in extruded amaranth and rye grains (Queiroz *et al.*, 2009; Dorota *et al.*, 2010) but decreased activity in sorghum (Dlamini *et al.*, 2007). Antioxidant activity during extrusion processing mainly depends on parameters such as moisture content and temperature (Queiroz *et al.*, 2009). According to Dorota *et al.* (2010), phenolic compounds, particularly ferulic acid formation, contributed significantly to the increase in total antioxidants in extruded rye grains. The highest antioxidant activity was found in extrudates prepared under conditions of 14% moisture and 180°C, and the lowest at 20% moisture and 120°C (Dorota *et al.*, 2010). Sensoy *et al.* (2006) roasted and extruded buckwheat flour in order to estimate changes in phenolic compounds. The results showed that roasting at 200°C for 10 min caused degradation of antioxidant activity, but this was not the case with extrusion at 170°C. The level of antioxidant activity changes during extrusion processing as a result of Maillard reactions and the transformation of inactive antioxidants into active antioxidants as a result of non-enzymatic browning (Porkorny and Schmidt, 2006). The Maillard reaction has been studied widely due to its effect on food properties such as flavour, colour and nutrition. The reaction takes place in heated foods. Amines react with carbonyl compounds, mainly reducing sugars, resulting in a number of complex products known as Maillard reaction products.

19.3.4 Retention of vitamins

Cereal grains are important sources of vitamins, which exhibit poor stability during extrusion processing (Riaz *et al.*, 2009). The most sensitive fat-soluble vitamins are A and E, while the vitamins C and B_1 are the most sensitive water-soluble ones. Reported results showed that vitamin retention during extrusion processing varies between 44 and 62% for B vitamins (Athar *et al.*, 2006), 56 and 79.2% for L-ascorbic acid (Plunkett and Ainsworth, 2007) and 76 and 130% for tocopherols (Lin *et al.*, 2003). An example of vitamin B retention in extruded samples is given in Table 19.5, with riboflavin and niacin having the highest stability and thiamin the lowest. Retention of vitamins mainly depends on cereal type and parameters used during extrusion, including higher temperature (Lin *et al.*, 2003; Athar *et al.*, 2006), and shorter time treatment (Lin *et al.*, 2003; Plunkett and Ainsworth, 2007). These observations were verified in a review

Table 19.5 Vitamin levels in the cereals before extrusion processing and vitamin retention (% retained) after extrusion

	Oats	Maize	Maize and peas
Vitamins before extrusion processing (mg/100 g)			
Thiamin	0.11	0.09	0.22
Riboflavin	0.06	0.04	0.08
Niacin	1.35	0.63	1.85
Pyridoxine	0.1	0.04	0.06
Vitamins (% retained)			
Thiamin	23	44	61
Riboflavin	100	86	70
Niacin	100	75	60
Pyridoxine	35	100	18

Source: adapted from Athar *et al.* (2006).

paper by Killeit (1994), who reported that the retention of vitamins generally decreases with increasing temperature, screw speed and specific energy input, and with decreasing moisture, throughput and die diameter. These parameters are difficult to optimize, and so it is not easy to ensure minimal loss of vitamins.

19.4 Cereal by-products as a new source of dietary fibre

Most manufacturers of wholegrain cereal foods may simply prefer to make their products from flours and grains. However, innovative sources of dietary fibre, such as cereal by-products, could be beneficial for businesses and consumers due to their low cost. Significant progress has been made in utilizing new fibre sources, including by-products of barley, wheat, corn and durum, in ready-to-eat extruded snacks (Ainsworth *et al.*, 2007; Stojceska *et al*, 2008; 2009; Rosentrater *et al.*, 2005; Esposito *et al.*, 2005; Yağci and Göğüş, 2008).

Esposito *et al.* (2005) used durum wheat bran while Rosentrater *et al.* (2005) used various levels of soybean corn by-product to produce extruded snacks with higher levels of dietary fibre. Combining corn bran with corn meal in extrudates significantly affected 'the radial expansion ratio, appearance and general acceptability levels' (Mendonya *et al.*, 2000). This challenge was overcome by changing the process conditions and establishing an optimum level of corn bran used, moisture content, and temperature, and the inclusion of glycerol monostearate.

Yağci and Göğüş (2008) incorporated durum clear flour into a formulation made from fruit by-products, using a single-screw extruder to produce expanded snack products. A model was developed using response surface methodology, in order to estimate the best physical and functional properties of extruded foods in terms of components and process variables.

Ainsworth *et al.* (2007) and Stojceska *et al.* (2008; 2009) used different levels of brewer's spent grain (BSG), and found that the maximum acceptable level that can be incorporated into extruded snacks is 30%. Increasing the level of corn starch and playing with the process conditions improved the sensorial characteristics of extruded products. Moreover, BSG has a beneficial effect on health (Stojceska, 2011) that may help prevent certain diseases, including constipation (Odes *et al.*, 1986), improve the physiological function of the colon (Zhang *et al.*, 1991), and lower cholesterol (Hassona, 1993).

Ingredients such as rice flour, wheat and starches are usually used to combine these potential functional ingredients and, with appropriate process conditions, could produce snack products with higher levels of dietary fibre.

19.5 Improving the quality of extruded products

A nutritional snack is only of value if it is acceptable to consumers. The quality of extruded snack products mainly depends on their organoleptic properties, and is measured by expansion ratio, density, texture, appearance and flavour (Dehghan-Shoar *et al.*, 2010), which are mainly influenced by moisture content, barrel temperature, screw speed, screw configuration and die geometry (Singh *et al.*, 2007). Those characteristics are related to the proportion and type of starch available, because the starch level affects the number and size of air cells developed during extrusion, which in turn affects expansion, density and texture. The presence of components other than starch may interfere with air cell expansion and limit the starch gelatinization necessary for expansion, resulting in an undesirably hard texture (Ainsworth *et al.*, 2007; Yanniotis *et al.*, 2007). Efforts to produce expanded high fibre snacks have generally resulted in products that are tough in texture and unable to hold their expansion upon extrusion.

Several authors have applied image analysis techniques (Mezreb *et al.*, 2003; Stojceska *et al.*, 2008; Arhaliass *et al.*, 2009) or developed predictive models (Lei *et al.*, 2005) in order to determine the structure of the extrudates and obtain useful information. Mezreb *et al.* (2003) studied the structural properties of extrudates using a digital image technique, and found that sectional and longitudinal expansion mainly depended on screw speed, water solubility and material used for extrusion.

Stojceska *et al.* (2008) observed the addition of fibre into a wheat–corn starch system, and found that different screw speeds had a major effect on the organization of cells in the extrudates, which contributed considerably to the final quality of extrudates in terms of appearance and expansion. Arhaliass *et al.* (2009) analysed sectional, longitudinal and volumetric expansion indices of wheat and maize extrudates under constant moisture and specific mechanical energy. They found that radial expansion was due to apparent viscosity, while axial expansion was dependent on the type of material used.

In order to estimate extruder performance, Lei *et al.* (2005) developed a predictive model for rice extrudates that considered different screw geometries. The model integrated process parameters including shear rate, barrel temperature, moisture content, flow rate and screw geometry. It was found that die pressure is a function of moisture content, product temperature and flow rate, while product temperature and shaft torque are functions of shear rate, moisture content, flow rate, barrel temperature and screw configuration.

The expansion of extruded products might be improved by injecting carbon dioxide as a puffing agent (Schmid *et al.*, 2005; Jeong and Toledo, 2004). Schmid *et al.* (2005) extruded wheat flour with 0.3% thiamin using a twin-screw extruder at temperatures between 40 and 80°C. Jeong and Toledo (2004) extruded pre-gelatinized rice flour using CO_2 injection in a twin-screw extruder at temperatures between 40 and 60°C. Satisfactory expansion in a highly porous product was obtained at injection pressures less than 0.6 MPa (Jeong and Toledo, 2004). However, expansion of the extruded products could also be improved by increasing screw speed and energy input and decreasing moisture content speed (Schmid *et al.*, 2005).

The importance of aerated snack consumption in terms of energy intake was highlighted in a study by Osterholt *et al.* (2007). It was found that the degree of aeration of snacks had a significant effect on weight, energy consumption and volume consumed when an equal volume of snacks was served. Energy consumed was reduced by 21% for the less aerated snacks.

In order to improve textural properties of extrudates, several researchers have used additives such as monoglycerides, sodium bicarbonate, gums and hydrocolloids (Lai *et al.*, 1989; Singh *et al.*, 2000; Miladinov and Hanna, 1995; Ravindran *et al.*, 2011; Yanniotis *et al.*, 2007; Thakur and Saxena, 2000). These additives tend to improve textural properties and act as stabilizers. The most commonly used gyms or hydrocolloids are gum arabic, pectins, alginates and guar gums. The addition of sodium bicarbonate to wheat extrudates improved the expansion of the final product but weakened the structure and caused browning (Lai *et al.*, 1989).

Singh *et al.* (2000) observed changes of maize grit product characteristics when a combination of sodium bicarbonate and glycerol monostearate was added, using various extrusion temperatures. Results indicated that the viscosity decreased when glycerol monostearate quantity increased, but increased with the increase of sodium bicarbonate levels. However, sodium bicarbonate at lower extrusion temperatures increased expansion, while at higher temperatures a reverse effect was detected.

Thakur and Saxena (2000) used response surface methodology to analyse the effect of xanthan, guar gum and arabic gum on the expansion ratio of extrudates, using a twin-screw extruder at a temperature of 160°C and a feed rate of 70 g/min. The stepwise variable selection showed that responses were most affected by changes in guar gum levels and to a lesser degree by xanthan and gum arabic. This model could be effective in resolving the difficulty of preparing gum-based ready-to-eat snacks under different extrusion process conditions.

Miladinov and Hanna (1995) produced extrudates with high apparent viscosity by adding equal amounts of xanthan gum and starch, and injecting adipoyl chloride. Viscosity increased with an increase of temperature up to 95°C, but disappeared at 110°C. Key parameters were amylose content, nozzle diameter and barrel temperature.

Yanniotis *et al.* (2007) used pectins to reduce hardness, while Fishman *et al.* (2000) used a mixture of pectin/starch/glycerol to improve the mechanical properties of extrudates. The results revealed that the degree of starch gelatinization could be controlled by extrusion temperatures and the amount of water used. Pectins improved the emulsifying properties of soybean proteins, and extrusion processing brought additional advantages to the interfacial properties of this combination (Bueno *et al.*, 2009).

Recently, Ravindran *et al.* (2011) improved pea–rice-based extruded products by incorporating different gums, including guar gum, locust bean gum and fenugreek gum. It was found that a good degree of expansion was obtained when these gums were added to the formulation mix at the level of 20%. The same result was detected in terms of colour and texture, and the snacks produced were good sources of protein and dietary fibre, and low in fat and glycaemic index (GI).

19.6 Conclusion

The popularity of nutritionally improved snack foods as part of the daily diet continues to rise, perhaps due to increasing customer awareness of its role in maintaining health. The addition of whole grains to ready-to-eat snacks as a source of dietary fibre, phenolic compounds and vitamins has been discussed, with a particular emphasis on the use of extrusion as a process for improving nutritional and textural properties. Factors such as formulation and process conditions affect the quality of the final products. Extrusion processing increases dietary fibre levels due to the formation of resistant starch. However, extrusion conditions such as moisture content, feed rate and screw speed could potentially improve the properties of extruded ready-to-eat snacks. In addition, the expansion of extruded snacks could be improved through the use of additives and puffing agents.

19.7 Future trends

There is increasing proof that whole grains provide significant health benefits. Dietary fibre consumption around the world fails to meet daily recommendations, and snacking could make an important contribution to TDF intake and energy. The growth in snacking, particularly high fat, high sugar and high salt snacks, has been seen as a contributing factor to poor diet quality. Initiatives to improve the human diet have highlighted the nutritional content of snack products and created demand for more nutritious options. Future research into extruded ready-to-eat snacks should focus on improving the nutritional quality of snack products while maintaining good sensorial properties. Whole grains are an excellent source of dietary fibre, antioxidants and vitamins, all of which are vital parts of a healthy diet. Whole grains have therefore been incorporated into various snack foods. Extrusion might be a suitable means of producing expanded and crunchy products that do not suffer from the heavier structure of traditional wholegrain formulations. The advantage of using extrusion is in its ability to create products with an open structure and desirable texture, which could be achieved by manipulating extrusion process conditions and reformulating products.

When whole grains undergo extrusion processing, vitamin levels are reduced as a result of chemical reactions that occur due to high temperatures, high pressures and screw speeds. Extruded snacks may therefore need to be fortified with vitamins through the use of post-extrusion applications such as spraying or coating, lowering the residence time, using short barrel extruders, or micro-encapsulation.

Furthermore, future research should also highlight the use of cereal by-products as potential sources of dietary fibre, proteins and antioxidants that could easily be incorporated into ready-to-eat extruded snacks. This might be of particular interest to manufacturers in terms of using cheaper or non-cost ingredients.

19.8 References

ADOM, K.K. and LIU, R.H. (2002). Antioxidant activity of grains. *Journal of Agricultural and Food Chemistry*, **50**, 6182–7.

AINSWORTH, P., IBANOĞLU, Ş., PLUNKETT, A., IBANOĞLU, E. and STOJCESKA, V. (2007). Effect of brewers spent grain addition and screw speed on the selected physical and nutritional properties of an extruded snack. *Journal of Food Engineering*, **81**, 702–9.

ARHALIASS, A., LEGRAND, J., VAUCHEL, P., FODIL-PACHA, P., LAMER, T. and BOUVIER, J.M. (2009). The Effect of Wheat and Maize Flours Properties on the Expansion Mechanism During Extrusion Cooking. *Food and Bioprocess Technology*, **2**, 186–93.

ATHAR, N., HARDACRE, A., TAYLOR, G., CLARK, S., HARDING, R. AND MCLAUGHLIN, J. (2006). Vitamin retention in extruded food products. *Journal of Food Composition and Analysis*, **19**, 379–83.

BELLISLE, F., DALIX, A.M., MENNEN, L., GALAN, P., HERCBERG, S. *et al.* (2003). Contribution of snacks and meals in the diet of French adults: a diet-diary study. *Physiology and Behavior*, **79**, 183–9.

BJÖRCK, I., NYMAN, M. and ASP, N. G. (1984). Extrusion cooking and dietary fibre: effects on dietary fiber content and on degradation in the rat intestinal tract. *Cereal Chemistry*, **61**, 174–9.

BRITISH NUTRITION FOUNDATION (2004). *Dietary Fibre*. British Nutrition Foundation. Available at: http://www.nutrition.org.uk/ (accessed 20 October 2012).

BUENO, A.S., PEREIRA, C.M., MENEGASSI, B., ARÊAS, G.J.A. and CASTRO, I.A. (2009). Effect of extrusion on the emulsifying properties of soybean proteins and pectin mixtures modelled by response surface methodology. *Journal of Food Engineering*, **90**, 504–10.

CAPREZ, A., ARRIGONI, E., AMADÒ, R. and NEUKOM, H. (1986). Influence of different types of thermal treatment on the chemical composition and physical properties of wheat bran. *Journal of Cereal Science*, **4**, 233–9.

CHÁVEZ-JÁUREGUI, R.N., SILVA, M.E.M.P. and ARÊAS, J.A.G. (2000). Extrusion cooking process for amaranth (*Amaranthus caudatus* L.). *Journal of Food Science*, **65**, 1009–15.

CHANVRIER, H., UTHAYAKUMARANA, S. and LILLFORDA, P. (2007). Rheological properties of wheat flour processed at low levels of hydration: Influence of starch and gluten. *Journal of Cereal Science*, **45**, 263–74.

CHEFTEL, J.C. (1986). Nutritional Effects of Extrusion Cooking. *Food Chemistry*, **20**, 263–83.

CHILLO, S., CIVICA, V., IANNETTI, M., MASTROMATTEO, M., SURIANO, N. and DEL NOBILE, M.A. (2010). Influence of repeated extrusions on some properties of non-conventional spaghetti. *Journal of Food Engineering*, **100**, 329–35.

COOKE, S. (2002). *The World's Top 500 Food Markets*. Leatherhead Food RA: Surrey.

DATAMONITOR (2004). Savoury snacks in the United Kingdom: Industry profile (Reference code 0183–0199). February, Datamonitor Europe: London.

DAVIS, D.A. and ARNOLD, C.R. (1995). Effects of two extrusion processing conditions on the digestibility of four cereal grains for *Penaeus vannamei*. *Aquaculture*, **133**, 287–94.

DEHGHAN-SHOAR, Z., HARDACRE, A.K. and BRENNAN, C.S. (2010). The Physico-chemical Characteristics of Extruded Snacks Enriched with Tomato Lycopene. *Food Chemistry*, **123**, 1117–22.

DELLA VALLE, G., VERGNES, B., COLONNA, P. and PATRIA, A. (1997). Relations between rheological properties of molten starches and their expansion behaviour in extrusion. *Journal of Food Engineering*, **31**, 277–95.

DESRUMAUX, A., BOUVIER, J.M. and BURRI, J. (1999). Effect of Free Fatty Acids Addition On Corn Grits Extrusion. *Cereal Chemistry*, **76**, 699–704.

DLAMINI, N.R., TAYLOR, J.R.N. and ROONEY, L.W. (2007). The effect of sorghum type and processing on the antioxidant properties of African sorghum-based foods. *Food Chemistry*, **105**, 1412–19.

DOROTA, G., KORUS, J., CZECHOWSKA, K., BARTOŃ, H. and FOŁTA, M. (2010). The impact of extrusion on the content of polyphenols and antioxidant activity of rye grains. *Acta Scientiarum Polonorum Technologia Alimentaria*, **9**, 319–30.

ENGLYST, H.N., BINGHAM, S.A., RUNSWICK, S.A., COLLINSON, E. and CUMMINGS, J.H. (1989). Dietary fibre (non-starch polysaccharides) in cereal products. *Journal of Nutrition Diet*, **2**, 253–71.

ESCARPA, A., GONZÁLEZ, M.C., MAÑAS, L.E., GARCÍA, D.F. and SAURA, C. (1996). Resistant starch formation: Standardization of high-pressure autoclave process. *Journal of Agricultural and Food Chemistry*, **44**, 924–8.

ESPOSITO, F., ARLOTTI, G., BONIFATI, A.M., NAPOLITANOA, A., VITALEC, D. and FOGLIANO, V. (2005). Antioxidant activity and dietary fibre in durum wheat bran by-products. *Food Research International*, **38**, 1167–73.

FABRY, P. and TEPPERMAN, J. (1970). Meal Frequency – A Possible Factor in Human Pathology. *American Journal of Clinical Nutrition*, **23**, 1059–68.

FARAJ, A., VASANTHAN, T. and HOOVER, R. (2004). The effect of extrusion cooking on resistant starch formation in waxy and regular barley flours. *Food Research International* **37**, 517–25.

FISHMAN, M.L., COFFIN, D.R., KONSTANCE, R.P. and ONWULATA, C.I. (2000). Extrusion of pectin/next term starch blends plasticized with glycerol. *Carbohydrate Polymers*, **41**, 317–25.

HAGENIMANA, A., DING, X. and FANG, T. (2006). Evaluation of rice flour modified by extrusion cooking. *Journal of Cereal Science*, **43**, 38–46.

HASSONA, H.Z. (1993). High fiber bread containing brewer's spent grains and its effect on lipid metabolism in rats. *Nahrung*, **37**, 576–82.

HUXLEY, R. (2003). *A Review of the UK Food Market. For Cornwall Agricultural Council and Cornwall Taste of the West.* Available at: http://www.investincornwall.co.uk/uploads/reports/the_uk_food_market.pdf (accessed 20 October 2012).

ILO, S. and BERGHOFER, E. (1999). Kinetics of Colour Changes During Extrusion Cooking of Maize Grits. *Journal of Food Engineering*, **39**, 73–80.

JACOBSEN, S.E. and SHERWOOD, S. (2002). *Cultivo de Granos Andinos en Ecuador: Informe Sobre los Rubros Quinua, Chocho y Amaranto*. United Nations Food and Agriculture Organization, Rome.

JEONG, H.S. and TOLEDO, R.T. (2004). Twin-screw extrusion at low temperature with carbon dioxide injection to assist expansion: extrudate characteristics. *Journal of Food Engineering*, **63**, 425–32.

KILLEIT, U. (1994). Vitamin retention in extrusion cooking. *Food Chemistry*, **49**, 149–55.

KOKINI, J., CHANG, C. and LAI, L. (1992). The role of rheological properties on extrudate expansion. In J.L. KOKINI, C.T. HO and M.V. KARWE (Eds), *Food extrusion, science and technology*, New York: Dekker, pp. 631–52.

KURPAD, A.V., VAN KLINKEN, J.W., OWEN, G. and DE BRUIN, E.A. (2007). Consumption of a mid-morning snack improves memory but not attention in school children. *Physiology and Behavior*, **90**, 142–50.

LAI, C.S., GUETZLAFF, J. and HOSENEY, R.C. (1989). Role of Sodium Bicarbonate and Trapped Air in Extrusion. *Cereal Chemistry*, **66**, 69–73.

LASEKAN, O.O., LASEKAN, W., IDOWU, M.A. and OJO, O.A. (1996). Effect of Extrusion Cooking Conditions on the Nutritional Value, Storage Stability and Sensory Characteristics of a Maize-Based Snack Food. *Journal of Cereal Science*, **24**, 79–85.

LEI, H., FULCHER, G.R., RUAN, R. and VAN LENGERICH, B. (2005). Empirical modelling of die pressure, shaft torque, SME, and product temperature of rice flour in a corotating twin-screw extruder. *Cereal Chemistry*, **82**(5), 582–7.

LIN, Y.H., YEH, C.S. and LU, S. (2003). Extrusion Processing of Rice-Based Breakfast Cereals Enhanced with Tocopherol from a Chinese Medical Plant. *Cereal Chemistry*, **80**, 491–4.

MAZUMDER, P., ROOPA, B.S. and BHATTACHARYA, S. (2007) Textural attributes of a model snack food at different moisture contents. *Journal of Food Engineering*, **79**, 511–16.

MENDONYA, S., GROSSMANN, M.V.E. and VERHE, R. (2000). Corn Bran as a Fibre Source in Expanded Snacks. *LWT – Food Science and Technology*, **33**, 2–8.

MEZREB, K., GOULLIEUX, A., RALAINIRINA, R. and QUENEUDEC, M. (2003). Application of image analysis to measure screw speed influence on physical properties of corn and wheat extrudates. *Journal of Food Engineering*, **57**, 145–52.

MILADINOV, V. D. and HANNA, M. A. (1995). Apparent viscosity of starch and xanthan gum extruded with cross linking agents. *Crops and Products*, **4**, 261–71.

MINTEL (2004). *Snacking and drinking on the go-UK*. April. London: Mintel International Group Ltd.

MINTEL (2010). *Cereal, energy and snack bars in Europe: Mintel marketing report*. Available at: http://store.mintel.com/cereal-energy-and-snack-bars-europe-july-2011.html (accessed 20 October 2012).

NEUHOUSER, M.L., PATTERSON, R.E., KRISTAL, A.R., ROCK, C.L., SZTAINER, D.N. *et al.* (2000). Do Consumers of Savory Snacks Have Poor-quality Diets? *Journal of the American Dietetic Association*, **100**, 576–9.

ODES, H.S., MADAR, Z., TROP, M., NANIR, S., GROSS, J. and COHEN, T. (1986). Pilot study of the efficacy of spent grain dietary fiber in the treatment of constipation. *Israel Journal of Medical Sciences*, **22**, 12–15.

ØSTERGÅRD, K., BJÖRCK, I. and VAINIONPÄÄ, J. (1989). Effects of extrusion cooking on starch and dietary fibre in barley. *Food Chemistry*, **34**, 215–27.

OSTERHOLT, K.M., ROE, L.S. and ROLLS, B.J. (2007). Incorporation of air into a snack food reduces energy intake. *Appetite*, **48**, 351–8.

PARKER, R. and RING, S.G. (2001). Aspects of the physical chemistry of starches. *Journal of Cereal Science*, **34**(1), 1–17.

PLATE, A.Y.A. and ARÊAS, J.A.G. (2002). Cholesterol-lowering effect of extruded amaranth (*Amaranthus caudatus* L.) in hypercholesterolemic rabbits. *Food Chemistry*, **76**, 1–6.

PLUNKETT, A. and AINSWORTH, P. (2007). The influence of barrel temperature and screw speed on the retention of L-ascorbic acid in an extruded rice based snack product. *Journal of Food Engineering*, **78**, 1127–33.

POKORNY, J. and SCHMIDT, S. (2006). Natural antioxidant functionality during food processing. In: J. POKORNY, N. YANISHLIEVA and M. GORDON (Eds), *Antioxidants in food*, Vol. 380, CRC Press, Washington, DC, pp. 331–51.

QUEIROZ, Y.S., MANÓLIOSOARES, R.A., CAPRILES, V.D., TORRES, E.A. and AREAS, J.A. (2009). Effect of processing on the antioxidant activity of amaranth grain, *Arch Latinoam Nutr*, **59**, 419–24.

RAVINDRAN, G., CARR, A. and HARDACRE, A. (2011). A comparative study of the effects of three galactomannans on the functionality of extruded pea–rice blends. *Food Chemistry*, **124**, 1620–6.

RIAZ, M.N., ASIF, M. and ALI, R. (2009). Stability of vitamins during extrusion. *Critical Reviews in Food Science and Nutrition*, **49**, 361–8.

ROSENTRATER, K.A., RICHARD, T.L., BERN, C.J. and FLORES, R.A. (2005). Small-Scale Extrusion of Corn Masa By-Products, *Cereal Chemistry*, **82**, 436–46.

SAJILATA, M.G. and SINGHAL, R.S. (2005). Specialty starches for snack foods. *Carbohydrate Polymers*, **59**, 131–51.

SCHMID, A.H., DOLAN, K.D. and NG, P.K.W. (2005). Effect of extruding wheat flour at lower temperatures on physical attributes of extrudates and on thiamin loss when using carbon dioxide gas as a puffing agent. *Cereal Chemistry*, **82**, 305–13.

ŞENSOY, Í, ROSEN, R.T., HO, C.T. and KARWE, M.V. (2006). Effect of processing on buckwheat phenolics and antioxidant activity. *Food Chemistry*, **99**, 388–93.

SINGH, N. and SMITH, A.C. (1997). A comparison of wheat starch, whole wheat meal and oat flour in the extrusion cooking process. *Journal of Food Engineering*, **34**, 15–32.

SINGH, N., SHARMA, S. and SINGH, B. (2000). The effect of sodium bicarbonate and glycerol monostearate addition on the extrusion behaviour of maize grits. *Journal of Food Engineering*, **46**, 61–6.

SINGH, B., SEKHON, K.S. and SINGH, N. (2007). Effects of moisture, temperature and level of pea grits on extrusion behaviour and product characteristics of rice. *Food Chemistry*, **100**, 198–202.

STOJCESKA, V. (2011). Dietary fiber from Brewer's Spent Grain as a functional ingredient in bread making technology. In V.R. PREEDY, R.R. WATSON and V.B. PATEL (Eds), *Flour and breads and their fortification in health and disease prevention*, London, Burlington, San Diego: Academic Press, Elsevier, pp. 171–81.

STOJCESKA, V., AINSWORTH, P., PLUNKETT, A. and IBANOĞLU, Ş. (2008). The recycling of brewer's processing by-product into ready-to-eat snacks using extrusion technology. *Journal of Cereal Science*, **47**, 469–79.

STOJCESKA, V., AINSWORTH, P., PLUNKETT, A. and IBANOĞLU, Ş. (2009). The effect of extrusion cooking using different water feed rates on the quality of ready-to-eat snacks made from food by-products. *Food Chemistry*, **114**, 226–32.

STOJCESKA, V., AINSWORTH, P., PLUNKETT, A. and IBANOĞLU, Ş. (2010). The advantage of using extrusion processing for increasing dietary fibre level in gluten-free products. *Food Chemistry*, 156–64.

THAKUR, S. and SAXENA, D.C. (2000). Formulation of Extruded Snack Food (Gum Based Cereal–Pulse Blend): Optimization of Ingredients Levels Using Response Surface Methodology. *Lebensmittel-Wissenschaft und-Technologie*, **33**, 354–61.

THANE CW, JONES AR, STEPHEN AM, SEAL CJ and JEBB SA. (2005). Whole-grain intake of British young people aged 4–18 years. *British Journal of Nutrition*, **94**, 825–31.

THYMI, S., KROKIDA, M.K., PAPPA, A. and MAROULIS, Z.B. (2005). Structural properties of extruded corn starch. *Journal of Food Engineering*, **68**, 519–26.

VASANTHAN, T., GAOSONG, J., YEUNG, J. and LI, J. (2002). Dietary fiber profile of barley flour as affected by extrusion cooking. *Food Chemistry*, **77**, 35–40.

XIE, F., YU, L., SUA, B., LIUA, P., WANG, J., *et al.* (1995). Rheological properties of starches with different amylose/amylopectin ratios. *Journal of Cereal Science*, **49**, 371–7.

YAĞCI, S. and GÖĞÜŞ, F. (2008). Response surface methodology for evaluation of physical and functional properties of extruded snack foods developed from food-by-products. *Journal of Food Engineering*, **86**, 122–32.

YANNIOTIS, S., PETRAKI, A. and SOUMPASI, E. (2007). Effect of pectin and wheat fibers on quality attributes of extruded cornstarch. *Journal of Food Engineering*, **80**, 594–9.

ZHANG, J.X., LUNDIN, E., ANDERSSON, H., BOSAEUS, I., DAHLGREN, S. and HALLMANS, G. (1991). Brewer's spent grain, serum lipids and fecal sterol excretion in human subjects with ileostomies. *Journal of Nutrition*, **121**, 778–84.

20

Companion animal nutrition as affected by dietary fibre inclusion

M. C. Rossoni Serão and G. C. Fahey Jr, University of Illinois, USA

DOI: 10.1533/9780857095787.4.407

Abstract: Dietary fibre has been a subject of study in companion animal nutrition for approximately 25 years, recently focusing on its benefits for dog and cat health and well-being. Pet animal diets contain significant amounts of carbohydrates, including dietary fibre. Depending on the properties of carbohydrates and their level in the diet, different physiological effects occur. High concentrations of dietary fibre affect appetite regulation and, potentially, gastric emptying, intestinal transit time and nutrient digestibility. Other effects include changes in faecal consistency and volume, increased production of short chain fatty acids, and alterations in the microbial population. Recent work on prebiotics and the benefits of a healthful large bowel microbiota has increased interest in dietary fibres and their potential value in clinical nutrition. This chapter is an update of the Fahey *et al.* (2004) comprehensive review of the effect of dietary fibre on companion animal nutrition and health. Studies conducted since 2004 will be emphasised.

Key words: dogs, cats, dietary fibre, pet foods, prebiotics, faeces, gut health.

20.1 Introduction

The use of dietary fibres in companion animal nutrition has been studied in earnest since the mid-1980s. Dogs and cats traditionally ingest high protein, high fat diets, and each has a gastrointestinal (GI) tract with modest colonic capacity but containing a robust population of anaerobic microbiota ($\sim 10^{10}$ colony-forming units (CFU)/ml digesta). Domesticated pet animals ingest diets containing significant amounts of carbohydrates that can reach as high as 30–40% dietary concentration, a portion of which is dietary fibre.

In contrast to the situation with farm animals, companion animal nutritionists do not formulate diets with a concern about animal performance, but rather longevity and health. A pet is, in many instances, a member of the family, and its well-being is a major concern to its owner. The inclusion of dietary fibre may result in health benefits to the animal. A decrease in the incidences of chronic diseases of humans, such as cardiovascular disease, GI disorders, diabetes, obesity, and various types of cancers, has been reported with elevated intakes of dietary fibre (Anderson *et al.*, 2009). Much less research has been conducted on the role of dietary fibres in enhancing pet animal nutrition and health (Fahey *et al.*, 2004).

Depending on the physicochemical properties of potentially fermentable carbohydrates and their level of inclusion in the diet, different physiological effects on the body will occur. Consumption of potentially fermentable carbohydrates may affect regulation of food intake, intestinal transit time, nutrient absorption, faecal volume and quality, and intestinal microbiota populations (Kritchevsky, 1988; Zentek, 1996). Carbohydrates entering the large bowel (dietary fibre, resistant starch (RS), non-digestible oligosaccharides) may exert their effects as a result of their physicochemical characteristics, the end-products of their fermentation (i.e. short-chain fatty acids (SCFA) and lactate), and (or) their ability to modulate the colonic microbiota.

Select dietary fibres also may function as prebiotics for dogs and cats. A prebiotic is 'a food ingredient that is resistant to enzymatic digestion in the small intestine and that beneficially affects the host by stimulating growth and (or) activity of specific species of bacteria in the lower gut, thus improving host health' (Gibson and Roberfroid, 1995). Beneficial bacteria (e.g. bifidobacteria and lactobacilli) are increased in concentration as a result of prebiotic feeding (Buddington, 2001), whereas pathogenic bacteria (e.g. *Clostridium perfringens* and *E. coli*) are decreased in concentration. This occurs as a result of reduced pH caused by increased production of SCFA and lactate, and competition for nutrients when prebiotics are present (Fuller and Gibson, 1997).

This chapter is an update of the Fahey *et al.* (2004) comprehensive review of the inclusion of dietary fibre on companion animal nutrition and health. Studies conducted since 2004 will be emphasised. Readers are referred to the 2004 chapter for details of studies conducted prior to that year.

20.2 Effects of dietary fibre on food intake and gastric and small intestinal function in companion animals

As regards the effects of dietary fibres on the GI system of companion animals, Fahey *et al.* (2004) elaborated on regulation of food intake, intestinal rate of passage, and nutrient digestibility when animals were fed select fibre sources. These same topics are relevant today.

20.2.1 Effects of dietary fibre on food intake

Inclusion of high concentrations of dietary fibre appears to affect appetite regulation as a result of an energy dilution mechanism inducing the dog to increase food intake (Fahey *et al.*, 2004). More recent research by Bosch *et al.* (2009) tested the effects of dietary fibre type on satiety-related hormones and voluntary food intake by dogs. The hypothesis that fibre fermentability might affect food intake was tested with 16 healthy adult beagles that were assigned to one of two dietary treatments (low fermentable fibre and high fermentable fibre). Dietary levels of fibre addition were 8.5% beet pulp + 2% inulin (high fermentable fibre diet) and 8.5% cellulose (low fermentable fibre diet). Dogs fed the high fermentable fibre diet tended ($p = 0.06$) to ingest less food compared with dogs fed the low fermentable fibre diet. This response could be explained by the significant increase in large intestinal fibre degradation in the former treatment, with a consequent increased rate of SCFA production, suggesting that SCFA served as an energy source and induced satiety in animals fed the combination of beet pulp + inulin.

20.2.2 Rate of digesta passage

Fahey *et al.* (2004) suggested that fibres from different sources, and with different characteristics (e.g. viscosity, solubility), and when fed at different dietary concentrations, could affect gastric emptying and intestinal transit time differently. Comparing results from different studies, Fahey *et al.* (2004) inferred that transit time was increased by dietary fibres with higher viscosity. This was confirmed in a human study by Shimoyama *et al.* (2007), who tested inclusion of a high-viscosity (pectin) liquid meal on gastric emptying in adult humans and concluded that the high viscosity caused by the addition of pectin to the enteral nutritional solution prevented the sudden overflow of nutrients from the stomach into the duodenum, thereby avoiding the inhibition of gastric motility by the duodenal brake. A similar mechanism is plausible for pet animals.

20.2.3 Nutrient digestibility

It is important to understand how animals respond to novel ingredient inclusion in select diet matrices. One of the most important outcomes in this regard is nutrient digestibility. Fahey *et al.* (2004) noted that not only digestibility but also absorption of nutrients may be affected by the presence of fibre in the diet. This occurs as a result of alterations in mixing, motility, and convection of digesta; intraluminal digestion rates; thickness of the unstirred water layer; inhibition of maximal transport capacity; pH; and, over a longer time period, changes in intestinal morphology.

Fibre fermentability and solubility will determine how a specific fibre will affect nutrient digestibility. Soluble fibres, in general, provide greater energy for gut microorganisms than do insoluble fibres, due to an increased fermentation capacity of the soluble fibre (Fahey *et al.*, 2004).

In Table 20.1, a summary of results of digestibility studies conducted since 2004 is presented. A general conclusion that can be drawn from these results is that soluble fibres appear to improve nutrient digestibility. However, total tract crude protein digestibility is nearly always lower when pet animals are fed soluble

Table 20.1 Summary of results of fibre digestibility studies conducted since 2004 with dogs and cats

Reference	Fibre source/inclusion level (%)	Animal/gender/age	Digestibility coefficients
Gajda *et al.* (2005)	High amylose corn hybrid/~33% Amylomaize/~33% Normal corn hybrids/~33%	Five dogs/female/ 2 years Hound bloodlines	Ileal starch digestibility was lower for dogs fed high amylose corn (64%) and amylomaize (63%) compared with the mean value for the normal corn hybrids (87.2%). Corresponding apparent total tract starch digestibility values were 72.8, 76.5, and 98%, respectively.
Spears *et al.* (2005)	Maltodextrin/30.0% High-molecular weight pullulan/30.0% Low-molecular weight pullulan/30.0% γ-cyclodextrin/30.0%	Eight dogs/female/ 2.0 years Hound bloodlines	High-MW pullulan had lower DM (70.2%), OM (73.0%), CP (79.8%), and carbohydrate (63.7%) ileal digestibilities compared with all other treatments.
Middelbos *et al.* (2007)	Control diet (0% supplemental fibre) Control + 1% cellulose + 1.5% FOS Control + 1% cellulose + 1.2% FOS + 0.3% YCW Control + 1% cellulose + 0.9% FOS + 0.6% YCW Control + 2.5% beet pulp	Six dogs/female/ 4.5 years Hound bloodlines	Total tract DM (83.2%) and OM (88.7%) digestibilities were lowest for the cellulose treatment. CP digestibility was lower for treatments containing carbohydrate blends (2.5% unit decrease compared with beet pulp treatment).
Guevara *et al.* (2008)	Native corn fibre/7% Native corn fibre with fines/7% Hydrolysed corn fibre/7% Hydrolysed extracted corn fibre/7%	Fifteen dogs/female/ 6.4 years Beagles	Apparent DM digestibility coefficient (82.3%) was higher with native corn fibre compared with beet pulp (78.4%), hydrolysed corn fibre (79.0%) and hydrolysed extracted corn fibre (79.2%), but not with native corn fibre with fines (80.9%). No differences in apparent CP digestion were noted.

Barry *et al.* (2009)	Cellulose/4.0% Cellulose + 0.2% inulin Cellulose + 0.4% inulin Cellulose + 0.2% scFOS Cellulose + 0.4% scFOS	Five dogs/female/ 5.5 years Hound bloodlines	Ileal digestibility of DM, OM, and CP increased linearly for dogs consuming inulin (2.7, 2.4, and 3.1% units, respectively) and scFOS treatments (2.0, 2.0, and 2.6% units, respectively).
Faber *et al.* (2011)	Galactoglucomannan/arabinoxylan complex/0, 0.5, 1.0, 2.0, 4.0 and 8.0%	Six dogs/female/ 3.4 years Hound bloodlines	Total tract DM and OM apparent digestibilities increased linearly, with a 3.8% unit increase in DM digestibility and a 3.9% unit increase in OM digestibility, while apparent CP digestibility decreased linearly (2.5% unit decrease) with supplementation of fibre source.
Barry *et al.* (2010)	Cellulose/4.0% Inulin-OF/4.0% Pectin/4.0%	Twelve cats/male/ 1.7 years Domestic shorthair	DM (90.5%), OM (88%), and CP (87.4%) digestibility coefficients were higher with inulin-OF supplementation.
Kanakupt *et al.* (2011)	Control scFOS/0.5% GOS/0.5% scFOS + GOS/0.5%; 0.5%	Eight cats/male/ 2.8 years Domestic shorthair	Decreased apparent CP total tract digestibility (2.4%) when cats were fed 0.5% scFOS + 0.5% GOS.

Notes: DM, dry matter; OM, organic matter; CP, crude protein; YCW, yeast cell wall; FOS, fructooligosaccharide; OF, oligofructose; scFOS, short-chain fructooligosaccharide; GOS, galactooligosaccharide; MW, molecular weight.

dietary fibres because they stimulate microbial protein synthesis in the large bowel, resulting in greater faecal excretion of nitrogen, thus lowering the apparent total tract crude protein digestion coefficient.

One study compared three normal corn hybrids with one high in amylose. Amylomaize, a commercially available RS, was also tested in the study as a positive control. Data indicate fibre-like behaviour of the high amylose corn hybrid in terms of both ileal and total tract starch digestibility, indicating that perhaps a natural dietary ingredient of this type could substitute for a portion of the traditional dietary fibre commonly added to pet animal diets (Gajda *et al.*, 2005).

20.3 Effects of dietary fibre on intestinal function of companion animals

Fibre fermentation in the large intestine may alter stool characteristics as well as large bowel microbiota composition and function. In this section, the production of SCFA and lactate as end-products of fermentation of indigestible carbohydrates reaching the large bowel will be discussed, and an update provided regarding prebiotic use in pet animal diets.

Fahey *et al.* (2004) outlined the intestinal characteristics of pet animals often affected by dietary fibres. These include an increase in wet stool bulk, number of defecations per day, and the acetate:propionate ratio, and a decrease in faecal moisture when animals are fed insoluble-non-viscous-low fermentable fibre sources. An increase in number of defecations (cats only), total SCFA concentration, colonic weight/length, colonic absorptive area, and glucose uptake, and a decrease in the acetate:propionate ratio occur when pet animals are fed soluble-viscous-partially fermentable fibre sources.

20.3.1 Stool quality

Stool quality reflects volume and consistency score of the stool produced. Use of dietary ingredients that are not digestible contributes to stool output, as does water-holding capacity of the resulting digesta (Fahey *et al.*, 2004). Since 2004, several studies have been conducted evaluating the effects of different fibres on stool quality of pet animals. Observations of stool quality are commonly used as a research outcome to assess the effect of a fibre on bowel function. A summary of these studies is presented in Table 20.2.

20.3.2 Prebiotic effects

Use of prebiotics in companion animal nutrition was reviewed by Swanson and Fahey (2006) and was updated by Vester and Fahey (2010). Chicory (a natural source of long-chain fructans), inulin (a long-chain fructan), oligofructose (OF) (fructan chains with 8 to 10 units), and short-chain

Table 20.2 Summary of results of studies conducted since 2004 that measured stool characteristics of dogs and cats

Ref.	Fibre source/inclusion level (%)	Animal/gender/age	Stool characteristics
Hesta *et al.* (2005)	Control Control + 3.11% OF	Four cats/female/above 7 years	14% increase in faecal output when cats were fed OF and 10% increase in faecal moisture.
Spears *et al.* (2005)	Maltodextrin/30.0% High-MW pullulan/30.0% Low-MW pullulan/30.0% γ-cyclodextrin/30.0%	Eight dogs/female/ 2.0 years Hound bloodlines	Faecal output increased over sevenfold on an as-is basis when animals were fed high-MW pullulan.
Middelbos *et al.* (2007)	Control diet (no supplemental fibre) Control + 1% cellulose + 1.5% FOS Control + 1% cellulose + 1.2% FOS + 0.3% YCW Control + 1% cellulose + 0.9% FOS + 0.6% YCW Control + 2.5% beet pulp	Six dogs/female/ 4.5 years Hound bloodlines	Animals fed beet pulp treatment had more wet faecal output (12.3% increase) compared with control + 1% cellulose + 1.5% FOS treatment.
Barry *et al.* (2009)	Cellulose/4.0% Cellulose + 0.2% inulin Cellulose + 0.4% inulin Cellulose + 0.2% scFOS Cellulose + 0.4% scFOS	Five dogs/female/ 5.5 years Hound bloodlines	Faecal score was not affected by the inclusion of fermentable carbohydrates in diets.
Faber *et al.* (2010)	Galactoglucomannan/arabinoxylan complex/0, 0.5, 1.0, 2.0, 4.0 and 8.0%	Six dogs/female/ 3.4 years Hound bloodlines	Faecal score increased (i.e. looser stool) when dogs were fed higher concentrations (4.0 and 8.0%) of fibre source.
Barry *et al.* (2010)	Cellulose/4.0% FOS/4.0% Pectin/4.0%	Twelve cats/male/ 1.7 years Domestic shorthair	Faecal score was greater when animals were fed FOS (2.8) and pectin (2.7) treatments compared with cellulose treatment (2.0); 5-point scale.
Kanakupt *et al.* (2011)	Control scFOS/0.5% GOS/0.5% scFOS + GOS/0.5%; 0.5%	Eight cats/male/ 2.8 years Domestic shorthair	Increase in faecal output (11%) on as-is basis was observed with the combination treatment, while faecal score was not affected.

Notes: DM, dry matter; OM, organic matter; CP, crude protein; OF, oligofructose; YCW, yeast cell wall; FOS, fructooligosaccharide; scFOS, short-chain fructooligosaccharide; GOS, galactooligosaccharide; MW, molecular weight.

fructooligosaccharides (scFOS) (fructan chains with three to five units) have been studied extensively (Hernot *et al.*, 2008). Other oligosaccharides have been tested, such as yeast cell wall (YCW), mannanoligosaccharide (MOS), α-galactooligosaccharide (GOS), isomaltooligosaccharide (IMO), lactosucrose, lactulose, maltodextrin-like oligosaccharide (MD), transgalactooligosaccharide (TGOS), and xylooligosaccharides (XOS), but not all satisfy the strict definition of a prebiotic as per Roberfroid (1998; a non-digestible food ingredient that beneficially affects the host by selectively stimulating the growth and/or activity of one or a limited number of bacteria in the colon and that improves host health).

The research reviewed by Swanson and Fahey (2006) and Vester and Fahey (2010) utilised a variety of outcomes to assess efficacy of prebiotics for dogs and cats: food intake, faecal output, stool consistency, macronutrient digestibility, fermentative end-product concentration, immune indices, and intestinal microbiota composition and function. A general conclusion from these reviews is that use of prebiotics by the companion animal industry is increasing, but, even with the advances made in recent years, more information is needed, especially for cats.

Two studies used cats to evaluate the effects of fructans (Barry *et al.*, 2010; Hesta *et al.*, 2005) on select nutritional outcomes. During a 2-week study, Hesta *et al.* (2005) observed that cats fed 3.1% OF tended to have an increase in faecal moisture (6%), dry matter (DM) output (27%), and faecal nitrogen excretion (36%), and a decrease in urinary nitrogen excretion (−48%). When Barry *et al.* (2010) supplemented feline diets with cellulose, inulin-OF, or pectin, it was concluded that a 4% level of supplementation of the fermentable fibres (inulin-OF and pectin) increased stool protein catabolite concentrations and microbial populations. When cats were fed inulin-OF and pectin compared with cellulose, an increase in stool odour caused by an increase in protein catabolite production was observed. Faecal ammonia and biogenic amine concentrations were higher. Short-chain fatty acid concentrations also increased. Even though inulin-OF treatments resulted in a more beneficial microbial population than did pectin, both fibre sources affected intestinal health indices of cats, but in different ways. Also, very different responses are noted when fructans are fed at 4% levels of dietary inclusion compared with levels < 1% of the diet. Lower concentrations are much more effective in decreasing large bowel concentrations of potentially toxic protein catabolites. This result highlights the undesirability of using prebiotics as the major dietary fibre source in pet animal diets.

20.3.3 *In vitro* evaluations of dietary fibres

In vitro models are relatively inexpensive, rapid methods of predicting fibre digestion in the human and animal gastrointestinal tract (Faber and Fahey, 2010). Determination of microbial digestion with the evaluation and quantification of fermentative end-products is possible using *in vitro* methods. It is possible to evaluate either a pure substrate or its interaction within a diet matrix. *In vitro* systems also provide a means of evaluating the efficacy of potential prebiotics (Gibson and Fuller, 2000). There are many different systems that vary in level of complexity and capability, some able to simulate both hydrolytic and fermentative digestion processes.

One of the most common measurements of an *in vitro* fermentation assay is gas production (rate, amount produced). Cutrignelli *et al.* (2009) used two dog breeds (German shepherd and Neapolitan mastiff) as faecal donors and evaluated the fermentation of a variety of carbohydrates. The authors observed that both sources of inocula exhibited low cellulolytic activity, resulting in low organic matter digestibility (OMD; 2.5%) and low gas production (3.53 ml/g) for the cellulose treatment, whereas the percentage OMD for FOS, inulin, and substrates rich in starch (potato, corn, spelt, and rice) was higher (ranging from 82.83 to 99.14%), demonstrating robust microbial activity with these substrates.

Bosch *et al.* (2008) compared *in vitro* fermentative activity in the canine distal gastrointestinal tract and fermentation kinetics of select fibre sources. By collecting samples from different sites in the gastrointestinal tract of dogs, using them as sources of inocula, and then comparing the results with an *in vitro* system using faecal samples as the source of inocula, the authors concluded that faeces is an appropriate inoculum source for *in vitro* fermentation studies, but may slightly overestimate the actual fermentation responses measured more proximally in the large intestine.

Biagi *et al.* (2008) studied *in vitro* fermentation responses of beet pulp, lactitol, citrus pulp, and chicory using dog faecal microbiota. Dogs were capable of digesting soluble fibres, as evidenced by total gas volume for all tested fibres (28% increase for beet pulp, 29% for citrus pulp, 33% for chicory, 48% for lactitol) when compared with control. Also, a significant decrease in ammonia concentration was noted for chicory (−9%), beet pulp (−12%), and citrus pulp (−16%). Lactitol increased acetic acid (+54%), n-butyric acid (+84%), and total SCFA production (+34%) when compared with the control. A significant increase of 0.3 log CFU lactobacilli/ml was observed as a result of lactitol and chicory fermentation.

According to Faber and Fahey (2010), *in vitro* assays may be used first to pre-screen test substrates, preventing unnecessary use of animals if no substrate effect exists. An animal model then may be used to confirm promising *in vitro* responses.

20.4 Clinical significance of dietary fibres in companion animal diets

The inclusion of dietary fibre in companion animal diets with the objective of ameliorating diseases was reported by Fahey *et al.* (2004), and effects were observed for attenuation of diabetes, small intestinal bacterial overgrowth, obesity, and renal disease.

20.4.1 Diabetes and glycaemic control

The idea of manipulating diet composition to influence postprandial glycaemia and attenuate blood glucose response as a nutritional strategy for management and prevention of diabetes was discussed by Fahey *et al.* (2004), the main conclusion being that high concentrations of inulin (approximately 80 g/kg) would help modulate blood metabolites, and that this would be useful in diets for dogs that are diabetic.

Recent studies have focused on the use of 'novel carbohydrates' as substitutes for traditional dietary fibres in human nutrition; the same trend is being followed in companion animal nutrition. Novel carbohydrates usually are derived from a source of starch that is modified physically or chemically to be incorporated into food. The possibility of incorporating into foodstuffs ingredients that result in laxation effects, faecal bulking, and reduced glycaemic response, and with a reduced energy value, has led to an increasing demand for carbohydrates that are easy to incorporate into foods but that mimic the physiological effects of dietary fibres (Murphy, 2001).

Using the dog model to assess glycaemic and insulinaemic responses, Knapp *et al.* (2008) evaluated select carbohydrates varying widely in chemical composition and functionality for physiological properties that could impact health. Polydextrose, pullulan, RS, and xanthan gum demonstrated varying degrees of resistance to digestion in the small intestine, but all of them resulted in an attenuated postprandial glycaemic response when compared with maltodextrin. Polyols, RS, non-starch polysaccharides, and other oligosaccharides are usually referred to as low digestible carbohydrates (Marteau and Flourie, 2001), and health benefits could result from their inclusion in companion animal diets since they often have lower energy concentrations due to their decreased rate of small intestinal digestion and absorption (Knapp *et al.*, 2008).

20.4.2 Obesity and weight control

Obesity may be defined as a clinical state of excessive accumulation of body fat (Kil and Swanson, 2010). Considered one of the most important health concerns for humans, obesity is highly associated with type 2 diabetes mellitus, hypertension, hyperlipidaemia, and heart disease (Sikaris, 2004). But these concerns do not apply only to the human, since 50% of the dog and cat population in the United States is considered obese or overweight, caused mainly by excess energy intake relative to energy expenditure.

Major issues regarding weight management (or weight loss) using dietary fibre centre on the manipulation of a state of 'fullness' or the 'satiety effect'. Fahey *et al.* (2004) addressed this in their discussion of the effect of dietary fibre on increasing eating time, slowing gastric emptying, and decreasing serum insulin concentration. Also, the possibility that fibre might decrease food intake and nutrient absorption, increase rate of dietary thermogenesis, decrease food intake mediated by SCFA, and stimulate the release of peptides that modify eating behaviour were considered. Nevertheless, the authors found inconclusive evidence to support fibre as an essential dietary component in weight reduction programs.

Currently available diets in the market for dogs include high fibre – moderate protein or high protein – moderate fibre diets. Weber *et al.* (2007) hypothesised that both protein and fibre can influence satiety, and observed that a high protein – high fibre diet reduced voluntary food intake compared with a high protein or a high fibre diet fed separately. Similar results were observed by German *et al.* (2010), who observed faster and greater weight loss when animals were fed high protein – high fibre diets compared with high protein – medium fibre diets. These studies evaluated different fibre sources, so it is difficult to conclude precisely how fibres act on satiety mechanisms.

Bosch *et al.* (2009) evaluated the effect of fibre fermentability on physiological satiety-related metabolites and voluntary food intake. Even without treatment effects in postprandial plasma glucose, peptide YY, glucagon-like peptide-1, and ghrelin responses, dogs fed a high fermentable fibre diet (8.5% beet pulp + 2% inulin) tended to eat less than dogs fed a low fermentable fibre diet (8.5% cellulose). Diets containing highly fermentable fibres may contribute in a positive way to the weight management of dogs. Respondek *et al.* (2008), after feeding 1% scFOS to a group of obese dogs, observed a decrease in insulin resistance and an apparent modulation of the transcription of genes involved in fatty acid and glucose metabolism.

20.5 Strategies for incorporating fibre into companion animal diets

The optimal fibre concentration has yet to be established for companion animals. The concentration in diets will depend on food intake, energy density of the food, and animal energy requirements (Meyer and Kienzle, 1991). Diet matrix, too, will dictate, in part, how much supplemental fibre should be added to the diet. Since the review published in 2004 by Fahey *et al.*, a number of studies have been conducted to evaluate the impacts of dietary fibre in companion animal nutrition, but the upper limit of fibre that may be included remains unknown. Not all fibre sources produce the same physiological effects. According to Fahey *et al.* (2004), an ideal dietary fibre would provide good stool characteristics (i.e. amount excreted, score) without affecting nutrient digestibility significantly and would contain both insoluble and soluble fibre components in a desirable ratio (80:20 to 70:30).

Recommendations regarding use of dietary fibres with prebiotic effects are also inconclusive. However, indications of beneficial effects have been observed in recent studies. In dogs, beneficial microbiota modulation was observed when animals were fed dietary scFOS and inulin concentrations between 0.2 and 0.4%, whereas concentrations as high as 3% did not negatively impact digestion or faecal scores (Verlinden *et al.*, 2006; Barry *et al.*, 2009). In cats, a dietary concentration greater than 0.5% of scFOS or GOS was needed to increase butyrate concentration (Kanakupt *et al.*, 2011). Higher concentrations of inulin-OF (4%) are tolerable for cats (Barry *et al.*, 2010), but a decrease in stool quality was observed with 6% levels of oligofructose (Hesta *et al.*, 2001). Middelbos *et al.* (2007) and Bosch *et al.* (2008) demonstrated the prebiotic effect of beet pulp *in vitro* and *in vivo* as indicated by comparable production of SCFA for both beet pulp and FOS. Also, dogs fed a diet containing 2.5% beet pulp had increased faecal butyrate and *Bifidobacteria* spp. concentrations compared with dogs fed a diet containing 2.5% cellulose (Middelbos *et al.*, 2007).

20.6 Conclusion

Evidence of the benefits of dietary fibre inclusion in pet animal nutrition has been established, but further research will reveal the full potential of the many dietary fibre ingredients that exist in the marketplace. Consideration of how to include these carbohydrates in select diet matrices must be carefully evaluated, since different dietary fibres vary in their physiological effects. Not all work well in all diets. Development of knowledge of optimal dietary fibre concentrations, the roles of novel carbohydrates, the activities of prebiotic fibres, and the potential health and behavioural benefits of dietary fibre, broadly defined, would allow the nutritionist to develop diets for companion animals to achieve optimal health and well-being. It is clear from the lack of studies published in this area that the role of dietary fibre in feline nutrition still needs to be established.

20.7 References

ANDERSON, J.W., BAIRD, P., DAVIS, R.H., JR, FERRERI, S., KNUDTSON, M., *et al.*, 2009. Health benefits of dietary fiber. *Nutrition Reviews*, **67**(4), pp. 188–205.

BARRY, K.A., HERNOT, D.C., MIDDELBOS, I.S., FRANCIS, C., DUNSFORD, B., *et al.*, 2009. Low-level fructan supplementation of dogs enhances nutrient digestion and modifies stool metabolite concentrations, but does not alter fecal microbiota populations. *Journal of Animal Science*, **87**(10), pp. 3244–52.

BARRY, K.A., WOJCICKI, B.J., MIDDELBOS, I.S., VESTER, B.M., SWANSON, K.S. and FAHEY, G.C., JR., 2010. Dietary cellulose, fructooligosaccharides, and pectin modify fecal protein catabolites and microbial populations in adult cats. *Journal of Animal Science*, **88**(9), pp. 2978–87.

BIAGI, G., CIPOLLINI, I. and ZAGHINI, G., 2008. In vitro fermentation of different sources of soluble fiber by dog faecal inoculum. *Veterinary Research Communications*, **32** (Suppl 1), pp. S335–S337.

BOSCH, G., PELLIKAAN, W.F., RUTTEN, P.G., VAN DER POEL, A.F., VERSTEGEN, M.W. and HENDRIKS, W.H., 2008. Comparative in vitro fermentation activity in the canine distal gastrointestinal tract and fermentation kinetics of fiber sources. *Journal of Animal Science*, **86**(11), pp. 2979–89.

BOSCH, G., VERBRUGGHE, A., HESTA, M., HOLST, J.J., VAN DER POEL, A.F., *et al.*, 2009. The effects of dietary fibre type on satiety-related hormones and voluntary food intake in dogs. *The British Journal of Nutrition*, **102**(2), pp. 318–25.

BUDDINGTON, R.K., 2001. The use of nondigestible oligosaccharides to manage the gastrointestinal ecosystem. *Microbial Ecology in Health and Disease*, **13**, pp. 9–15.

CUTRIGNELLI, M.I., BOVERA, F., TUDISCO, R., D'URSO, S., MARONO, S., *et al.*, 2009. In vitro fermentation characteristics of different carbohydrate sources in two dog breeds (German shepherd and Neapolitan mastiff). *Journal of Animal Physiology and Anïmal Nutrition*, **93**(3), pp. 305–12.

FABER, T.A. and FAHEY, G.C., JR, 2010. Animal, in vitro, and cell culture models to study the role of dietary fibers in the gastrointestinal tract of humans. In: T.M. PAESCHKE and W.R. AIMUTIS, eds, *Nondigestible Carbohydrates and Digestive Health*. Ames, IA: Blackwell Publishing and Institute of Food Technologists.

FABER, T.A., HOPKINS, A.C., MIDDELBOS, I.S., PRICE, N.P. and FAHEY, G.C., JR., 2011. Galactoglucomannan oligosaccharide supplementation affects nutrient digestibility, fermentation end-product production, and large bowel microbiota of the dog. *Journal of Animal Science*, **89**(1), pp. 103–12.

FAHEY, G.C., JR, FLICKINGER, E.A., GRIESHOP, C.M. and SWANSON, K.S., 2004. The role of dietary fibre in companion animal nutrition. In: VAN DER KAMP, J.W., ed., *Dietary Fibre: Bio-active Carbohydrates for Food and Feed*. Wageningen, the Netherlands: Wageningen Academic Publishers, pp. 295–328.

FULLER, R. and GIBSON, G.R., 1997. Modification of the intestinal microflora using probiotics and prebiotics. *Scandinavian Journal of Gastroenterology* (Supplement), **222**, pp. 28–31.

GAJDA, M., FLICKINGER, E.A., GRIESHOP, C.M., BAUER, L.L., MERCHEN, N.R. and FAHEY, G.C., JR, 2005. Corn hybrid affects in vitro and in vivo measures of nutrient digestibility in dogs. *Journal of Animal Science*, **83**(1), pp. 160–71.

GERMAN, A.J., HOLDEN, S.L., BISSOT, T., MORRIS, P.J. and BIOURGE, V., 2010. A high protein high fibre diet improves weight loss in obese dogs. *Veterinary Journal*, **183**(3), pp. 294–7.

GIBSON, G.R. and FULLER, R., 2000. Aspects of in vitro and in vivo research approaches directed toward identifying probiotics and prebiotics for human use. *The Journal of Nutrition*, **130**(2S Suppl), pp. 391S–395S.

GIBSON, G.R. and ROBERFROID, M.B., 1995. Dietary modulation of the human colonic microbiota: Introducing the concept of prebiotics. *The Journal of Nutrition*, **125**(6), pp. 1401–12.

GUEVARA, M.A., BAUER, L.L., ABBAS, C.A., BEERY, K.E., HOLZGRAEFE, D.P., *et al.*, 2008. Chemical composition, in vitro fermentation characteristics, and in vivo digestibility responses by dogs to select corn fibers. *Journal of Agricultural and Food Chemistry*, **56**(5), pp. 1619–26.

HERNOT, D.C., ORGUÉ, E., FAHEY, G.C., JR and RASTALL, R.A., 2008. Prebiotics and synbiotics in companion animal science. In: J. VERSALOVIC and M. WILSON, eds, *Therapeutic Microbiology; Probiotics and Related Strategies*. Washington, DC: ASM Press.

HESTA, M., JANSSENS, G.P., DEBRAEKELEER, J. and DE WILDE, R., 2001. The effect of oligofructose and inulin on faecal characteristics and nutrient digestibility in healthy cats. *Journal of Animal Physiology and Animal Nutrition*, **85**(5–6), pp. 135–41.

HESTA, M., HOORNAERT, E., VERLINDEN, A. and JANSSENS, G.P., 2005. The effect of oligofructose on urea metabolism and faecal odour components in cats. *Journal of Animal Physiology and Animal Nutrition*, **89**(3–6), pp. 208–14.

KANAKUPT, K., VESTER BOLER, B.M., DUNSFORD, B.R. and FAHEY, G.C., JR, 2011. Effects of short-chain fructooligosaccharides and galactooligosaccharides, individually and in combination, on nutrient digestibility, fecal fermentative metabolite concentrations, and large bowel microbial ecology of healthy adult cats. *Journal of Animal Science*, **89**(5), pp. 1376–84.

KIL, D.Y. and SWANSON, K.S., 2010. Endocrinology of obesity. *Veterinary Clinics of North America: Small Animal Practice*, **40**(2), pp. 205–19.

KNAPP, B.K., PARSONS, C.M., SWANSON, K.S. and FAHEY, G.C., JR, 2008. Physiological responses to novel carbohydrates as assessed using canine and avian models. *Journal of Agricultural and Food Chemistry*, **56**(17), pp. 7999–8006.

KRITCHEVSKY, D., 1988. Dietary fiber. *Annual Reviews of Nutrition*, **8**, pp. 301–28.

MARTEAU, P. and FLOURIE, B., 2001. Tolerance to low-digestible carbohydrates: Symptomatology and methods. *The British Journal of Nutrition*, **85** (Suppl 1), pp. S17–S21.

MEYER, H. and KIENZLE, E., 1991. Dietary protein and carbohydrates: Relationship to clinical disease. In: *Proceedings Purina International Symposium*, Orlando, FL, 1991, pp. 13–26.

MIDDELBOS, I.S., FASTINGER, N.D. and FAHEY, G.C., JR, 2007. Evaluation of fermentable oligosaccharides in diets fed to dogs in comparison to fiber standards. *Journal of Animal Science*, **85**(11), pp. 3033–44.

MURPHY, O., 2001. Non-polyol low-digestible carbohydrates: Food applications and functional benefits. *The British Journal of Nutrition*, **85** (Suppl 1), pp. S47–S53.

RESPONDEK, F., SWANSON, K.S., BELSITO, K.R., VESTER, B.M., WAGNER, A., *et al.*, 2008. Short-chain fructooligosaccharides influence insulin sensitivity and gene expression of fat tissue in obese dogs. *The Journal of Nutrition*, **138**(9), pp. 1712–18.

ROBERFROID, M.B., 1998. Prebiotics and synbiotics: concepts and nutritional properties. *The British Journal of Nutrition*, **80**(4), pp. 197–202.

SHIMOYAMA, Y., KUSANO, M., KAWAMURA, O., ZAI, H., KURIBAYASHI, S., *et al.*, 2007. High-viscosity liquid meal accelerates gastric emptying. *Neurogastroenterology and Motility: The Official Journal of the European Gastrointestinal Motility Society*, **19**(11), pp. 879–86.

SIKARIS, K.A., 2004. The clinical biochemistry of obesity. *The Clinical Biochemist Reviews*, **25**(3), pp. 170–81.

SPEARS, J.K., KARR-LILIENTHAL, L.K., GRIESHOP, C.M., FLICKINGER, E.A., WOLF, B.W. and FAHEY, G.C., JR, 2005. Pullulans and gamma-cyclodextrin affect apparent digestibility and metabolism in healthy adult ileal cannulated dogs. *The Journal of Nutrition*, **135**(8), pp. 1946–52.

SWANSON, K.S. and FAHEY, G.C., JR, 2006. Prebiotic impacts on companion animals. In: G.R. GIBSON and R.A. RASTALL, eds, *Prebiotics: Development and Application*. West Sussex, UK: John Wiley & Sons.

VERLINDEN, A., HESTA, M., HERMANS, J.M. and JANSSENS, G.P., 2006. The effects of inulin supplementation of diets with or without hydrolysed protein sources on digestibility, faecal characteristics, haematology and immunoglobulins in dogs. *The British Journal of Nutrition*, **96**(5), pp. 936–44.

VESTER, B.M. and FAHEY, G.C., JR, 2010. Prebiotics and probiotics in companion animal nutrition. In: S. CHO and E.T. FINOCCHIARO, eds, *Handbook of Prebiotics and Probiotics Ingredients: Health Benefits and Food Applications*. Washington, DC: CRC Press.

WEBER, M., BISSOT, T., SERVET, E., SERGHERAERT, R., BIOURGE, V. and GERMAN, A.J., 2007. A high-protein, high-fiber diet designed for weight loss improves satiety in dogs. *Journal of Veterinary Internal Medicine / American College of Veterinary Internal Medicine*, **21**(6), pp. 1203–8.

ZENTEK, J., 1996. Cellulose, pectins, and guar gum as fiber sources in canine diets. *Journal of Animal Physiology and Animal Nutrition*, **75**, pp. 36–45.

21

Soluble and insoluble fibre in infant nutrition

G. Boehm, Danone Research, Centre for Specialised Nutrition, Germany

DOI: 10.1533/9780857095787.4.421

Abstract: Dietary fibre recommendations currently exclude infants of less than 1 year. Dietary fibre intake studies have previously excluded non-digestible carbohydrates from human milk and the prebiotics used to replace them in infant formulas, and have focused on plant fibres deriving from weaning foods. However, they can be fermented by intestinal microbiota, contribute to changes in intestinal microbiota, and influence stool consistency. The intestinal microbiota interact with different cells in the intestine, and contribute to postnatal development and the immune system. Direct interactions with glycan structures on the cellular surface of the intestine have also been observed, and there is increasing evidence that these interactions have long-lasting effects. Thus, non-digestible carbohydrates could offer protection against immune-mediated diseases and metabolic disturbances later in life.

Key words: dietary fibre, infant nutrition, non-digestible carbohydrates, intestinal microbiota, glycan, human milk, prebiotic.

21.1 Introduction

Recommendations for dietary fibre in childhood commonly exclude infants of less than 1 year,[1–3] mainly due to a lack of information on the physiological effects and health benefits of dietary fibre in infancy, particularly compared with that available for adolescents and the elderly.[4–6] As a result, most recommendations are based on data obtained from adults, measured on the basis of body weight, age or energy intake.[7,8] These approaches do not give sufficient consideration to the enormous structural and functional developmental changes that occur in the gastrointestinal tract during the first year,[9,10] which may cause the physiological functions of dietary fibre to be different from those seen later in life. This is particularly relevant with regard to the specific impact of dietary fibre on the development of the intestinal microbiota after birth.[11,12]

One factor that leads to confusion in the discussion of dietary fibre in infancy is the definition of fibre itself. In 1972, Trowell published the first definition of fibre as 'that proportion of food which is derived from the cellular walls of plants which is digested very poorly by human beings'.[13] At that stage, it was mainly non-starch polysaccharides (NSPs) and lignin that were considered as sources of fibre. Over the next two decades the definition expanded to include a whole range of non-digestible carbohydrates other than NSP, such as resistant starch, fructo-oligosaccharides (FOS), galacto-oligosaccharides (GOS) and some synthetic non-digestible carbohydrates.[14,15] Since these substances can reach the colon and can be fermented by the colonic microbiota, many of them have been introduced into dietary products due to their prebiotic effect. Although they are usually called prebiotics, they also fulfil the criteria of the new definition of fibre.

During the first month, the natural diet for infants is breast milk. It has been known for more than a century that breast-fed infants develop intestinal microbiota dominated by bifidobacteria.[16] In the 1950s, human milk oligosaccharides (HMOS) were identified as an important growth factor for intestinal microbiota.[17] The development of new analytical techniques[18–21] has led to the identification of several new complex HMOS structures.[18–22] Modern microbiological techniques[11,23] have also offered insights into the role of HMOS in the metabolism of intestinal microbiota.[24] Over the past two decades, an increasing amount of evidence has revealed that the intestinal microbiota interact strongly with the intestinal tissue.[25] This interaction plays an important role in the postnatal development of the intestinal tract, the regulation and stimulation of the immune system, and the metabolic regulation of the growing infant.[26–30] HMOS can also act as receptor analogues for filaments of pathogenic bacteria, preventing the adhesion of these bacteria onto the intestinal epithelial surface. Since that adhesion is the first stage of bacterial infection, they can thus be said to provide an anti-infective effect.

Glycoconjugates play an important role as parts of signalling molecules on the surface of the epithelial, dendritic and neuronal cells of the intestine. Since HMOS share a number of features with these glycoconjugates, the two cell types can directly interact, and the HMOS can affect the functions of the glycoconjugates. Although the structural–functional relationship is still poorly understood, it is most likely that the specific nature of this interaction is one reason for the great structural variety of HMOS. The structural and functional aspects of HMOS and prebiotic oligosaccharides of non-milk origin have been intensively reviewed by Bode,[31] Vos *et al.*,[32] Boehm and Moro,[33] and most recently by a Task Force of The Institute of Life Sciences.[34]

The complex structures of HMOS have made them difficult to synthesize for the development of dietary products. They are similar in some respects to the oligosaccharides found in the milk of domestic animals, but human milk contains up to 100 times as many oligosaccharides as animal milk.[19,20] As a consequence, several carbohydrate structures of non-milk origin with the potential to at least partially mimic HMOS functions are currently being investigated.[34,35]

In the most relevant studies of dietary intake during infancy, HMOS and the prebiotics used as a substitute in infant formulas were not considered to be fibre and were consequently excluded from the data analysis,[36–39] with only fibre derived from weaning food taken as relevant.[37] When solid food is introduced into an infant's diet, the morphological and functional development of the gastrointestinal tract and intestinal microbiota are not yet complete. Since dietary fibre deriving from weaning foods can also be fermented by intestinal microbiota, this type of fibre does contribute to the transition of the intestinal microbiota towards the composition seen in adults, and also exerts several other effects traditionally referred to as fibre effects, such as influencing stool consistency.[4,5]

This chapter considers the HMOS and their prebiotic substitutes of non-milk origin as soluble fibres, along with the dietary fibre derived from weaning foods. Their physiological functions will be discussed, with particular focus on the developmental aspects of the gastrointestinal tract, the intestinal microbiota, and the immune system during the first year. Since there is increasing evidence that diet during infancy has an impact on metabolic and immune programming, the possible effects of dietary fibre intake during infancy on health in later life will also be briefly discussed.

21.2 Non-digestible carbohydrates in human milk

The main carbohydrate in human milk is lactose, which provides approximately 50% of the total energy consumed by the infant. In addition, human milk also contains up to 1.2 g per litre of complex carbohydrates, commonly referred to as HMOS. The term 'oligosaccharides' reflects the fact that these substances were initially discovered only as very small molecules.[17] In 1980, the Joint Commission on Biochemical Nomenclature (JCBN) defined oligosaccharides as carbohydrates with a degree of polymerization of up to 10,[40] but advances in analytical techniques have led to the detection of structures with over 50 monomers.[18–22,41] In 1990, the British Nutrition Foundation defined the limit between oligosaccharides and polysaccharides at a degree of polymerization of 20;[42] however, since there is no physiological reason for the definition to be based on a specific degree of polymerization, in 1997 the JCBN came to the conclusion that no definitive distinction between oligosaccharides and polysaccharides can be drawn. It has been concluded that the term 'oligosaccharides' should be used for clearly defined structures, whereas the term 'polysaccharides' should refer to polymers of unspecified length.[43]

21.2.1 Structure of non-digestible carbohydrates in human milk

The structure of HMOS is very complex: they have a core structure carrying lactose (Lac) at the reducing end, which is glycosidically bonded to lacto-N-biose units (Galβ1–3GlcNAc) in type 1 structures or to lactosamine structures (Galβ1–4GlcNAc) in type 2 structures. The monomers are either β1,3-linked, resulting in elongated linear structures, or β1,6-linked, building branched oligosaccharides. Various fucosyltransferases and sialyltransferases link these core structures to fucose (α1–2, α1–4, or α1–6 linkages) and to sialic acid (N-acetyl neuraminic acid) (α2–3 or α2–6 linkages) at different positions in the core molecule.[18–22]

The milk of domestic animals also contains oligosaccharides, but, in comparison to human milk, the concentrations of oligosaccharides in these milks are much lower and their structure is less complex.[23,24] However, the β-glycosidically bonded galactose is also characteristic of many of these oligosaccharides, protecting them – like HMOS – from digestion during passage through the human intestine. In contrast to HMOS, though, linkages to fucose are very rare, and linkages of galactose and N-acetylglucosamine are dominant. The exact structure and nature of the linkages vary between species. The oligosaccharides found in the milk of domestic animals are extensively reviewed by Urashima *et al.*[20] Based on the structure of these oligosaccharides, it can be assumed that they can also provide functional benefits in humans. However, the isolation of these compounds is difficult, and large-scale preparations have therefore not been commercially available as yet. Consequently, no human clinical trial has been published to date using fractions of animal milk oligosaccharides.

Little is known about the effect of the maternal diet on the expression of oligosaccharide structures in human milk. Since these structures are effectively absent from a normal adult diet, and are poorly absorbed, they are wholly synthesized by the breast tissue.[20] The genetic background of the lactating mother therefore plays an important role in the composition of the HMOS in any one individual. Several studies have been carried out on the effect of the secretor status (based on the Lewis blood groups) of the mother and the composition of the HMOS fractions,[22,44,45] with significant variation observed between individuals. In addition, significant qualitative and quantitative changes can be observed over the period of lactation.[22,46]

21.2.2 Functions of non-digestible carbohydrates from human milk

The physiological consequences of the broad variation between individuals are not yet fully understood. However, there is increasing evidence that HMOS provide a wide spectrum of specific biological functions to the developing infant, which might explain the high number of different structures in the HMOS fraction.

Prebiotic function

In the human intestine, there are no enzymes able to digest HMOS.[47] They can pass through the small intestine and reach the colon as intact molecules; the new definition means that they are therefore considered to be fibres. Since the closure of the gut is not complete,[48] a small portion can be absorbed[49] and is excreted by the kidneys.[50] Several intestinal microorganisms are able to metabolize HMOS,[51–56] indicating that one part of their function is to stimulate the selective growth of beneficial colonic bacteria.[11,12] In fact, the intestinal microbiota of breast-fed infants differ significantly from those of formula-fed infants.[23]

The selective fermentation of HMOS by the colonic microbiota not only results in the characteristic composition of intestinal microbiota in breast-fed infants but is also accompanied by low faecal pH and a specific short chain fatty acid (SCFA) pattern. The faecal SCFA are characterized by a high proportion of acetate (87%), while propionate (11%) and butyrate (2%) can also be detected.[57,58] *In vitro*, the SCFA and low pH depress the growth of several pathogens,[59] as well as specifically stimulating the synthesis of Mucin 2, which in turn influences the protective effect of the intestinal epithelium.[60] These *in vitro* data are in line with the observation that infants with low faecal pH and the SCFA pattern described above have reduced numbers of faecal pathogens.[33]

In summary, there is evidence that human milk is an important source of prebiotic compounds, which play a crucial role in the development of intestinal microbiota after birth. Since evidence also shows that the intestinal microbiota play a key role in the postnatal development of the immune system of the infant, breast feeding is considered to be the best protection against infection and immune-related diseases.[61–72]

Interactions with glycoconjugates on biological surfaces

Since glycoconjugates are very important components of the surface structures of human cells, bacterial ligands and several toxic substances, it can be hypothesized that HMOS with a similar structure can directly interact with the respective surface structures. Acidic HMOS might play a particularly important role in this function of HMOS.

One aspect of these interactions is the role of HMOS as receptor analogues for pathogens. The structure of several ligands of pathogens (both bacteria and viruses) and pathogenic substances consist of glycol structures which are also found in the HMOS fraction.[19,20] There is evidence that these structures act as receptor analogues that compete with the ligands on the surface of the intestine, thereby preventing the adhesion of the pathogens on the epithelial surface. Since the adhesion of these pathogens is the first important step of the infection cascade, its prevention results in protection against intestinal infection. In fact, this type of anti-adhesion effect has been demonstrated for clinically relevant pathogens such as *Streptococcus pneumoniae*,[73] different strains of enteropathogenic *Escherichia coli*[74] and their toxins,[75] *Campylobacter jejuni*[76,77] and *Helicobacter pylori*,[78] and is considered an important part of the anti-infective and protective function of breast feeding.[63,73,74] There are many different target structures,[20] which might in part explain the great variation observed in HMOS structures.

The structural analogy between HMOS and glycoconjugates on cellular surfaces is probably the basis for direct interactions with intestinal and immune cells. Such direct interactions have been described for oligosaccharide-specific induction of inflammatory cytokines in schistosoma-infected mice,[79,80] binding of selectins,[81] dendritic cell-specific C-type lectin,[82] integrins[83] and Toll-like receptors.[34] In an *in vitro* study with separated white blood cells from cord blood, incubation with HMOS separated from human milk samples[84,85] resulted in a decrease of regulatory T cells.[86] In this experiment, the acidic fraction of HMOS was more effective than the neutral fraction, indicating that acidic HMOS has a specific role to play in direct interactions with immune cells.[87]

In addition, initial results from data analysis indicate that HMOS are part of the ingredient set that promotes mineral absorption, influences lipid metabolism, and might be important for the supply of amino acids like lysine and for optimal brain development.[88–90] These properties are partially linked to their prebiotic effect, but early indications suggest that direct interactions with epithelial cells also play a role. The latter hypothesis is mainly based on animal experiments or human data in adults.[34] Further research is therefore required to prove this fascinating hypothesis of direct functional influence of HMOS on different cell types during infancy.[19,21,31]

In summary, a number of questions still remain regarding the relationship between the structure of oligosaccharides and their biological function. Further research is needed in the future in order to identify which structural elements in HMOS are most important for their function.

21.3 Soluble non-digestible carbohydrates of non-human milk origin

The complexity of the structure of HMOS has so far made it impossible to produce identical structures for inclusion in infant formulas. The structure of the oligosaccharides found in the milk of domestic animals indicates that they might at least partially mimic the functions of HMOS, being able to act as prebiotics, and possibly also to directly interact with immune and epithelial cells, as extensively reviewed by Urashima *et al.*[20] However, isolating these oligosaccharides from milk or milk products requires extensive technological effort; thus none of these substances has so far been used as a component of commercially available infant formulas.

There has consequently been a great deal of research carried out with the aim of identifying non-milk substances that might at least exert a prebiotic function. Such substances can be found in bacteria, fungi and plants, can be derived from the hydrolysis of natural polymers by enzymatic cleavage and can be synthesized from monomers or small oligosaccharides. As mentioned above for HMOS, the term oligosaccharides is used for defined structures independent of molecular size, whereas the term polymers is used for structures of unspecified length.[40]

21.3.1 Structure of non-digestible carbohydrates of non-human milk origin

The use of prebiotics was not initially designed for infants, as the first data were obtained in adults and the elderly.[34,91,92] The selection of structures with prebiotic effects was mainly based on two factors: resistance against intraluminal digestion, or at least low digestibility during passage through the small intestine; and selective metabolization by the beneficial intestinal microbiota, like that observed in HMOS.[93–102] In the early 1990s, when the prebiotic concept was adapted for use in infant nutrition, prebiotic substances already identified in previous studies on adult nutrition were considered and tested for use in infancy.[35,103] More recently, acidic oligosaccharides deriving from the degradation of pectin (pectin-derived

Table 21.1 Soluble non-digestible carbohydrates tested for prebiotic effects in human infants

Ingredient	Source	Studies in infants	No. of tested infants
GOS	Enzymatic synthesis from lactose	2	112
FOS /inulin	Extraction from natural sources	11	714
Lactosucrose	Enzymatic synthesis from sucrose	2	18
GOS + lactosucrose		1	150
scFOS + inulin		1	20
GOS + lcFOS		20	1511
GOS + lcFOS + pAOS		4	548

Notes: OS, oligosaccharides; GOS, galacto-oligosaccharides; FOS, fructo-oligosaccharides; pAOS, pectin-derived acidic oligosaccharides; lc, long chain; sc, short chain.

acidic oligosaccharides, pAOS) have been investigated as new soluble fibres.[32,34,87,103,104] These oligosaccharides have been specifically developed for infants on the basis of the use of carrot soup as a traditional dietary treatment for diarrhoea.[105] Table 21.1 shows the available non-digestible oligosaccharides which have demonstrated prebiotic effects in infants.

The most extensively studied prebiotic oligosaccharides in humans are GOS and inulin/FOS.[34–36] There is a consensus that both of these exert prebiotic effects in humans at every stage of life. In infancy, a specific mixture consisting of 90% GOS and 10% long chain FOS (lcFOS) at a concentration of up to 0.8 g/100 ml is the only prebiotic ingredient included in the EU directive for compounds in infant formulas.[106]

The inulin-type fructans are linear or branched fructose polymers, which are either β2–1-linked inulins or β2–6-linked levans (Table 21.1).[107] They can easily be extracted from plant sources and have been widely used as ingredients in dietary products. In their natural state, the size of the molecule varies significantly (from a polymerization degree of 2 to over 60). Because biological activity varies according to molecule size,[97,98] they are separated from natural inulin divided into short chain FOS (scFOS) with a degree of polymerization of up to 10 monomers, and lcFOS with a degree of polymerization above 10 monomers.

GOS are synthesized from lactose via enzymatic transgalactosylation using a β-galactosidase of mainly bacterial origin.[108] These GOS consist of a chain of galactose monomers, usually with a glucose monomer on the reducing terminus. The degree of polymerization is up to 10 monomers. In some studies they are defined as short chain GOS, but this term is used inconsistently used: in practice, GOS and scGOS can be considered to be synonymous.

21.3.2 Functions of non-digestible carbohydrates of non-human milk origin

In vitro experiments demonstrate that intestinal bacteria can metabolize several sugar structures, and, provided that they can pass the small intestine undigested, they can theoretically be used as prebiotic ingredients.[51–56] There is some initial evidence to suggest that they, like HMOS, might also adhere to the cellular surface, resulting in direct cellular responses.[32,60,86,87]

Prebiotic function

As it is widely accepted that the intestinal microbiota play an important physiological role in the host, a number of attempts have been made to influence the intestinal microbiota through dietary intervention.[11,33,34,91,92] As mentioned above, the composition of the intestinal microbiota of breast-fed infants differs significantly from that found in formula-fed infants. There is strong evidence that the intestinal microbiota that develop during breast feeding support a healthy postnatal development of the infant.[33,34] The aim of adding prebiotic ingredients in infant formula is therefore to make the intestinal microbiota of formula-fed infants closer to those found in breast-fed infants.

In principle there are two major strategies that can be used to influence the intestinal microbiota. One is the use of living bacteria added to food, which must survive the gastrointestinal tract to be active in the colon: these are known as probiotics.[109] The second strategy is the use of dietary ingredients that are non-digestible, reach the colon and can be used by health-promoting colonic bacteria: it is these that are known as prebiotics.[91]

During the past decade, significant advances in microbiological methods have provided important insights into the physiology of the microbiota and their contribution to the functionality of the host.[11] Based on these insights, the first approach to prebiotics, published in 1995, has recently been updated.[92] The authors conclude that prebiotics have to be resistant until they are fermented by the intestinal (i.e. not only colonic) microbiota. The balanced stimulation of growth and/or activity of the health-promoting microbiota in the gastrointestinal tract is only useful if changes in the composition of the intestinal microbiota provide any health benefit for the infant.[92]

There is evidence that different microbiota metabolize specific prebiotic structures, indicating that the effect of a prebiotic compound (whether a single ingredient or a mixture) is dependent on its structure, the quantity reaching the colon and the existing composition of the colonic microbiota. The prebiotic effect must therefore be demonstrated for all new ingredients, mixtures and dosages.[106] To date, the results of a number of clinical studies in infants have been published, using GOS,[110,111] scFOS,[112–121] inulin,[122,123] lactulose,[124,125] a mixture of GOS/lactulose,[126] a mixture of scFOS/inulin,[127] a mixture of GOS/lcFOS[128–158] and a mixture of GOS/lcFOS/pAOS[159–162] as the prebiotic compound (see Table 21.2).

The faecal bifidobacteria count and the percentage of total bacteria composed of faecal bifidobacteria are the generally accepted markers of a prebiotic effect. However, for a compound to be definitively classified as a prebiotic, it must demonstrate resistance to intestinal digestion and absorption, fermentation by intestinal microbiota and the selective stimulation of growth and/or activities of intestinal microbiota beneficial to the health or well-being of the infant.[92]

Table 21.2 Clinical trials with prebiotic oligosaccharides in term infants (nutritional intervention during the first year of life)

Prebiotic	Duration of intervention	*N* (active)	Main outcome	Author
Part A: Supplementation with single prebiotic ingredients				
GOS	6 months	43	Increased counts of bifidobacteria and lactobacilli.	Yahiro *et al.*[110]
GOS	6 months	69	Increased counts of bifidobacteria and lactobacilli, decreased faecal pH.	Ben *et al.*[111]
scFOS	6–24 months	57	Increased counts of bifidobacteria after antibiotic treatment.	Brunser *et al.*[112]
scFOS	4–24 months	63	Decreased severity of diarrhoeal diseases (no microbiology).	Saarveeda *et al.*[113] Tschernis *et al.*[114]
scFOS	2–12 weeks	58	No clear effect on counts of bifidobacteria, softer stools (dose dependent).	Euler *et al.*[115]
scFOS	4–12 months	27	Softer stools, no effect on faecal pH (no microbiology).	Moore *et al.*[116]
scFOS	6–12 months	239	No influence on clinical course and incidence of diarrhoea, no effect on vaccination response (no microbiology).	Duggan *et al.*[117]
scFOS	6–24 months	10	Trend for higher counts of bifidobacteria and decrease in potential pathogens, no persistence after intervention.	Waligora-Dupriet *et al.*[118]
scFOS	6 weeks	36	Increased number of stools, no bifidogenic effect, no influence on faecal pH.	Guesry *et al.*[119]
scFOS	14 weeks	146	Safe and less complication (no microbiology).	Bettler and Euler[120]
scFOS	21 days	36	Increased counts of bifidobacteria within 1 week of intervention.	Kapiki *et al.*[121]
Inulin	5–24 weeks	14	Increased counts of bifidobacteria and lactobacilli.	Kim *et al.*[122]
Inulin	5–12 months	28	Tendency of increased short chain fatty acid production, significant influence on mineral absorption (no microbiology).	Yap *et al.*[123]
Lactulose	6 months	6	Increased counts of bifidobacteria, reduced faecal pH.	Nagendra *et al.*[124]
Lactulose	1–36 months	12	Increased counts of bifidobacteria, reduced allergic symptoms.	Rinne *et al.*[125]

(*Continued overleaf.*)

Table 21.2 (Continued)

Prebiotic	Duration of intervention	*N* (active)	Main outcome	Author
Part B: Supplementation with prebiotic mixtures				
GOS/Lactulose	6 months	150	Softer stools and increased stool frequency (no microbiology).	Ziegler *et al.*[126]
scFOS/inulin	12 months	24	Increased postvaccination IgG plasma levels (measles).	Firmansyah *et al.*[127]
GOS/lcFOS	3–20 weeks	20	Reduced hardness of stool (no microbiology).	Bongers *et al.*[128]
GOS/lcFOS	4 months	56	Increased counts of bifidobacteria and lactobacilli, decreased faecal pH, effect dose-dependent.	Moro *et al.*[129] Moro *et al.*[130]
GOS/lcFOS	6 months	28	Increased counts of bifidobacteria, softer stools.	Schmelze *et al.*[131]
GOS/lcFOS	6 months	21	Increased counts of bifidobacteria and lactobacilli, dominance of *B. infantis*, short chain fatty acid pattern like breast-fed infants.	Knol *et al.*[132] Haarman and Knol[133] Haarman and Knol[134]
GOS/lcFOS	1–12 weeks	34	Trend for higher counts of bifidobacteria, reduced counts of clostridia.	Costalos *et al.*[135]
GOS/lcFOS	9–12 months	604	Reduction of gastrointestinal problems (no microbiology).	Savino *et al.*[136]
GOS/lcFOS	9–12 months	55	Reduction of gastrointestinal problems (no microbiology).	Savino *et al.*[137]
GOS/lcFOS	4–12 months	10	Increased counts of bifidobacteria.	Scholtens *et al.*[138]
GOS/lcFOS	4 months	19	Reduced faecal pH, increased faecal short chain fatty acids, increased faecal sIgA; no significant higher counts of bifidobacteria compared with controls.	Bakker-Zierikzee *et al.*[139] Bakker-Zierikzee *et al.*[140]
GOS/lcFOS	6 months	102	Increased counts of bifidobacteria, reduced incidence of atopic dermatitis, reduced incidence of infections, anti-allergic serum antibodies.	Moro *et al.*[141] Arslanoglu *et al.*[142] Garssen *et al.*[143] Arslanoglu *et al.*[144] van Hoffen *et al.*[145]

GOS/lcFOS	26 weeks	86	Increased counts of bifidobacteria, increased faecal sIgA, no effect on plasma immune parameters, no effect on cholesterol absorption.	Alliet *et al.*[146] Scholtens *et al.*[147] Raes *et al.*[148]
GOS/lcFOS	12 weeks	14	Increased counts of bifidobacteria.	Desci *et al.*[149]
GOS/lcFOS	6 months	8	Increased counts of bifidobacteria, *Bifidobacterium* microbiota close to breast-fed infants.	Rinne *et al.*[150]
GOS/lcFOS	4 weeks	20	Increased counts of bifidobacteria and lactobacilli.	Penders *et al.*[151]
GOS/lcFOS	12 months	162	Decreased rates of infections (no microbiology).	Bruzzese *et al.*[152]
GOS/lcFOS	6 days	54	No treatment effect on acute diarrhoea.	Vaisman *et al.*[153]
GOS/lcFOS	2–12 weeks	77	Improved tolerance to oral feeding in very low birth weight infants.	Modi *et al.*[154]
GOS/lcFOS	21 days	15	Increasing counts of bifidobacteria, reduction of hardness of stools, reduction of counts of faecal pathogens.	Boehm *et al.*[155] Knol *et al.*[156]
GOS/lcFOS	21 days	10	Reduction of gastrointestinal transit time; reduction of stool viscosity (no microbiology).	Mihatsch *et al.*[157]
GOS/lcFOS	21 days	10	Statistically significant but small effect on reduction of gastric emptying time (no microbiology).	Indrio *et al.*[158]
GOS/lcFOS/pAOS	6 months	31	Increasing counts of bifidobacteria, decreased faecal pH.	Fanaro *et al.*[159]
GOS/lcFOS/pAOS	2 months	49	Increased counts of bifidobacteria and lactobacilli.	Magne *et al.*[160]
GOS/lcFOS/pAOS	32 days	54	Tendency for lower bacterial infection rate.	Westerbeek *et al.*[161]
GOS/lcFOS/pAOS	12 months	414	Reduction of cumulative incidence of atopic dermatitis during the first year of life.	Grüber *et al.*[162]

Notes: GOS, galacto-oligosaccharides; FOS, fructo-oligosaccharides; pAOS, acidic oligosaccharides deriving from pectin; lc, long chain; sc, short chain; IgA, Immunoglobin A; IgA, Immunogolbin G; slgA, Secrfetary Iga;

Low digestibility has been demonstrated for GOS and lcFOS through the detection of these two structures in the faeces of term infants fed with a formula supplemented with a mixture of both.[130] The fermentation of prebiotics has been demonstrated by analysing the faecal SCFA pattern and faecal pH, which was found to be reduced in infants fed GOS,[111] lactulose,[124] a specific mixture of GOS/lcFOS[129,132,139,141] and a mixture of GOS/lcFOS/pAOS.[159] In contrast, there are two studies that demonstrate that scFOS has no effect on faecal pH.[116,119] A SCFA pattern close to that found in breast-fed infants was observed in infants fed scFOS,[123] and a mixture of GOS/lcFOS also resulted in a similar pattern.[132,139] The similarity in the pH and SCFA pattern between breast-fed infants and those fed using a formula containing a specific mixture of GOS/lcFOS indicates that both diets selectively stimulate comparable or similar parts of the intestinal microbiota.[48,60] The selective stimulation of the growth of intestinal bacteria has also been demonstrated by analysing the composition of the faecal microbiota. Increased bifidobacteria counts have been found in infants fed GOS,[110,111] scFOS,[112,118,121] inulin,[122] lactulose,[125] a specific mixture of GOS/lcFOS[129,131–135,138,141,146,149–151,155] or a mixture of GOS/lcFOS/pAOS.[159,160] The stimulation of *Lactobacillus* microbiota was achieved with GOS,[110,111] a specific mixture of GOS/lcFOS,[129,132,134,151] and a mixture of GOS/lcFOS/pAOS.[160] In two studies with the specific mixture of GOS/lcFOS, the *Bifidobacterium* microbiota were very similar to those found in breast-fed infants.[132,133,150] A reduction in pathogenic bacteria was found in infants fed scFOS[118] or a specific mixture of GOS/lcFOS.[132,135,150]

There is some evidence to suggest that the specific stimulation of growth of a limited number of bacteria has clinical relevance, since early intestinal colonization with specific microbiota is thought to be associated with the development of allergic symptoms later in life. Bjorksten *et al.*[163] found that allergic infants in Estonia – a country with a low prevalence of allergies – were colonized by lactobacilli and bifidobacteria to a lesser extent than allergic infants in Sweden, which has a high prevalence of allergies. In contrast, the Estonian infants were more frequently colonized with aerobic pathogenic micro-organisms, particularly coliforms and *Staphylococcus aureus*, compared with the Swedish infants. It was also found that allergic infants had more adult-like species in their faecal flora, including *B. adolescentis*, compared with healthy infants, in whom *B. bifidum, B. infantis* and *B. breve* predominated.[164] Similar findings have also been reported in Japanese infants suffering from atopic dermatitis.[165] This suggests that different bacterial species may have different functional effects on the immunological reaction of the host. Specific modulation of the composition of the intestinal microbiota through the use of prebiotics is therefore expected to have an impact on the correct functioning of the immune system.

In summary, the bifidogenic effect during infancy has been demonstrated using different prebiotics but has been shown to be particularly effective with a specific mixture of GOS/lcFOS (ratio 9:1, maximal dosage 0.8 g/100 ml, corresponding to the concentration of neutral HMOS in mature breast milk). Due to the very complex composition of the intestinal microbiota, and considering the great variety of structures found in HMOS, it is possible that mixtures of different types of oligosaccharides and different chain lengths which are combined to meet the metabolic requirements of different bacteria will be better able to mimic the prebiotic effect of breast feeding than individual compounds.

Effect on intestinal physiology

The SCFA play an important role in the regulation of intestinal motility,[166,167] and *in vitro* data provide evidence that they interact with different intestinal cells. The influence of a specific mixture of GOS/lcFOS on intestinal motility has been measured in two studies in preterm infants. Infants fed a formula supplemented with these prebiotics had significantly faster gastric emptying time[158] and a significantly reduced gastrointestinal transit time[157] compared with infants fed a formula with a placebo. The data from the infants fed with prebiotic formula were similar to those observed in breast-fed infants. Feeding formula supplemented with prebiotics resulted in softer stools: this is documented for short fructo-oligosaccharide (sFOS),[115,119,120] a mixture of GOS/lactulose[126] and a specific mixture of GOS/lcFOS.[128,129,131,154,155,157,161] In a few studies, this was also accompanied by an increased number of stools per day, when GOS/lactulose[126] or a specific mixture of GOS/lcFOS[155] was used.

The effect of the prebiotics on the transit time and the viscosity of the stool results in better gastrointestinal tolerance of formula feeding. An improved tolerance (particularly fewer cases of constipation and gastrointestinal colic) has been described in infants fed on formula containing scFOS[120] and a mixture of GOS/lcFOS.[136,137,154,155] This effect could be of clinical relevance, particularly for preterm infants.[154,157,158]

There is evidence that prebiotics improve mineral absorption in adults.[168,169] This effect has been little studied in infants, with the exception of one small study in preterm infants using a mixture of GOS/lcFOS.[170] The results of this study do suggest that prebiotics have a positive effect in this regard, but the small sample number and the indirect nature of the measured parameter (namely the proportions of calcium/phosphorus in urine) do not allow any firm conclusion to be drawn.

Finally, SCFA have been shown *in vitro* to stimulate mucin 2 secretion and to improve intestinal barrier integrity,[60] indicating that they have the potential to influence the physiological role of intestinal cells. In combination with a pH of below 6, they slow the growth of several pathogens,[59] which could contribute to the anti-infective effect of prebiotics (see *Effect on immune system*).

Effect on immune system

In the first weeks/months of life, an infant's intestinal barrier is still not complete and the immune system is imbalanced, leading to the risk of developing allergies to food antigens.[171,172] The avoidance of food antigens early in life is therefore often recommended.[173,174] However, there is also evidence that early presentation of antigens might play an important role in stimulating the maturation of the mucosal immune system, causing increased tolerance to food antigens.[175,176] The intestinal microbiota also play an important role in the stimulation and maturation of the immune system.[26–30,177–179] Since soluble fibres contribute to the quantity and quality of the intestinal microbiota, prebiotics therefore influence the development of the immune system.[180]

The relationship between prebiotics and the immune system is very complex and not fully understood. The complexity of these relationships is a result of the fact that the intestinal microbiota consist of more than 800 species,[181] which might all play distinct individual roles in the stimulation of the immune system. Moreover, the immune system also consists of several different layers, which are affected differently by intestinal microbiota.[71,180] Ethical limitations make it practically impossible to perform clinical studies in humans to obtain insights into the mechanisms by which prebiotics affect the immune system. Studies in animals, particularly mice, are therefore used as an alternative,[182] but systematic data from animal studies are available only for the prebiotic mixture of scGOS and lcFOS.[32,33]

The effect of the mixture of scGOS/lcFOS on the vaccination response and the stimulation of Type 1 T helper cell (Th1) in mice has been investigated.[183] The animals were vaccinated against influenza, with a booster vaccination given 21 days after the first. Thirty days after the first vaccination, different parameters were measured to identify the response to the vaccination (ear swelling after local testing with the vaccine, plasma titres of specific antibodies, T-cell proliferation, cytokine production, natural killer cell activity, and *ex vivo* lymphocyte stimulation). All data demonstrated a modulation of the immune system towards Th1. Evidence from different studies has shown that the effect of the prebiotics on the immune function is mainly mediated by their influence on the intestinal microbiota,[183] which clearly indicates the significance of these data for humans.

In order to evaluate the possible influence of prebiotics on any allergic reaction, a mouse model has been developed using ovalbumin as an antigen.[184] After several inhalation tests (21, 24 and 27 days after first sensitization), the effect of dietary fibres on the allergic reaction was evaluated on the basis of several parameters (airway responsiveness, lymphocyte profile in bronchial lavage fluid, different antibody levels in plasma). All the data obtained from these experiments indicate that the specific prebiotic mixture reduces the allergic reaction to ovalbumin.[184,185]

The data from the animal experiments allow us to conclude that prebiotics are able to modulate the immune system, mainly through changes in the intestinal microbiota. Some data could also be interpreted as a direct effect of the studied prebiotics on intestinal immune cells,[32,87] but this hypothesis requires further investigation. Although the mechanisms by which the prebiotics carry out their function are not fully understood, the animal data lead to the conclusion that prebiotics might indeed have an impact on the prevention of infection and allergic diseases.

Following international recommendations,[182] several clinical trials have been performed on the basis of the data obtained from the animal experiments, and are discussed below. Since evidence from animal studies suggested that prebiotics might reduce the risk of the occurrence of allergic diseases and might stimulate defences against infection, the trials were designed to focus on these two clinical outcomes. As a secondary aim, attention was also paid to the immunological biomarkers which might be useful in evaluating the impact of prebiotics on the immune system.

The first study to measure clinical outcomes was performed in a cohort of 210 infants at risk of developing allergies, assessed on the basis of family history. The infants were randomized and fed a hypoallergenic cow's milk formula (the cow's milk protein was extensively hydrolysed to avoid antigen overload) supplemented with either 0.8 g scGOS/lcFOS (ratio: 9.1) or the same quantity of maltodextrin as a placebo. After six months, the first allergic symptom – atopic dermatitis – was significantly lower in the group fed the prebiotic formula than in the group fed the placebo formula.[141] This effect was accompanied by a reduction in some infectious episodes.[144] Both the reduction in the allergic symptoms and the reduction of the infection rate support the hypothesis that the animal data are indeed relevant to humans. The cohort was followed up to the age of 5, and the effect was observed over the whole period even though supplementation was halted after 6 months. This indicates that the effects of intestinal microbiota on the immune system established during the first few months remain relatively stable over a longer period: this observation is also supported by other studies.[163–165]

The effect of the prebiotic mixture scGOS/lcFOS (0.4 g/100 ml formula) on the occurrence of infectious episodes during the first year was studied in a cohort of healthy infants. The concentration of prebiotics in this study was only half of that used in previous studies to obtain a reduced rate of infectious episodes during the first year.[152]

More recently, the specific mixture scGOS/lcFOS was enhanced using acidic oligosaccharides derived from pectin degradation.[153] These pectin-derived oligosaccharides have an acidic load, enabling these molecules to adhere to the epithelial surface as first described by Guggenbichler *et al.*[104] This therefore suggests that they inhibit the adherence of pathogens, thereby directly reducing the risk of infection, in addition to their prebiotic effect.[159,160] In fact, a study of preterm infants fed this mixture (80% scGOS/lcFOS + 20% pAOS) resulted in a generally lower infection rate.[161] In a large multicentre trial, approximately 1200 healthy term infants without familial risk of developing allergies were fed the same prebiotic mixture, resulting in a reduction of the cumulative incidence of infection from 11.2% to 6.5% after 1 year of observation.[162] These results clearly provide support for the data observed in the study of infants considered at risk of developing allergies.

A challenge facing all clinical studies is that, due to the complexity of the immune system, it has no single biomarker. Several different markers of the immune system must therefore be taken into account. A group of experts recently classified the biomarkers for immune modulation into three categories: high, medium and low suitability.[186] Vaccine-specific serum antibody production, vaccine-specific or total secretory IgA and the response to attenuated pathogens were all classified as markers with high suitability. Markers with medium suitability were judged to include natural killer cell cytotoxicity, oxidative burst of phagocytes, lymphocyte proliferation and the assessment of the cytokine pattern produced by activated immune cells. Since no single marker allows firm conclusions to be drawn about the modulation of the whole immune system, combining markers with high and medium suitability is currently the best approach for the measurement of immune modulation in human nutrition intervention studies. Most recently, results from animal tests and initial human studies have indicated that immunoglobulin-free light chains are involved in triggering the allergic process[187,188] and might be suitable as a sensitive biomarker of the immune system in infants.[189]

As outlined in Table 21.2, several of these biomarkers have been investigated with inconsistent results. In healthy infants without risk of developing allergies, many of the described biomarkers remain unchanged during exposure to prebiotics,[148,190] which might indicate that a normal and balanced immune system cannot be further 'improved'. On the other hand, the stability of the immune system against prebiotics can be seen as an argument in favour of the safety of prebiotics.[34,148]

In summary, the data clearly indicate that soluble fibres acting as prebiotics can positively influence the postnatal development of the immune system and can contribute to better health during infancy. Epidemiological data indicate that this positive influence exerted by prebiotics on the immune system will have long-term consequences.[163–165] Prebiotics may therefore be included among the recommended strategies to prevent immune-mediated diseases later in life.

21.4 Insoluble non-digestible carbohydrates

Dietary fibres are traditionally defined as a portion of plant material that human gastrointestinal enzymes cannot digest. They consist of polysaccharides, which are structural[191] or storage components[192] of the plant cell wall. Some disperse in water and appear as soluble fibres, but the majority of plant cell polysaccharides constitute insoluble fibres. In its natural form, plant material contains a mixture of soluble and insoluble fibres. In the following sections of the chapter, the main plant structures and their possible physiological functions during infancy will be explained.

21.4.1 Structure and functions of insoluble non-digestible carbohydrates

A wide range of complex polysaccharide compounds make up the structural or storage components of the plant cell wall. During the division of plant cells, a pectin-rich membrane is built. On the inner surface the primary cell wall develops, which consists mainly of celluloses, hemicelluloses and pectins. The external secondary cell wall is composed of different layers of celluloses and hemicelluloses, and a small part is based on pectins. The secondary cell wall is also stabilized by the incorporation of lignin.[193]

Celluloses consist of approximately 150 unbranched helical structured polymers formed by 2000–8000 (1–4)-linked β-D-glucose units. Hemicelluloses of the xylan type vary significantly according to the botanical source. Their structures are based on (β1–4)-linked xylose monomers. Hemicelluloses of the xyloglucan type consist of cellulose-like backbones, but up to 75% of the glucose residues are substituted by (1–6)-linked β-D-xylose monomers. Pectic polysaccharides consist of galacturonic acid and rhamnose main chains with side chains containing arabinose, galactose and some other monomers in lower quantities. In general, the cell walls of growing dicotyledon plants consist of approximately 30% celluloses, 25% xyloglucans, 5% glucans, 15% homogalacturonans, 15% rhamnogalacturonans, and 5% glycoproteins.[193]

During the weaning period, the infant mainly receives fibres from bran flakes, precooked cereal grains, leafy green vegetables and legumes, and fruits.[37] The weaning diet therefore provides the infant's gastrointestinal tract with a very complex pattern of insoluble fibres.

One important aspect of the possible functions of dietary fibres is their fermentability by intestinal microbiota. The complexity of the structure and the molecule size define the rate of metabolization by the intestinal microbiota. The part that can be fermented has physiological consequences similar to those described for the soluble oligosaccharides. The remaining non-fermented part plays a role in determining the viscosity of the intestinal intra-luminal phase and is responsible for stool bulking. Since the fermentation by intestinal microbiota has a significant effect on the physiological role played by dietary fibres, the soluble and insoluble fractions of plant fibres are linked even though their dietary effects are different.

During breast feeding, the infant has no dietary intake of plant material. In developed countries, the introduction of weaning food begins at the age of 4 to 6 months. The World Health Organization recommends breast feeding for the first 6 months.[3] After the period of exclusive breast milk or milk formula feeding, the infant's diet changes and begins to more closely resemble the usual diet of the family. During weaning, plant material from different sources is introduced into the infant's diet. Although human clinical trials exist that focus on soluble fibres with prebiotic effects in infants, there have been no equivalent clinical trials studying the physiological effects of insoluble fibres during the weaning period. No valid data, therefore, exist regarding any specific function of insoluble fibres during the first year.

However, the data from studies relating to later stages of life demonstrate the impact of these insoluble fibres on intestinal physiology and health; these findings might also prove relevant for infants. There is increasing evidence that specific plant polysaccharide structures might be able to modulate the immune system.[194] However, in animal studies, no immune modulator effect could be observed when a mixture of unchanged dietary fibres was used.[32] Links have also been found between the consumption of insoluble fibres and a lower risk of cardiovascular diseases and diabetes, and improved gastrointestinal health and weight control.[4] Since these data are not obtained during the first year, no definitive conclusion can be drawn from these data with regard to the effect of insoluble dietary fibre in infants. However, the results should encourage further research in the area, since the impact of early feeding on long-term health effects is evident.[195]

21.4.2 Dietary recommendations for insoluble non-digestible carbohydrates in infants

Although intervention studies of soluble fibre in human infants have been published, no similar studies exist for insoluble fibre. Dietary recommendations are therefore necessarily based on a small number of epidemiological studies and not on conclusive intervention studies in the target group. Even then, there is a limited amount of epidemiological data available about the intake of dietary fibres during the first year. The most commonly used method to estimate the intake of dietary fibres is based on a 3-day record of a weighed diet. The calculation of the individual nutrients is performed on the basis of a calculation using nutrient databases. These data, therefore, allow no conclusion to be drawn regarding specific polysaccharide structures.

In a German cohort study based on 537 observed infants, the overall intake of dietary fibre increased from 6 months to 12 months (4.45 ± 2.92 g/day vs. 8.88 ± 2.86 g/day or 0.58 ± 0.38 g/kg x day vs. 1.01 ± 0.33 g/kg x day, respectively). Oligosaccharides such as prebiotics or nutritional supplements were not included in the analysis.[8] These data are comparable to the results of the Institute of Medicine's 2002 study[196] and of the Feeding Infants and Toddlers Study performed in US infants and toddlers in 2004,[38] which also excluded soluble fibres in the pre-weaning period. The data are somewhat higher than those suggested for Italian infants (12 months: 3.3 ± 1.9 g/day) by Agostoni *et al.*[37]

Since the data provide no insight into physiological mechanisms or functions, the practical outcomes of these studies are somewhat limited. The American Dietetic Association stated in 2008 that the dietary reference intakes for infants aged from 0 to 12 months have still not been determined.[4] Consequently, specific recommendations regarding dietary fibre intakes are very imprecise. The American Dietetic Association recommended a variety of plant food between 6 and 12 months,[4] while Agostoni *et al.*[37] recommended up to 5 g fibres/day, which can be easily achieved through adequate intake of fruits and vegetables. In conclusion, due to the lack of data, only non-evidence based pragmatic recommendations would be possible.

21.5 Conclusion

The non-digestible carbohydrates found in human milk have highly complex structures and have a positive impact on the gastrointestinal tract of infants. HMOS are known to stimulate the growth of good bacteria, leading to a lower level of pathogenic bacteria, and act as receptor analogues for pathogens, thereby blocking the first stage of infection. Breast milk can therefore be considered the best method of protecting against infection and immune-related diseases. Further research is required, however, in order to identify which structural elements in HMOS are most important for their function and to establish the nature of the relationship between oligosaccharides and their specific biological functions.

The complexity of HMOS means that they cannot be easily reproduced for use in infant formulas; studies have shown that a specific mixture of GOS and inulin/FOS has a prebiotic effect, and can be added to formula to at least partially mimic the effect of the HMOS found in breast milk. A connection has been observed between the growth of specific beneficial bacteria (promoted by prebiotics) and patterns of allergy development in infants; the same prebiotic mixture has also been shown to have physiological effects on the gastrointestinal tract, including improved gastric emptying time, greater tolerance of formula feeding, and possibly improved mineral absorption. The effect of prebiotics on the immune system has been largely tested on animals, but clinical trials on infants have indicated long-lasting effects in terms of reducing allergy risk and occurrence of infection.

Finally, the effects of insoluble fibre intake during the weaning stage (in the form of bran flakes, leafy green vegetables, and so on) have been little studied in infants, but in adults insoluble dietary fibre has been connected with a number of positive effects, including improvements in the immune system and lower risk of cardiovascular disease and diabetes. Further research is required in this area in order to draw up accurate recommendations for insoluble dietary fibre intake for infants.

21.6 References

1. WILLIAMS CL, BOLELLA M, WYNDER EL (1995), 'A new recommendation for dietary fiber in childhood', *Pediatrics*, **96**, 985–8.
2. PAVLOVIC M, PRENTICE A, THORSDOTTIR I, WOLFRAM G, BRANCA F (2007), 'Challenges in harmonizing energy and nutrient recommendations in Europe', *Ann Nutr Metab*, **51**,108–14.
3. UNITED NATIONS CHILDREN'S FUND (2006), 1990–2005. 'Celebrating the Innocent declaration on the protection, promotion and support of breastfeeding. Past achievements, present challenges and priority actions for infant and young child feeding'. Second edition, United Nations Childrens Fund (UNICEF).
4. SLAVIN JL (2008), 'Position of the American Dietetic Association: Health implications of dietary fiber', *J Am Diet Assoc*, **108**, 1716–31.
5. ANDERSON JW, BAIRD P, DAVIS RH, FERRERI S, KNUDTSON M, *et al.* (2009), 'Health benefits of dietary fiber', *Nutr Rev*, **67**, 188–205.
6. DONINI LM, SAVINA C, CANELLA C (2009), 'Nutrition in the elderly: Role of fiber', *Arch Geront Geriatr*, (suppl. 1), 61–9.
7. PRENTICE A, BRANCA F, DECSI T, MICHAELSEN KF, FLETCHER RJ, *et al.* (2004), 'Energy and nutrient dietary reference values for children in Europe: methodological approaches and current nutritional recommendations', *Br J Nutr*, **92**, 83–146.
8. ALEXY U, KERSTING M, SICHERT-HELLERT W (2006), 'Evaluation of dietary fibre intake from infancy to adolescence against various references – results of the DONALD study', *Europ J Clin Nutr*, **60**, 909–14.
9. BERSETH CL (1996), 'Gastrointestinal motility in the neonate', *Clin Perinatol*, **23**,179–90.
10. LEBENTHAL E, LEE PC, HEITLINGER LA (1983), 'Impact of development of the gastrointestinal tract on infant feeding', *J Pediatr*, **102**, 1–9.
11. MORELLI L (2008), 'Postnatal development of intestinal microflora as influenced by infant nutrition', *J Nutr*, **138**, 1791S–1795S.
12. ORRHAGE K, NORD CE (1999), 'Factors controlling the bacterial colonisation of the intestine in breastfed infants', *Acta Paediatr*, **88**, 47–57.

13. TROWELL H (1972), 'Dietary fibre and coronary heart disease', *Rev Eur Etud Clin Biol*, **17**, 345–9.
14. ANNON I (2001), 'The definition of dietary fibre. Report of the Dietary Fibre Definition Committee of the American Association of Cereal Chemists', *Cereal Food World*, **46**, 112–29.
15. WHO/FAO (2008), 'Codex Alimentarius Commission (CNFSDU): 29th Session 2007 and 30th Session', *ALINORM*, 08/31/26 and 09/32/26.
16. TISSIER HCR (1899), 'La vécation chromophile d'Escherich et la Bacterium coli', *Soc Biol*, **51**, 943–5.
17. GYÖRGY P, NORRIS RF, ROSE CS (1954), 'A variant of *Lactobacillus bifidus* requiring a special growth factor', *Arch Biochem Biophys*, **48**, 193–201.
18. NEWBURG DS, NEUBAUER SH (1995), 'Carbohydrates in milk', in *Handbook of milk composition*, Robert G. Jenson (eds) Academic Press, San Diego, pp. 34–123.
19. BOEHM G, STAHL B (2003), 'Oligosaccharides', in MATTILA-SANDHOLM T and SAARELA M (eds) *Functional dairy products*, Woodhead Publishing Ltd, Cambridge, UK, pp. 203–43.
20. URASHIMA T, ASAKUMA S, MESSER M (2007), 'Milk oligosaccharides', in KAMERLING JP (ed.) *Comprehensive glycoscience*, Elsevier Ltd, Oxford, UK, pp. 695–723.
21. KUNZ C, RUDLOFF S, BEIER W, KLEIN N, STROBEL S (2000), 'Oligosaccharides in human milk: structural, functional and metabolic aspects', *Annu Rev Nutr*, **20**, 699–722.
22. THURL S, MUNZERT M, HENKER J, BOEHM G, MÜLLER-WERNER B, *et al.* (2010), 'Variation of human milk oligosaccharides in relation to milk groups and lactational periods', *Br J Nutr*, **104**, 1261–71.
23. HARMSEN HJ, WILDEBOER-VELOO AC, RAANGS GC, WAGENDORP AA, KLIJN N, *et al.* (2000), 'Analysis of intestinal flora development in breast fed and formula fed infants by using molecular identification and detection methods', *J Pediatr Gastroenterol Nutr*, **30**, 61–70.
24. COPPA GV, ZAMPINI L, GALEAZZI T, GABRIELLI O (2006), 'Prebiotics in human milk: a review', *Dig Liver Dis*, **38** (suppl. 2), S291–S294.
25. TURRONI F, BOTTACINI F, FORONI E, MULDER I, KIM JH, *et al.* (2010), 'Genome analysis of *Bifidobacterium bifidum* PRL2010 reveals metabolic pathways for host-derived glycan foraging', *Proc Natl Acad Sci USA*, **107**, 19514–19.
26. POSSEMIERS S, GROOTAERT C, VERMEIREN J, GROSS G, MARZORATI M, *et al.* (2009), 'The intestinal environment in health and disease – recent insights on the potential of intestinal bacteria to influence human health', *Curr Pharm Des*, **14**, 2051–65.
27. CONROY ME, SHI HN, WALKER WA (2009), 'The long-term health effects of neonatal microbial flora', *Current Opin Allergy Clin Immunol*, **9**, 197–201.
28. BARBOSA T, RESCIGNO M (2010), 'Host–bacteria interactions in the intestine: homeostasis to chronic inflammation', *Wiley Interdiscip Rev Syst Biol Med*, **2**, 80–97.
29. SALZMAN NH (2011), 'Microbiota–immune system interaction: an uneasy alliance', *Curr Opin Microbiol*, **14**, 99–105.
30. SEKIROV I, RUSSELL SL, ANTUNES LC, FINLAY BB (2010), 'Gut microbiota in health and disease', *Physiol Rev*, **90**, 859–904.
31. BODE L (2006), 'Recent advances on structure, metabolism, and function of human milk oligosaccharides', *J Nutr*, **136**, 2127–30.
32. VOS AP, M'RABET L, STAHL B, BOEHM G, GARSSEN J (2007), 'Immune modulatory effects and potential working mechanisms of orally applied non-digestible carbohydrates', *Crit Rev Immunol*, **27**, 97–140.
33. BOEHM G, MORO G (2008), 'Structural and functional aspects of prebiotics used in infant nutrition', *J Nutr*, **138**, 1818S–1828S.
34. ROBERFROID M, GIBSON GR, HOYLES L, MCCARTNEY AL, RASTALL R, *et al.* (2010), 'Prebiotic effects: metabolic and health benefits', *Br J Nutr*, **104** (suppl. 2), S1–63.
35. BOEHM G, STAHL B, VAN LAERE K, KNOL J, FANARO S, *et al.* (2004), 'Prebiotics in infant formulas', *J Clin Gastroenterol*, **38** (suppl. 2), S76–S79.

36. EDWARDS CA, PARRETT AM (2003), 'Dietary fibre in infancy and childhood', *Proc Nutr Soc*, **62**,17–23.
37. AGOSTONI C, RIVA E, GIOVANNINI M (1995), 'Dietary fiber in weaning foods of young children', *Pediatrics*, **96**, 1002–5.
38. BRIEFEL RR, REIDY K, KARWE V, JANKOWSKI L, HENDRICKS K (2004), 'Toddlers' transition to table foods: Impact on nutrient intakes and food patterns', *J Am Diet Assoc*, **104**, 38–44.
39. ALEXY U, KERSTING M, SICHERT-HELLERT W, MANZ F, SCHÖCH G (1999), 'Macronutrients intake of 3- to 36-months-old German infants and children: Results of the DONALD study', *Ann Nutr Metab*, **43**, 14–22.
40. IUB-IUPAC JOINT COMMISSION ON BIOCHEMICAL NOMENCLATURE (JCBN) (1980), 'Abbreviated terminology of oligosaccharide chains. Recommendations', *J Biol Chem*, **257**, 334.
41. BOEHM G, BEERMANN C, GEORGI G, STAHL B (2007), 'Infant formulas', in HUI YH (ed.) *Handbook of food products manufacturing*. John Wiley & Sons Inc., Hoboken, New Jersey, pp. 677–714.
42. BRITISH NUTRITION FOUNDATION (1990), *Complex carbohydrates in foods: Report of the British Nutrition Foundation's Task Force*, Chapman and Hall, London.
43. IUB-IUPAC JOINT COMMISSION ON BIOCHEMICAL NOMENCLATURE (JCBN) (1997), 'Nomenclature of carbohydrates. Recommendations', *Carbohydr Res*, **297**, 9–23.
44. THURL S, HENKER J, SIEGEL M, TOVAR K, SAWATZKI G (1997), 'Detection of four human milk groups with respect to Lewis blood group dependent oligosaccharides', *Glycoconj J*, **14**, 795–9.
45. WATKINS WM, GREENWELL P, YATES AD, JOHNSON PH (1988), 'Regulation of expression of carbohydrate blood group antigens', *Biochemie*, **70**, 1597–611.
46. COPPA GV, GABRIELLI O, PIERANI P, CATASSI C, CARLUCCI A, GIORGI PL (1993), 'Changes in carbohydrate composition in human milk over 4 months of lactation', *Pediatrics*, **91**, 637–41.
47. ENGFER MB, STAHL B, FINKE B, SAWATZKI G, DANIEL H (2000), 'Human milk oligosaccharides are resistant to enzymatic hydrolysis in the upper gastrointestinal tract', *Am J Clin Nutr*, **71**, 1589–96.
48. BOEHM G, JAKOBSSON I, MANSSON M, RÄIHÄ NCR (1992), 'Macromolecular absorption in small-for-gestational-age infants', *Acta Paediatr*, **81**, 864–7.
49. GNOTH MJ, KUNZ C, KINNE-SAFRANE E, RUDLOFF S (2000), 'Human milk oligosaccharides are minimally digested in vitro', *J Nutr* **130**, 3014–20.
50. COPPA GV, PIERANI P, ZAMPINI L, BRUNI S, CARLONI I, GABRIELLI O (2001), 'Characterization of oligosaccharides in milk and feces of breast-fed infants by high performance anion exchange chromatography', *Adv Exp Med Biol*, **501**, 307–14.
51. HILL MJ (1995), 'Bacterial fermentation of complex carbohydrate in the human colon', *Eur J Can Prev*, **4**, 353–8.
52. SCHELL MA, KARMIRANTZOU M, SNEL B, VILANOVA D, BERGER B, *et al.* (2002), 'The genome sequence of *Bifidobacterium longum* reflects its adaptation to the human gastrointestinal tract', *Proc Natl Acad Sci USA*, **99**, 14422–7.
53. VENTURA M, CANCHAYA C, FITZGERALD GF, GUPTA RS, VAN SINDEREN D (2007), 'Genomics as a means to understand bacterial phylogeny and ecological adaptation: the case of bifidobacteria', *Antonie Van Leeuwenhoek*, 351–72.
54. KLIJN A, MERCENIER A, ARIGONI F (2005), 'Lessons from the genomes of bifidobacteria', *FEMS Microbiol Rev*, **29**, 491–509.
55. WARD RE, NINONUEVO M, MILLS DA, LEBRILLA CB, GERMAN JB (2006), 'In vitro fermentation of breast milk oligosaccharides by *Bifodobacterium infantis* and *Lactobacillus gasseri*', *Appl Environ Microbiol*, **72**, 4497–9.
56. GOVERS M, BUCO A, HENDRICH T, STAHL B, BOEHM G (2005), 'Comparison of human milk oligosaccharides with oligosaccharides for use in infant nutrition on *in vitro* fermentation using faeces from breast-fed and formula-fed infants', *J Pediatr Gastroenterol Nutr*, **40**, 694.

57. KNOL J, SCHOLTENS P, KAFKA C, STEENBAKKERS J, GROß S, *et al.* (2005), 'Colon microflora in infants fed formula with galacto- and fructo-oligosaccharides: more like breast fed infants', *J Pediatr Gastroenterol Nutr*, **40**, 36–42.
58. SIIGUR U, ORMISSON A, TAMM A (1993), 'Faecal short-chain fatty acids in breast-fed and bottle-fed infants', *Acta Paediatr*, **82**, 536–8.
59. VAN LIMPT C, CRIENEN A, VRIESEMA A, KNOL J (2004), 'Effect of colonic short chain fatty acids, lactate and pH on the growth of common gut pathogens', *Pediatr Res*, **56**, 487.
60. BURGER VAN PASSEN N, VINCENT A, PUIMAN PJ, VAN DER SLUIS M, BOUMA J, *et al.* (2009), 'The regulation of intestinal mucin MUC2 expression by short-chain fatty acids: implications for epithelial protection', *Biochem J*, **420**, 211–19.
61. FIELD CJ (2005), 'The immunological components of human milk and their effect on immune development in infants', *J Nutr*, **135**, 1–4.
62. ODDY WH (2002), 'The impact of breast milk on infant and child health', *Breastfeed Rev*, **10**, 5–18.
63. HAMOSH M (1996), 'Breastfeeding: Unravelling the mysteries of mother's milk', *Medscape Womens Health*, **16**, 4–9.
64. DAVIS MK (2001), 'Breastfeeding in chronic disease in childhood and adolescence', *Pediatr Clin North Am*, **48**, 125–41.
65. GAROFALO RP, GOLDMAN AS (1999), 'Expression of functional immunomodulatory and anti-inflammatory factors in human milk', *Clin Perinatol*, **26**, 361–78.
66. HALKEN S, HOST A (2001), 'Prevention', *Curr Opin Allergy Clin Immunol*, **1**, 229–36.
67. KELLY D, COUTTS AG (2000), 'Early nutrition and the development of immune function in the neonate', *Proc Nutr Soc*, **59**, 177–85.
68. HOWIE PW, FORSYTH JS, OGSTON SA, CLARK A, DU FLOREY VC (1990), 'Protective effect of breast feeding against infection', *Br Med J*, **300**, 11–18.
69. HANSON LA, KOROTKOVA M (2002), 'The role of breastfeeding in prevention of neonatal infection', *Semin Neonatol*, **7**, 275–81.
70. CHIEN PF, HOWIE PW (2001), 'Breast milk and the risk of opportunistic infection in infancy in industrialized and non-industrialized settings', *Adv Nutr Res*, **10**, 69–104.
71. M'RABET L, VOS AP, BOEHM G, GARSSEN J (2008), 'Breast-feeding and its role in early development of the immune system in infants: consequences for health later in life', *J Nutr*, **138**, 1782S–1790S.
72. CHIRICO G, MARZOLLO R, CORTINOVIS S, FONTE C, GASPARONI A (2008), 'Antiinfective properties of human milk', *J Nutr*, **138**, 1801S–1806S.
73. ANDERSSON B, PORRAS O, HANSON LA, LAGERGARD T, SVAMBERG-EDEN C (1986), 'Inhibition of attachment of *Streptococcus pneumoniae* and *Haemophilus influenzae* by human milk and receptor oligosaccharides', *J Infect Dis*, **153**, 232–7.
74. NEWBURG DS, PICKERING LK, MCCLUER RM, CLEARY TG (1990), 'Fucosylated oligosaccharides of human milk protect suckling mice from heat-stable enterotoxin of *Escherichia coli*', *J Infect Dis*, **162**, 1075–80.
75. ZOPF D, ROTH S (1996), 'Oligosaccharide anti-infective agents', *Lancet*, **347**, 1017–21.
76. CERVANTES LE, NEWBURG DS, RUIZCIOS GM (1995), 'Fucosylated chains (H–2 and Lewis) are the main human milk receptor analogs for campylobacter', *Pediatr Res*, **37**, 171A.
77. RUIZ-PALACIOS GM, CERVANTES LE, RAMOS P, CHAVEZ-MUNGUIA B, NEWBURG DS (2003), '*Campylobacter jejuni* binds intestinal H(O) antigen (Fuc α 1, 2Gal β 1, 4GlcNAc), and fucosyloligosaccharides of human milk inhibit its binding and infection', *J Biol Chem*, **278**, 14112–20.
78. SHARON N, OFEK I (2000), 'Safe as mother's milk: carbohydrates as future anti-adhesion drugs for bacterial diseases', *Glycoconj J*, **17**, 659–64.
79. VELUPILLAI P, HARN DA (1994), 'Oligosaccharide-specific induction of interleukin 10 production by B220+ cells from schistosome-infected mice: a mechanism for regulation of CD4+ T-cell subsets', *Proc Natl Acad Sci USA*, **91**, 18–22.
80. TERRAZAS LI, WALSH K, PISKORSKA D, MCGUIRE E, HARN DA (2001), 'The schistosome oligosaccharide lacto-N-neotetraose expands Gr1(+) cells that secrete anti-inflammatory

cytokines and inhibit proliferation of naive CD4(+) cells: a potential mechanism for immune polarization in helminth infections', *J Immunol*, **167**, 5294–303.
81. SCHUMACHER G, BENDAS G, STAHL B, BEERMANN C (2006), 'Human milk oligosaccharides affect P-selectin binding capacities: in vitro investigation', *Nutrition*, **22**, 620–7.
82. NAARDING MA, LUDWIG IS, GROOT F, BERKHOUT B, GEIJTENBEEK, TB, *et al.* (2005), 'Lewis X-component in human milk binds DC-SIGN and inhibits HIV–1 transfer to CD4+ lymphocytes', *J Clin Invest*, **115**, 3256–64.
83. BODE L, RUDLOFF S, KUNZ C, STROBEL S, KLEIN N (2004), 'Human milk oligosaccharides reduce platelet-neutrophil complex formation leading to a decrease in neutrophil β2 integrin expression', *J Leukoc Biol*, **76**, 820–6.
84. FINKE B, STAHL B, PRITSCHET M, FACIUS D, WOLFGANG J, BOEHM G (2002), 'Preparative continuous annular chromatography (P-CAC) enables the large-scale fractionation of fructans', *J Agric Food Chem*, **50**, 4743–8.
85. GEISSER A, HENDRICH T, BOEHM G, STAHL B (2005), 'Separation of lactose from human milk oligosaccharides with simulated moving bed chromatography', *J Chromatography A*, **1092**, 17–23.
86. EIWEGGER T, STAHL B, SCHMITT JJ, BOEHM G, GERSTMAYR M, *et al.* (2004), 'Human milk derived oligosaccharides and plant derived oligosaccharides stimulate cytokine production of cord blood T-cells in vitro', *Pediatr Res*, **56**, 536–40.
87. EIWEGGER T, STAHL B, HAIDL P, SCHMITT J, BOEHM G, *et al.* (2010), 'Prebiotic oligosaccharides: In vitro evidence for gastrointestinal epithelial transfer and immunomodulatory properties', *Pediatr Allergy Immunol*, **21**, 1179–88.
88. HODDINOTT P, TAPPIN D, WRIGHT C (2008), 'Breast feeding', *BMJ*, **336**, 881–7.
89. HORTA BL, BAHL R, MARTINEZ JC, *et al.* (2007), 'Evidence on the long-term effects of breast-feeding: systematic reviews and meta-analyses', *WHO Library Cataloguing-in-Publication*, World Health Organisation.
90. METGES CC, EBERHARD M, PETZKE KJ (2006), 'Synthesis and absorption of intestinal microbial lysine in humans and non-ruminant animals and impact on human estimated average requirements of dietary lysine', *Curr Opin Clin Nutr Metab Care*, **9**, 37–41.
91. GIBSON GR, ROBERFROID MB (1995), 'Dietary modulation of the human colonic microbiota: introducing the concept of prebiotics', *J Nutr*, **125**, 1401–12.
92. GIBSON GR, PROBERT HM, VAN LOO JAE, RASTALL RA, ROBERFROID MB (2004), 'Dietary Modulation of the Human Colonic Microbiota: Updating the Concept of Prebiotics', *Nutr Res Rev*, **17**, 259–75.
93. GOVERS M, BUCO A, HENDRICH T, STAHL B, BOEHM G (2005), 'Comparison of human milk oligosaccharides with oligosaccharides for use in infant nutrition on in vitro fermentation using faeces from breast-fed and formula-fed infants', *J Pediatr Gastroenterol Nutr*, **40**, 694.
94. PEREZ-CONES AD, LOPES G, ROS G (2005), 'Fermentation capabilities of bifidobacteria using nondigestible oligosaccharides, and their viability as probiotics in commercial powder infant formula', *J Food Sci*, **70**, M279–M285.
95. GOPAL PK, SULLIVAN PA, SMART JB (2001), 'Utilisation of galacto-oligosaccharides as selective substrates for growth by lactic acid bacteria including *Bifidobacterium lactis* DR10 and *Lactobacillus rhamnosus* DR20', *Int Dairy J*, **11**, 19–25.
96. ROSSI M, CORRADINI C, AMARETTI A, NICOLINI M, POMPEI A, *et al.* (2005), 'Fermentation of fructooligosaccharides and inulin by bifidobacteria: a comparative study of pure and fecal cultures', *Appl Environ Microbiol*, **71**, 6150–8.
97. PERRIN S, FOUGNIES C, GRILL JP, JACOBS H, SCHNEIDER F (2002), 'Fermentation of chicory fructo-oligosaccharides in mixtures of different degrees of polymerisation by three strains of bifidobacteria', *Can J Microbiol*, **48**, 759–63.
98. HILL MJ (1995), 'Bacterial fermentation of complex carbohydrate in the human colon', *Eur J Can Prev*, **4**, 353–8.

99. SCHELL MA, KARMIRANTZOU M, SNEL B, VILANOVA D, BERGER B, *et al.* (2002), 'The genome sequence of *Bifidobacterium longum* reflects its adaptation to the human gastrointestinal tract', *Proc Natl Acad Sci USA*, **99**, 14422–7.
100. VENTURA M, CANCHAYA C, FITZGERALD GF, GUPTA RS, VAN SINDEREN D (2007), 'Genomics as a means to understand bacterial phylogeny and ecological adaptation: the case of bifidobacteria', *Antonie Van Leeuwenhoek*, **36**, 351–72.
101. KLIJN A, MERCENIER A, ARIGONI F (2005), 'Lessons from the genomes of bifidobacteria', *FEMS Microbiol Rev*, **29**, 491–509.
102. WARD RE, NINONUEVO M, MILLS DA, LEBRILLA CB, GERMAN JB (2006), 'In vitro fermentation of breast milk oligosaccharides by *Bifidobacterium infantis* and *Lactobacillus gasseri*', *Appl Environ Microbiol*, **72**, 4497–9.
103. BOEHM G, FANARO S, JELINEK J, STAHL B, MARINI A (2003), 'Prebiotic concept for infant nutrition', *Acta Paediatrica*, Suppl. **441**, 64–7.
104. GUGGENBICHLER JP, DE BETTIGNIES-DUTZ A, MEISSNER P, SCHELLMOSER S, JURENITSCH J (1997), 'Acidic oligosaccharides from natural sources block adherence of *Escherichia coli* on uroepithelial cells', *Pharm Pharmacol Lett*, **7**, 35–8.
105. MORO E (1908), 'Karottensuppe bei Ernährungsstörungen der Säuglinge', *Münchener Medizinische Wochenzeitschrift*, **31**, 1637–40.
106. EU (2006), Commission Directive 2006/141/EC on infant formula and follow-on formula and amending Directive 1999/21/EC (2006), *Official Journal of the European Union*, **L401**, 1–3.
107. ROBERFROID MB (2005), 'Introducing inulin-type fructans', *Br J Nutr*, **93**, 13–25.
108. KINSELL JE, TAYLOR SL (eds) (1995), Commercial β-galactosidase, in *Food Processing. Advances in Food and Nutrition Research*. San Diego, Academic Press.
109. FULLER R (1989), 'Probiotics in man and animals', *J Appl Bacteriol*, **66**, 365–78.
110. YAHIRO M, NISHIKAWA I, MURAKAMI Y, YOSHIDA H, AHIKO K (1998), 'Studies on application of galactosyl lactose for infant formula. II. Changes of fecal characteristics on infant fed galactosyl lactose', *Reports of Research Laboratory, Snow Brand Milk Products*, **78**, 27–32.
111. BEN X, ZHOU X, ZHAO W, YU W, PAN W, *et al.* (2004), 'Supplementation of milk formula with galacto-oligosaccharides improves intestinal micro-flora and fermentation in term infants', *Chin Med J*, **117**, 927–31.
112. BRUNSER O, GOTTELAND M, CRUCHET S, FIGUEROA G, GARRIDO D, STEENHOUT P (2006), 'Effect of a milk formula with prebiotics on the intestinal microbiota of infants after an antibiotic treatment', *Pediatr Res*, **59**, 451–6.
113. SAARVEDA J, TSCHERINA A, MOORE N, ABI-HANNA A, COLETTA F, *et al.* (1999), 'Gastrointestinal function in infants consuming a weaning food supplemented with oligofructose, a prebiotic', *J Pediatr Gastroenterol Nutr*, **29**, 95.
114. TSCHERNIS A, MOORE N, ABI-HANNA A, YOLKEN R, COLERTS F, *et al.* (1999), 'Effects of long-term consumption of a weaning food supplemented with oligofructose, a prebiotic, on general infant health status', *J Pediatr Gastroenterol Nutr*, **29**, 58.
115. EULER AR, MITCHELL DK, KLINE R, PICKERING LK (2005), 'Prebiotic effect of fructo-oligosaccharide supplemented term infant formula at two concentrations compared with unsupplemented formula and human milk', *J Pediatr Gastroenterol Nutr*, **40**, 157–64.
116. MOORE N, CHAO C, YANG L, STORM H, OLIVA-HEMKER M, SAARVEDRA JM (2003), 'Effects of fructo-oligosaccharide-supplemented infant cereal: A double-blind, randomized trial', *Br J Nutr*, **90**, 581–7.
117. DUGGAN C, PENNY ME, HIBBERD P, GIL A, HUAPAYA A, *et al.* (2003), 'Oligofructose-supplemented infant cereal: 2 randomised, blinded, community-based trials in Peruvian infants', *Am J Clin Nutr*, **77**, 937–42.
118. WALIGORA-DUPRIET AJ, CAMPEOTTO F, NICOLIS I, BONET A, SOULAINES P, *et al.* (2007), 'Effect of oligofructose supplementation on gut microflora and well-being in young children attending a day care centre', *Int J Food Microbiol*, **113**, 108–13.

119. GUESRY PR, BODANSKI H, TOMSIT E, AESCHLIMANN JM (2000), 'Effect of 3 doses of fructo-oligosaccharides in infants', *J Pediatr Gastroenterol Nutr*, **31**, S252.
120. BETTLER J, EULER AR (2006), 'An evaluation of the growth of term infants fed formula supplemented with fructo-oligosaccharides', *Int J Probiotics Prebiotics*, **1**, 19–26.
121. KAPIKI A, COSTALOS C, OIKONOMIDOU C, TRIANTAFYLLDOU A, LOUKATOU E, PERTROHILOU V (2007), 'The effect of a fructo-oligosaccharide supplemented formula on gut flora of preterm infants', *Early Hum Develop*, **83**, 335–9.
122. KIM SH, LEE DH, MEYER D (2007), 'Supplementation of infant formula with native inulin has a prebiotic effect in formula-fed babies', *Asia Pacific J Clin Nutr*, **16**, 172–7.
123. YAP KW, MOHAMED S, YAZID AM (2005), 'Dose-response effects of inulin on fecal short-chain fatty acids content and mineral absorption of formula fed infants', *Nutr Food Science*, **35**, 208–19.
124. NAGENDRA R, VISWANATHA S, ARUM KS, KRISHNA MB, VENKAT RS (1995), 'Effect of feeding milk formula containing lactulose to infants on faecal bifidobacterial flora', *Nutr Res*, **15**, 14–24.
125. RINNE M, KIRJAVAINEN P, SALMINEN S, ISOLAURI E (2003), 'Lactulose – any clinical benefits beyond constipation relief? A pilot study in infants with allergic symptoms', *Biosci Microflora*, **22**, 155–7.
126. ZIEGLER E, VANDERHOOF JA, PETSCHOW B, MITMESSER SH, STOLZ SI, *et al.* (2007), 'Term infants fed formula supplemented with selected blends of prebiotics grow normally and have soft stools similar to those reported for breast-fed infants', *J Pediatr Gastroenterol Nutr*, **44**, 359–64.
127. FIRMANSYAH A, PRAMITA GD, FASSLER CARRIÈ AL, HASCKE F, LINK-AMSTER H (2000), 'Improved humoral immune response to measles vaccine in infants receiving cereal with fructooligosaccharides', *J Pediatr Gastroenterol Nutr*, **31**, suppl. 2, s134.
128. BONGERS MEJ, DE LORIJN F, REITSMA JB, GROENEWEG M, TAMINIAU JAJM, BENNINGA MA (2007), 'The clinical effect of a new infant formula in term infants with constipation: a double-blind, randomized cross-over trial', *Nutr J*, **6**, 8–15.
129. MORO G, MINOLI I, MOSCA M, JELINEK J, STAHL B, BOEHM G (2002), 'Dosage-related bifidogenic effects of galacto- and fructo-oligosaccharides in formula-fed term infants', *J Pediatr Gastroenterol Nutr*, **34**, 291–5.
130. MORO G, STAHL B, JELINEK J, BOEHM G, COPPA GV (2005), 'Dietary prebiotic oligosaccharides are detectable in faeces of formula-fed infants', *Acta Paediatr Suppl*, **94**, 27–30.
131. SCHMELZE H, WIRTH S, SKOPNIK H, RADKE M, KNOL J, *et al.* (2003), 'Randomized double-blind study on the nutritional efficacy and bifidogenicity of a new infant formula containing partially hydrolysed protein, a high β-palmitic acid level, and nondigestible oligosaccharides', *J Pediatr Gastroenterol Nutr*, **36**, 343–51.
132. KNOL J, SCHOLTENS P, KAFKA C, STEENBAKKERS J, GROß S, *et al.* (2005), 'Colon microflora in infants fed formula with galacto- and fructo-oligosaccharides: more like breast-fed infants', *J Pediatr Gastroenterol Nutr*, **40**, 36–42.
133. HAARMAN M, KNOL J (2005), 'Quantitative real-time PCR assays to identify and quantify fecal *Bifidobacterium* species in infants receiving a prebiotic infant formula', *Appl Environmental Microbiol*, **71**, 2318–24.
134. HAARMAN M, KNOL J (2006), 'Quantitative real-time PCR analysis of fecal *Lactobacillus* species in infants receiving a prebiotic infant formula', *Appl Environ Microbiol*, **71**, 2359–65.
135. COSTALOS C, KAPIKI A, APOSTOLOU M, PAPATHOMA E (2008), 'The effect of a prebiotic supplemented formula on growth and stool microbiology of term infants', *Early Hum Dev*, **84**, 45–9.
136. SAVINO F, CRESCI F, MACCARIO S, CAVALLO F, DALMASSO P, *et al.* (2003), ' "Minor" feeding problems during the first months of life: effect of a partially hydrolysed milk formula containing fructo- and galacto-oligosaccharides', *Acta Paediatr Suppl*, **92**, 86–90.

137. SAVINO F, MACCARIO S, CASTANGNO E, CRESCI F, CAVALLO F, *et al.* (2005), 'Advances in the management of digestive problems during the first months of life', *Acta Paediatr Suppl*, **94**, 120–4.
138. SCHOLTENS P, ALLES M, BINDELS J, LINDE VAN DER E, TOOLBOM JJM, KNOL J (2006), 'Bifidogenic effect of solid weaning foods with added prebiotic oligosaccharides: a randomized controlled clinical trial', *J Pediatr Gastroenterol Nutr*, **42**, 553–9.
139. BAKKER-ZIERIKZEE AM, TOL EA, KROES H, ALLES MS, KOK FJ, BINDELS JG (2006), 'Faecal sIgA secretion in infants fed on pre- or probiotic infant formula', *Pediatr Allergy Immunol*, **17**, 134–140.
140. BAKKER-ZIERIKZEE AM, ALLES M, KNOL J, KOK FJ, TOLBOOM JJM, BINDELS JG (2005), 'Effects of infant formula containing a mixture of galacto- and fructo-oligosaccharides or viable *Bifidobacterium animalis* on the intestinal microflora during the first 4 months of life', *Br J Nutr*, **94**, 783–90.
141. MORO G, ARSLANOGLU S, STAHL B, JELINEK J, WAHN U, BOEHM G (2006), 'A mixture of prebiotic oligosaccharides reduces the incidence of atopic dermatitis during the first six months of age', *Arch Dis Child*, **91**, 814–19.
142. ARSLANOGLU S, MORO G, SCHMITT J, BOEHM G (2008), 'Early dietary intervention with a mixture of prebiotic oligosaccharides reduces the allergy associated symptoms and infections during the first 2 years of life', *J Nutr*, **138**, 1091–5.
143. GARSSEN J, ARSLANOGLU S, BOEHM G, FABER J, KNOL J, *et al.* (2007), 'A mixture of short chain galacto-oligosaccharides and long chain fructo-oligosaccharides induces an anti-allergic immunoglobulin profile in infants at risk for allergy', *Allergy*, **62**, 47–8.
144. ARSLANOGLU S, MORO GE, BOEHM G (2007), 'Early supplementation of prebiotic oligosaccharides protects formula-fed infants against infections during the first 6 months of life', *J Nutr*, **137**, 2420–4.
145. VAN HOFFEN E, RUITER B, FABER J, M'RABET L, KNOL EF, *et al.* (2009), 'A specific mixture of short-chain galacto-oligosaccharides and long-chain fructo-oligosaccharides induces a beneficial immunoglobulin profile in infants at high risk for allergy', *Allergy*, **64**, 484–7.
146. ALLIET P, SCHOLTENS P, RAES M, HENSEN K, JONGEN H, *et al.* (2007), 'Effect of prebiotic galacto-oligosaccharide, long-chain fructo-oligosaccharide infant formula on serum cholesterol and triacylglycerol levels', *Nutrition*, **23**, 719–23.
147. SCHOLTENS PAMJ, ALLIET P, RAES M, ALLES MA, KROES H, *et al.* (2008), 'Fecal secretory immunoglobulin A is increased in healthy infants who receive a formula with short-chain galacto-oligosaccharides and long-chain fructo-oligosaccharides', *J Nutr*, **138**, 1141–7.
148. RAES M, SCHOLTENS PAMJ, ALLIET P, HENSEN K, JONGEN H, *et al.* (2009), 'Exploration of basal immune parameters in healthy infants receiving an infant milk formula supplemented with prebiotics', *Pediatr Allergy Immunol*, Jon Wiley & Sons A/S, PMID: 20003064.
149. DESCI T, ARATO A, BALOGH M, DOLINARY T, KANJO AH, *et al.* (2005), 'Randomized placebo controlled double blind study on the effect of prebiotic oligosaccharides on intestinal flora in healthy term infants (translation from Hungarian language)', *Orvosi Heliap*, **146**, 2445–50.
150. RINNE MM, GUEIMONDE M, KALLIOMÄKI M, HOPPU U, SALMINEN SJ, ISOLAURI E (2005), 'Similar bifidogenic effects of prebiotic-supplemented partially hydrolyzed infant formula and breastfeeding on infant gut microbiota', *FEMS Immunol Med Microbiol*, **43**, 59–65.
151. PENDERS J, THIS C, VINK C, STELMA FF, SNIJDERS B, *et al.* (2006), 'Factors influencing the composition of the intestinal microbiota in early infancy', *Pediatrics*, **118**, 511–21.
152. BRUZZESE E, VOLPICELLI M, SALVINI F, BISCEGLIA M, LIONETTI P, *et al.* (2009), 'Early administration of GOS/FOS prevents intestinal and respiratory infections in infants', *Clin Nutr*, **18**, 326–34.

153. VAISMAN N, PRESS J, LEIBOVITZ E, BOEHM G, BARAL V (2010), 'Short-term effect of prebiotics administration on stool characteristics and serum cytokines dynamics in very young children with acute diarrhea', *Nutrients*, **2**, 683–92.
154. MODI N, UTHAYA S, FELL J, KULINSKAYA E (2010), 'A randomized, double-blind, controlled trial of the effect of prebiotic oligosaccharides on enteral tolerance in preterm infants (ISRCTN77444690)', *Pediatr Res*, **68**, 440–5.
155. BOEHM G, LIDESTRI M, CASETTA P, JELINEK J, NEGRETTI F, *et al.* (2002), 'Supplementation of an oligosaccharide mixture to a bovine milk formula increases counts of faecal bifidobacteria in preterm infants', *Arch Dis Child Fetal Neonatal Ed*, **86**, F178–F181.
156. KNOL J, BOEHM G, LIDESTRI L, NEGRETTI F, JELINEK J, *et al.* (2005), 'Increase of faecal bifidobacteria due to dietary oligosaccharides induces a reduction of clinically relevant pathogen germs in the faeces of formula-fed preterm infants', *Acta Paediatr Suppl*, **449**, 31–3.
157. MIHATSCH WA, HOEGEL J, POHLANDT F (2006), 'Prebiotic oligosaccharides reduce stool viscosity and accelerate gastrointestinal transport in preterm infants', *Acta Paediatr*, **95**, 843–8.
158. INDRIO F, RIEZZO G, MONTAGNA O, VALENZANO E, MAUTONE A, BOEHM G (2009), 'Prebiotics improve gastric motility and gastric electrical activity in preterm newborns', *J Pediatr Gastroenterol Nutr*, **49**, 258–61.
159. FANARO S, JELINEK J, STAHL B, BOEHM G, KOCK R, VIGI V (2005), 'Acidic oligosaccharides from pectin hydrolysate as new component for infant formulae: effect on intestinal flora, stool characteristics, and pH', *J Pediatr Gastroenterol Nutr*, **41**, 186–90.
160. MAGNE F, HACHELAF W, SUAU A, BOUDRAA G, BOUZIANE-NEDJADI K, *et al.* (2008), 'Effects on faecal microbiota of dietary and acidic oligosaccharides in children during partial formula feeding', *J Pediatr Gastroenterol Nutr*, **46**, 580–8.
161. WESTERBEEK EAM, VAN DEN BERG JP, LAFEBER HN, FETTER WPF, BOEHM G, *et al.* (2010), 'Neutral and acidic oligosaccharides in preterm infants: a randomized, double-blind, placebo-controlled trial', *Am J Clin Nutr*, **91**, 679–86.
162. GRÜBER C, VAN STUIJVENBERG M, MOSCA F, MORO G, CHIRICO G, *et al.* (2010), 'Reduced occurrence of early atopic dermatitis because of immunoactive prebiotics among low-atopy risk infants', *J Allergy Clin Immunol*, **126**, 791–7.
163. BJORKSTEN B, SEPP E, JULGE K, VOOR T, MIKELSAAR M (2001), 'Allergy development and the intestinal microflora during the first year of life', *J Allergy Clin Immunol*, **108**, 516–20.
164. OUWEHAND AC, ISOLAURI E, HE F, HASHIMOTO H, BENNO Y, SALMINEN S (2001), 'Differences in Bifidobacterium flora composition in allergic and healthy infants', *J Allergy Clin Immunol*, **108**, 144–5.
165. WATANABE S, NARISAWA Y, ARASE S, OKAMATSU H, IKENAGA T, *et al.* (2003), 'Differences in fecal microflora between patients with atopic dermatitis and healthy control subjects', *J Allergy Clin Immunol*, **111**, 587–91.
166. DASS NB, JOHN AK, BASSIL AK, CRUMBLEY CW, SHEHEE WR, *et al.* (2007), 'The relationship between the effects of short-chain fatty acids on intestinal motility in vitro and GPR43 receptor activation', *Neurogastroenterol Motil*, **19**, 66–74.
167. GRIDER JR, PILAND BE (2007), 'The peristaltic reflex induced by short-chain fatty acids is mediated by sequential release of 5-HT and neuronal CGRP but not BDNF', *Am J Physiol Gastrointest Liver Physiol*, **292**, G429–37.
168. ABRAMS SA, GRIFFIN JJ, HAWTHORNE KM, *et al.* (2005), 'A combination of prebiotic short- and long-chain inulin-type fructans enhances calcium absorption and bone mineralization in young adolescents', *Am J Clin Nutr*, **82**, 471–6.
169. CASHMAN KDA (2006), 'A prebiotic substance persistently enhances intestinal calcium absorption and increases bone mineralization in young adolescents', *Nutr Rev*, **64**, 189–96.
170. LIDESTRI M, AGOSTI M, MARINI A, BOEHM G (2003), 'Oligosaccharides might stimulate calcium absorption in formula-fed preterm infants', *Acta Paediatr Suppl*, **441**, 91–2.

171. GROSCHWITZ KR, HOGAN SP (2009), 'Intestinal barrier function: molecular regulation and disease pathogenesis', *J Allergy Clin Immunol*, **124**, 3–20.
172. O'CONNELL EL (2003), 'Pediatric allergy: a brief review of risk factors associated with developing allergic disease in childhood', *Ann Allergy Asthma Immunol*, **90**, 53–8.
173. WAHN HU (2008), 'Strategies for atopy prevention', *J Nutr*, **138**, 1770–25.
174. ARSHAD SH, BATEMAN B, SADEGHNEJAD A, GANT C, MATTHEWS SM (2007), 'Prevention of allergic disease during childhood by allergen avoidance: the Isle of Wight prevention study', *J Allergy Clin Immunol*, **119**, 307–13.
175. STROBEL S (2001), 'Immunity induced after a feed of antigen during early life: oral tolerance v. sensitisation', *Proc Nutr Soc*, **60**, 437–42.
176. MENEZES JS, MUCIDA DS, CARA DC, ALVAREZ-LEITE JI, RUSSO M, *et al.* (2003), 'Stimulation by food proteins plays a critical role in the maturation of the immune system', *Int Immunol*, **15**, 447–55.
177. CORTHÈSY B, GASKINS HR, MERCENIER A (2007), 'Cross talk between probiotic bacteria and the host immune system', *J Nutr*, **137**, 781–90.
178. NEU J, DOUGLAS-ESCOBAR M, LOPEZ M (2007), 'Microbes and the developing gastrointestinal tract', *Nutr Clin Pract*, **22**, 174–82.
179. ROOK GAW, BRUNET LR (2005), 'Microbes, immunoregulation and the gut', *Gut*, **54**, 317–20.
180. BOEHM G, STAHL B, GARSSEN J, BRUZZESE E, ARSLANOGLU S (2005), 'Prebiotics in infant formulas: immune modulators during infancy', *Nutrafoods*, **4**, 51–7.
181. MORELLI L (2008), 'Postnatal development of intestinal microflora as influenced by infant nutrition', *J Nutr*, **138**, 1791–5.
182. MURARO A, DREBORG S, HALKEN S, HOST A, NIGGEMANN B, *et al.* (2004), 'Dietary prevention of allergic diseases in infants and small children. Part II: Evaluation of methods in allergy prevention studies and sensitization markers. Definitions and diagnostic criteria for allergic diseases', *Pediatr Allergy Immunol*, **15**, 196–205.
183. VOS AP, HAARMAN M, VAN GINKEL JWH, KNOL J, GARSSEN J, *et al.* (2007), 'Dietary supplementation of neutral and acidic oligosaccharides enhances Th1-dependent vaccination responses in mice', *Pediatr Allergy Immunol*, **18**, 304–12.
184. VOS AP, VAN ESCH B, M'RABET L, FOLKERTS G, GARSSEN J (2007), 'Dietary supplementation with specific oligosaccharide mixtures decreases parameters of allergic asthma in mice', *Int Immunopharmacol*, **7**, 1582–7.
185. SCHOUTEN B, VAN ESCH BC, VAN THUIJL AO, BLOKHUIS BR, GROOT KORMELINK T, *et al.* (2010), 'Contribution of IgE and immunoglobulin free light chain in the allergic reaction to cow's milk proteins', *J Allergy Clin Immunol*, **125**, 1308–14.
186. ALBERS R, ANTOINE JM, BOURDET-SICARD R, CALDER PC, GLEESON M, *et al.* (2005), 'Markers to measure immunomodulation in human nutrition intervention studies', *Br J Nutr*, **94**, 452–81.
187. REDEGELD FA, VAN DER HEIJDEN W, KOOL M, HEIJDRA BM, GARSSEN J, *et al.* (2002), 'Immunoglobulin-free light chains elicit immediate hypersensitivity-like responses', *Nat Med*, **8**, 694–701.
188. POWE DG, KORMELINK TG, SISSON M, BLOKHUIS BJ, KRAMER MF, *et al.* (2010), 'Evidence for the involvement of free light chain immunoglobulins in allergic and nonallergic rhinitis', *J Allergy Clin Immunol*, **125**, 139–45.
189. SCHOUTEN B, VAN ESCH BC, KORMELINK TG, MORO GE, ARSLANOGLU S, *et al.* (2011), 'Non-digestible oligosaccharides reduce immunoglobulin free light-chain concentrations in infants at risk for allergy', *J Pediatr Allergy Immunol*, **22**, 537–42.
190. SALVINI F, RIVA E, SALVARICI E, BOEHM G, JELINEK J, *et al.* (2011), 'A specific prebiotic mixture added to starting infant formula has long-lasting bifidogenic effects', *J Nutr*, **141**, 1335–9.
191. WALDRON KW and FAULDS CB (2007), 'Cell wall polysaccharides: Composition and structure', in *Comprehensive Glycoscience*, Vol. **1**, Elsevier, pp. 181–201.

192. NISHINARI K, TAKEMASA M, ZHANG H, TAKAHASHI R (2007), 'Storage plant polysaccharides: Xyloglucans, galactomannans, glucomannans', in *Comprehensive Glycoscience*, Vol. 2, Elsevier, pp. 613–52.
193. JACOBASCH G, DONGOWSKI G (2000), 'Ballaststoffe mit spezifischen Wirkungen', in *Praxishandbuch Functional Food*, B. Behr's Verlag, pp. 1–49.
194. YAMADA H, KIYOHARA H (2007), 'Immunomodulating activity of plant polysaccharide structures', in *Comprehensive Glycoscience*, Vol. 4, Elsevier, pp. 663–94.
195. LE HUEROU-LURON I, BLAT S, BOUNDRY G (2010), 'Breast- v. formula feeding: impacts on the digestive tract and immediate and long-term health effects', *Nutr Res Rev*, **23**, 23–36.
196. INSTITUTE OF MEDICINE, FOOD AND NUTRITION BOARD (2002), *Dietary Reference Intakes for Energy, Carbohydrate, Fiber, Fat, Fatty Acids, Cholesterol, Protein, and Amino Acids*, National Academic Press, Washington.

Index

acacia gums, 373–4
sensory properties, 374
solubility, 373
stability, 374
tolerance, 374
viscosity, 373–4
adequate intake (AI), 64
agar, 107–8
aleurone, 156, 177
alginates, 107, 300, 302
alkylresorcinol, 11–12
Amylomaize, 412
animal nutrition
clinical significance, 415–17
diabetes and glycaemic control, 415–16
obesity and weight control, 416–17
dietary fibre inclusion, 407–18
food intake, gastric and small intestinal function, 408–12
effects of dietary fibre, 408–9
nutrient digestibility, 409–12
rate of digesta passage, 409
intestinal function, 412–15
prebiotic effects, 412, 414
stool quality, 412
in vitro evaluations of dietary fibres, 414–15
strategies for incorporating into diets, 417–18
antioxidant, 396–8
total antioxidant activity of grains, 397
AOAC 985.29, 10–11, 17, 26, 32, 56
AOAC 991.43, 10, 26, 32, 56, 57
AOAC 995.16, 32
AOAC 997.08, 32
AOAC 999.03, 56
AOAC 2000.11, 32
AOAC 2001.02, 32
AOAC 2001.03, 32, 57
AOAC 2002.02, 32, 57
AOAC 2009.01, 11, 17–18, 34, 53
AOAC 2011.25, 11, 53
arabinoxylan (AX), 104, 213, 222–3
agronomy and environment effect, 162–3
DF content correlations in wheat lines, 162
genetic variation, 157–61
amount and composition, 157–60
contents reported for whole grains, flour and wheat, 158–9
dietary fibre components in wheat lines, 161
fibre content in flour and bran of wheat cultivar, 160
structure, 160–1
heritability and genetic analysis, 163–5
Asphaerocephala, 303
autoclaving, 201

β-glucan, 102–4, 223–6, 292, 319, 325
agronomy and environment effect, 162–3
DF content correlations in wheat lines, 162
bread making effect on molecular weight and extractability, 224
heritability and genetic analysis, 163–5
molecular weight distribution profile, 225
barley, 395
barley bran, 178–9, 181, 183
barley flour, 297
beverages, 322
bran, 217–18
breads
different types, 212–13
fibre-enriched and wholegrain, 211–30
fibre enrichment, 216–21
bran, 217–18
bread enriched with fructan and/or fructo-oligosaccharides, 218–19
composite flour, 218
dietary fibre content of major cereal brans, 217
fortification with fibre concentration, 219–20
gluten-free bread, 220–1
milling fractions, 218
resistant starch, 219
whole grains and their dietary fibre content, 216
wholegrain, 216
major DF components in flour, 213–15

rye and wheat fructan molecular weight distribution profile, 215
processing, 221–8
arabinoxylan, 222–3
β-glucan, 223–6
β-glucan and arabinoxylan molecular weight distribution profile, 223
β-glucan molecular weight distribution profile, 225
bread making effect on molecular weight and extractability of β-glucan, 224
fructan, 226
fructan molecular weight distribution profile, 226
resistant starch, 226–8
total DF, 221–2
properties of dietary fibre-enriched dough and breads, 228–30
dough properties, 228–9
organoleptic properties of bread, 229–30
brewer's spent grain (BSG), 399
buckwheat, 297

Cannaedulluls starch, 302
carbohydrate polymers, 5, 31
carboxymethylcellulose (CMC), 358
cardiovascular disease (CVD), 68, 77
carrageenan, 107, 333
cellotetraosyl, 214
cellotriosyl, 214
cellulose, 63, 99–100, 214
cereal β-glucans, 374–6
organoleptic properties, 376
solubility, 375
stability, 375–6
viscosity, 375
cereal bran, 181, 183
production technology, 172–80, 180–1
rye, oat and wheat bran produced from non-peeled grains, 173
cereal cell walls, 171–2
cereal dietary fibre, 77, 80–1
intake showing a decreased risk of type 2 diabetes, 80
cereal dietary fibres, 354–8
other cellulose DFs used as ingredients in minced fish products, 357–8
other cellulose DFs used as ingredients in surimi products, 357
wheat dietary fibre in minced fish products, 356–7
sensory evaluation of samples with wheat dietary fibre, 357
wheat dietary fibre in surimi and surimi gels, 354–6
WDF arrangement in squid surimi gels, 355
cereal grains, 8
cheese, 324–5
chitin, 101
chitosan, 101, 353–4
coalescence, 238
Codex Alimentarius, 53, 56–8
composite flour, 218
constipation, 66–7
consumer behaviour
external factors, 132–6
convenience, 135–6
cost, 134–5
food availability and environments, 132–4
future trends, 139–42
wholegrain foods and consumer demands, 139–41
wholegrain foods stakeholder collaboration, 141–2
interpersonal factors, 125–32
familiarity and sensory attributes, 130–2
knowledge of wholegrains and fibres in relation to disease prevention, 129–30
US whole grain and fibre related health claims, 127
wholegrain and high fibre identification, 125–9
introduction approach to wholegrain foods, 136–9
consumption of partial and 100% wholegrain foods by elementary school children, 137
wholegrain foods, 120–42
cooked meat products, 337–40
enriched with different dietary fibres and fibre-rich materials, 338–9
crispbread, 213
curdlan, 109, 301, 361

dairy desserts, 313
diabetes, 415–16
dietary fibre, 3–22, 212, 316, 329, 370
agronomy and environment effect on arabinoxylan (AX) and β-glucan, 162–3
arabinoxylan (AX) genetic variation, 157–61
characterisation and digestive impact, 64–7
calorific content, 67
physiological characterisation, 64–6
transit time and constipation, 66–7
companion animal nutrition, 407–18
clinical significance, 415–17
food intake, gastric and small intestinal function, 408–12
intestinal function, 412–15
strategies for incorporating into diets, 417–18
components measurement by AOAC 985.29 and 991.43, 32
content and composition in wheat, 153–67
definition, 4–5
definition, measurement and intake, 62–4
disease, 67–8
bowel health, 68
extruded products, 256–68

effects of DF on extrusion process and product quality, 260–5
effects of extrusion on dietary fibre properties, 265–7
extrusion cooking, 257–60
future trends, 267–8
fibre-enriched beverage, 369–85
adding fibres into drinks, 370–2
fructans and glucose products, 378–83
future trends, 384–5
gums and beta-glucans, 373–7
rationale for fibre addition in beverage, 370
troubleshooting, 384
typical beverage formulation, 383–4
food analysis, 25–58
food content analysis, 10–11
future trends, 72–3
genetic variation exploitation in plant breeding, 165–6
health claims, 18–22
EFSA scientific opinions on fibre-related health claims, 19–20
health outcome, 61–73
heritability and genetic analysis of arabinoxylan (AX) and β-glucan, 163–5
ingredients and technical functionality, 96–115
components interaction, 99
gel-forming capacity, 98
water holding capacity, 97–8
insoluble ingredients, 99–101
integrated TDF assay procedure, 33
interlaboratory evaluation of integrated total dietary fibre procedure, 52–3
labelling, 12–16
mature wheat grain structure, 154
methodology acceptance by Codex Alimentarius, 53, 56–8
methods approved by CCMAS, 27–9
microbiota, 71–2
obesity, 68–71
origin, source and major techno-functionalities and applications in food, 112–15
original integrated total dietary fibre procedure, 47–52
ready-to-eat snacks, 389–402
cereal by-products, 399
extrusion processing, 390, 392
future trends, 401
improving quality of extruded products, 399–401
nutritional benefits of extruded whole grains, 392–9
recommendations and guidelines, 16–18
resistant starch, 111
resistant starch and non-digestible oligosaccharides measurement, 34–47
resistant starch values determined by AOAC 2002.02 and 2009.01, 34
soluble and insoluble, in infant nutrition, 421–39
insoluble non-digestible carbohydrates, 436–8
non-digestible carbohydrates in human milk, 423–6
soluble non-digestible carbohydrates of non-human milk origin, 426–36
soluble high molecular weight ingredients, 101–9
soluble low molecular weight ingredients, 109–11
wheat fractions, 154–7
grain outer layer, 156
dietary fibre intake, 16–18, 62–4
recommended for adults, 17
dietary fibre labelling, 12
Dietary Reference Intake (DRI), 69
digestive tolerance, 372
dry white Chinese noodles (DWCN), 296
durum, 274–6, 399

emulsification, 99
enzyme digestion, 41–3
blanks, 41
samples, 42–3
enzyme purity, 41
euglycaemic hyperinsulinaemic clamp technique, 86
extruded products, 256–68
effects of DF on extrusion process and product quality, 260–5
effect of fibre type on extrudate quality, 262–2
extrudates with different percentages of corn starch, wheat fibre and pectin, 265
fibre-enriched ingredients used in extrusion, 263
fibre-induced changes in extrusion, 260–2
role of other ingredients in fibre-enriched extrusion, 263–5
effects of extrusion on dietary fibre properties, 265–7
changes in associated compounds, 266–7
changes in DF polymers, 265–6
changes in nutritional properties, 267
extrusion cooking, 257–60
extruders in cereal processing, 257–8
operational parameters important for product properties, 258–60
operational variables controlling extruded product quality, 259
sections of extruder and expansion mechanism, 258
single and twin screw extruders, 258
future trends, 267–8
extruders, 257
extrusion, 257
extrusion cooking, 202
extrusion processing

improving quality of products, 399–401
ready-to-eat snacks, 390, 392
extrusion technology, 257

fat replacement, 99
fermentation, 200
fermented meat products, 341–2
enriched with different dietary fibres and fibre rich materials, 341
fibre, 422
fibre concentration, 219–20
fibre consumption
future trends, 139–42
wholegrain foods and consumer demands, 139–41
wholegrain foods stakeholder collaboration, 141–2
introduction approach to wholegrain foods, 136–9
consumption of partial and 100% wholegrain foods by elementary school children, 137
wholegrain foods, 120–42, 121–5
consumption data, 121–5
definitions, 121
socio-demographic differences, 125
fibre-enriched beverage, 369–85
adding fibres into drinks, 370–2
digestive tolerance, 372
formulating dietary fibres into drinks, 371–2
physical properties, 371
stability, 371–2
fructans and glucose products, 378–83
inulin and fructo- oligosaccharides, 378–80
polydextrose, 380–2
resistant maltodextrins, 382–3
future trends, 384–5
gums and beta-glucans, 373–7
acacia gums, 373–4
cereal β-glucans, 374–6
guar gum, 376–7
rationale for fibre addition in beverage, 370
troubleshooting, 384
typical beverage formulation, 383–4
juice drink containing fibre, 383
powdered mix containing fibre, 384
water with fibre, 384
fibre-enriched dairy products, 311–25
challenges of fibre enrichment, 314–16
bioavailability of other nutrients, 315–16
protein and polysaccharide incompatibility and phase separation, 314–15
rheology and texture, 315
dairy product categories and formulation, 312–14
future trends, 325
potential dietary fibre supplements for dairy products, 316–19
insoluble fibre, 317
soluble fibre, 317–19
potential product applications, 319–25
applications of dietary fibres in dairy products, 320–1
beverages, 319, 322
cheese, 324–5
frozen dairy desserts, 324
gelled products, 322–3
fibre-enriched meat products, 329–43
dietary fibre in meat products, 333–42
cooked meat products, 337–40
cooked products enriched with different dietary fibres and fibre-rich materials, 338–9
fermented meat products, 341–2
fermented products enriched with different dietary fibres and fibre rich materials, 341
fresh meat products, 333–7
fresh meat products enriched with different dietary fibres and fibre-rich materials, 334–5
fibre as an ingredient in meat product formulation, 332–3
fibre technological properties for meat processing, 332–3
healthy properties of fibre for meat-based functional foods, 333
future trends, 342–3
strategies for healthier meat products development, 331–2
illustration, 331
fibre-enriched seafood, 348–63
fortification with dietary fibres of aquatic origin, 349–54
hardness of blue whiting minced gel, 351
seafood waste polysaccharides, 353–4
seaweed hydrocolloids, 350–3
seaweeds, 349–50
water-holding capacity of blue whiting, 353
fortification with dietary fibres of terrestrial origin, 354–62
blue whiting minced gels containing guar gum, 355
cereal dietary fibres, 354–8
fancy brochette with added wheat DF and *Fucus* DF, 360
fruits, 358–9, 360
others, 361–2
polysaccharide produced by microbial fermentation, 359, 361
seeds, 354, 355
sensory evaluation of samples with wheat dietary fibre, 357
WDF arrangement in squid surimi gels, 355
future trends, 362–3
fibre-enriched wheat flour noodles, 297–301
addition of specific fibre materials, 299

high-fibre flours addition, 297–9
Fibruline, 361
filtering flask, 37
flatbread, 213
flaxseed gum, 104–5
food analysis
dietary fibre, 25–58
components measurement by AOAC 985.29 and 991.43, 32
integrated TDF assay procedure, 33
interlaboratory evaluation of integrated total dietary fibre procedure, 52–3
methodology acceptance by Codex Alimentarius, 53, 56–8
methods approved by CCMAS, 27–9
original integrated total dietary fibre procedure, 47–52
resistant starch and non-digestible oligosaccharides measurement, 34–47
resistant starch values determined by AOAC 2002.02 and 2009.01, 34
food availability, 132–4
food content, 10–12
dietary fibre analysis, 10–11
wholegrain analysis, 11–12
food descriptor, 128
food deserts, 133
food environment, 132–4
food intake, 70
effects of dietary fibre, 408–9
food labelling, 126
frequently sampled intravenous glucose tolerance test (FSIGTT), 86
fresh meat products, 333–7
enriched with different dietary fibres and fibre-rich materials, 334–5
frozen dairy desserts, 313, 324
fructan, 214, 218–19, 226
molecular weight distribution profile, 226
fructo-oligosaccharides, 218–19, 378–80
sensory properties, 379
solubility, 378
stability, 378–9
tolerance, 379–80
viscosity, 378
fruits, 193–203, 358–9, 360
effects of processing on fruit and vegetable dietary fibre, 198–203
chemical processing, 198–9
enzymatic processing, 199–200
mechanical processing, 198
grape dietary fibre, 358–9
pectin, 359
as sources of dietary fibre, 194–7
chemistry of cell wall components, 195–7
composition of cell wall polysaccharides, 196–7
definitions and dietary fibre recommendations, 194–5
thermal processing effect on fruit and vegetable dietary fibre, 200–3
content and composition, 201–2
functional properties, 202–3
fucoidan, 350
Fucus vesiculosus L., 350
functional fibre, 62, 316

galactoglucomannan, 103
galacturonic acid, 195
gastrointestinal transit time, 66–7
gel-forming fibre, 65
gellan gum, 108–9
gelled products, 322–3
genetic analysis, 164–5
genetic variation
arabinoxylan (AX) genetic variation, 157–61
exploitation in grain dietary fibre in plant breeding, 165–6
ghrelin, 71
glass transition (Tg) property, 260
Glucagel, 219
glucagon-like peptide-1 (GLP-1), 71
glucomannan, 361–2
glucuronoarabinoxylan (GAX), 156
gluten, 220
gluten-free bread, 220–1
glycaemic control, 415–16
grain fibre, 88, 89
green banana flour, 299
guar gum, 354, 376–7
sensory properties, 377
solubility, 377
stability, 377
tolerance, 377
viscosity, 377
gum arabic, 106, 318
gums, 401

hard-bite noodle, 294
Healthy Eating Index 2005, 256
hemicellulose, 63
heritability, 163–4
variance components of dietary fibre of wheat grain, 164
high hydrostatic pressure (HHP), 202
high molecular weight dietary fibre (HMWDF)
calculation, 47
determination, 35–6, 43–4
total dietary fibre values determination, 36
high molecular weight soluble dietary fibre (HMWSDF), 33
homeostatic model assessment (HOMA), 86
human milk oligosaccharides, 422
hydration, 97–8
hydrothermal treatment, 225

image analysis techniques, 400
in vitro models, 414–15

infant nutrition
insoluble non-digestible carbohydrates, 436–8
dietary recommendations, 438
structure and functions, 436–7
non-digestible carbohydrates in human milk, 423–6
functions, 424–6
structure, 423–4
soluble and insoluble dietary fibre, 421–39
soluble non-digestible carbohydrates of non-human milk origin, 426–36
functions, 427–36
structure, 426–7
insoluble dietary fibre (IDF), 33
determination, 35, 44
insoluble fibre, 64–5
insoluble non-digestible carbohydrates, 436–8
dietary recommendations, 438
structure and functions, 436–7
insulin metabolism, 86
insulin sensitivity, 81, 86, 87
insulin sensitivity index (ISI), 86
integrated total dietary fibre
interlaboratory evaluation procedure, 52–3
collaborative study data for total dietary fibre, 55
HMWDF plus LMWSDF statistical data determination using AOAC 2009.01, 53
statistical details for various dietary fibre methods, 54
original procedure, 47–52
desalting of samples for HPLC, 50–1
difficult sample analysis, 51–2
elution of D-sorbitol and fructo-oligosaccharides, 51
incubation conditions, 48
internal standards, 48–50
maltodextrins, maltose, diethylene glycol and D-sorbitol chromatography, 50
shaking, suspended stirring and stirring effect, 49
sucrose and maltose hydrolysis with thermostable α-glucosidase, 52
inulin, 110–11, 318, 324, 337, 361, 378–80
sensory properties, 379
solubility, 378
stability, 378–9
tolerance, 379–80
viscosity, 378

junction zones, 315

κ-carrageenan, 314, 352
konjac flour, 339–40
konjac glucomannan, 106

label ingredients, 128
lactose, 423
legume fibre, 101
lignin, 99–100, 214
locust bean gum, 354
low molecular weight soluble dietary fibre (LMWSDF), 33

Maggi Tastylite Atta Whole Wheat Noodles, 292
Maillard reaction products, 244
Maillard reactions, 398
mechanical fractionation processing, 198
microbial polysacch, 108–9
microbiota, 71–2
milk beverages, 312–13
milling fractions, 218
mixed-bed ion exchange resins, 41
Raftilose P-95, 42
modern milling, 9
mucilages, 104–6
muffins
batter, 238–44
consistency index and flow behaviour index, 239
elastic and viscous modulus evolution, 241–2
flow properties, 238–9
frequency dependence of elastic modulus and viscous modulus, 244
frequency of elastic modulus and viscous modulus, 240
influence of RS level replacing flour on muffin batter flow properties, 239
loss tangent values evolution, 243
viscoelastic properties, 239–44
colour properties, 244–5
performance of resistant starches use in bakery products, 237–8
properties, 244–9
sensory characteristics, 250–2
sensory shelf life, 249–50
texture analysis, 245–9
different RS concentrations effect on TPA parameter values for muffins, 246
freshly baked muffins, 245–6
textural changes during storage, 246–9
mustard mucilage, 105
MyPyramid, 256

6-*n*-propylthiouracil (PROP), 131
non-digestible carbohydrates, 5, 423–6
functions, 424–6
interactions with glycoconjugates on biological surfaces, 425–6
prebiotic function, 424–5
structure, 423–4
non-digestible oligosaccharides, 109–10
non-viscous fibre, 65
non-wheat cereal dietary fibre
cereal bran production technology, 172–80, 180–1
cereal cell walls, 171–2
future trends, 183
ingredients, 170–83

ingredients food applications, 181–3
studies on effects of bran addition to food products, 182
nonstarch polysaccharides (NSP), 30
noodles
fibre-enriched and wholewheat, 291–304
fibre-enriched wheat flour noodles, 297–301
wheat flour noodles and resistant starch, 301
wholewheat noodles, 295–7
quality attributes, 293–5
composite flour noodles quality assessment, 295
noodles from other botanical sources, 294–5
wheat flour noodles, 293–4
wholegrain and fibre-enriched noodles from other botanical sources, 302–4
rice noodles fibre enrichment, 302–3
starch noodles fibre enrichment, 303–4
novel carbohydrates, 416
nutrient digestibility, 409–12
results of fibre digestibility studies, 410–11
Nutrim, 219, 299
Nutrition and Health Claims directive, 256
Nutrition Labeling and Education Act (1990), 256

oat bran, 100, 176–8, 181, 183, 217
oat kernel, 181
OatWell, 219
obesity, 68–71, 416–17
oligofructose, 318
oral glucose tolerance test, 86

partially hydrolysed guar gum (PHGG), 376–7
pasta
durum wheat flour characteristics, 274–6
enrichment with whole grains or dietary fibre, 281–3
effect of dietary fibre addition on cooked pasta digestion characteristics, 282
fibre-enriched and wholewheat, 273–85
future trends, 285
ingredient selection, processing and nutrition, 283–5
nutritional quality, 276–7
chemical composition of cooked pasta, 276
comparative glycaemic index and glycaemic loading of pasta, 277
process variables affecting production, 277–80
effects of dietary fibre addition to textural attributes of cooked pasta, 280
process variables, and sensorial and textural properties, 278–80
pectin, 101–2, 194, 195, 401, 409
pectin methylesterase (PME), 199
peptide YY3-36 (PYY3-36), 71
percent whole grain, 128
pericarp, 156, 177
phytic acid, 217–18
plant breeding, 165–6
polydextrose, 318–19, 380–2
sensory properties, 381
solubility, 380
stability, 381
tolerance, 381–2
viscosity, 380
polygalacturanase, 199
polyphenol oxidase (PPO), 293
polypropylene columns
Bio-Rad, Econo-Pac Disposable Chromatography Columns, 38
polysaccharide
produced by microbial fermentation, 359, 361
polysaccharides, 301
power-law equation, 238
prebiotics, 72, 408
effects in animal nutrition, 412, 414
pseudo-cereal grains, 8
psyllium gum, 105–6
puddings, 313

quantitative insulin sensitivity check index (QUICKI), 86

ready-to-eat snacks
cereal by-products, 399
dietary fibre, 389–402
extrusion processing, 390, 392
health benefits, 389–90
nutritional composition of some processed breakfast cereals and snacks, 391
improving quality of extruded products, 399–401
nutritional benefits of extruded whole grains, 392–9
antioxidant activity, 396–8
differences of dietary fibre levels before and after extrusion, 394
formation of dietary fibre, 393
nutrient and caloric content, 393
physicochemical changes in starches, 395–6
resistant starch content of native and extruded barley flours, 393
retention of vitamins, 398–9
recombination, 9
resistant maltodextrins, 382–3
organoleptic properties, 382
solubility, 382
stability, 382
tolerance, 382–3
viscosity, 382
resistant starch, 111, 219, 226–8, 236, 317, 323
performance in baking, 236–53
muffin batter, 238–44
muffin properties, 244–9

sensory characteristics of muffins, 250–2
sensory shelf life of muffins, 249–50
uses in bakery products, 237–8
response surface methodology, 401
rice bran, 179–80, 183, 339
rice noodles
fibre enrichment, 302–3
and resistant starch, 302–3
rubber policeman spatulas, 38
schematic diagram, 37
rubber ring adaptor, 37
rye bran, 176, 183

satiation, 69–70
satiety, 69–70
SDFP, 33
determination, 35, 44
SDFS, 33
calculation, 47
determination, 35–6, 45–6
HPLC chromatography of maltodextrins, maltose, glycerol and D-sorbitol, 46
total dietary fibre values determination, 36
seafood waste polysaccharides, 353–4
seaweed hydrocolloids, 350–3
seaweed polysaccharides, 107–8
seaweeds, 349–50
seeds, 354, 355
sheet and cut process, 293
short chain fatty acids (SCFA), 87, 89
small amplitude oscillator shear (SAOS), 239
sodium bicarbonate, 401
soft-bite noodle, 294
Solka Floc, 357
soluble dietary fibre, 33
soluble fibre, 64–5
soluble non-digestible carbohydrates, 426–36
functions, 427–36
effect on immune system, 433–6
effect on intestinal physiology, 433
prebiotic function, 428–33
structure, 426–7
tested for prebiotic effects in human infants, 427
sour cream, 314
starch noodles
fibre enrichment, 303–4
and resistant starch, 304
starches
physicochemical changes, 395–6
flow behaviour of wheat flours in molten state, 397
starchy endosperm cells, 154–6
arabinoxylan structure, 155
β-D-glucan molecule structure and distribution, 155
sterilisation, 201
stool quality, 412
study results measuring stool characteristics of dogs and cats, 413
subaleurone, 177
Subexi noodles, 293
supercritical fluid extrusion (SCFX), 265
Swelite, 357

tamarind gum, 354
Teff flour, 395
texture profile analysis (TPA), 245
thermal pasteurisation, 201
thermo-irreversible gels, 332
total colour difference, 245
total dietary fibre (TDF), 221–2, 236
integrated measurement, 34–47
apparatus, 36–9
arrangements for mixing or stirring of suspensions, 35
integrated calculations, 47
principle, 34–6
reagents, 39–41
test sample preparation, 41
total fibre, 62, 316
type 2 diabetes, 68, 81, 86, 90

UltraTrim, 219

vegetables, 193–203
effects of processing on fruit and vegetable dietary fibre, 198–203
chemical processing, 198–9
enzymatic processing, 199–200
mechanical processing, 198
as sources of dietary fibre, 194–7
chemistry of cell wall components, 195–7
composition of cell wall polysaccharides, 196–7
definitions and dietary fibre recommendations, 194–5
thermal processing effect on fruit and vegetable dietary fibre, 200–3
content and composition, 201–2
functional properties, 202–3
Viscofibre, 219
viscosity, 98
viscous fibre, 65
Vitacel, 355
vitamins, 398–9
levels in cereals before and after extrusion, 398

water-soluble soybean polysaccharide (SSPS), 318, 323
weight control, 416–17
wheat
content and composition dietary fibre, 153–67
agronomy and environment effect on arabinoxylan (AX) and β-glucan, 162–3
arabinoxylan (AX) genetic variation, 157–61
genetic variation exploitation in plant breeding, 165–6

heritability and genetic analysis of arabinoxylan (AX) and β-glucan, 163–5
mature wheat grain structure, 154
wheat fractions, 154–7
wheat bran, 100–1, 174–5, 181, 217
layers, 175
wheat embryo, 156–7
wheat fibre, 262
wheat flour noodles, 293–4
and resistant starch, 301
wheat germ, 156–7
wheat kernel, 180
wheying off, 314
white flour, 154–6
arabinoxylan structure, 155
β-D-glucan molecule structure and distribution, 155
Whole Grain Council (WGC), 216
wholegrain flour, 137
wholegrain foods, 3–22
consumption and consumer challenges, 120–42
external factors, 132–6
future trends, 139–42
interpersonal factors, 125–32
introduction approach, 136–9
definition, 5–8
characteristics, 6–7
development, 10
epidemiological studies, 77–81
cereal dietary fibre, 77, 80–1
consumption showing decreased risk of type 2 diabetes and metabolic syndrome, 78–9
protective effects, 77
food content analysis, 11–12
food factors important for health, 87–9
chemical composition, 88
structure, 88–9
future trends, 89–90
health, 76–90
health claims, 18–22, 21–2
EFSA scientific opinions on fibre-related health claims, 19–20
human interventions, 81–7
whole *vs.* refined grains, 82–5
labelling, 12–16
new product launches by category, 4
processing, 8–9
recommendations and guidelines, 16–18
wholegrain intake, 18, 122–5, 138
wholegrain labelling, 12–16
food qualification, 13–15
wholegrains, 216
extruded, nutritional benefits, 392–9
wholemeal, 8
wholewheat noodles, 295–7

xanthan gum, 108, 302, 359, 401
xyloglucan, 103, 195

yoghurt, 313, 323